MEDICAL RADIOLOGY

Diagnostic Imaging

Editors:
A. L. Baert, Leuven
K. Sartor, Heidelberg

Springer
Berlin
Heidelberg
New York
Hong Kong
London
Milan
Paris
Tokyo

A. M. Davies · R.W. Whitehouse · J. P. R. Jenkins (Eds.)

Imaging of the Foot & Ankle

Techniques and Applications

With Contributions by

T. D. Berg · T. H. Berquist · S. Bianchi · S. L. Burrows · V. N. Cassar-Pullicino
V. P. Chandnani · M. Cobby · A. M. Davies · B. J. DeMichaelis · G. Y. El-Khoury
J. M. Elliott · S. J. Erickson · J. Garcia · H. K. Genant · A. Gentili · A. J. Grainger
J. W. Helgason · S. Hofmann · H. Imhof · J. P. R. Jenkins · F. Kainberger · A. Katz
J. Kramer · G. Lavis · H. P. Ledermann · C. Martinoli · E. G. McNally · W. B. Morrison
S. Nehrer · M. Recht · P. Renton · D. A. Ritchie · L. L. Seeger · M. E. Schweitzer
B. Tins · P. N. M. Tyrrell · D. Vanel · H. Vogel · I. Watt · R. W. Whitehouse · J. S. Yu

Foreword by

A. L. Baert

With 451 Figures in 753 Separate Illustrations, 11 in Color and 35 Tables

Springer

A. Mark Davies, MD
Consultant Radiologist
The MRI Centre
Royal Orthopaedic Hospital
Birmingham B31 2 AP
UK

Jeremy P. R. Jenkins, MBChB, FRCP, DMRD, FRCR
Department of Clinical Radiology
Manchester Royal Infirmary
Oxford Road
Manchester, M13 9WL
UK

Richard William Whitehouse, MD
Department of Clinical Radiology
Manchester Royal Infirmary
Oxford Road
Manchester, M13 9WL
UK

Medical Radiology · Diagnostic Imaging and Radiation Oncology
Series Editors: A. L. Baert · L. W. Brady · H.-P. Heilmann · M. Molls · K. Sartor

Continuation of
Handbuch der medizinischen Radiologie
Encyclopedia of Medical Radiology

ISBN 3-540-67294-X Springer-Verlag Berlin Heidelberg New York

Library of Congress Cataloging-in-Publication Data

Imaging of the foot & ankle : techniques and applications / A. M. Davies, R. W. Whitehouse, J. P. R. Jenkins (eds.); with contributions by T. Berg ... [et al.] ; foreword by A. L. Baert.
p. ; cm. -- (Medical radiology)
Includes bibliographical references and index.
ISBN 354067294X (hardcover : alk. paper)
1. Foot--Imaging. 2. Ankle--Imaging. 3. Foot--Diseases--Diagnosis. 4. Ankle--Diseases--Diagnosis. I. Title: Imaging of the foot and ankle. II Davies, A. M. (Arthur Mark), 1954- III. Whitehouse, Richard W. IV. Jenkins, J. P. R. (Jeremy P. R.) V. Berg, T. (Thomas) VI. Series.
[DNLM: 1. Foot Diseases--diagnosis. 2. Ankle Injuries--diagnosis. 3. Diagnostic Imaging--methods. 4. Foot Injuries--diagnosis. WE 880 I31 2002]
RC951 .I434 2002
617.5′850757--dc21

2002070776

Springer-Verlag Berlin Heidelberg New York
a member of BertelsmannSpringer Science+Business Media GmbH

http//www. springer.de

Printed in Germany

Cover-Design and Typesetting: Verlagsservice Teichmann, 69256 Mauer

21/3150 – 5 4 3 2 1 0 – Printed on acid-free paper

Foreword

This volume provides a multimodality imaging approach to the pathology of the foot and the ankle, covering both the various imaging techniques and all clinical aspects of diseases of these anatomic areas.

The chapters on technique are compact but still deal comprehensively with all specific facets of the problem. The clinical chapters are well written, detailed and superbly illustrated.

The editors succeeded in assembling an excellent group of international experts from the European continent as well as from the USA to cover all commonly held modern views and concepts on the topic.

This outstanding volume will serve the needs not only of general radiologists dealing in their daily practice with the frequently occurring traumatic conditions of the ankle and foot but also of specialised musculoskeletal radiologists looking for guidance in their management of patients suffering from arthritis, osteochondritis, infectious or metabolic diseases or even the rare tumoral and tumour-like conditions of this part of the lower limb. It can be recommended highly as invaluable reading not only to radiologists but also to orthopaedic surgeons and rheumatologists.

I am confident that this excellent book will meet the same success as the volume on the knee already published in this series by Dr. Mark Davies.

Leuven

Albert L. Baert

Preface

As our understanding of the disease processes and biomechanics of foot and ankle disorders improves there is a need to continuously update the radiologists, orthopaedic surgeons and other professions working in this field. Several recent texts on the foot and ankle have concentrated on a single imaging technique such as MR imaging. This book, in common with several others published in this series, takes a dual approach to the subject. The first section acquaints the reader with the full range of techniques available for imaging the ankle and foot pathology, emphasising indications and contraindications. The seven chapters include contributions on radiography, computed tomography, MR imaging and ultrasound. The remaining fifteen chapters discuss the optimal application of these techniques to specific pathologies, highlighting practical solutions to everyday clinical problems.

The editors are grateful to the international panel of authors for their contributions to this book, which aims to provide a comprehensive overview of current imaging of the foot and ankle.

Birmingham	A. Mark Davies
Manchester	Richard William Whitehouse
Manchester	Jeremy P. R. Jenkins

Contents

Imaging Techniques and Procedures

1 Radiography

A. Gentili and L. L. Seeger

CONTENTS

A. Gentili, MD
Professor of Radiology, UCSD Thornton Hospital, Department of Radiology, 9300 Campus Point Drive, 7756, La Jolla, CA 92037, USA

L.L. Seeger, MD
Professor, Dept. of Radiological Sciences, 200 UCLA Medical Plaza, Suite 165-57, Los Angeles, CA 90095-6952, USA

In this chapter, after covering the basic radiographic techniques used in the imaging of the foot and ankle, the standard line, axes, and angles are reviewed, and normal variants are presented.

1.1 Radiographic Technique

Radiographs should be the first imaging study obtained for the evaluation of foot and ankle pathology. Proper radiographic techniques are essential for high-quality radiographs. This chapter covers the most common radiographic projections used to image the foot and ankle. It does not attempt to review all specialized projections that have been described in the past. Most specialized projections are infrequently used nowadays, and only when routine projections are inconclusive. Most of the time, computed tomography or magnetic resonance imaging is used as the next step.

1.1.1 Radiographic Projections of the Ankle

Standard projections for the evaluation of ankle pathology are anteroposterior, mortise, and lateral (Ballinger and Frank 1999; Bontager and Lampignano 1997).

1.1.1.1 Anteroposterior Projection of the Ankle

1.1.1.1.1 Technique

Nonweight-Bearing. The patient is supine or sitting with the knee extended. The foot is dorsiflexed with the plantar surface of the foot perpendicular to the cassette. The central ray is perpendicular to the cassette and directed between the medial and lateral malleolus (Fig. 1.1).

Weight-Bearing. The patient is upright and stands on wood blocks or on a platform with a slot for the cassette. The cassette is position vertically. The central ray is directed horizontally, perpendicular to the cassette, between the medial and lateral malleoli (Fig. 1.2).

1.1.1.1.2 Radiographic Evaluation

On this projection, the tibiotalar joint and the medial mortise are visualized. The lateral aspect of the ankle mortise is obscured due to superimposition of the distal fibula on the talus.

a
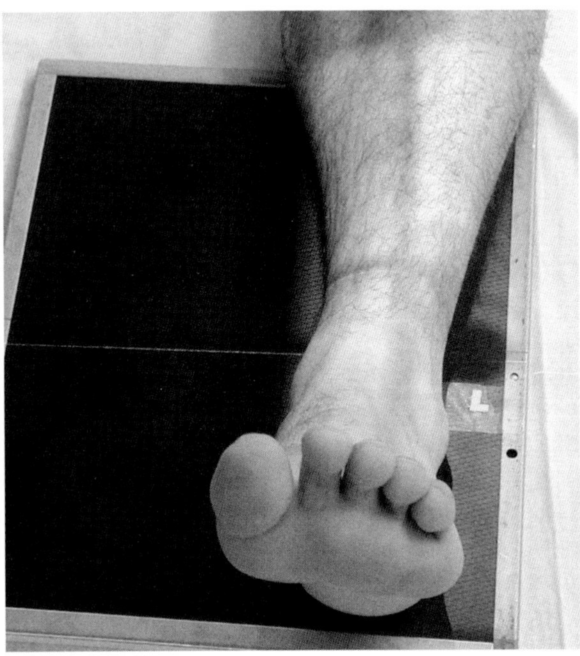

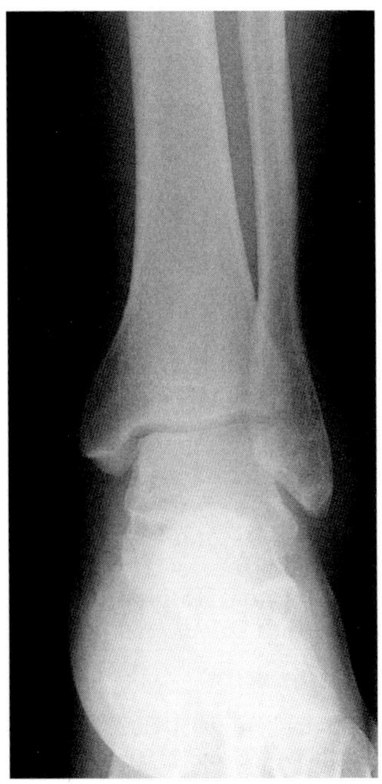
b

Fig. 1.1a. Patient positioning for anteroposterior (AP) nonweight-bearing ankle radiograph. **b** AP nonweight-bearing ankle radiograph

a b

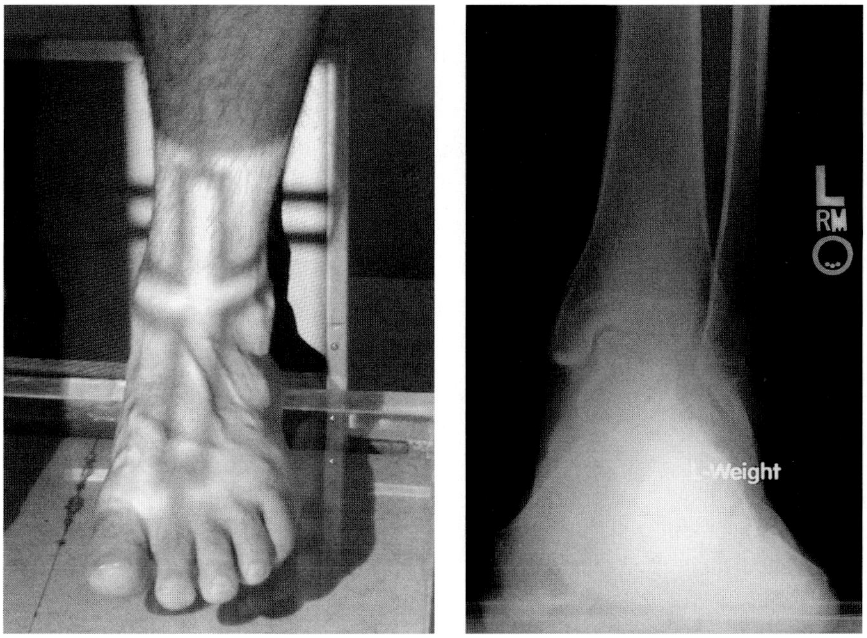

Fig. 1.2a. Patient positioning for AP weight-bearing ankle radiograph. **b** AP weight-bearing ankle radiograph

1.1.1.2
Lateral Projection of the Ankle

1.1.1.2.1
Technique

Nonweight-bearing (Mediolateral). The patient is recumbent on the affected side. The knee is adjusted so that the transverse axis of the patella is vertical. The ankle is dorsiflexed, and the plantar surface is perpendicular to the cassette. The central ray is directed perpendicular to the cassette, towards the medial malleolus (Fig. 1.3).

Weight-Bearing (Lateromedial). The patient is upright and stands on wood blocks or on a platform with a central slot for the cassette. The cassette is position vertically between the ankles. The central ray is directed horizontally, perpendicular to the cassette, towards the lateral malleolus (Fig. 1.4).

1.1.1.2.2
Radiographic Evaluation

On this projection, the tibiotalar, subtalar, calcaneocuboid, and talonavicular joints are well seen. The base of the 5th metatarsal should be included on this projection, as a fracture of the 5th metatarsal base may mimic an ankle sprain. The pre-Achilles' fat pad appears as a triangular radiolucency sharply demarcated posteriorly by the anterior surface of the Achilles' tendon, anteriorly by the deep muscles of the lower leg, and inferiorly by the superior surface of the tuberosity of the calcaneus. An Achilles' tendon tear, ankle and calcaneal fractures may obscure the pre-Achilles' fat pad. Ankle joint effusions (Fig. 1.5) have a characteristic tear drop appearance on this projection, with soft-tissue densities anterior and posterior to the ankle joint (Towbin et al. 1988).

1.1.1.3
Mortise Projection of the Ankle

1.1.1.3.1
Technique

Nonweight-Bearing. The patient is supine or sitting with the knee extended. The foot is dorsiflexed, with the plantar surface of the foot perpendicular to the cassette. The entire leg and foot are internally rotated 15°–20° until the malleoli are parallel to the cassette. The central ray is perpendicular to the cassette and directed midway between the medial and lateral malleoli (Fig. 1.6).

Weight-Bearing. The patient is upright and stands on wood blocks or on a platform with a slot for the cassette. The entire leg and foot are internally rotated 15°–20° until the malleoli are parallel to the cassette. The cassette is position vertically. The central ray is directed horizontally, perpendicular to the cassette, and directed midway between the medial and lateral malleoli (Fig. 1.7).

a 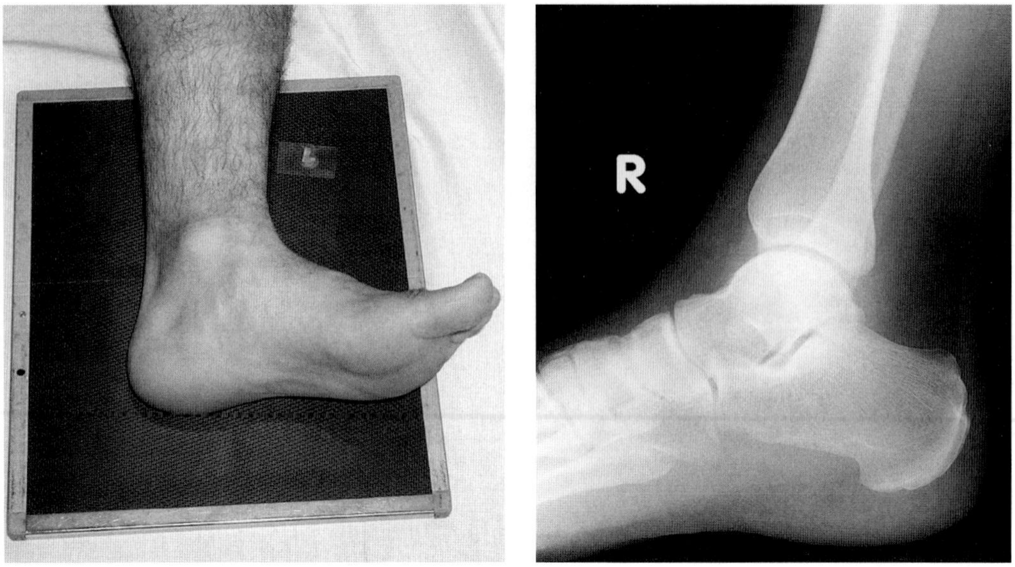

b

Fig. 1.3a. Patient positioning for a lateral nonweight-bearing ankle radiograph. **b** Lateral nonweight-bearing ankle radiograph

a 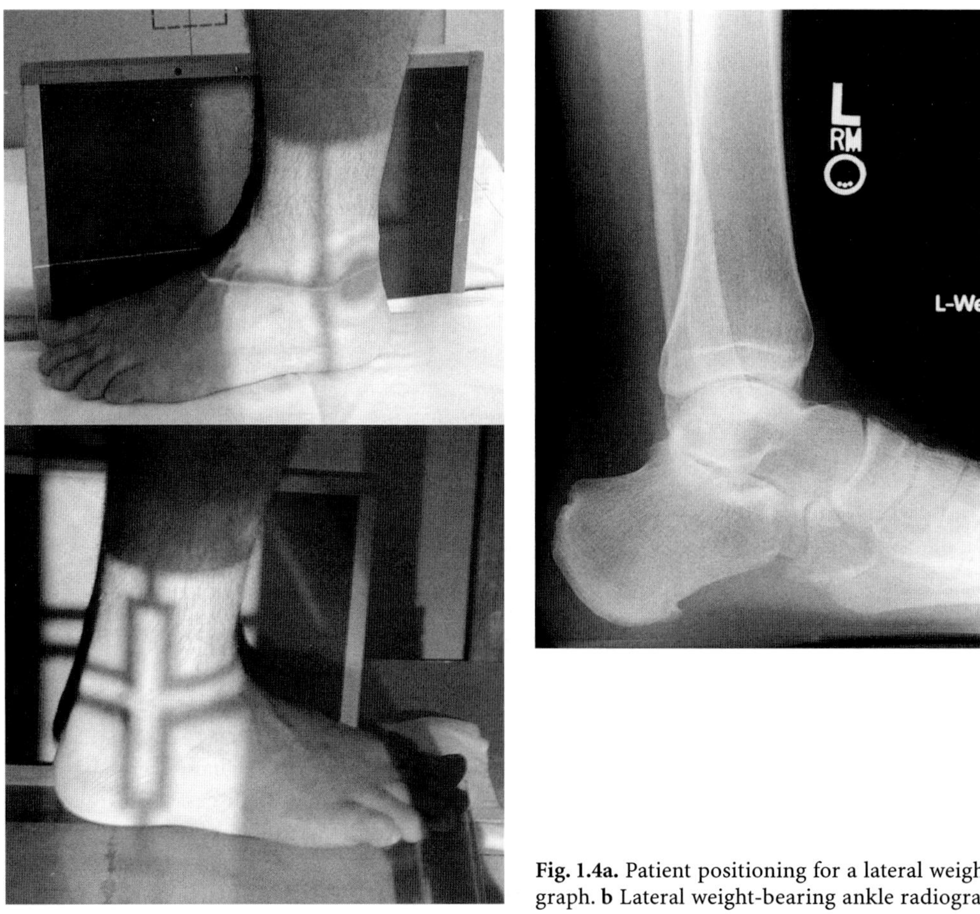

b

Fig. 1.4a. Patient positioning for a lateral weight-bearing ankle radiograph. **b** Lateral weight-bearing ankle radiograph

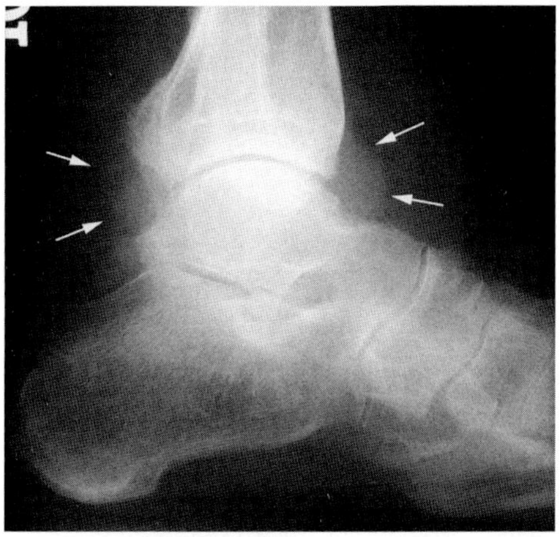

Fig. 1.5. Lateral radiograph of the ankle. The teardrop-shaped densities seen extending anteriorly and posteriorly from the ankle joint have been referred to as the 'teardrop sign' of ankle effusion (*arrows*)

a b

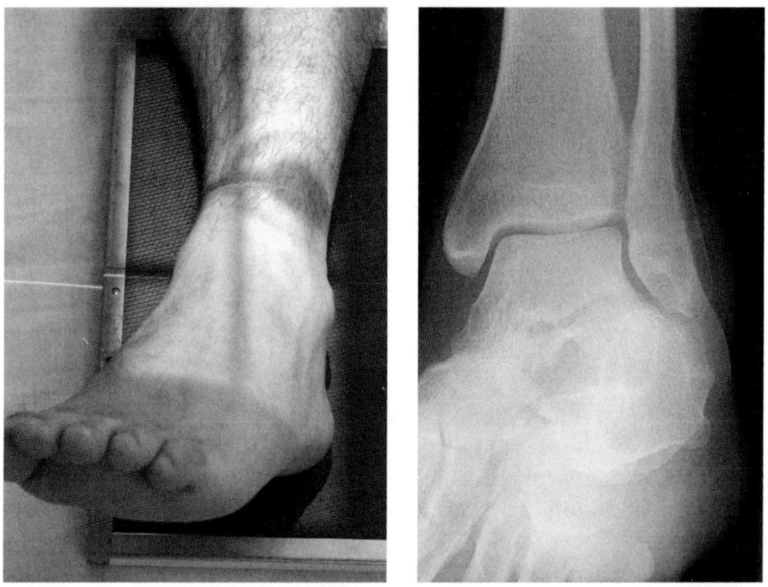

Fig. 1.6a. Patient positioning for a mortise nonweight-bearing ankle radiograph. **b** Mortise nonweight-bearing ankle radiograph

a b

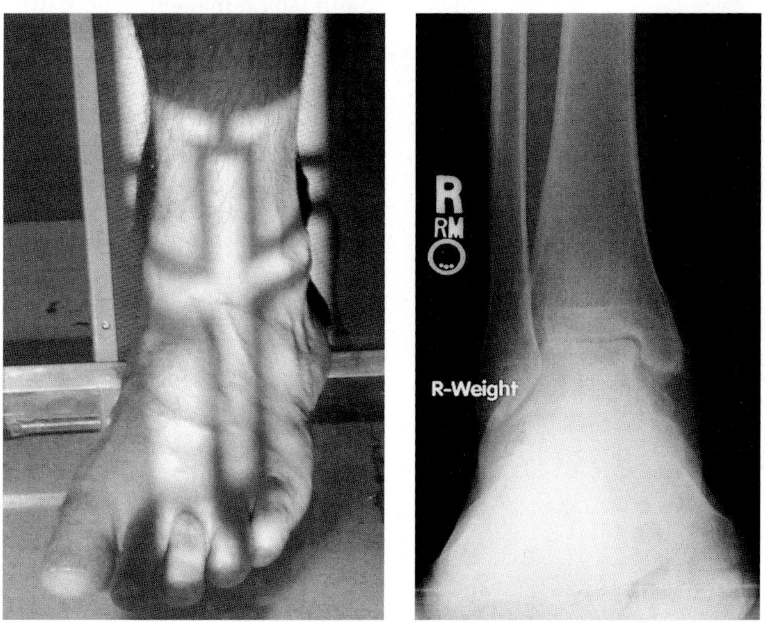

Fig. 1.7a. Patient positioning for a mortise weight-bearing ankle radiograph. **b** Mortise weight-bearing ankle radiograph

1.1.1.3.2 Radiographic Evaluation

This projection gives a true AP projection of the tibiotalar joint. The talar dome is visualized in its entirety, free of superimpositions. The medial and lateral talomalleolar articulations are open. The ankle joint space should be uniform and measure approximately 3–4 mm. Asymmetry greater than 2 mm is abnormal.

1.1.1.4 45° Medial and Lateral Oblique Projections of the Ankle

1.1.1.4.1 Technique

The patient is supine with the knee extended. The foot is dorsiflexed, with the plantar surface of the foot perpendicular to the cassette. The entire leg and foot are rotated 45° internally for the medial oblique or 45° externally for the lateral oblique. The central ray is perpendicular to the cassette and directed midway between the medial and lateral malleoli (Fig. 1.8).

1.1.1.4.2 Radiographic Evaluation

The medial oblique view is often replaced by the mortise view. On the medial oblique, there is superimposition of the fibula on the talus. The lateral oblique is used in trauma to delineate the medial malleolus better.

1.1.1.5 'Off' Lateral or 'Poor' Lateral Projection of the Ankle

1.1.1.5.1 Technique

The patient is positioned as for a lateral projection of the foot, the foot is rotated 15° with the heel elevated 5 cm from the tabletop and with the toes pointing toward the table. The central ray is vertically oriented and is directed to the lateral malleolus (Fig. 1.9).

1.1.1.5.2 Radiographic Evaluation

This projection is used to evaluate fractures of the posterior lip of the tibia. On this projection, the posterior lip of the tibia is superimposed on the fibula, but is well seen.

1.1.1.6 Anteroposterior Stress Projections (Inversion – Varus and Eversion – Valgus Stress)

1.1.1.6.1 Technique

The patient is supine with the knee extended. The foot is dorsiflexed, with the plantar surface of the foot perpendicular to the cassette. Stress is applied either manually or with a special stressing apparatus. If this is too painful, local anesthetic may be injected. The central ray is directed perpendicular to the cassette between the medial and lateral malleoli (Fig. 1.10).

a

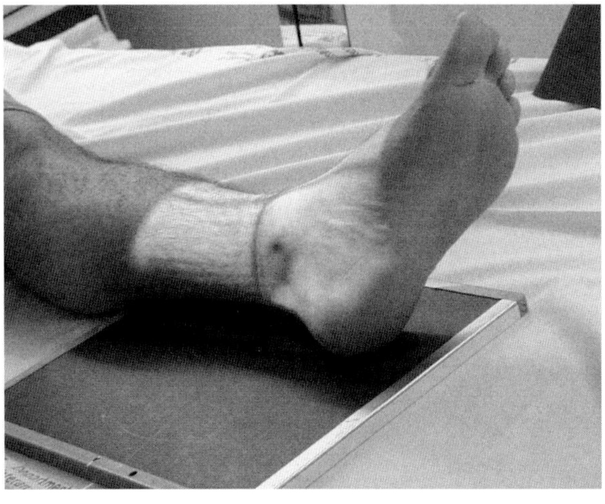

b

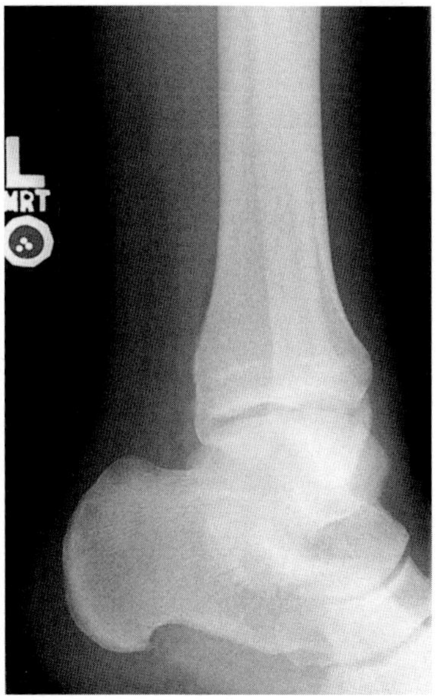

Fig. 1.8a. Patient positioning for a 45° medial oblique nonweight-bearing ankle radiograph. **b** The 45° medial oblique nonweight-bearing ankle radiograph

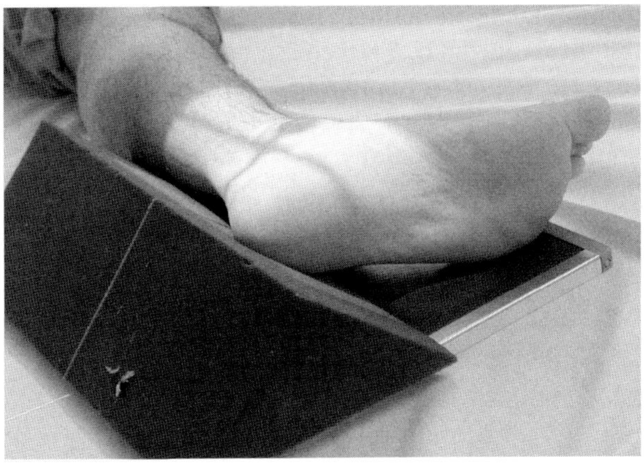

a

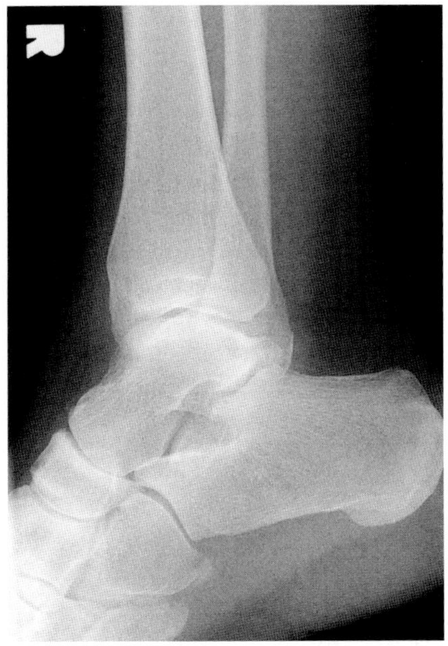

b

Fig. 1.9a. Patient positioning for an 'off' lateral nonweight-bearing ankle radiograph. **b** 'Off' lateral nonweight-bearing ankle radiograph

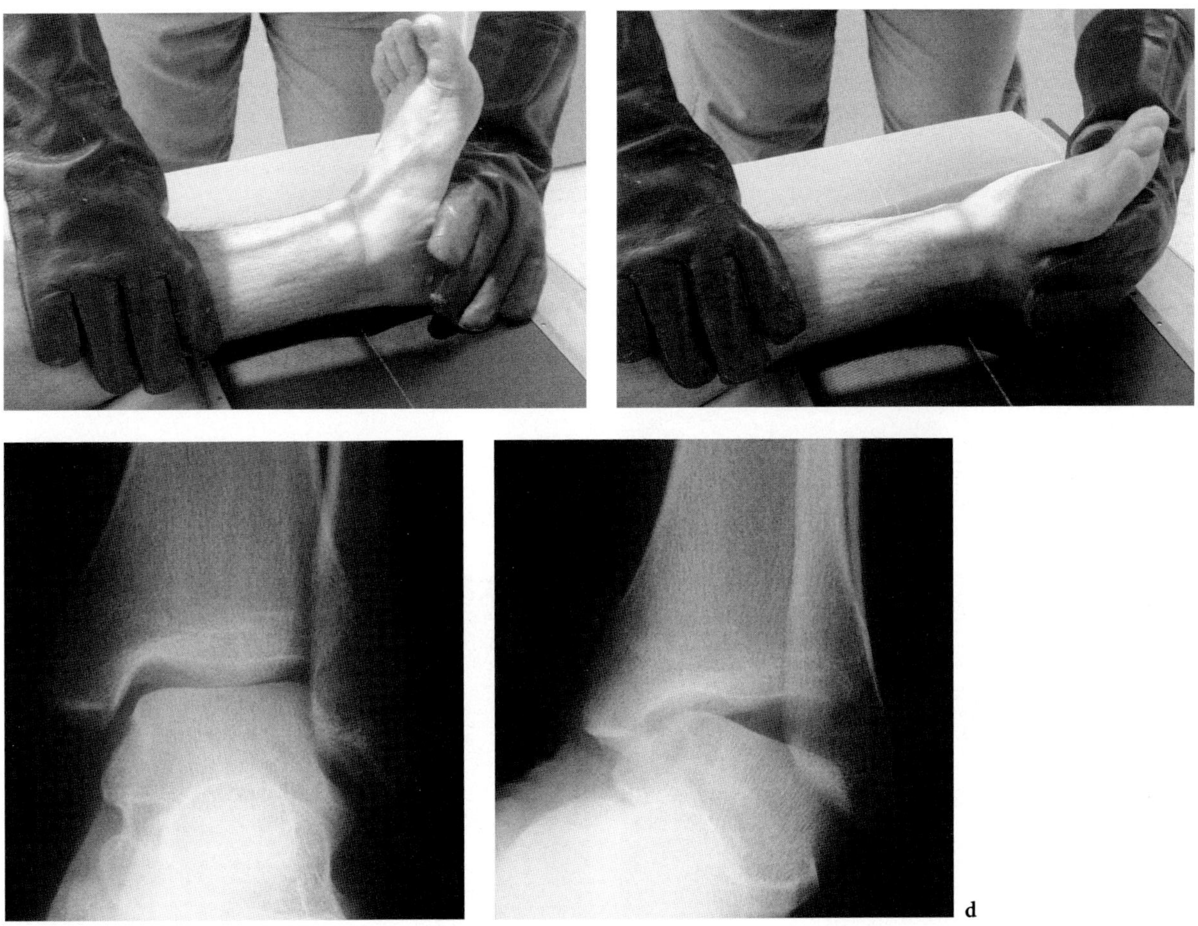

Fig. 1.10a. Patient positioning for AP eversion-valgus stress ankle radiograph. **b** Patient positioning for AP inversion-varus stress ankle radiograph. **c** Normal AP stress radiograph of the ankle. **d** Abnormal AP varus stress radiograph of the ankle, with widening of the lateral mortise

1.1.1.6.2
Radiographic Evaluation

These projections are used to assess injury of the ankle ligaments in the absence of bone abnormalities. When stress radiographs are obtained, comparison radiographs of the unaffected ankle are necessary, as up to 25° talar tilt has been described in the asymptomatic ankle. More than 10° difference in talar tilt or more than 3 mm difference in widening of the ankle joint between the injured and asymptomatic sites is considered indicative of ligamentous injury.

1.1.1.7
Lateral Stress Views

1.1.1.7.1
Technique

The patient is supine. The knee is extended. The foot is dorsiflexed, and the plantar surface is perpendicular to the table. The foot is supported with the heel elevated 5–10 cm above the table. The cassette is perpendicular to the table and touches the lateral aspect of the foot and ankle. Stress is applied either manually or with a sandbag placed on the anterior aspect of the distal leg above the ankle. The central ray is directed perpendicular to the cassette towards the medial malleolus (Fig. 1.11) (Haupfauer 1970).

1.1.1.7.2
Radiographic Evaluation

This projection is used to assess injuries of the anterior talofibular ligament. When stress radiographs are obtained, comparison radiographs of the unaffected ankle are necessary. More than 2 mm difference in translation of the ankle joint between the injured and asymptomatic sites is considered indicative of ligamentous injury (positive anterior drawer sign).

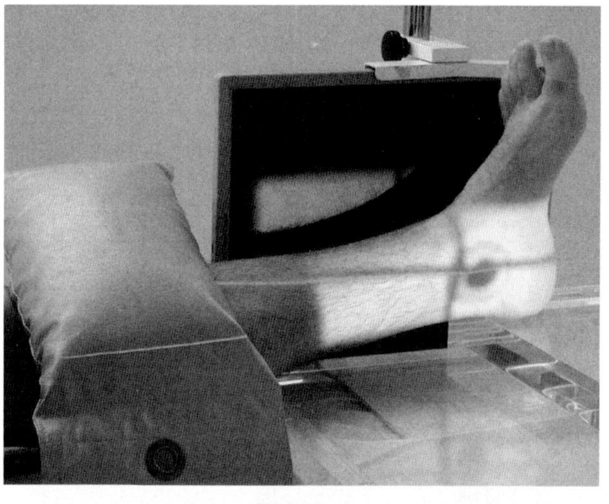
a

Fig. 1.11a. Patient positioning for lateral stress ankle radiograph. **b** Lateral radiograph of the ankle with no stress. **c** Lateral stress radiograph of the ankle demonstrates a positive anterior drawer sign, consistent with an anterior talofibular ligament tear

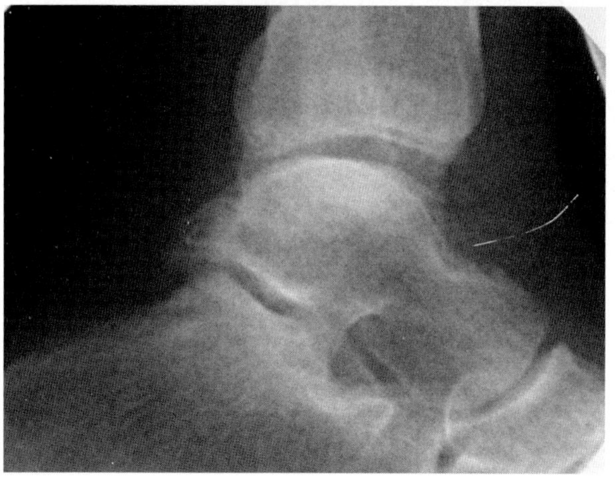
b

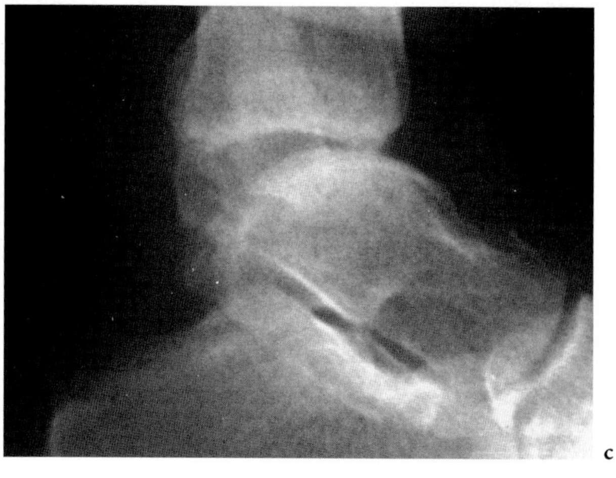
c

1.1.2
Radiographic Projections of the Foot

Standard projections for the evaluation of foot pathology are anteroposterior, medial oblique, and lateral (Ballinger and Frank 1999, Bontager and Lampignano 1997). If possible, the anteroposterior and lateral projections are obtained in weight-bearing mode to evaluate structural changes not evident on nonweight-bearing projections. The lateral oblique projection is infrequently used as it does not provide significant additional information except for the assessment of the medial aspect of the navicular and medial cuneiform.

1.1.2.1
Anteroposterior (Dorsoplantar) Projection of the Foot

1.1.2.1.1
Technique

Nonweight-Bearing. The patient is supine or sitting with the knee flexed. The plantar surface of the foot is in contact with the cassette. The central ray is angled 10° posteriorly (toward the calcaneus) and is directed to the third metatarsal base (Fig. 1.12).

Weight-Bearing. The patient is upright and stands on the cassette. The plantar surface of the foot is in contact with the cassette. The central ray is angled 15° posteriorly (toward the calcaneus) and is directed to the second metatarsal base (Fig. 1.13).

1.1.2.1.2
Radiographic Evaluation

On this projection, the metatarsophalangeal joints appear open. The interphalangeal joints may appear narrowed due to divergence of the X-ray beam. The bases of the first and second metatarsals are usually separated. The medial cortex of the 2nd metatarsal should align with the medial cortex of the middle cuneiform. This is the best view to detect subtle Lisfranc's injury. The bases of the 2nd to 5th metatarsals often overlap. The navicular, cuneiform, and cuboid bones are visible with some overlap. With sufficient exposure, the talonavicular and calcaneocuboid joints are also visible. The weight-bearing view is used when angular measurements are to be performed.

a b

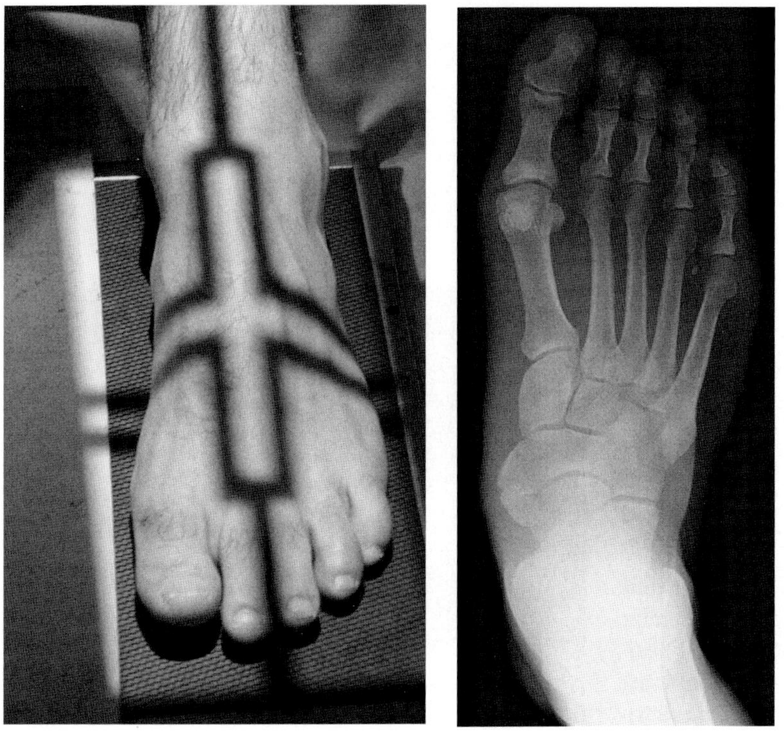

Fig. 1.12a. Patient positioning for AP nonweight-bearing foot radiograph. **b** AP nonweight-bearing foot radiograph

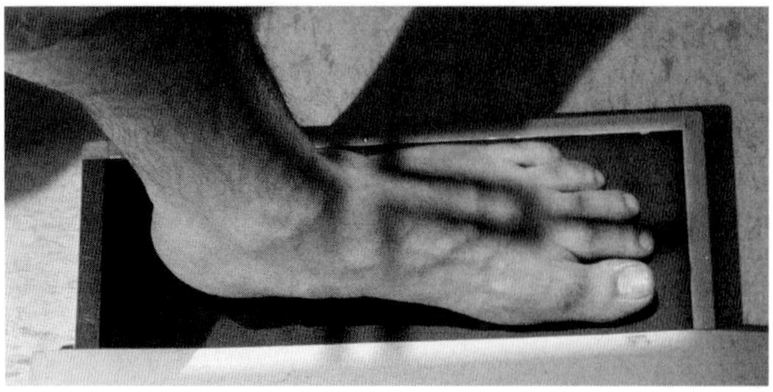

a

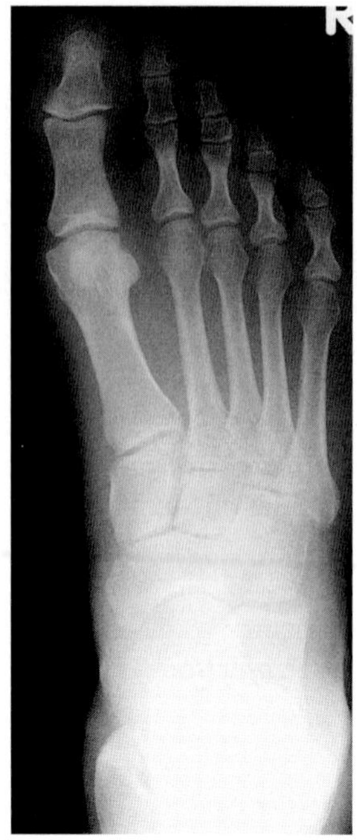

b

Fig. 1.13a. Patient positioning for AP weight-bearing foot radiograph. b AP weight-bearing foot radiograph

1.1.2.2 Lateral Projection of the Foot

1.1.2.2.1 Technique

Nonweight-bearing (Mediolateral). The patient is recumbent on the affected side, and the knee is flexed 45°. The foot is dorsiflexed, and the plantar surface is perpendicular to the cassette. The central ray is directed perpendicular to the cassette towards the third metatarsal base (Fig. 1.14).

Weight-Bearing (Lateromedial). The patient is upright and stands on a wood block or a platform with a central slot for the cassette. The patient's weight should be equally distributed between both feet. The cassette is positioned vertically between the feet, low enough to include the plantar surface. The central ray is directed horizontally, perpendicular to the cassette, towards the base of the 5th metatarsal (Fig. 1.15).

1.1.2.2.2 Radiographic Evaluation

On this projection, the entire foot and the distal tibia and fibula should be visualized. The ankle, subtalar, calcaneocuboid, and talonavicular joint are well seen. The tarsometatarsal and metatarsophalangeal joint are superimposed. The pre-Achilles' fat pad appears as a tri-

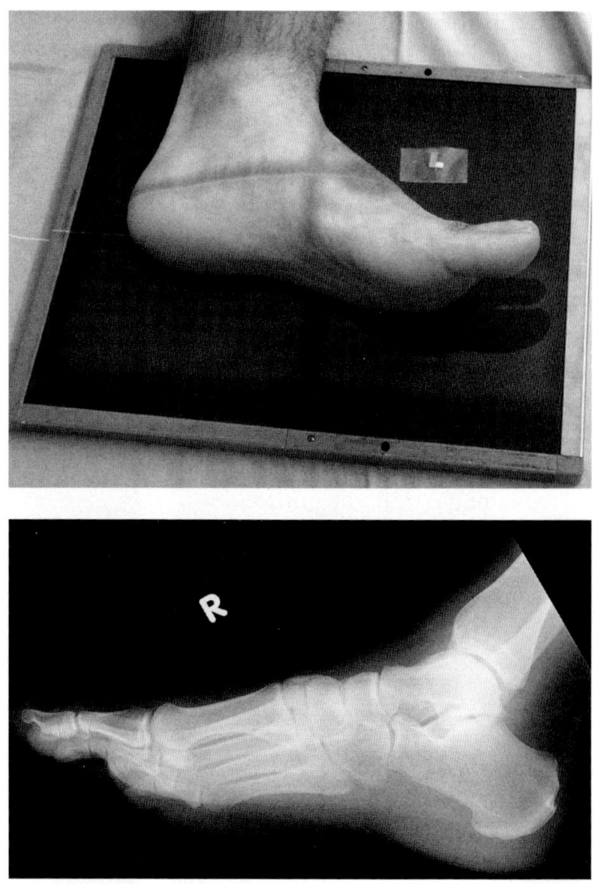

Fig. 1.14a. Patient positioning for a lateral nonweight-bearing foot radiograph. b Lateral nonweight-bearing foot radiograph

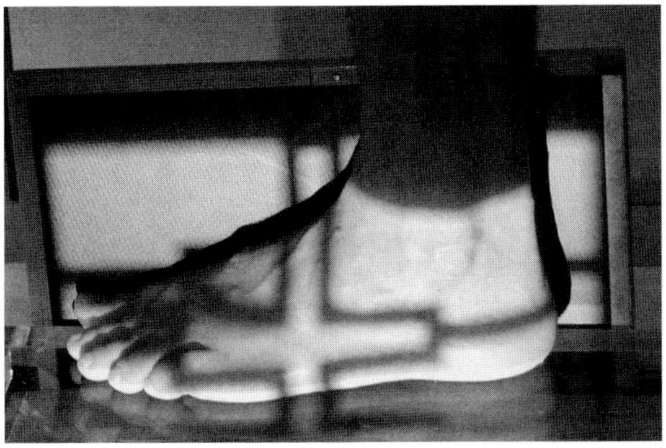

a

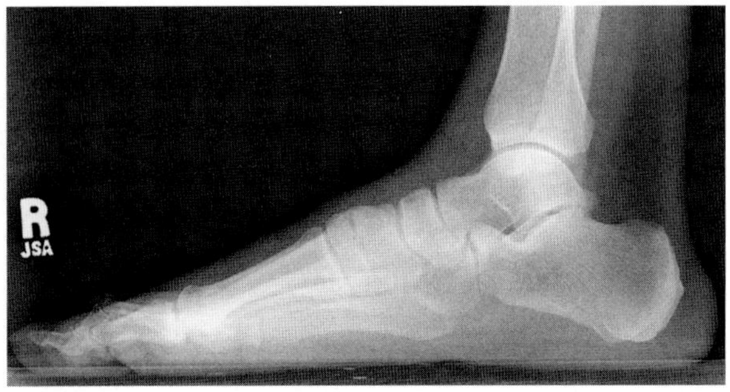

b

Fig. 1.15a. Patient positioning for a lateral weight-bearing foot radiograph. **b** Lateral weight-bearing foot radiograph

angular radiolucency sharply demarcating the anterior surface of the Achilles' tendon. The weight-bearing view is used to evaluate pes planus/cavus deformities.

1.1.2.3
Medial Oblique Projection of the Foot

1.1.2.3.1
Technique

Different techniques are used for the oblique projection. Some departments use 30°, while others use 45° obliquity. The patient is supine or sitting with the knee flexed. The plantar surface of the foot is 30°–45° to the plane of the cassette, with the medial aspect of the foot in contact with the cassette. A radiolucent block may be use to stabilize the foot. The central ray is directed perpendicular to the cassette towards the 3rd metatarsal base (Fig. 1.16).

1.1.2.3.2
Radiographic Evaluation

On this projection, the entire foot is visualized. The 3rd–5th metatarsal bones are demonstrated without superimposition. The navicular, cuboid, talar head, sinus tarsi, and calcaneus are well seen. The bone bar of the calcaneonavicular coalition is best seen on this projection.

1.1.2.4
Lateral Oblique Projection of the Foot

1.1.2.4.1
Technique

The patient is supine or sitting with the knee flexed. The plantar surface of the foot is 30° to the plane

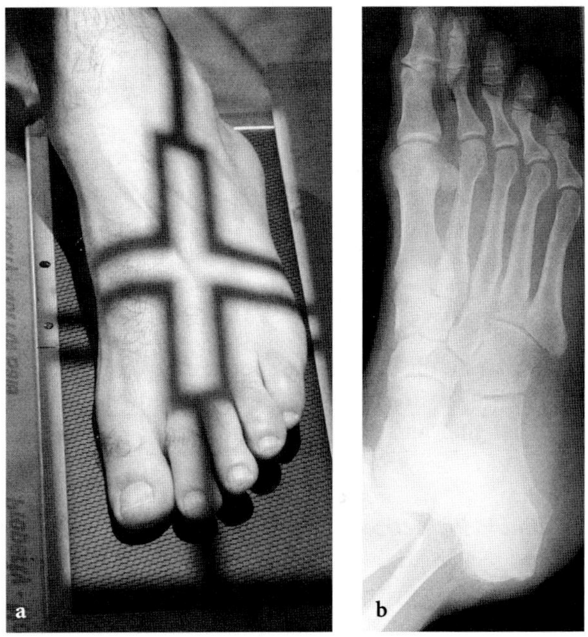

Fig. 1.16a. Patient positioning for a medial oblique foot radiograph. **b** Medial oblique foot radiograph

of the cassette with the lateral aspect of the foot in contact with the cassette. A radiolucent block may be use to stabilize the foot. The central ray is directed perpendicular to the cassette towards the 3rd metatarsal base (Fig. 1.17).

1.1.2.4.2
Radiographic Evaluation

On this projection, the entire foot is visualized. The 3rd–5th metatarsal bones are partially superimposed. The navicular, cuboid, talar head, sinus tarsi, and calcaneocuboid joint are well seen. This

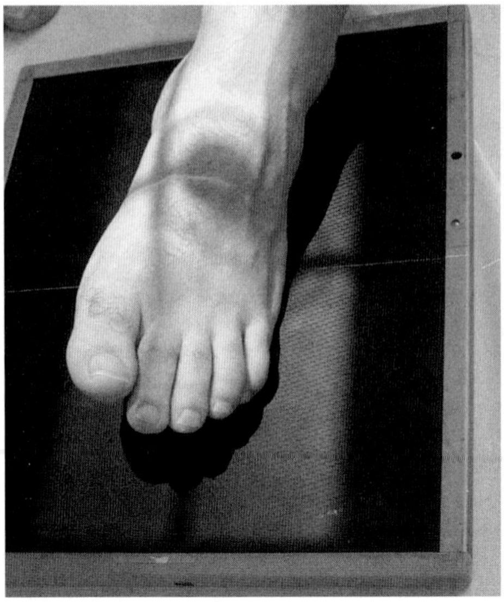

a

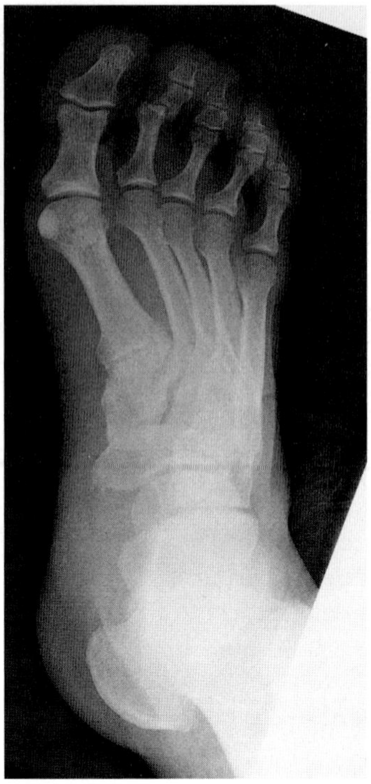

b

Fig. 1.17a. Patient positioning for a lateral oblique foot radiograph. b Lateral oblique foot radiograph

projection is infrequently used because it does not demonstrate the most common fractures of the foot. It is, however, useful to evaluate the medial aspect of the navicular and medial cuneiform.

1.1.2.5
Sesamoid Projection

1.1.2.5.1
Technique

Two different techniques are used to radiograph the sesamoid bones:

1. The patient is supine or sitting with the heel in contact with the cassette. The toes are dorsiflexed using a strap. The plantar surface of the 1st metatarsophalangeal joint is positioned perpendicular to the cassette. The central ray is directed perpendicular to the cassette and tangentially to the plantar surface of the 1st metatarsal head. This technique is usually more comfortable for the patient (Fig. 1.18a).
2. The patient is prone, and the toes are dorsiflexed and in contact with the cassette. The plantar surface is positioned to form a 70°–75° angle with the cassette. The central ray is directed perpendicular to the cassette and tangentially to the plantar surface of the 1st metatarsal head (Fig. 1.18b).

1.1.2.5.2
Radiographic Evaluation

This projection shows the sesamoid bones free from superimposition and the metatarsosesamoid joint in tangent. It is used for assessing sesamoid fractures, arthritis, and alignment of the metatarsosesamoid joint (Fig. 1.18c).

1.1.3
Radiographic Projections of the Toes

The anteroposterior, lateral, and oblique projections of the foot are usually adequate to demonstrate abnormalities of the toes. A dedicated toes projection can be obtained to better visualize the toes or when the area of interest is limited to the toes. Our routine toe series includes 3 projections: anteroposterior projection of the foot, medial oblique and lateral radiographs of the toe in question.

1.1.3.1
Anteroposterior (Dorsoplantar) Projection of the Toes

This projection is often replaced by the anteroposterior projection of the foot.

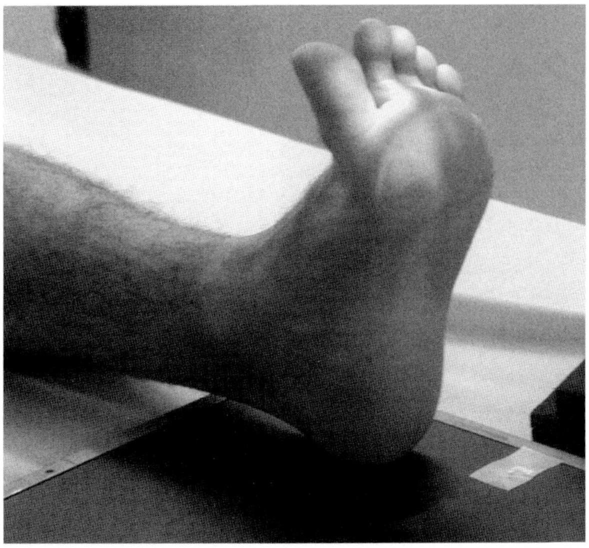

a

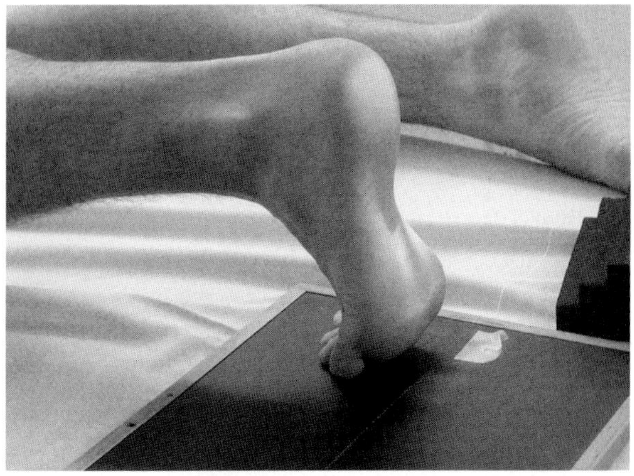

b

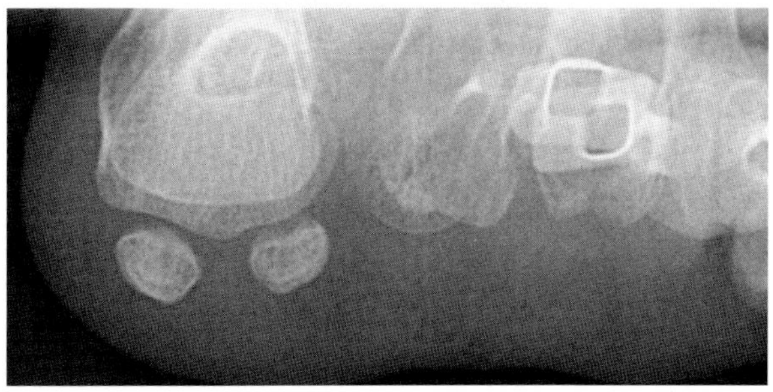

c

Fig. 1.18a. Patient positioning supine for a radiograph of the sesamoid bones. **b** . Patient positioning prone for a radiograph of the sesamoid bones. **c** Radiograph of the sesamoid bones

1.1.3.1.1 Technique

The patient is supine or sitting with the knee flexed. The plantar surface of the foot is in contact with the cassette. The central ray is angled 15° posteriorly (toward the calcaneus) and is directed to the metatarsophalangeal joint of the affected toe (Fig. 1.19).

1.1.3.1.2 Radiographic Evaluation

On this projection, the phalanges are separated without superimposition of soft tissues; the interphalangeal joints appear open.

1.1.3.2 Lateral Projection of the Toes

1.1.3.2.1 Technique

The patient is recumbent. The foot is dorsiflexed, and the plantar surface of the foot is perpendicular to the cassette. The medial surface of the foot is in contact with the cassette for radiographs of the 1st, 2nd, or 3rd toes, and the lateral surface of the foot is in contact with the cassette for radiographs of the 4th and 5th toes. The central ray is directed perpendicular to the cassette towards the interphalangeal joint for the 1st toe or the proximal interphalangeal joint for the 2nd–5th toes. Straps, gauze, sponge, or tape are used to separate the unaffected toes and prevent superimposition (Fig. 1.20).

1.1.3.2.2 Radiographic Evaluation

On this projection, the phalanges are displayed without superimposition, the interphalangeal joints appear open, and the nail is seen in profile.

1.1.3.3 Oblique Projection of the Toes

1.1.3.3.1 Technique

The patient is supine or sitting with the knee flexed. When imaging the 1st–3rd toes, a medial oblique projection is obtained with the plantar surface of the foot at 30°–45° to the plane of the cassette and with the medial aspect of the foot in contact with the cassette. When imaging the 4th or 5th toes, a lateral oblique view is obtained with the plantar surface of

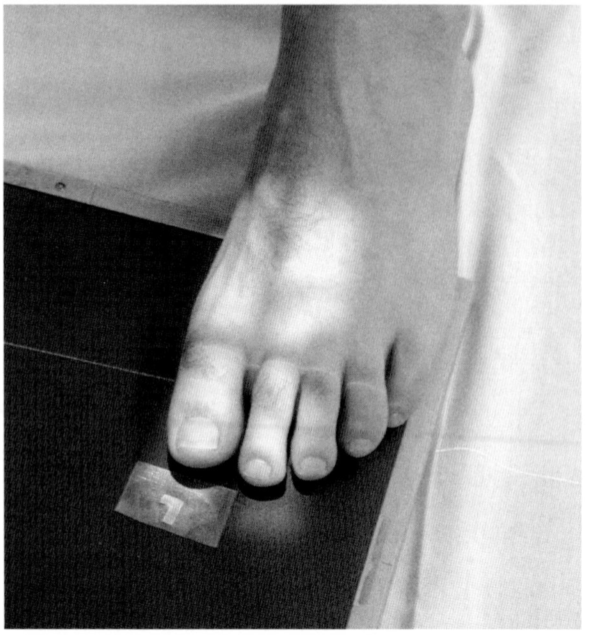
a

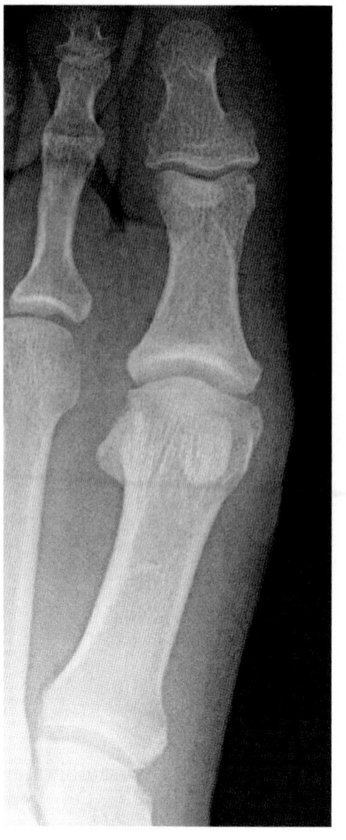
b

Fig. 1.19a. Patient positioning for AP radiograph of the great toe. b AP radiograph of the great toe

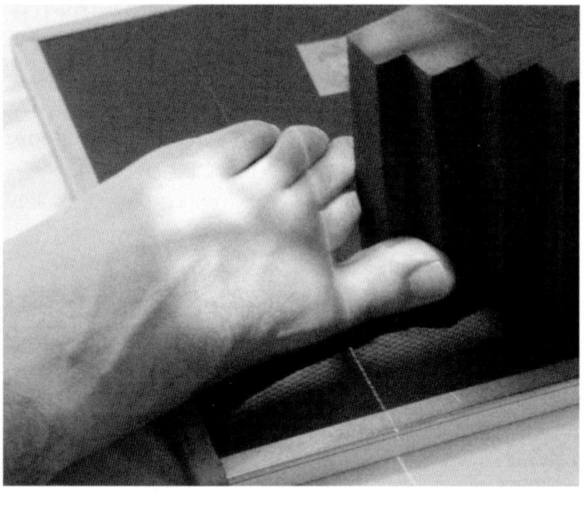
a

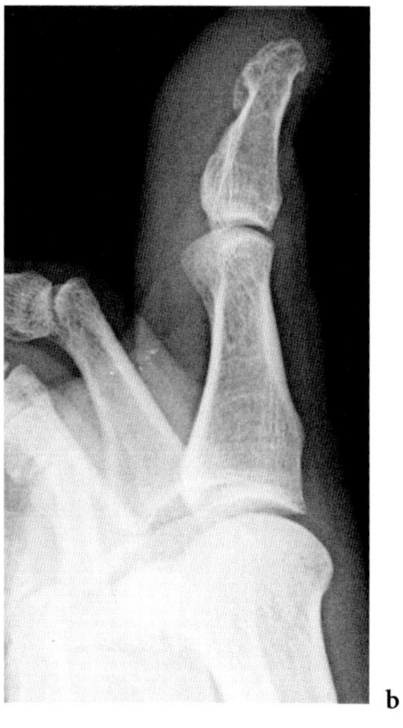
b

Fig. 1.20a. Patient positioning for a lateral radiograph of the great toe; notice the sponge used to prevent superimposition of the toes. b Lateral radiograph of the great toe

the foot at 30°–45° to the plane of the cassette and with the lateral aspect of the foot in contact with the cassette. A radiolucent block is used to stabilize the foot. The central ray is directed perpendicular to the cassette towards the metatarsal phalangeal joint of the affected toe (Fig. 1.21).

1.1.3.3.2 Radiographic Evaluation

On this projection, the phalanges are displayed without superimposition, the interphalangeal joints appear open, and the metatarsal heads show no or only minimal overlapping.

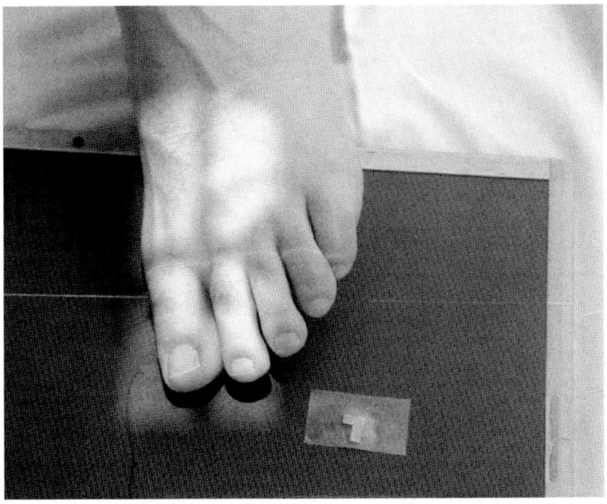

a

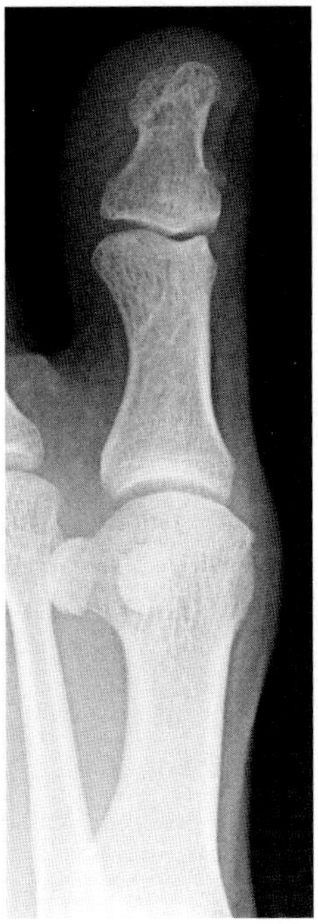

b

Fig. 1.21a. Patient positioning for an oblique radiograph of the great toe. **b** An oblique radiograph of the great toe

1.1.4
Calcaneal Projections

The calcaneus is well seen on the lateral projection of the foot or ankle, but better definition is obtained when the central ray is directed to the calcaneus. On the anteroposterior projection of the foot, the posterior portion of the calcaneus is not visualized. For this reason, an axial projection of the calcaneus is needed.

1.1.4.1
Axial Calcaneal Projection

1.1.4.1.1
Technique

The dorsoplantar projection is preferred because there is less distortion of the calcaneus. In trauma patients, the plantodorsal projection is used as it is easier to do.

Dorsoplantar. The patient is prone, with the affected ankle elevated, the toes just touching the tabletop, and the plantar surface perpendicular to the tabletop. The cassette is vertical, perpendicular to the tabletop, and is touching the plantar surface of the foot. The central ray is angled 40°caudad and is directed to the Achilles' tendon, 5 cm proximal to the plantar surface of the foot (Fig. 1.22a).

Plantodorsal. The patient is supine or seated on the table. The leg is extended. The foot is dorsiflexed, with the plantar surface perpendicular to the cassette. A strap can be used to keep the foot dorsiflexed. The central ray is angled 40° cephalic, and directed to the 3rd metatarsal base (Fig. 1.22b).

1.1.4.1.2
Radiographic Evaluation

On this projection, the entire calcaneus and the subtalar joint should be visualized (Fig. 1.22c).

1.1.4.2
Lateral Calcaneal Projection

1.1.4.2.1
Technique

Positioning for the lateral projection of the calcaneus is very similar to that for the lateral projection of the ankle. The patient is recumbent on the affected side. The knee is adjusted so that the transverse axis of the patella is vertical. The foot is

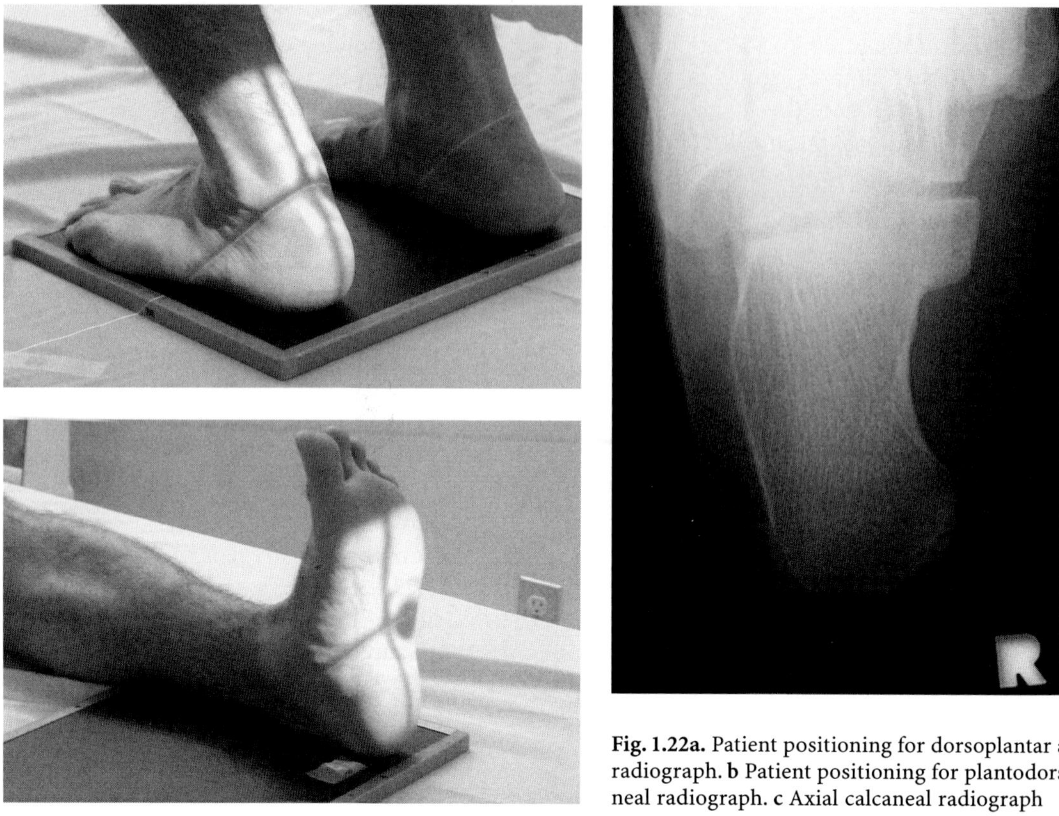

Fig. 1.22a. Patient positioning for dorsoplantar axial calcaneal radiograph. **b** Patient positioning for plantodorsal axial calcaneal radiograph. **c** Axial calcaneal radiograph

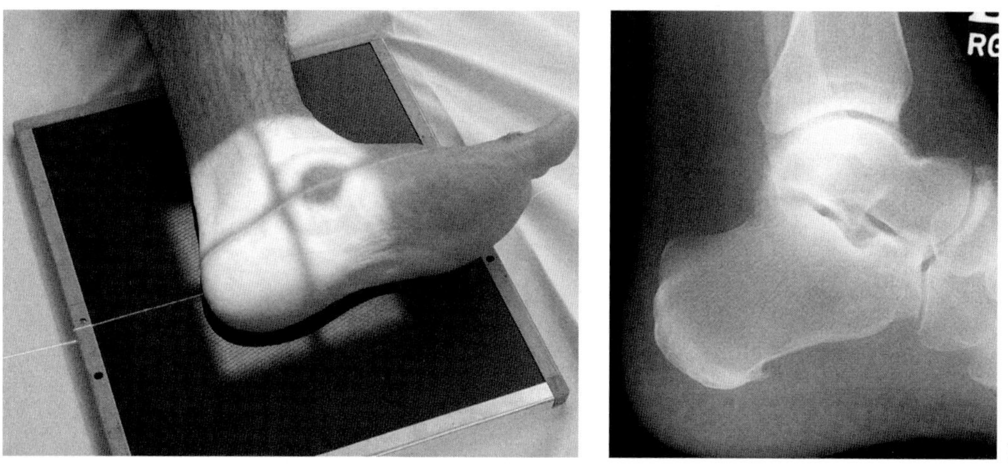

Fig. 1.23a. Patient positioning for a lateral radiograph of the calcaneus. **b** Lateral radiograph of the calcaneus

dorsiflexed, and the plantar surface is positioned perpendicular to the cassette. The main difference from the lateral projection of the ankle is that the central ray is perpendicular to the cassette and is directed 2 cm inferior to the medial malleolus (Fig. 1.23).

1.1.4.2.2 Radiographic Evaluation

On this projection, the tibiotalar, subtalar, calcaneocuboid, and talonavicular joints are well seen. The base of the 5th metatarsal should be included on this projection, as fracture of the 5th metatarsal base may mimic an ankle sprain. The pre-Achilles' fat pad appears as a triangular radiolucency sharply demarcated posteriorly by the anterior surface of the Achilles' tendon, anteriorly by the deep muscles of the leg, and inferiorly by the superior surface of the tuberosity of the calcaneus. Achilles' tendon tears, ankle and calcaneal fractures may obscure the pre-Achilles' fat pad.

1.2 Foot Angle and Axis

1.2.1 Axes and Angles on the Dorsoplantar Projection

The angles and axes are measured on the dorsoplantar and lateral weight-bearing radiographs obtained in the angle and base of gait. This provides an accurate representation of the foot in its functional position (Kashak and Laine 1988).

1.2.1.1 Longitudinal Axis of the Rearfoot

The longitudinal axis of the rearfoot (hindfoot) (LARF) is a line parallel to the distal portion of the lateral border of the calcaneus. In the normal foot, it is parallel to the axis of the 4th metatarsal bone.

1.2.1.2 Collum Tali Axis

The collum tali axis (CTA) is a line bisecting the head and neck of the talus (Fig. 1.24). Normally, this line extends through the center of the 1st metatarsal head. In the pronated foot, it passes medial to the 1st metatarsal head, and in the supinated foot it runs lateral to the 1st metatarsal head.

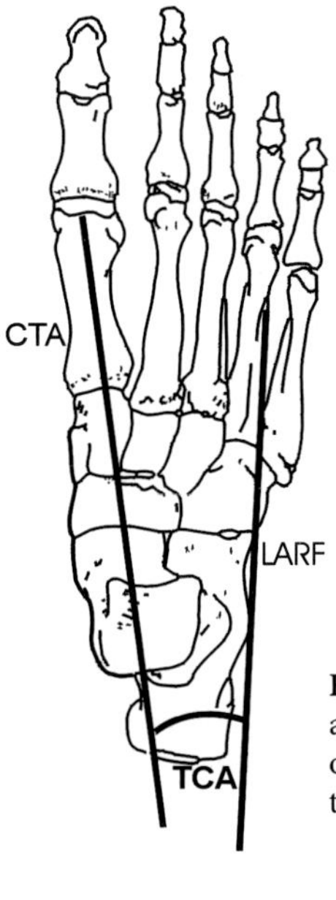

Fig. 1.24. Talocalcaneal angle (*TCA*): angle between the longitudinal axis of the rearfoot (*LARF*) and the collum tali axis (*CTA*)

1.2.1.3 Talocalcaneal Angle

The talocalcaneal angle is the angle between the CTA and the LARF (Fig. 1.24). The normal range is 17°–21°. With pronation, the talocalcaneal angle is greater than 21°; with supination it is less than 16°.

1.2.1.4 Cuboid Abduction Angle

The angle between LARF and a line tangent to the lateral surface of the cuboid ranges normally between 0° and 5° (Fig. 1.25). This angle increases above 5° with pronation of the midtarsal joint and decreases below 0° with supination and adduction.

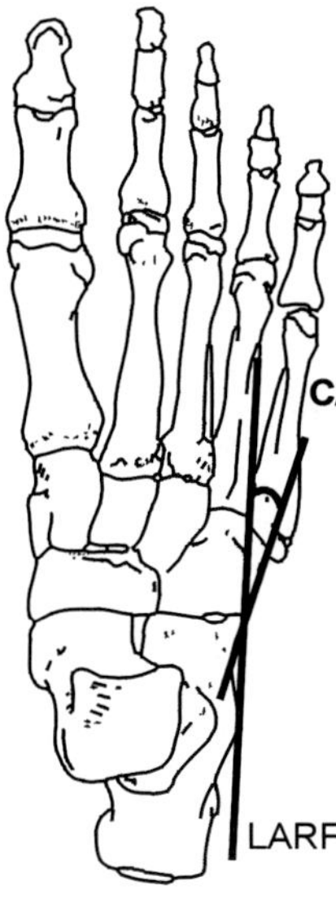

Fig. 1.25. Cuboid abduction angle (*CAA*): angle between *LARF* and the lateral surface of the cuboid

1.2.1.5 Longitudinal Axis of the Lesser Tarsus

The longitudinal axis of the lesser tarsus (LALT) is a line perpendicular to the line AB that transects the lesser tarsus (Fig. 1.26). A is one-half the distance between the medial aspect of the talonavicular joint and the medial aspect of the 1st tarsometatarsal joint. B is one-half the distance between the lateral aspect of the calcaneocuboid joint and the lateral aspect of the 5th tarsometatarsal joint.

1.2.1.6 Lesser Tarsus Angle

The lesser tarsus angle (LTA) is the angle between LALT and LARF (Fig. 1.26). This angle increases with pronation and decreases with supination.

1.2.1.7 Talonavicular Angle

The talonavicular angle (TNA) is the angle between the CTA and the bisection of the midfoot (Fig. 1.27). Normal values range between 60° and 80°. This angle is greater than 80° in the supinated foot and less than 60° in the pronated foot.

1.2.1.8 Longitudinal Axis of the Metatarsus

The longitudinal axis of the metatarsus is a line bisecting the neck and the proximal portion of the diaphysis of the 2nd metatarsal bone (Fig. 1.28).

1.2.1.9 Forefoot Adductus Angle

The forefoot adductus angle is the angle between the longitudinal axis of the metatarsus and LARF (Fig. 1.28). Normal values range between 4° and 12°. This angle decreases with pronation.

1.2.1.10 Metatarsus Adductus Angle

The metatarsus adductus angle (MAA) is the angle between the longitudinal axis of the metatarsus and LALT (Fig. 1.29). Normal values are less than 15°. A foot with a normal MAA is a 'rectus' foot; a foot with an increased MAA is an 'adductus' foot. Medial deviation of the 1st metatarsal increases as the MAA increases.

1.2.1.11 First Intermetatarsal Angle

The first intermetatarsal angle (IM) or metatarsus primus adductus angle is the angle between the longitudinal axis of the 1st and 2nd metatarsal bones (Fig. 1.30). Normal IM is 8°–12° in a rectus foot and 8°–10° in an adductus foot (Trepal 1989).

1.2.1.12 Hallux Valgus Angle

The hallux valgus or hallux abductus angle (HAV) is formed by the longitudinal axis of the 1st proximal phalanx and the longitudinal axis of the 1st metatarsus (Fig. 1.31). The normal range is 5°–15°. Hallux abductus valgus is mild when HAV is 16°–25°, moderate when HAV is 26°–35°, and severe when HAV is greater than 35°. In hallux varus or adductus, HAV is

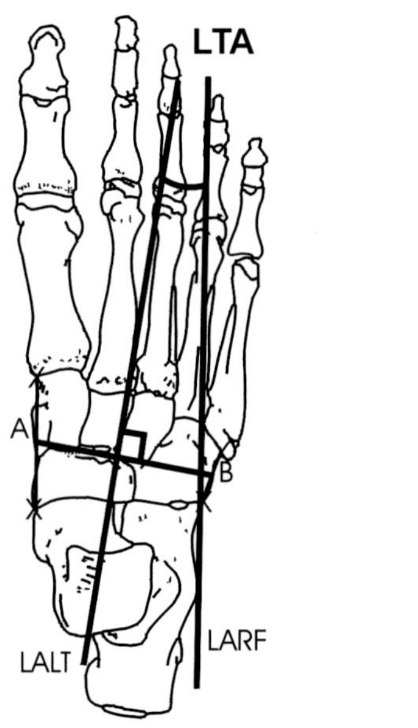

Fig. 1.26. Lesser tarsus angle (*LTA*): angle between *LARF* and the longitudinal axis of the lesser tarsus (*LALT*)

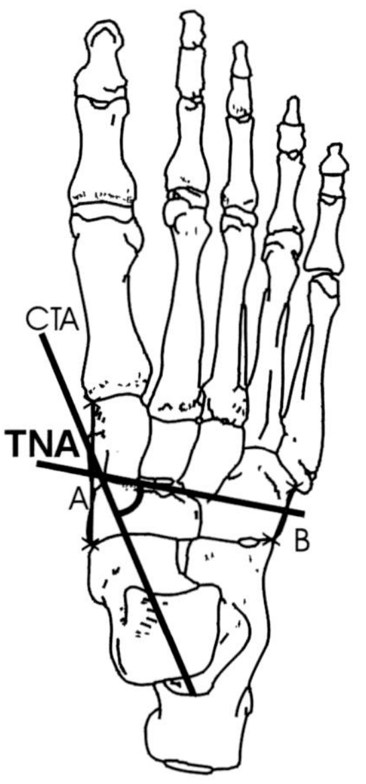

Fig. 1.27. Talonavicular angle (*TNA*): angle between *CTA* and the bisection of the lesser tarsum (*AB*)

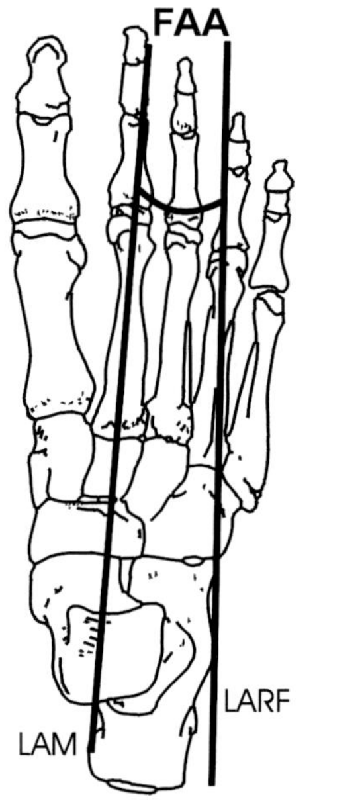

Fig. 1.28. Forefoot adductus angle (*FAA*): angle between the longitudinal axis of the metatarsus (*LAM*) and *LARF*

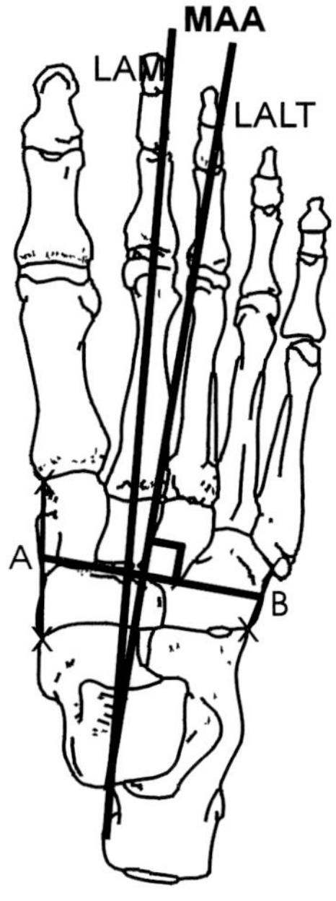

Fig. 1.29. Metatarsus adductus angle (*MAA*): angle between *LAM* and *LALT*

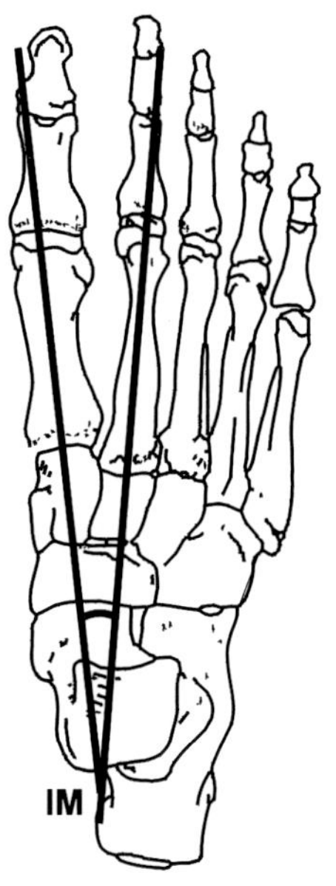

Fig. 1.30. First intermetatarsal angle (*IM*) angle between the longitudinal axes of the 1st and 2nd metatarsal bones

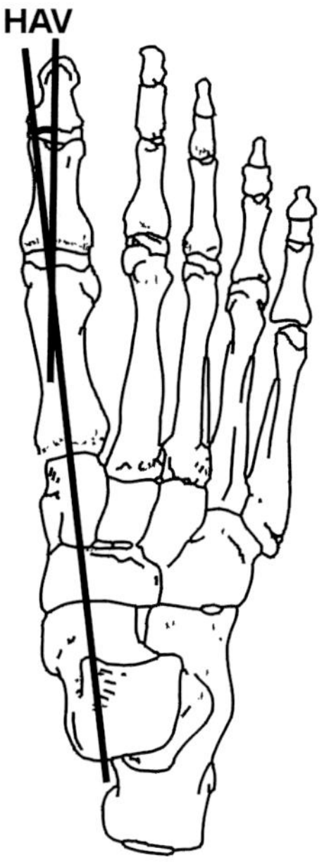

Fig. 1.31. Hallux valgus angle (*HAV*): angle between the longitudinal axis of the 1st proximal phalanx and the longitudinal axis of the 1st metatarsus

0°–5° (Karasick and Wapner 1990; Laporta et al. 1974; Mann 1989).

1.2.1.13
Proximal and Distal Articular Set Angles

The proximal articular set angle (PASA) is the angle between lines perpendicular to the effective articular surface of the 1st metatarsal head and the longitudinal axis of the 1st metatarsal bone (Fig. 1.32). The distal articular set angle (DASA) is the angle between lines perpendicular to the effective articular surface of the 1st proximal phalanx and longitudinal axis of 1st proximal phalanx (Fig. 1.32). The normal PASA is less than 10°. The normal DASA is 0°–6°.

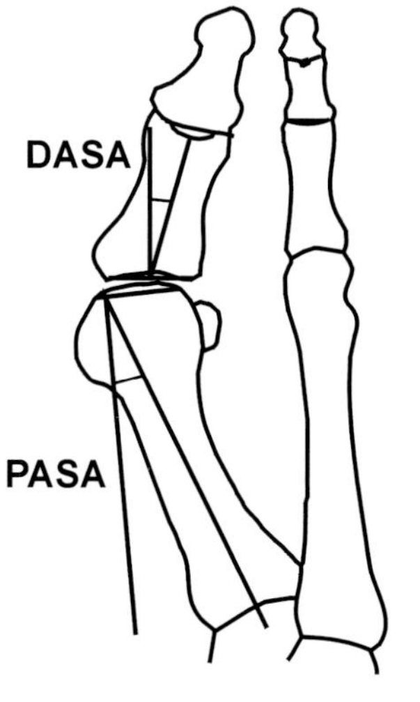

Fig. 1.32. Proximal and distal articular set angles (*PASA* and *DASA*)

1.2.1.14
Hallux Interphalangeal Angle

The hallux interphalangeal angle (HIA) is the angle formed between the longitudinal axes of the proximal and distal phalanges of the hallux (Fig. 1.33). Normal HIA is less than 10°.

1.2.2
Axes and Angles on the Lateral Projection

1.2.2.1
Plane of Support

The plane of support is defined by the line connecting the most inferior point of the tuberosity of the calcaneus with the most inferior point of the 5th metatarsal head (Fig. 1.34).

1.2.2.2
Collum Tali Axis

The collum tali axis bisects the head and neck of the talus (Fig. 1.34).

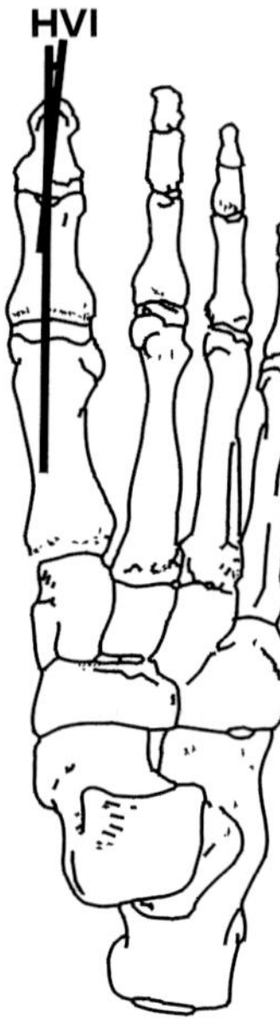

Fig. 1.33. Hallux interphalangeus angle (HIA): angle between the longitudinal axes of the proximal and distal phalanges of the hallux

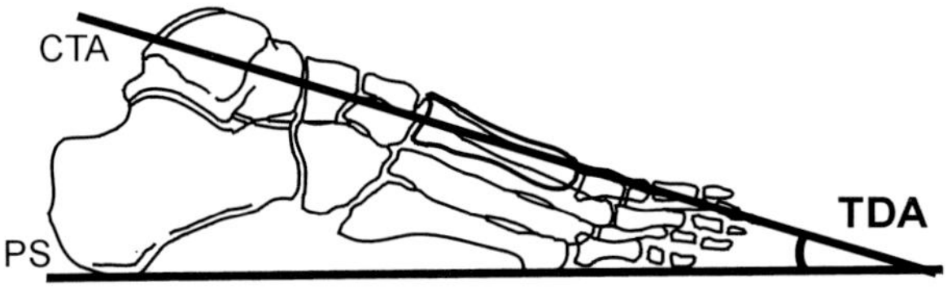

Fig. 1.34. Talar declination angle (*TDA*): angle between *CTA* and the plane of support (*PS*)

1.2.2.3 Talar Declination Angle

The talar declination angle is the angle between the plane of support and the collum tali axis (Fig. 1.34). The normal value is approximately 21°. It should be the same as the 1st metatarsal declination angle.

1.2.2.4 Calcaneal Axis or Calcaneal Inclination Axis

The calcaneal axis or calcaneal inclination axis is the line connecting the most inferior point of the tuberosity of the calcaneus with the most distal and inferior point of the calcaneus along the calcaneocuboid joint (Fig. 1.35).

1.2.2.5 Lateral Talocalcaneal Angle

The lateral talocalcaneal angle is formed by the calcaneal axis and the collum tali axis (Fig. 1.35). The normal value lies between 35° and 50°.

1.2.2.6 First Metatarsal Declination Axis

The first metatarsal declination axis is the line bisecting the neck and proximal shaft of the 1st metatarsal bone and is normally parallel to CTA (Fig. 1.36). In metatarsus primus elevatus, the 1st metatarsal declination axis angles above CTA. A plantarflexed 1st metatarsal is present when the 1st metatarsal declination axis angles below the CTA. Metatarsus primus elevatus contributes to the development of hallux limitus and hallux rigidus.

1.2.2.7 First Metatarsal Declination Angle

The first metatarsal declination angle is the angle between the plane of support and the first metatarsal declination axis. The normal value is approximately 21°. It should be the same as the talar declination angle (Fig. 1.36).

1.2.2.8 Calcaneal Inclination Angle

The calcaneal inclination angle is the angle between the plane of support and the calcaneal inclination axis (Fig. 1.37). The normal range is 20°–30°. This angle is decreased in pes planus and increased in rearfoot cavus (Fig. 1.38).

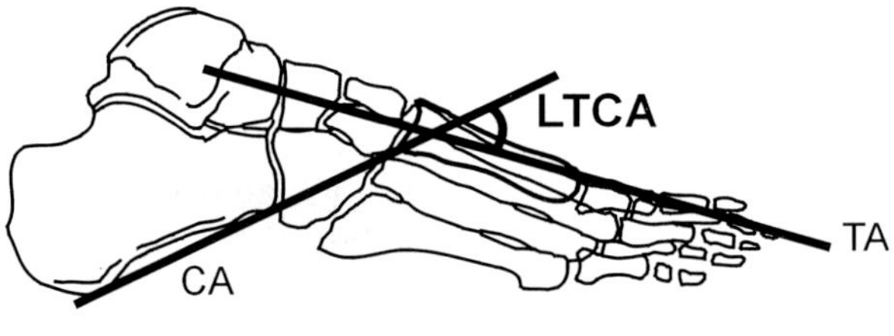

Fig. 1.35. Lateral talocalcaneal angle (*LTCA*): angle between the calcaneal axis (*CA*) and *CTA*

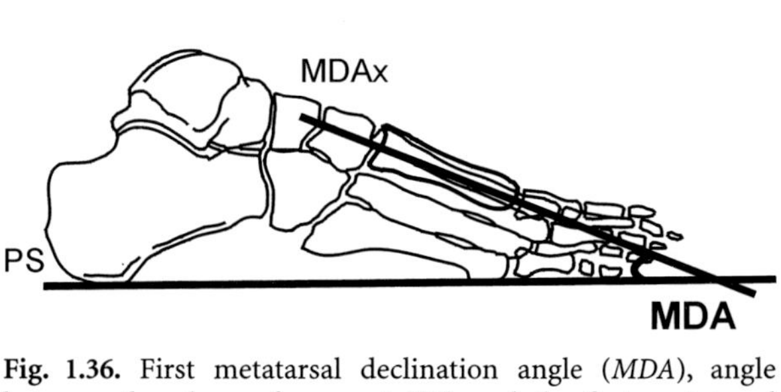

Fig. 1.36. First metatarsal declination angle (*MDA*), angle between the plane of support (*PS*) and the first metatarsal declination axis (*MDAx*). The longitudinal axis of the rearfoot is a line parallel to the distal portion of the lateral border of the calcaneus (Fig. 1.1). In the normal foot, this axis is parallel to the axis of the 4th metatarsal bone

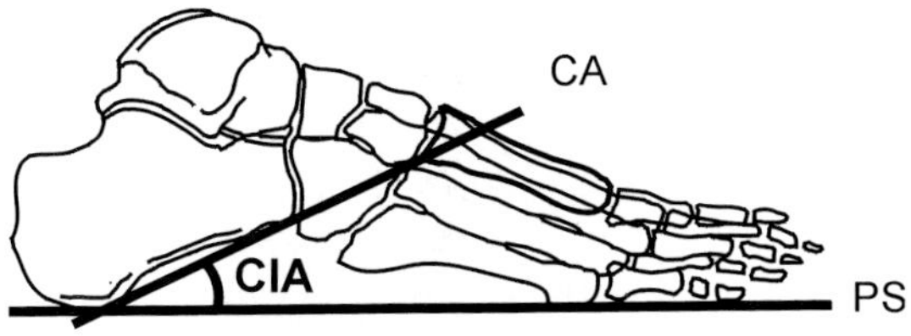

Fig. 1.37. Calcaneal inclination angle (*CIA*): angle between the plane of support (*PS*) and the calcaneal inclination axis (*CA*)

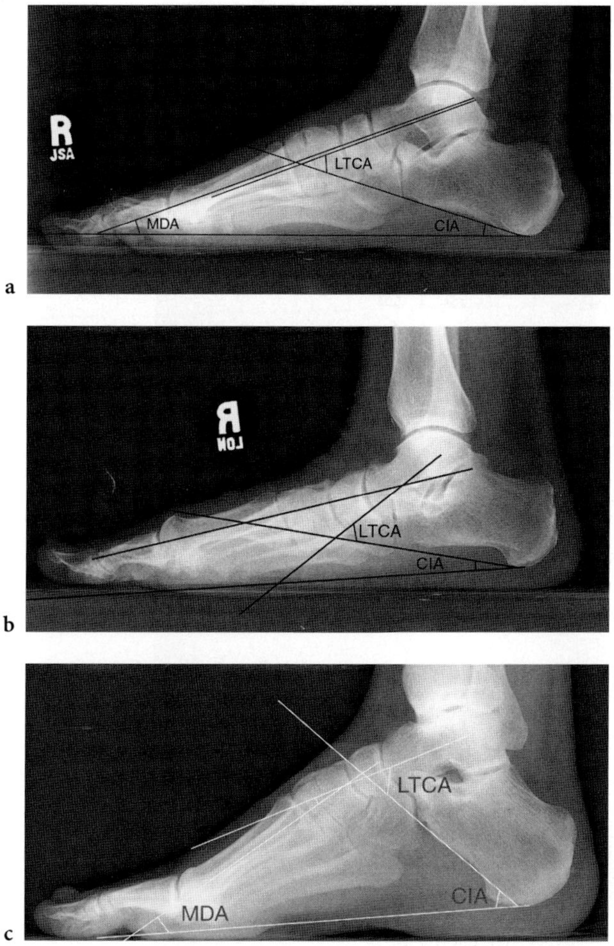

Fig. 1.38a. Normal foot. **b** Pes planus: the axis of the talus is more vertical than normal, the talocalcaneal angle is greater than 50°. **c** Pes cavus: the axis of the talus is more horizontal than normal, CIA is greater than 40°

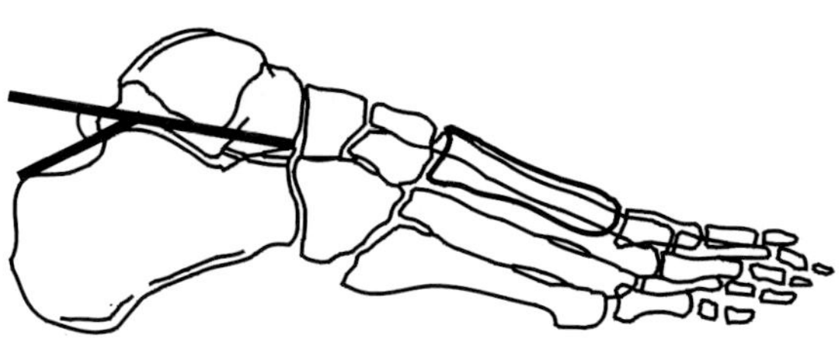

Fig. 1.39. Böhler's angle

1.2.2.9
Böhler's Angle

Böhler's angle is the angle between a line connecting the highest point of the posterior facet of the calcaneus with the highest point of the posterior tuberosity, and a second line connecting the highest point of the posterior facet with the dorsal aspect of the anterior process. The normal range is 25°–40°. It is decreased with calcaneal fractures (Fig. 1.39).

1.3
Normal Variants: Sesamoid Bones and Accessory Ossicles

Numerous sesamoid bones and accessory ossification centers may be present in the foot. Occasionally, these can be confused with fractures (Keats 1988; Keats and Anderson 2001). Figure 1.40 shows the most common location of these ossicles (Schmidt et al. 1993).

Sesamoid Bones. Two sesamoid bones are normally seen at the plantar surface of the 1st metatarsal head. Frequently, sesamoid bones are also present at the 2nd and 5th metatarsal heads and rarely at the 3rd and 4th metatarsal heads (Fig. 1.41). The sesamoid of the 1st metatarsal is bipartite in one-third of cases.

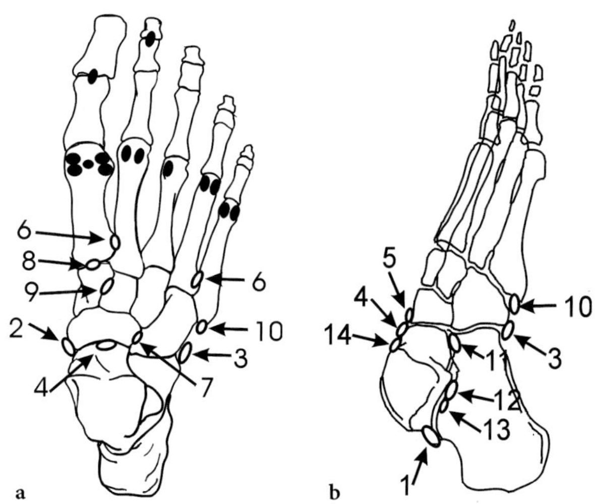

Fig. 1.40a,b. Accessory ossicles and sesamoid bones: 1 = os trigonum, 2 = os tibiale externum, 3 = os perineum, 4 = os supratalare, 5 = os supranaviculare, 6 = os intermetatarseum, 7 = cuboideum secundarium, 8 = os cubometatarseum, 9 = os cuneiforme, 10 = os vesalianum, 11 = calcaneus secundarius, 12 = os sustentaculum, 13 = talus accessories, 14 = os talotibiale

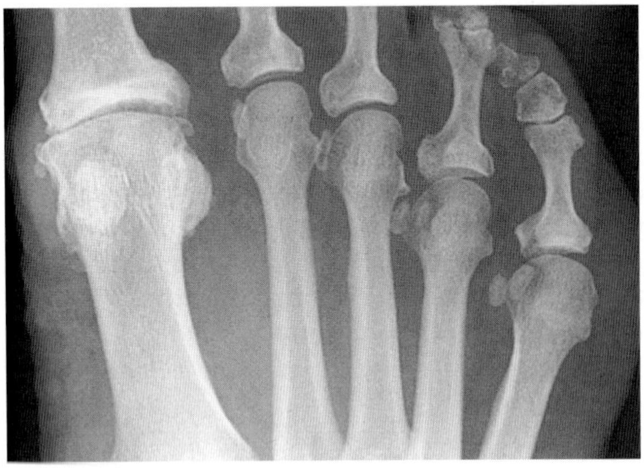

Fig. 1.41. Sesamoid bones

Occasionally, the first toe has a sesamoid plantar to the interphalangeal joint (Fig. 1.42).

Os Trigonum. The os trigonum is located in the lateral groove of the lateral tubercle of the posterior process of the talus (Fig. 1.43).

Os Subtibiale, Os Subfibulare. The os subtibiale (Fig. 1.44) and the os subfibulare (Fig. 1.45) are found inferior to the medial and lateral malleoli, respectively. They may represent unfused epiphyseal ossification centers, supernumerary ossicles, or post-traumatic ossicles.

Os Tibiale Externum. The os tibiale externum (Fig. 1.46) (os naviculare secondarium, accessory navicular bone) is the most common accessory ossicle of the foot. It is located medial and dorsal to the navicular bone and is connected to the navicular bone by hyaline or fibrocar-

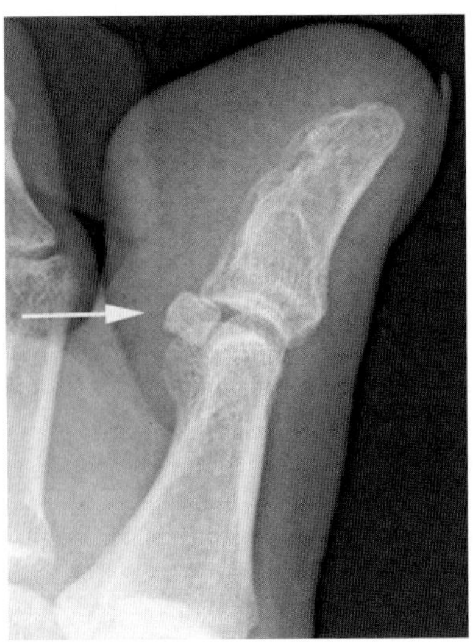

Fig. 1.42. Sesamoid bone (*arrow*) near proximal interphalangeal joint

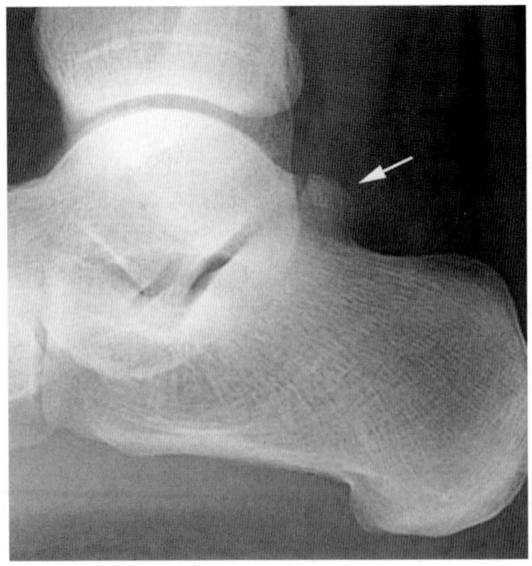

Fig. 1.43. Os trigonum (*arrow*)

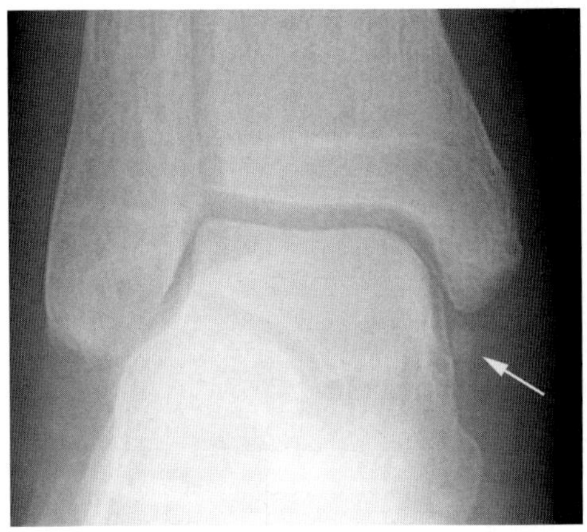

Fig. 1.44. Os subtibiale (*arrow*)

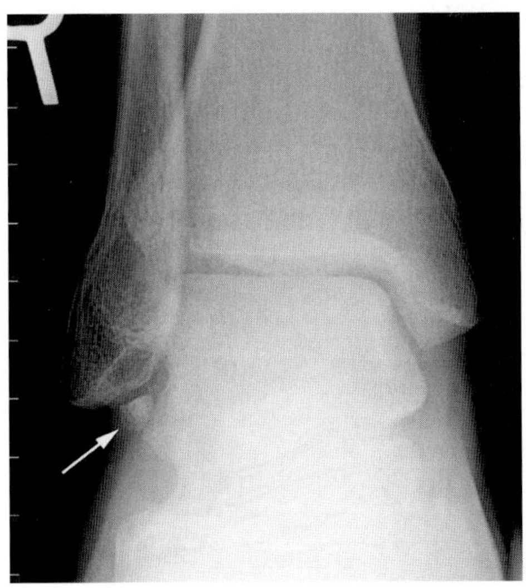

Fig. 1.45. Os subfibulare (*arrow*)

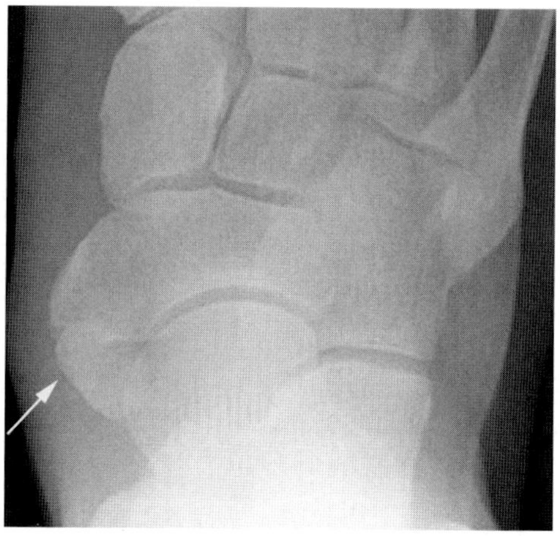

Fig. 1.46. Os tibiale externum (*arrow*)

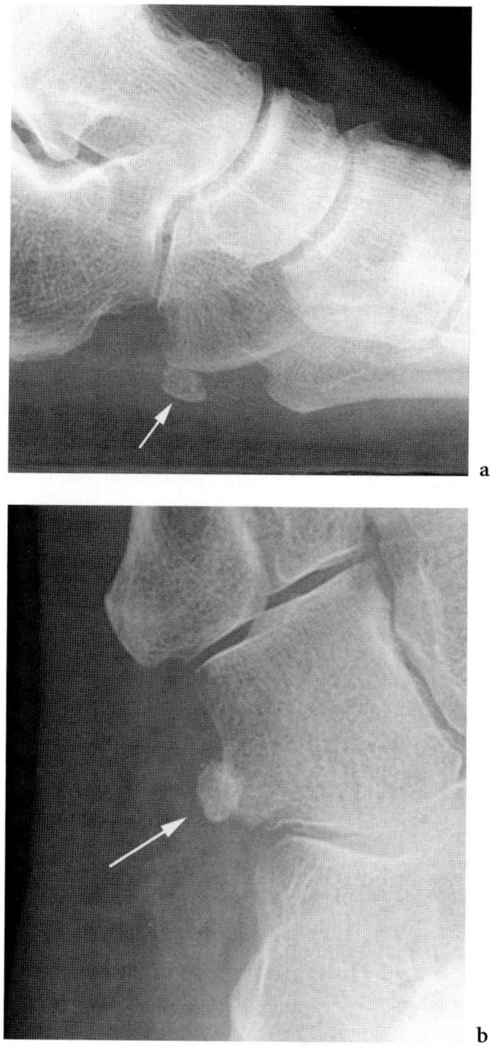

Fig. 1.47a,b. Os peroneum (*arrow*)

tilage. The posterior tibial tendon inserts on this ossicle in the majority of cases (Kiter et al. 1999).

Os Peroneum. The os peroneum (Fig. 1.47) is a sesamoid bone of the peroneus longus tendon. It is located adjacent to the lateral and inferior aspect of the cuboid, and occasionally can articulate with the cuboid.

Os Supratalare. The os supratalare (Fig. 1.48) is located dorsal to the talar neck.

Os Supranaviculare. The os supranaviculare (Fig. 1.49) is located dorsal to the talonavicular joint.

Os Intermetatarseum. The os intermetatarseum (Fig. 1.50) is located between the 1st and 2nd metatarsal bases. It can be confused with calcification of the intermetatarsal artery.

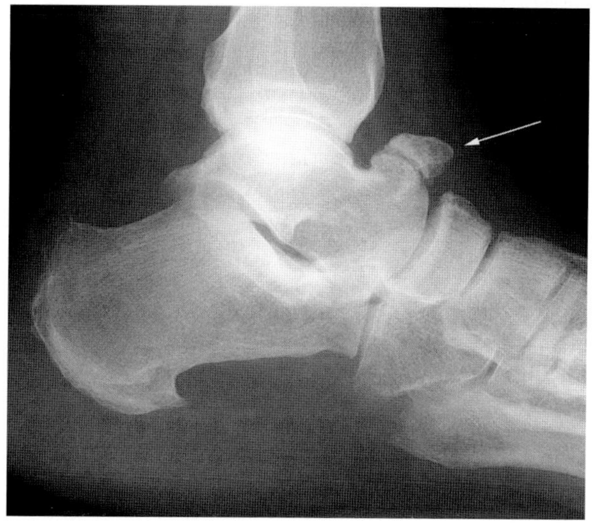

Fig. 1.48. Os supratalare (*arrow*)

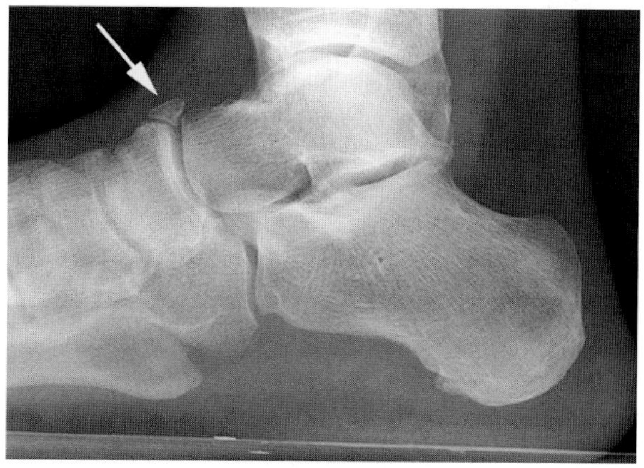

Fig. 1.49. Os supranaviculare (*arrow*)

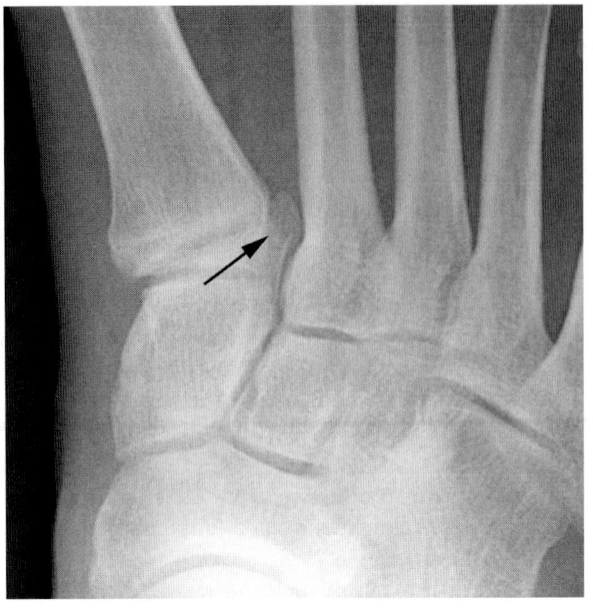

Fig. 1.50. Os intermetatarseum (*arrow*)

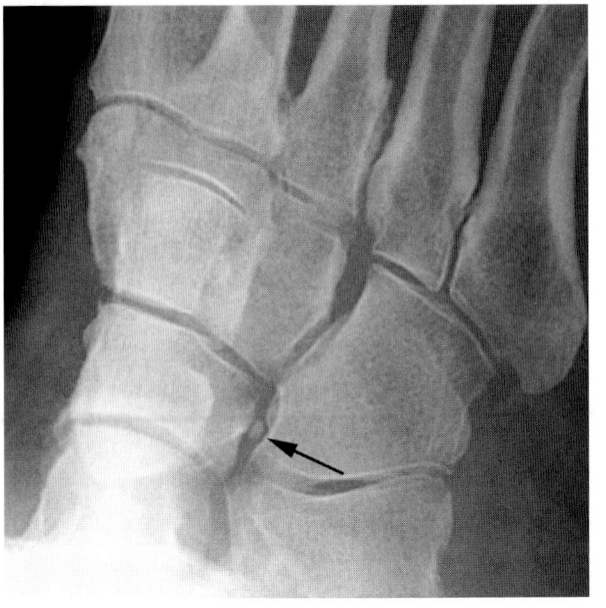

Fig. 1.51. Os cuboideum secondarium (*arrow*)

Os Intermetatarseum. The os intermetatarseum (Fig. 1.50) is located between the 1st and 2nd metatarsal bases. It can be confused with calcification of the intermetatarsal artery.

Os Cuboideum Secondarium. The os cuboideum secondarium (Fig. 1.51) is located dorsal and medial to the cuboid bone.

References

Ballinger WP, Frank ED (1999) Merrill's atlas of radiographic positions and radiologic procedures, 9th edn. Mosby, St Louis

Bontrager KL, Lampignano JP (1997) Radiographic positioning and related anatomy, 4th edn. Mosby, St Louis, pp 188–203

Haupfauer W (1970) A contribution to the diagnosis of fresh rupture of the fibular ligament. Monatsschr Unfallheilkd 73:178–184

Karasick D, Wapner KL (1990) Hallux valgus deformity: Preoperative radiologic assessment. AJR 155:119–123

Kashak TJ, Laine W (1988) Surgical radiology. Clin Pod Med Surg 5:797–829

Keats TE (1988) Normal roentgen variants of the foot and ankle that may simulate disease. Clin Podiatr Med Surg 5:777–795

Keats TE, Anderson MW (2001) Atlas of normal Roentgen variants that may simulate disease. Mosby, St Louis

Kiter E, Erdag N, Karatosun V, et al (1999) Tibialis posterior tendon abnormalities in feet with accessory navicular bone and flatfoot. Acta Orthop Scand 70:618–621

Laporta G, Melillo T, Olinsky D (1974) X-ray evaluation of hallux abducto valgus deformity. J Am Podiatr Assoc 64: 544–566

Mann RA (1989) The great toe. Orthop Clin 20:519–533

Schmidt H, Freyschmidt J, Holthusen W (1993) Borderlands of normal and early pathologic findings in skeletal radiography, 4th edn. Thieme, New York

Towbin R, Dunbar JS, Towbin J, Clark R (1980) Teardrop sign: plain film recognition of ankle effusion. AJR Am J Roentgenol 134:985–990

Trepal MJ (1989). Hallux valgus and metatarsus adductus: the surgical dilemma. Clin Pod Med Surg 6:103–113

2 Anatomy, Arthrography, Bursography and Tenography of the Ankle and Foot

V. N. Cassar-Pullicino and B. Tins

CONTENTS

2.1 Introduction

Arthrography, tenography and bursography of the ankle developed as a natural progression from the application of these techniques in other areas of the body. In the 1970s and 1980s these methods became well established, and single and double contrast techniques were both used. Currently, conventional arthrography of the ankle and foot joints in isolation has become uncommon. The main applications today are as part of CT- or MR-arthrography or in combination with direct diagnostic/therapeutic procedures. CT- and MR-arthrography are superior to non-arthrographic joint imaging in depicting the anatomy and pathology of the ankle joint in many clinical scenarios.

Diagnostic/therapeutic procedures of the ankle and foot involve the injection of a local anaesthetic or a glucocorticoid into an anatomical space to establish the origin of pain and as a form of treatment. Arthrography confirms which anatomical compartment is being injected. It also depicts abnormal communications, which can lead to misdiagnosis if not appreciated.

Similarly, the indications for tenography of the tendons around the ankle have become fewer, but tenography is still occasionally used in the diagnosis of disruption of the lateral ankle ligaments. More importantly, it is still the only method able to diagnose chronic and stenosing tenosynovitis. Tenography can also form part of a diagnostic and/or therapeutic injection of a local anaesthetic or glucocorticoid.

A clear understanding of the regional anatomy is an essential prerequisite to performing and interpreting these interventional techniques.

2.2 Anatomy

2.2.1 Bones, Joints and Ligaments

The tibia and fibula articulate with the talus to form the ankle joint. They are joined by a syndesmosis consisting of the interosseous membrane and the anterior and posterior tibiofibular ligaments. The anterior and posterior tibiofibular ligaments join the two bones just proximal to the ankle joint. On the lateral side of the ankle, the anterior talofibular ligament, the calcaneofibular ligament and the posterior talofibular ligament join the fibula to the hindfoot and reinforce the joint capsule. On the medial side, the deltoid ligament binds the tibia to the talus and calcaneus.

V. N. Cassar-Pullicino, LRCP, MRCS, MD, DMRD, FRCR
Department of Radiology, The Robert Jones & Agnes Hunt Orthopaedic & District Hospital, Oswestry, Shropshire, SY10 7AG, UK
B. Tins, MD, Dipl. Phys, FRCR
Department of Radiology, The Robert Jones & Agnes Hunt Orthopaedic & District Hospital, Oswestry, Shropshire, SY10 7AG, UK

The joint capsule of the ankle joint has an anterior and a posterior recess to allow for hinge joint mobility (Figs. 2.1, 2.5b, 2.6e, 2.4e). There is a further, usually small, syndesmotic recess (infundibulum) along the most distal part of the syndesmosis between the tibia and fibula (Table 2.1) (Fig. 2.1b). The insertion of the joint capsule onto the bone is largely identical with the cartilage-bone transition with the exception of the anterior recess, which extends over a bare area of bone on the talar neck. The ligaments in the ankle region are intimately related to the joint capsule and in sections form part of it.

Table 2.1. Location and relevance of contrast medium collections in ankle arthrography

Location	Area of extravasation	Significance
Lateral	Around tip of lateral malleolus	Anterior talofibular ligament tear
	Filling of peroneal tendon sheaths	Calcaneofibular ligament tear
Medial	Filling of post-tibial tendon sheath	Abnormal
	Around medial malleolus	Deltoid ligament tear
Cranial	Syndesmotic recess	Normal
	Cranial extravasation from syndesmotic recess	Anterior tibiofibular ligament tear
Caudal	Subtalar joint	Normal
Anterior	Anterior recess	Normal
Posterior	Posterior recess	Normal
	Flexor hallucis longus sheath (extending distally on medial side of foot)	Normal

The anterior talofibular ligament is the weakest of the three lateral ligaments. It extends anteromedially from the anterior surface of the distal fibula to the lateral side of the talar neck, sloping slightly downwards (Fig. 2.4g). This ligament is actually located within the joint capsule. The calcaneofibular ligament (Fig. 2.2) is located between the anterior and posterior talofibular

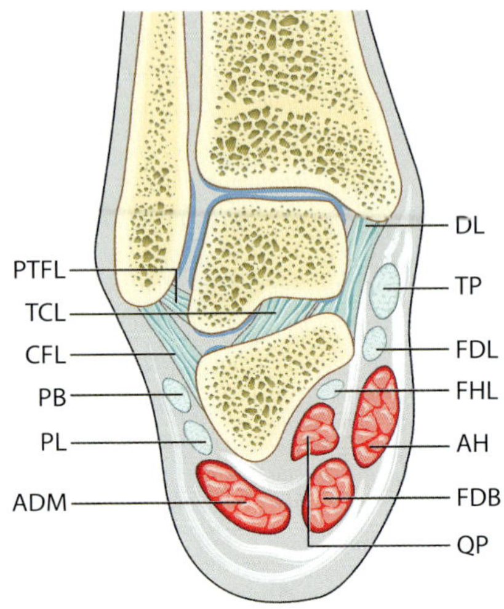

Fig. 2.2. Diagrammatic coronal view of the ankle joint. Medially, the deltoid ligament (*DL*) joins the tibia to the talus and calcaneus. Tibialis posterior (*TP*), flexor digitorum longus (*FDL*) and flexor hallucis longus (*FHL*) tendons are seen. Laterally, there are the posterior talofibular (*PTFL*) and calcaneofibular (*CFL*) ligaments. Peroneus brevis (*PB*) and longus (*PL*) tendons adjacent. Talocalcaneal ligament (*TCL*) in the sinus tarsi. Caudally, abductor digiti minimi (*ADM*), quadratus plantae (*QP*), flexor digitorum brevis (*FDB*) and abductor hallucis (*AH*) muscles

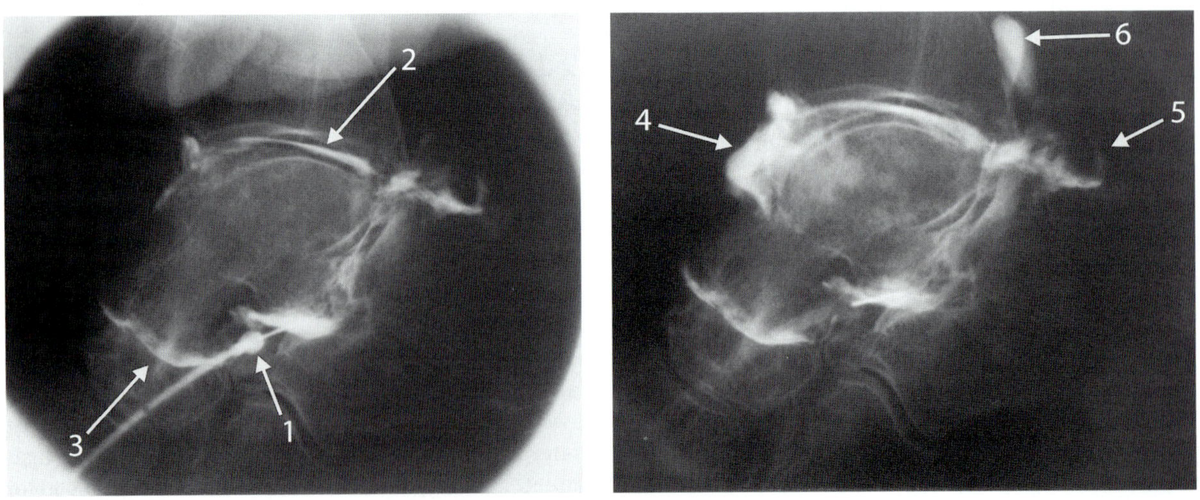

a b

Fig. 2.1a, b. Subtalar joint injection in a rheumatoid patient. The needle is demonstrated in the joint space (*1*). Spread of contrast medium into the ankle joint (*2*) (can be normal) and the talonavicular joint (*3*) (abnormal) is seen. Note the good depiction of cartilage thickness and surface. Injection of radiolucent local anaesthetic results in filling of the anterior (*4*), posterior (*5*) and syndesmotic recesses (*6*) of the ankle joint ligaments. From the posterior surface of the distal fibula it passes inferiorly, medially and slightly posteriorly to the calcaneus. This ligament is stronger than the anterior talofibular ligament. It is intimately related and in parts fused to the peroneal tendon sheath, which overlies it directly laterally (Fig. 2.6a).The posterior talofibular ligament runs from the medial and posterior surface of the fibular tip, the malleolar fossa, medially and posteriorly and slightly downwards (Figs. 2.2, 2.4g, 2.6a). In the neutral position it lies roughly in the same axial plane as the anterior talofibular ligament. It is strong and rarely injured.

The deltoid ligament lies on the medial side of the ankle joint. It fans broadly from the medial malleolus to the talus, navicular and calcaneus, assuming a roughly delta shape (Figs. 2.2, 2.4f). It divides into deep fibres to the talus and navicular and superficial fibres to the calcaneus. The deltoid ligament is quite strong and injured only by great force.

The talus and calcaneus form the basis of the hindfoot. The talus has a posterior bony protrusion, the posterior process. The posterior process has two dorsal tubercles, a medial and a lateral. In the groove between them runs the tendon of flexor hallucis longus (Fig. 2.3). The tubercles also serve as insertion areas for interosseous ligaments in the hindfoot area. The lateral tubercle is larger and develops from its own ossification centre. In about 13%–16% of the population it fails to form a bony union with the talus. The resulting extra ossicle is named the os trigonum.

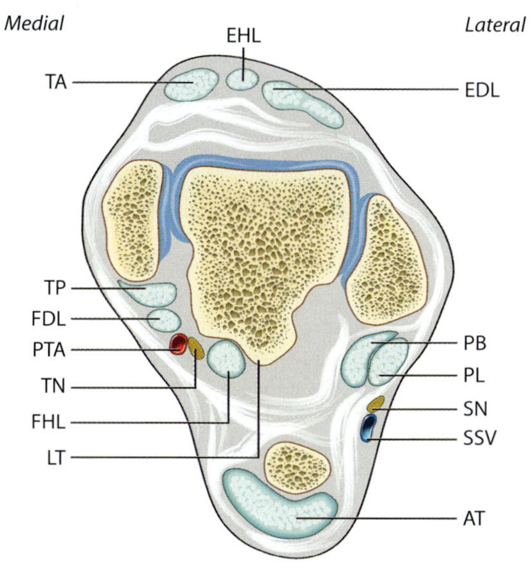

Fig. 2.3. Diagrammatic axial view of the ankle joint. Anteriorly, tendons of tibialis anterior (*TA*), extensor hallucis longus (*EHL*) and extensor digitorum longus (*EDL*) muscles. Medially, tendons of tibialis posterior (*TP*), flexor digitorum longus (*FDL*) and flexor hallucis longus (*FHL*) muscles. In between the FDL and FHL, the posterior tibial artery (*PTA*) and tibial nerve (*TN*). Lateral to the FHL tendon, the lateral tubercle (*LT*) of the talus. Posteriorly, the Achilles tendon (*AT*) with a small portion of the calcaneus just anterior. Laterally, tendons of peroneus brevis (*PB*) and longus (*PL*) muscles. Adjacent sural nerve (*SN*) and short saphenous vein (*SSV*)

The long axis of the talus and calcaneus are roughly sagittally aligned. Posteriorly, the talus rests directly on the calcaneus via the posterior talocalcaneal (subtalar) joint (Figs. 2.4e, 2.6a,d). The subtalar joint can normally communicate with the ankle joint (10%–20% of the population) (Fig. 2.6e). The long axis of the calcaneus points more laterally than that of the talus. To support the talus further distally, the calcaneus forms a medial bony ridge, the sustentaculum tali. Two further articular facets between the calcaneus and talus are located here. These two joint facets are part of the more complex anterior talocalcaneonavicular joint. This complex is contained in one joint capsule. Therefore, the posterior and the anterior talocalcaneal joints have separate joint capsules. These do not normally communicate. The joints are separated by fibrous tissue and the interosseous talocalcaneal ligament in a bony groove of the talus, the sulcus tali, and in a corresponding groove of the calcaneus, the sulcus calcanei (Fig. 2.2). The grooves widen laterally to form the sinus tarsi. Despite the complex anatomy, the anterior and posterior talocalcaneal joints are functionally part of a single joint.

The hindfoot articulates with the more distal tarsus, forming the talocalcaneonavicular joint medially and cranially to the more lateral and caudal calcaneocuboid joint (Fig. 2.7). In the former joint the main articulation is between the talus and navicular. The navicular bone in turn articulates with the three cuneiform bones, which in turn articulate with the first to third metatarsals. The cuboid articulates directly with the fourth and fifth metatarsals.

2.2.2 Ankle Tendons

The ankle joint is surrounded by tendons (Figs. 2.3, 2.4g). With the exception of the Achilles tendon they are all closely related to the ankle joint. The Achilles tendon is the common tendon of the triceps surae muscle, formed by the soleus and the two gastrocnemius muscles. It inserts into the dorsal calcaneus. Deep to the insertion, on top of the calcaneus, lies the small retrocalcaneal bursa. The Achilles tendon does not have a synovial tendon sheath but is surrounded by a connective tissue envelope, the so-called

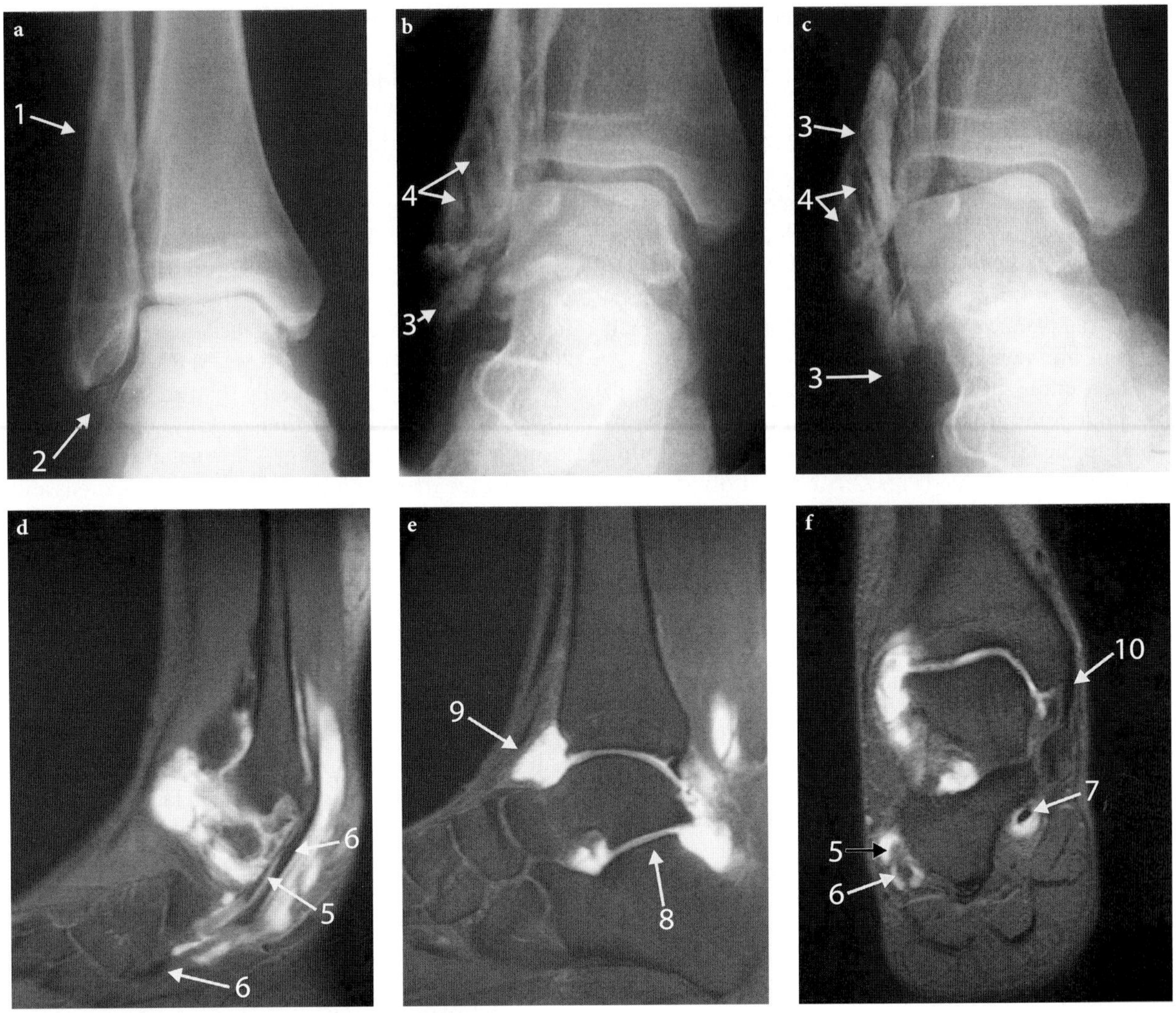

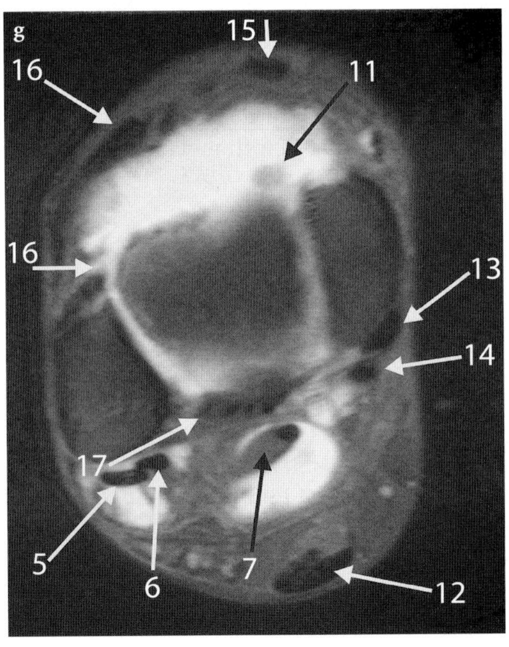

Fig. 2.4a–g. A 47-year-old lady with ankle instability and pain with a history of fibula fracture. **a** Anteroposterior (AP) view of the right ankle demonstrates a healed distal fibular shaft fracture (*1*) and separate ossicles adjacent to the tip of the fibula (*2*). AP (**b**) and AP stress view (**c**) post-arthrogram demonstrate gross lateral instability (**c**) and contrast medium in the peroneal tendon sheath (*3*) outlining the peroneal tendons (*4*). This indicates injury of the calcaneofibular ligament. **d–g** MR arthrogram (T1-weighted fat-saturated sequences) confirms these findings and demonstrates abnormal contrast medium collection in the peroneal tendon sheath surrounding the peroneus longus (*5*) and brevis (*6*) tendon (**d, f, g**). Contrast in the sheath around the flexor hallucis longus tendon (*7*) is normal (**f, g**). Contrast in the subtalar joint (*8*) is normal (**e**). Normal anterior recess of the ankle joint (*9*) (**e**). On the coronal image (**f**) the normal deltoid ligament (*10*) is well demonstrated. On the axial image (**g**) there is a loose body (*11*) evident anterior to the talus. Tendo achilles (*12*), posterior tibial tendon (*13*), flexor digitorum longus tendon (*14*), flexor hallucis longus tendon (*7*), anterior tibial tendon (*15*) and extensor digitorum longus tendon (*16*) are well demonstrated. Flexor hallucis longus is still part muscle (*7*). Note the disrupted anterior talofibular ligament (*16*) and the intact posterior talofibular ligament (*17*)

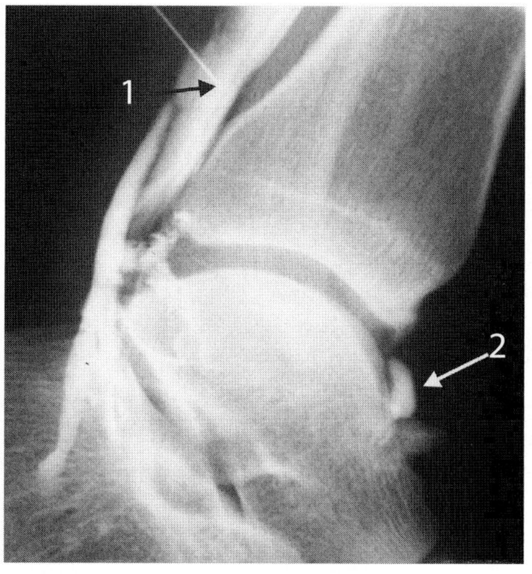

a

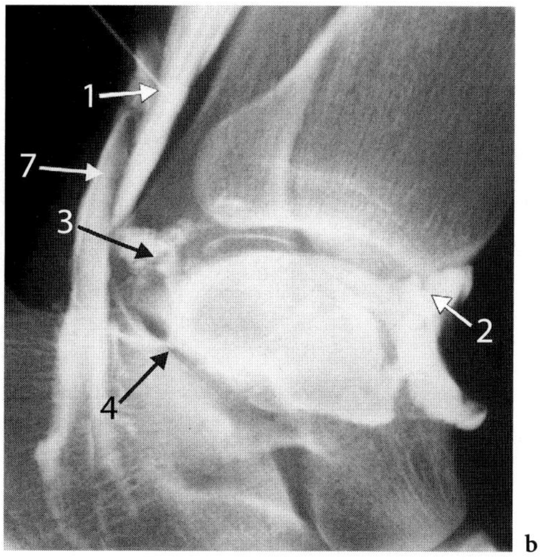

b

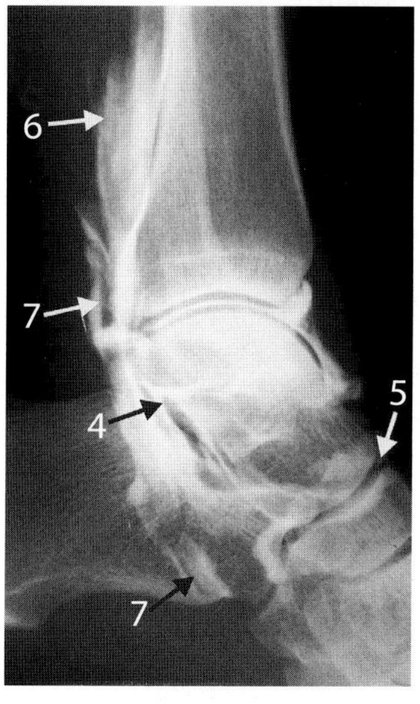

c

Fig. 2.5a–c. Peroneal tenogram. **a, b** Tendon sheath puncture (*1*) approximately 4 cm proximal to the fibula tip. Early abnormal communication with the ankle joint (**a**) indicating calcaneofibular ligament injury with contrast medium in the anterior (*2*) and posterior recess (*3*). Contrast medium is seen in the subtalar joint (*4*) (**b**) and also in the talonavicular joint (*5*) (**c**). Backspill of contrast medium into the peroneal muscles is seen (*6*) (**c**). The peroneal tendons are seen as filling defect (*7*)

paratenon. Tendon sheaths usually occur only around tendons that are exposed to compressive stress, commonly by not having a straight line of pull.

There are usually eight further tendons around the ankle joint, which are all closely related to the joint itself. These tendons all have tendon sheaths. The length of these sheaths is quite variable; they do, however, almost always cover the area of greatest stress to the tendon. Tendon sheaths consist of an outer fibrous covering with incorporation of adjacent periosteum where present and an inner synovial lining.

2.2.2.1 Peroneal Tendons

There are two peroneal tendons located on the lateral side of the ankle joint. The peroneus longus muscle arises from the lateral fibula and the neighbouring fasciae on the proximal two-thirds of the calf. In the ankle region its tendon lies dorsolateral to the peroneus brevis tendon, which is in-between the peroneus longus tendon and the posterior tip of the fibula (Figs. 2.2, 2.3). The peroneus brevis muscle arises from the distal two-thirds of the lateral fibula and adjacent septa. The two tendons are initially contained in a common tendon sheath. Rarely, the tendons can be conjoined. The common tendon sheath forms approximately 4 cm proximal to the lateral malleolus and usually separates into individual sheaths after the tendons have passed the lateral malleolus (Figs. 2.5, 2.8–2.10). Usually, the sheaths terminate at the level of the distal third of the calcaneus. The peroneus brevis inserts on the base of the fifth metacarpal, while the peroneus longus

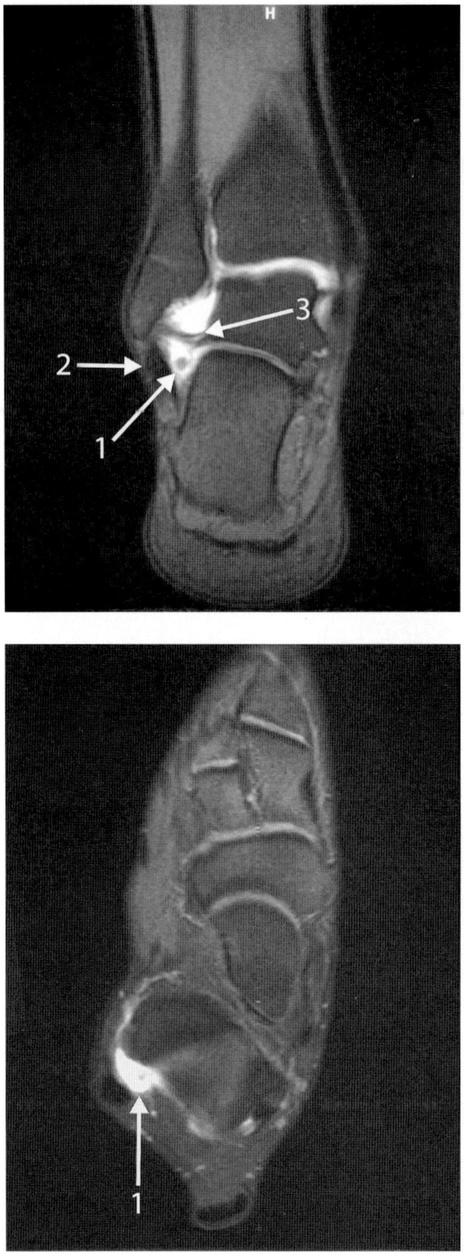

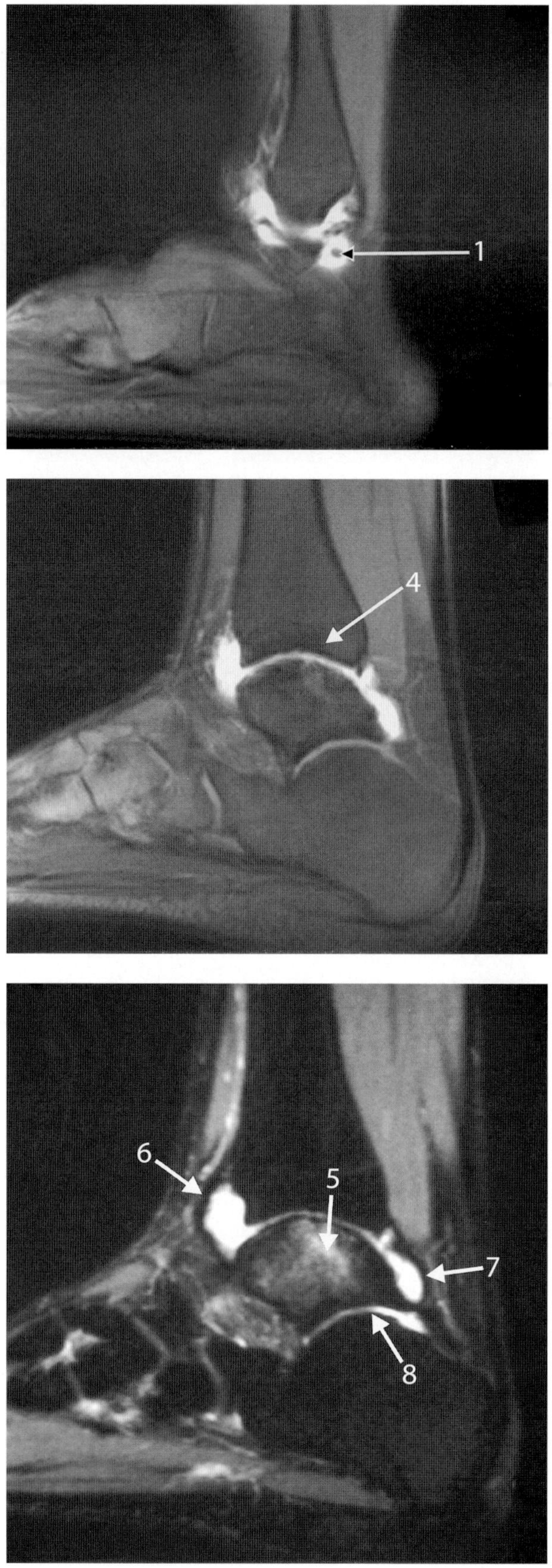

a b c d e

Fig. 2.6a–e. MR arthrogram of the right ankle for ankle pain. Fat-saturated T1-weighted (**a**–**d**) and STIR (**e**) sequences. A loose body is seen (*1*) in the lateral recess (**a**–**c**). **a** The intimate relation of the calcaneofibular ligament to the peroneal tendon sheath is demonstrated (*2*). The posterior talofibular ligament is seen (*3*). Imbibition of contrast medium into the talar and tibial surface (*4*) with loss of cartilage thickness is seen (**d**), the underlying talus shows bone marrow oedema (*5*) (**e**). Anterior (*6*) and posterior (*7*) articular recess are again noted, as is the subtalar joint (*8*)

a b c d

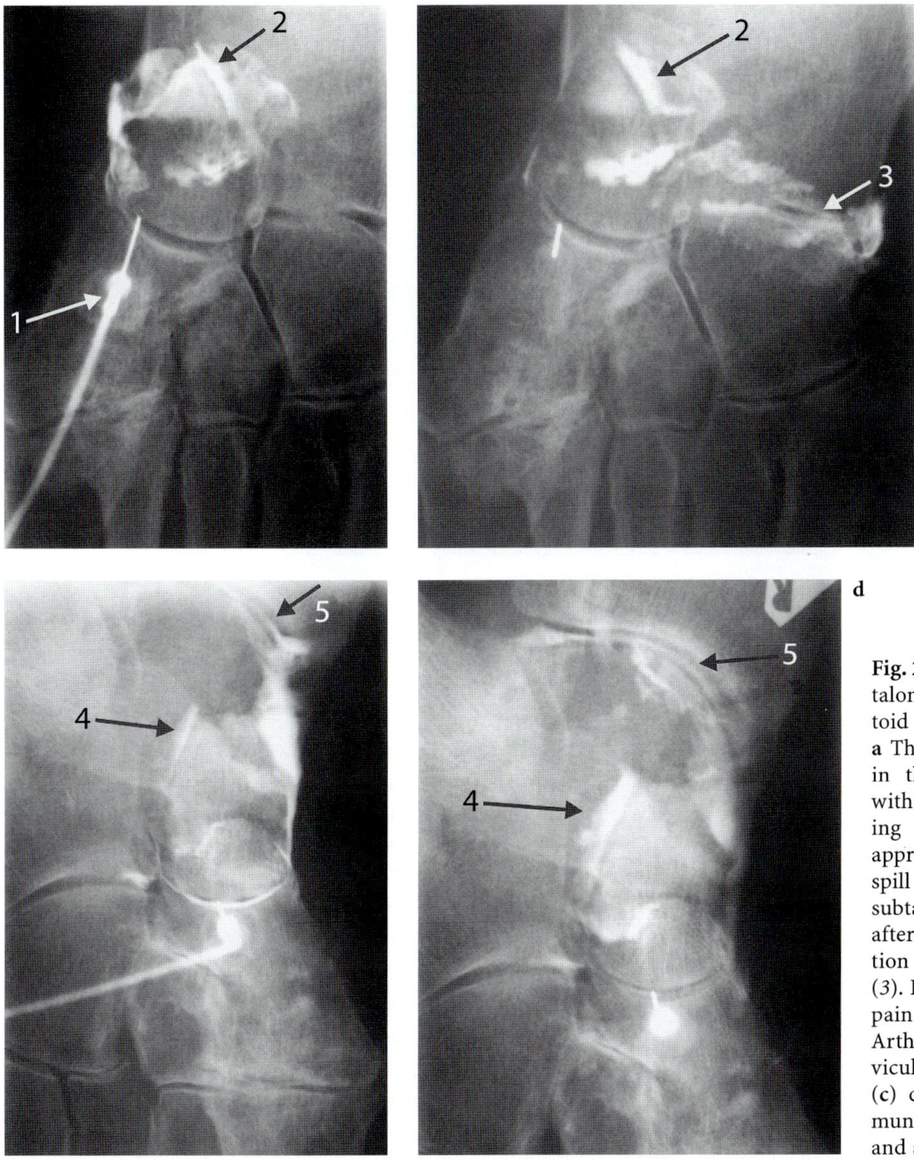

Fig. 2.7a–d. Arthrogram of the left talonavicular joint in a rheumatoid patient for pain localisation. **a** The injecting needle (*1*) is seen in the talonavicular joint space with the contrast-filled connecting tube attached. Dorsolateral approach. Immediate abnormal spill of contrast medium into the subtalar joint (*2*) is seen. **b** Shortly afterwards, abnormal communication with the calcaneocuboid joint (*3*). If pain relief occurs, the exact pain source cannot be determined. Arthrogram of the right talonavicular joint in the same patient (**c**) demonstrates abnormal communication with the subtalar (*4*) and ankle joints (*5*) (**d**)

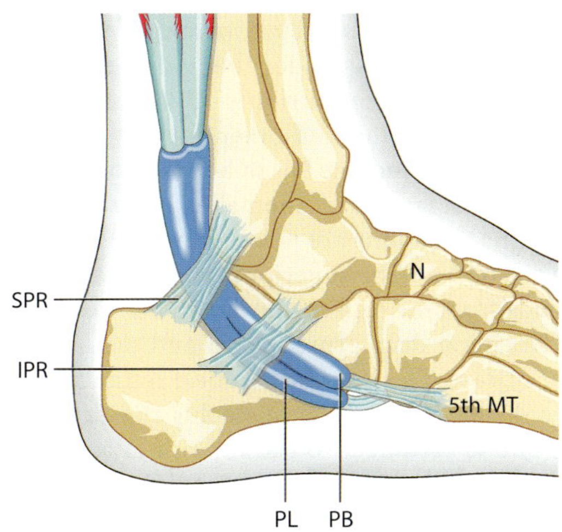

Fig. 2.8. Diagrammatic lateral view of the ankle. Peroneus brevis (*PB*) and longus (*PL*) tendons are seen with an initially common tendon sheath which then separates. The superior (*SPR*) and inferior (*IPR*) peroneal retinacula prevent tendon luxation. Base of the 5th metatarsal (*5th MT*)and navicular bone (*N*) are labelled

a b

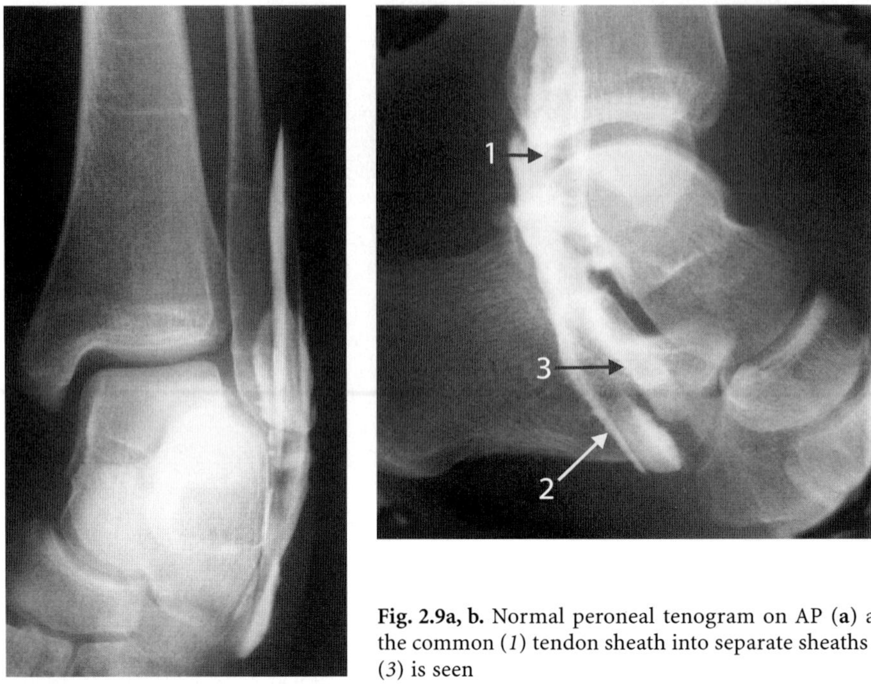

Fig. 2.9a, b. Normal peroneal tenogram on AP (**a**) and lateral view (**b**). Separation of the common (*1*) tendon sheath into separate sheaths for peroneus brevis (*2*) and longus (*3*) is seen

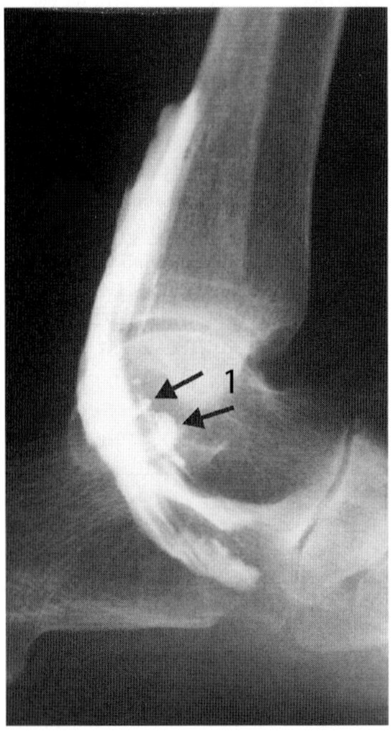

Fig. 2.10. Normal peroneal tenogram. Normal sacculations of the common tendon sheath due to the inferior peroneal retinaculum (*1*)

courses medially in a groove on the undersurface of the cuboid and inserts on the base of the first metatarsal, frequently sending some fibres to the neighbouring 2nd metatarsal and first cuneiform (Fig. 2.8). Underneath the cuboid a second, separate tendon sheath usually envelops the tendon. The common peroneal tendon sheath is usually fused with the underlying periosteum and the calcaneofibular ligament, which separates it from the ankle joint (Fig. 2.6a). Communication of the ankle joint and the peroneal tendon sheath is always abnormal and usually indicates an injury of the calcaneofibular ligament (Fig. 2.4c, 2.11, 2.12).

A common normal variant (13%) in the lateral ankle region is the presence of an accessory peroneus quartus muscle. This muscle arises off the posterior intermuscular septum and inserts on the fibular aspect of the calcaneus. It lies in the space usually only occupied by the pre-Achilles fat pad and can be mistaken as a pathological soft-tissue mass, particularly on radiographs. It can cause increased pressure on the peroneus brevis tendon behind the lateral malleolus and thereby contribute to degenerative change. There is a plethora of other normal variants in the ankle region, and one has to be aware of this in the differential diagnosis of 'anomalies' here.

The peroneal tendons are held in position by two retinacula (Fig. 2.8). The superior peroneal retinaculum extends from the back of the lateral malleolus to the posterolateral deep crural fascia and the lateral calcaneal surface. The inferior peroneal retinaculum is located distal to the lateral malleolus and extends from the lateral calcaneus to the anterior talus. Here it is partly continuous with the inferior extensor retinaculum. Functionally, both muscles evert and plantar flex the foot; the peroneus longus additionally supports the arch of the foot.

2.2.2.2
Flexor Tendons

There are three tendons on the medial side of the ankle joint: the posterior tibial, flexor hallucis longus and flexor digitorum longus tendons (Figs. 2.2–2.4g, 2.13). The tibialis posterior muscle arises on the posterolateral tibia and interosseous membrane and is sandwiched between the flexor digitorum longus muscle medially and the flexor hallucis longus muscle more laterally. Of these three, the flexor hallucis longus muscle extends furthest distally, and its muscle belly is often still seen just proximal to the ankle joint on MR imaging.

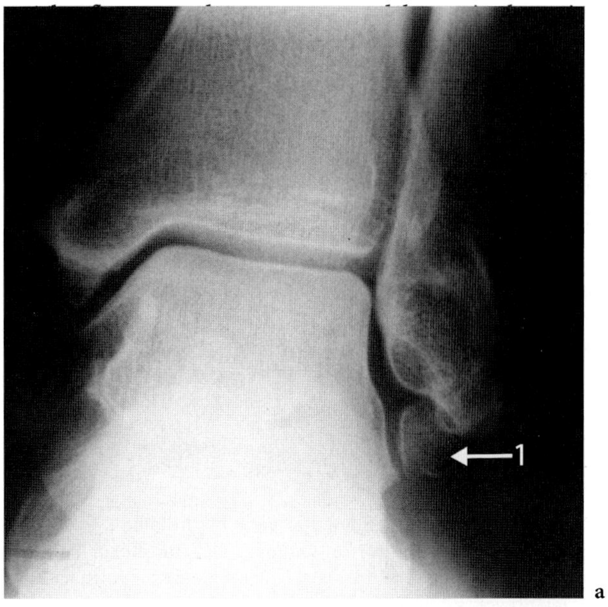

a

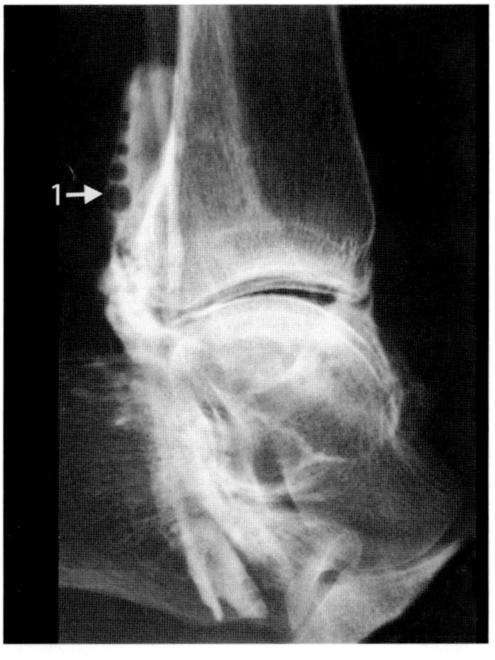

Fig. 2.11. Double contrast arthrogram of the left ankle resulting in spillage of contrast medium and air into the peroneal tendon sheath (*1*) indicating injury to the calcaneofibular ligament

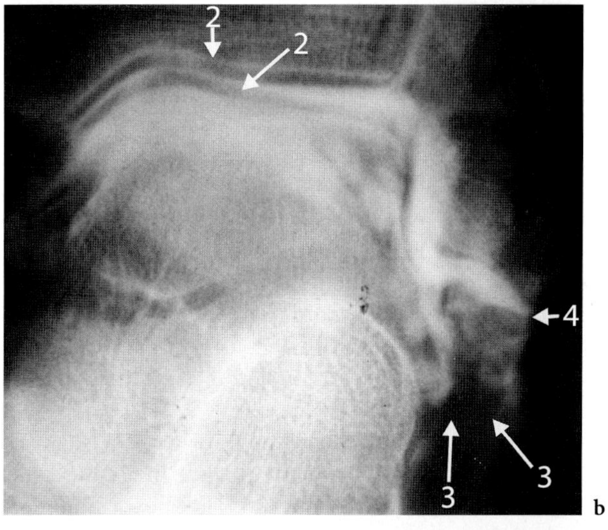

b

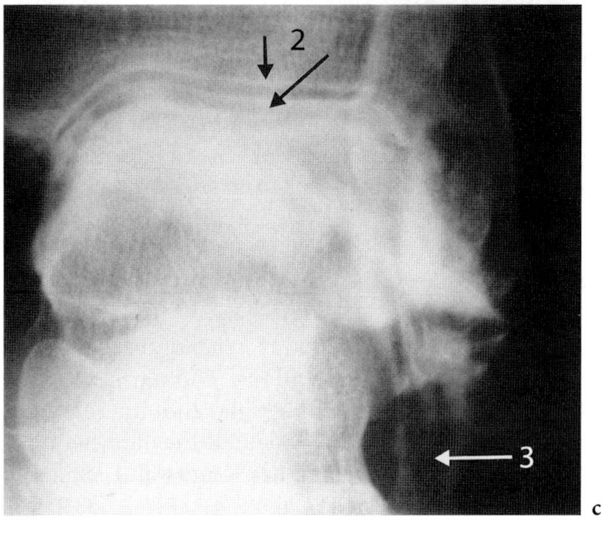

c

Fig. 2.12a–c. Right ankle arthrogram in a patient with recurrent subluxation of the ankle joint and history of distal fibula fracture. **a** AP view demonstrates detached bony fragment adjacent to the tip of the fibula (*1*). **b** Contrast medium is seen between the detached bone and the fibula (*4*). **b, c** Note the good demonstration of cartilage (*2*). The peroneal tendons (*3*) are outlined by contrast medium in their tendon sheath. This indicates abnormal communication with the joint due to an injury to the calcaneofibular ligament

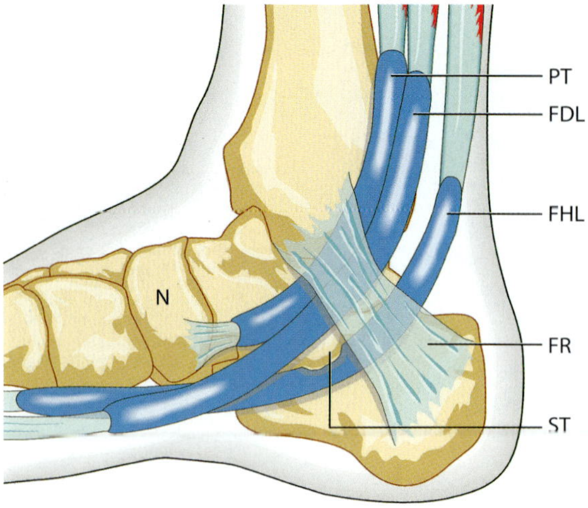

Fig. 2.13. Diagrammatic medial view of the ankle. Posterior tibial (*PT*), flexor digitorum longus (*FDL*) and flexor hallucis longus (*FHL*) tendons are seen. The single flexor retinaculum (*FR*) prevents luxation. Note the insertion of the posterior tibial tendon into the navicular bone (*N*) and the FHL tendon running in a groove underneath the sustentaculum tali (*ST*)

flexor hallucis longus tendon in the hindfoot area, coursing laterally, to end up the most lateral of the three tendons. It inserts in the 2nd to 5th toes on the plantar side.

The flexor hallucis longus tendon is the most dorsal of the three tendons in the malleolar area. It inserts on the plantar side of the big toe. It runs through a groove in the posterior process of the talus and through another groove underneath the sustentaculum tali (Figs. 2.2, 2.13).

All three tendons have separate tendon sheaths where they course round the medial malleolus and under the flexor retinaculum. The flexor hallucis and digitorum longus sheaths can normally communicate with each other and with the ankle joint; the prevalence is between 10% and 20% (Table 2.1) (Fig. 2.4f,g). There is no normal communication with the tibialis posterior tendon sheath. All three muscles plantar flex and invert the foot. The tibialis posterior additionally adducts the foot and supports the arch.

2.2.2.3
Extensor Tendons

The third group of tendons related to the ankle joint are the extensor tendons. They arise on the anterolateral aspect of the tibia and interosseous membrane. From medial to lateral they are the tibialis anterior, extensor hallucis longus and extensor digitorum longus muscle tendons (Figs. 2.3, 2.4g). The tendons run parallel to each other over the dorsum of the ankle joint. They are kept in place by the superior extensor retinaculum overlying the joint ventrally, extending from the distal fibula to the distal medial tibia. The inferior extensor retinaculum is shaped roughly like a 'y' lying on its side with the long limb arising from the lateral superior calcaneus (here contiguous with the insertion of the inferior peroneal retinaculum) and extending with one crus to the medial malleolus and the other crus to the sulcus calcanei medially. Communication between the extensor tendon sheaths and the ankle joint is abnormal.

2.3
Technique

2.3.1
Arthrography

Ankle arthrography is a relatively simple procedure. The most commonly used technique involves AP puncture with lateral fluoroscopy guidance. The anterior puncture site should be approximately 1.5 cm distal to the joint line, with the needle angled upward to the articular surface of the tibia (Fig. 2.14). The dorsalis pedis artery and the extensor tendons are

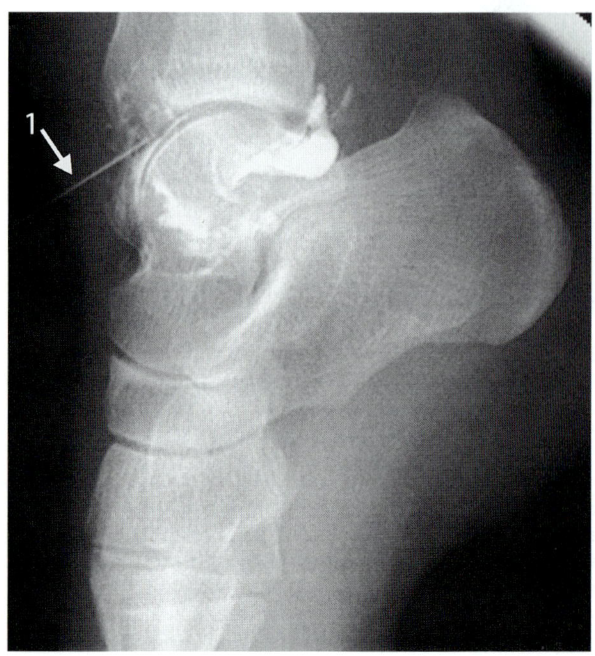

Fig. 2.14. Ankle arthrogram, lateral view. Needle (*1*) is seen angling slightly cranially to the undersurface of the tibia

avoided by puncturing medial to the anterior tibial tendon or between the anterior tibial and extensor hallucis longus tendons (Fig. 2.15). A 20 G needle and 6–10 ml of iodinated contrast medium are used (Haller et al. 1988; Resnick 1995).

The choice of concentration of the contrast medium will depend on the application and personal preference. Generally speaking, the concentration of iodinated contrast medium should be high enough to demonstrate even small joint capsule leakage and achieve good contrast in double-contrast techniques. It should, however, not obscure the bone–contrast medium interface, and non-calcified soft-tissue structures such as cartilage, synovium or loose bodies should be visible as negative contrast (Figs. 2.1, 2.11, 2.12).

Double-contrast techniques elegantly demonstrate the internal anatomy of the joint and articular surfaces (Figs. 2.11, 2.16). Negative contrast (air) arthrography is the method of choice in precisely locating the site of suspected loose bodies seen radiographically (Fig. 2.17).

The posterior subtalar joint is usually punctured from a postero-oblique or an antero-oblique approach, using a 4–5 cm, 21–22 G needle and about 2.5 ml of contrast, though the amount of contrast needed can vary from 1 to 7 ml (Figs. 2.1, 2.18, 2.19) (Haller et al. 1988; Sugimoto et al. 1998, 2002). Meticulous positioning of the patient's foot is crucial for this procedure. In the postero-oblique approach the peroneal tendon sheath should be avoided.

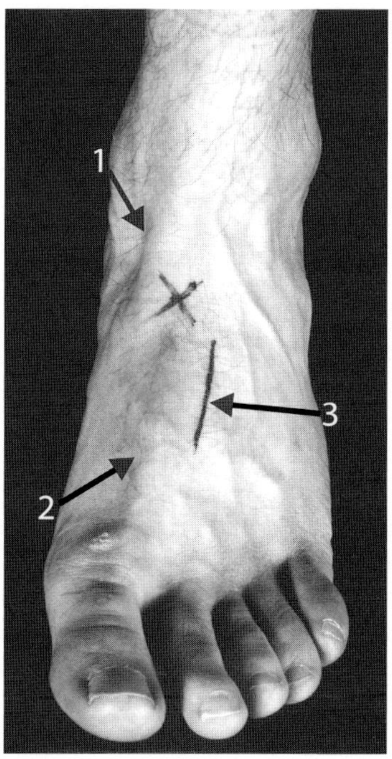

Fig. 2.15. Photograph of a foot. Anterior tibial (*1*) and extensor hallucis longus (*2*) tendons are visible. The course of the anterior tibial artery is marked (*3*). The *cross* marks the puncture site for an ankle arthrogram, anterior approach, between the palpable and visible tendons

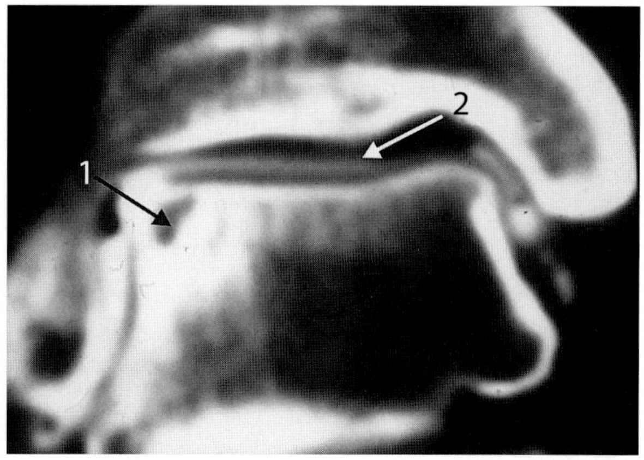

Fig. 2.16. Double-contrast CT-arthrogram of the ankle. Large osteochondral injury of the lateral talar convexity (*1*). Note the irregular bony contour and loss of the overlying cartilage. The ability of positive-contrast CT-arthrograms to outline normal cartilage (*2*) is demonstrated

The anterior subtalar (or talocalcaneonavicular) joint is punctured by a direct dorsal approach to the talonavicular articulation while avoiding the dorsalis pedis artery. A short 22 G needle and 3–5 ml of contrast medium are used (Fig. 2.7).

The calcaneocuboid joint can be reached from a lateral approach with the needle parallel to the joint space. A short 22 G needle and 1–2 ml of contrast are usually sufficient.

All other small joints of the foot can be punctured using a short 25 G needle with a direct dorsal or dorso-oblique approach (Fig. 2.20). They usually accommodate 1–2 ml of contrast medium (Haller et al. 1988).

2.3.2
Bursography

Bursography in the foot and ankle is normally limited to the retrocalcaneal bursa on top of the calcaneus. A short 22 G needle can be used. The approach is to either side of the Achilles tendon, angling forward towards the superior surface of the calcaneus. The bursa takes around 1 ml of contrast (Haller et al. 1988; Resnick 1995). The procedure can be performed blindly or using fluoroscopy or ultrasound guidance.

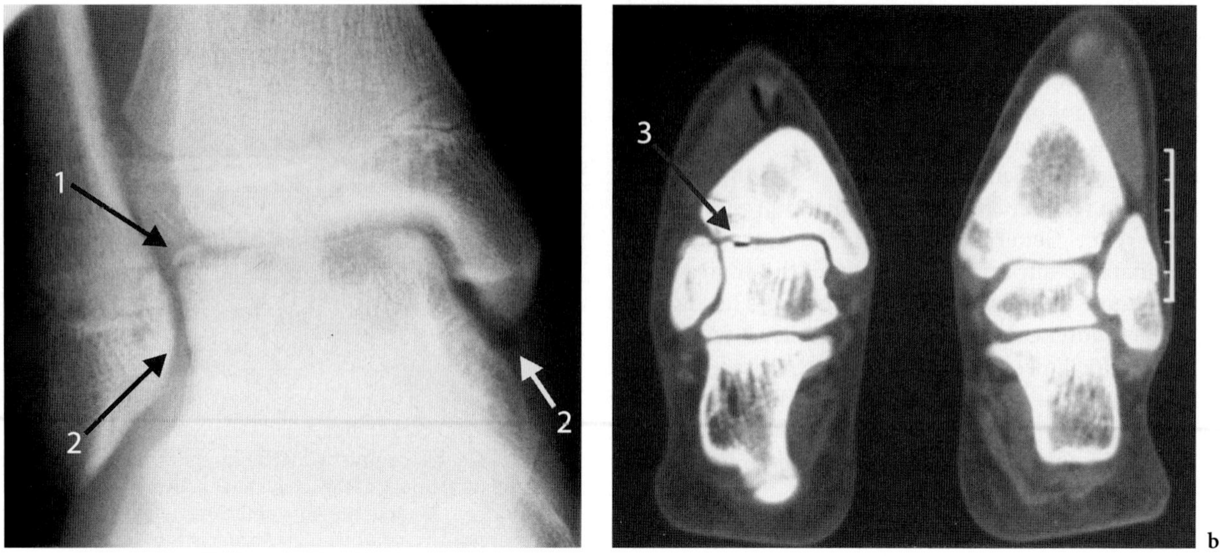

Fig. 2.17a, b. Osteochondral fracture of the lateral talar convexity in a 15-year-old boy demonstrated by air ankle arthrogram. **a** AP view demonstrates the fracture site (*1*) and gas in the joint (*2*). **b** The subsequent CT-arthrogram demonstrates detachment of the fragment (*3*)

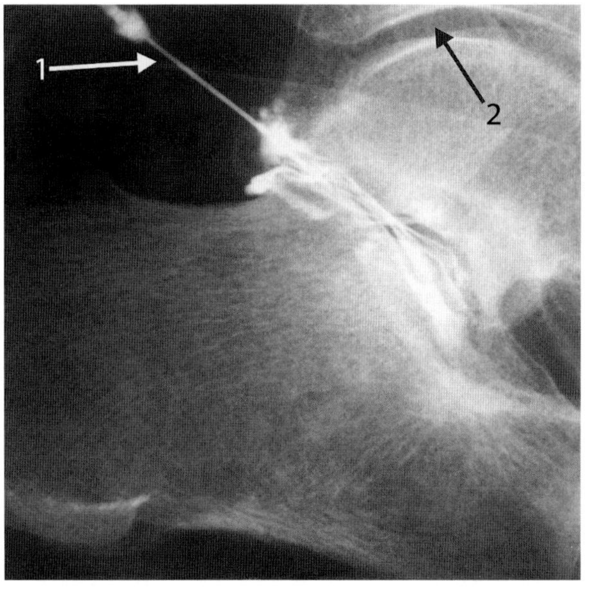

Fig. 2.18. Normal subtalar arthrogram. Dorsal approach. Note the oblique course of the needle (*1*). Meticulous positioning of the foot prior to the advance of the needle is paramount for this technique. No communication with the ankle joint (*2*)

2.3.3 Tenography

Tenography demonstrates the tendons as filling defects in their tendon sheaths after injection of the sheaths with a positive contrast medium (Figs. 2.9, 2.10). The tendon is usually located by palpation; ultrasound can be used for support. A 20–25 G needle is angled approximately 30° against the tendon (Fig. 2.5) and advanced until resistance caused by the tendon is felt or the underlying bone is reached. Most authors prefer 22 G or 25 G, though the smaller the needle bore, the more difficult it becomes to rely on feel for the assessment of correct positioning (Eichelberger and Brogdon 1982). When appropriate resistance is felt, the needle is slowly withdrawn, maintaining a constant pressure on the plunger of an attached syringe. Use of a connecting tube between the needle and syringe aids in manipulation. A 'give' in resistance indicates that the needle tip is in the tendon sheath and fluid is flowing freely.

Iodinated contrast medium and fluoroscopic control can be used for monitoring. This has the disadvantage of image degradation if extravasation occurs (Resnick 1995; Jaffee et al. 2001). Alternatively, normal saline solution can be used for the initial cannulation (Mu Huo Teng et al. 1984; Bleichrodt et al. 1989); ultrasound can here demonstrate free flow into the tendon sheath. A cutdown technique to the tendon sheath for 'heavy' patients is rarely required (Reinherz and Sheldon 1986). Inflating a blood pressure cuff around the distal calf can help reduce backflow (Fig. 2.5c) of contrast into the calf muscles (Reinherz and Sheldon 1986). The amount of contrast needed varies from 4 to 25 ml (Reinherz and Sheldon 1986; Haller et al. 1988).

The puncture site for the common peroneal sheath is approximately 4 cm proximal to the lateral malleolus (Fig. 2.5). The flexor tendon sheaths are cannulated approximately 1 cm proximal to the medial

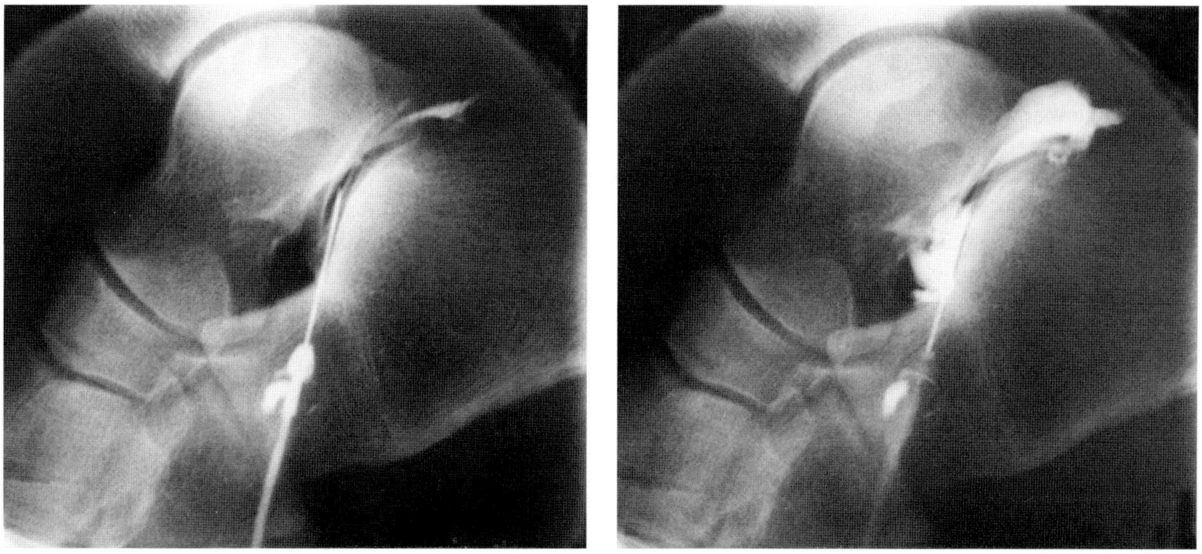

a b

Fig. 2.19a, b. Normal right subtalar joint arthrogram. Medial approach. Meticulous positioning is required before beginning the procedure

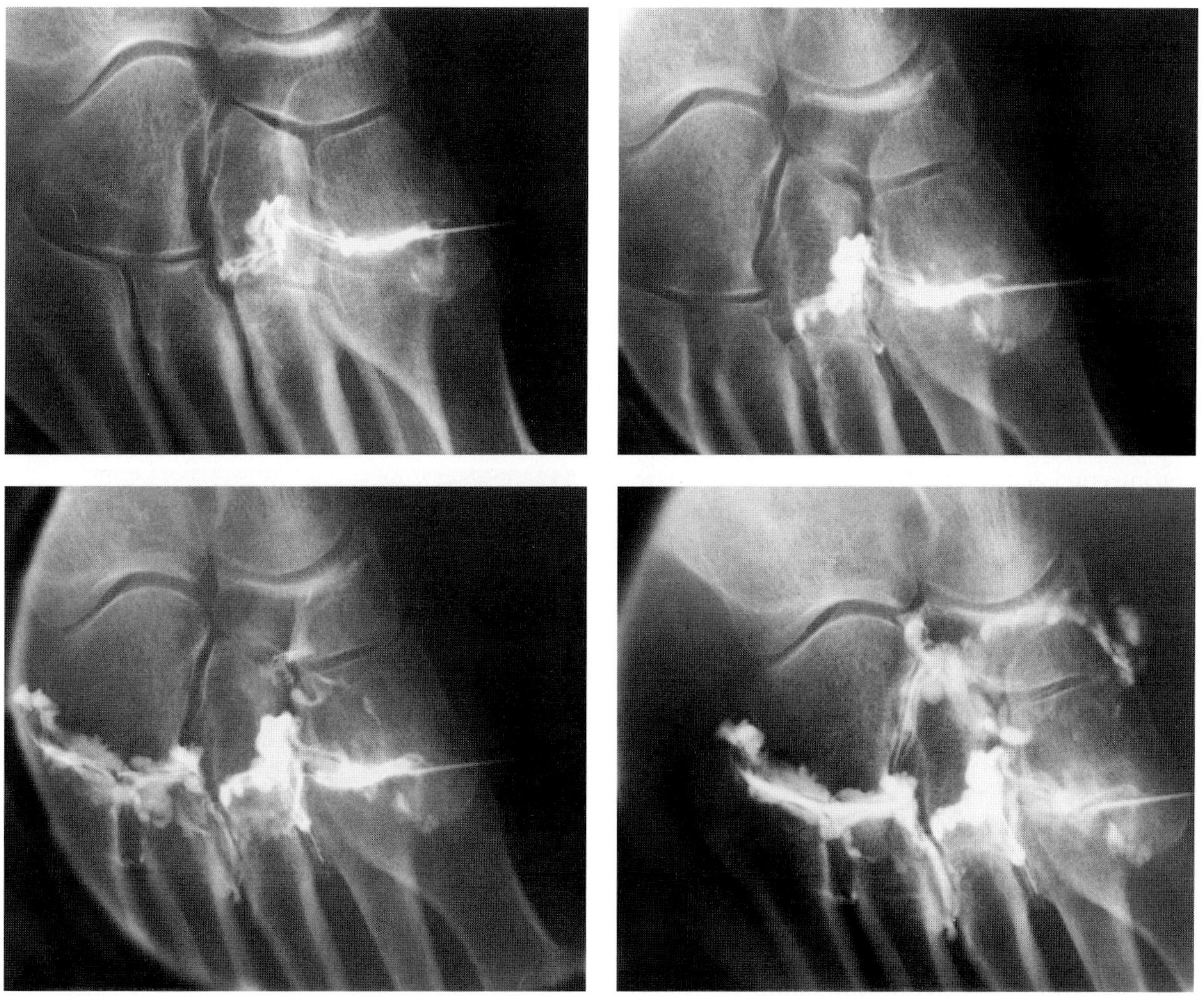

a b c d

Fig. 2.20a–d. Arthrogram of the right first tarsometatarsal joint. Dorsomedial approach. The series of films demonstrates virtually immediate abnormal spill of contrast medium into the 2nd and 3rd tarsometatarsal joint (**a, b**) and subsequently into all tarsometatarsal joints and intertarsal joints (**c, d**) malleolar tip and the extensor tendon sheaths dorsal to the navicular. If a particular tendon sheath cannot be cannulated, the high anatomic variability should be kept in mind, as the length and size of tendon sheaths vary greatly (Mu Huo Teng et al. 1984). Care should be taken to spare the dorsalis pedis and the posterior tibial artery when cannulating.

AP, lateral and oblique radiographs are taken. Additional tunnel views for the peroneal tendons with the forefoot inverted and the tube angled 45° cephalad have been proposed but are not common practice (Deyerle 1973).

2.3.4 CT Tenography

Tenography can be combined with a CT examination. After contrast medium injection into the tendon sheath, the ankle region is scanned in standard axial fashion, slice thickness 1 mm. Exact symmetrical positioning of both feet is recommended to aid image interpretation. Large window width is also advised (Wybier et al. 1997).

2.3.5 Complications

As with any contrast injection there is a risk of an anaphylactic reaction or other less severe adverse effects to contrast administration. There is also a risk of infection. For arthrography a 1:25,000 risk for infection and a 10:25,000 risk for a mild allergic reaction for ionic-type contrast media are quoted (Freiberger 1979). Contrast media can cause mild transient synovitis.

Tendon rupture due to injection of tendon sheaths with glucocorticoids can occur, especially if accidental intratendinous injection occurs or if the tendon was already damaged before the injection, e.g. by a partial tear (Jaffee et al. 2001).

2.4 Indications and Findings

Arthrography, tenography and bursography became popular in the 1970s, but as the non-invasive techniques of musculoskeletal ultrasound and MR imaging became widely available, these took over a large part of the diagnostic work.

2.4.1 Arthrography

Ankle arthrography was extensively used to diagnose acute injuries to the lateral collateral ligaments of the ankle. It proved unreliable in the diagnosis of calcaneofibular injuries; peroneal tenography proved more accurate (Fig. 2.5) (Eichelberger and Brogdon 1982; Reinherz and Sheldon 1986; Haller et al. 1988; Bleichrodt et al. 1989; Resnick 1995). Arthrography was also used to diagnose synovial disease, loose bodies, joint cartilage and osteochondral injuries and in the assessment of congenital anomalies (Haller et al. 1988). Today, arthrography plays only a role as part of CT- or MR-arthrography for the assessment of these conditions (Figs. 2.4, 2.6, 2.17, 2.21, 2.22). In isolation, arthrography is still being used on its own to assess chronic ankle instability where there is poor access to MR imaging (Fig. 2.4a–c), and it is still a reliable way of diagnosing lateral collateral ligament injuries in the acute phase (Table 2.1; Figs. 2.4c, 2.11, 2.12b,c) (Sugimoto et al. 1998, 2002; van Dijk et al. 1998). If more than 2–3 days pass between the injury and examination, there is a risk of missing a significant ligamentous injury due to a fibrinous plug in the capsular tear.

The assessment of lateral instability of the ankle can be part of an arthrographic examination, but it can only be reliably diagnosed when examined under general anaesthesia (Fig. 2.4c). A 10°–12° tilt is seen as the upper limit of normal for lateral opening of the ankle joint. A difference of more than 5°

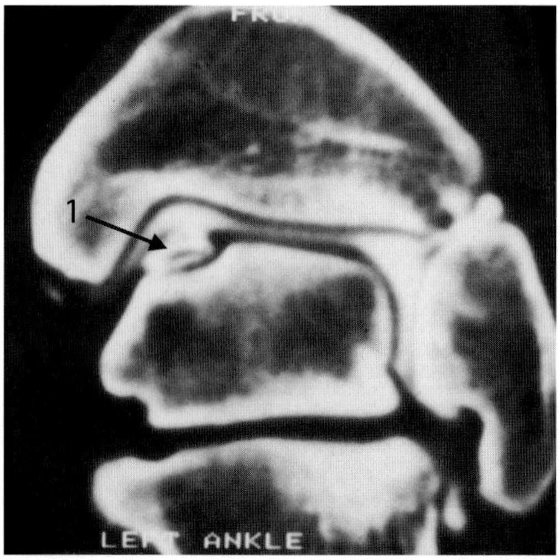

Fig. 2.21. Single-contrast CT-arthrogram of the left ankle demonstrating a large osteochondral defect of the talus medially (*1*). The residual fragment in the defect site is surrounded by contrast medium and therefore also detached

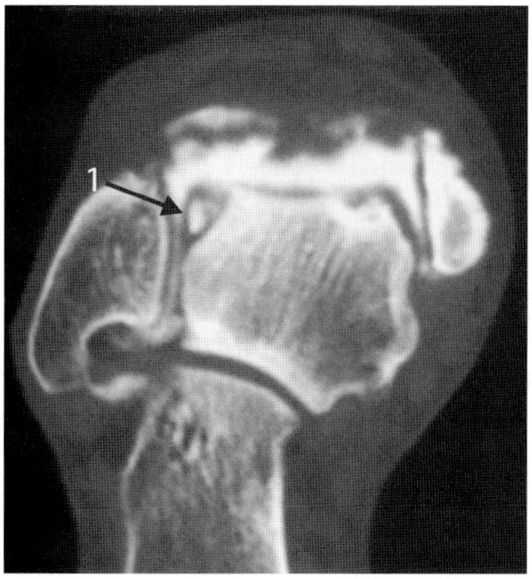

a

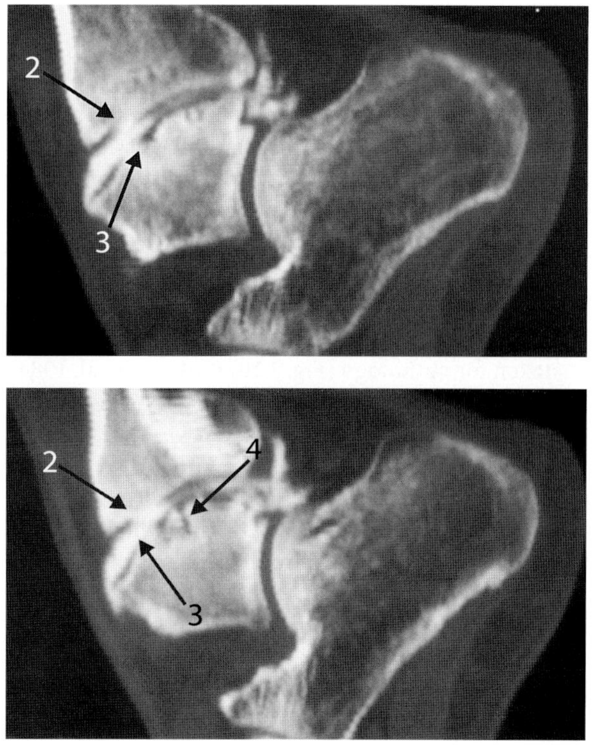

b

c

Fig. 2.22a–c. Single-contrast CT-arthrogram of a 26-year-old man with persisting ankle pain after severe trauma. **a** An osteochondral lesion of the lateral talus is demonstrated (*1*). The overlying cartilage is thinned but otherwise intact. Therefore, no loose body here. **b, c** On the sagittal reconstructions, corresponding cartilage defects of tibia (*2*) and talus (*3*) are seen. **c** A further large central osteochondral defect of the talus (*4*) is demonstrated

to the contralateral side is also considered abnormal (Sugimoto et al. 1998).

The other major indication for arthrography today is the localisation and treatment of joint-related pain as there is no reliable correlation of radiographic degenerative change and pain origin (Mitchell et al. 1995). Injections performed without imaging control have two main problems. The intended anatomical structure might not actually have been injected successfully, and the occurrence of abnormal communications cannot be appreciated (Figs. 2.1, 2.7, 2.11, 2.12b,c, 2.20). Under these circumstances a particular joint might wrongly be assumed to be the source of a patient's complaints, while leakage of a local anaesthetic into a neighbouring joint is responsible for subsidence of the symptoms.

A residual indication for conventional arthrography is the diagnosis of adhesive capsulitis. This condition is difficult to appreciate with any other imaging technique. Non-distension of the joint capsule is seen, combined with increased resistance to injection and subsequent leakage of contrast along the needle track.

2.4.2 Bursography

Bursography is rarely used today, particularly in the ankle region. The retrocalcaneal bursa can be injected with local anaesthetics or glucocorticoids to diagnose and/or treat local inflammation (Haller et al. 1988; Resnick 1995).

2.4.3 Tenography

Tenography used to be part of the diagnostic work-up for ankle ligament injuries as discussed above (Fig. 2.5). It should be remembered that the flexor hallucis and digitorum longus tendon sheaths can normally communicate with each other and the ankle joint. Communication of the peroneus sheath or the extensor sheaths with the ankle joint is, however, abnormal (Table 2.1; Figs. 2.5, 2.4d,f,g, 2.6b,c, 2.11).

Tenography did not prove reliable for the diagnosis of complete or partial tendon tears. Its role today is in the diagnosis and treatment of tenosynovitis. Tenosynovitis is a collective term for peritendinitis, chronic tenosynovitis and stenosing tenosynovitis. Only the latter two conditions can be diagnosed with tenography, but here tenography is superior to other imaging modalities including ultrasound and MR imaging (Wybier et al. 1997; Jaffee et al. 2001). Tenosynovitis is usually mechanically induced but also occurs in systemic inflammatory conditions. If long-standing, tendinitis leads to tendon degeneration and ultimately rupture.

On tenography, chronic tenosynovitis is recognised by an irregular outline of the tendon and tendon sheath with outpouchings, filling defects and possibly focal tendon enlargement. Obstruction of contrast medium flow in the tendon sheath can be due to a complete or partial tendon rupture, stenosing tenosynovitis or any mass lesion. Tenography cannot reliably differentiate between these aetiologies. The normal impression of the retinacula onto the tendon sheaths should not be mistaken for pathology (Fig. 2.10) (Gilula et al. 1984; Haller et al. 1988; Cheung et al. 1992; Wybier et al. 1997; Schreibman 1998).

Tenography can be combined with CT to aid the assessment of the tendons and adjacent structures (Wybier et al. 1997). A classification of tenosynovitis based on the number of outpouchings of the tendon sheath has been suggested, with 1–5 being mild, 6–10 moderate and >10 severe disease (Jaffee et al. 2001). Other authors suggests though that 1–2 outpouchings can still be normal (Mu Huo Teng et al. 1984).

In cases of suspected tenosynovitis, the injection of a local anaesthetic with or without a glucocorticoid can be used as a diagnostic test and as a therapeutic trial. The mechanical distension of the tendon sheath is assumed to have an additional beneficial effect by disrupting small adhesions. Care should be taken not to inject into the tendon substance, particularly when injecting a corticosteroid. Following posterior tibial tendon sheath injection, protection with a brace for 6 weeks has been suggested, though there are no conclusive studies on this subject. In the case of partial tendon tears, corticosteroids should not be injected (Jaffee et al. 2001).

In the ankle region the peroneus brevis and the posterior tibial tendons are the ones most commonly injured. The peroneus brevis tendon is compressed between the peroneus longus tendon and the lateral malleolus and is prone to longitudinal splitting and, if left untreated, to rupture. Injury to the retinacula with recurrent tendon subluxation is another cause for peroneus brevis tendon degeneration. The peroneus longus tendon tends to rupture more distally, at the level of the calcaneocuboid joint (Helgason 1998). The posterior tibial tendon can become compressed against the medial malleolus, leading to degeneration and ultimately rupture. Posterior tibial tendon ruptures are bilateral in 5% of cases, with women more often affected than men (Cheung et al. 1992).

Tendon tears can initially go unnoticed. Untreated tendon and ligament injury is likely to lead to bony instability and secondary articular problems. These then present as chronic pain and flatfoot deformity. Therefore, tendon injury should be included in the differential diagnosis for almost any patient presenting with flatfoot deformity, and ligament/tendon injury should be actively excluded in such cases.

References

Bleichrodt RP, Kingue LM, Binnendijk B, Klein J-P (1989) Injuries of the lateral ankle ligaments: classification with tenography and arthrography. Radiology 173:347–349

Cheung Y, Rosenberg ZS, Magee T, Chinitz L (1992) Normal anatomy and pathologic conditions of ankle tendons: current imaging technique. Radiographics 12:429–444

Deyerle WM (1973) Long term follow-up of fractures of the os calcis. Orthop Clin North Am 1973:213–227

Eichelberger RP, Lichtenstein P, Brogdon BG (1982) Peroneal tenography. JAMA 247:2587–2591

Freiberger RH, Kaye JJ, Spiller J (1979) Arthrography. Appleton-Century-Crofts, New York

Gilula LA, Oloff L, Caputi R, Destouet JM, Jacobs A, Solomon MA (1984) Ankle tenography: a key to unexplained symptomatology, part II. Diagnosis of chronic tendon disabilities. Radiology 151:581–587

Haller J, Resnick D, Sartoris D, Mitchell M, Howard B, Gilula L (1988) Arthrography, tenography and bursography of the ankle and foot. Clin Podiatr Med Surg 5:893–908

Helgason JW, Chandnani VP (1998) MR arthrography of the ankle. Radiol Clin North Am 36:729–738

Jaffee NW, Gilula LA, Wissman RD, Johnson JE (2001) Diagnostic and therapeutic ankle tenography: outcomes and complications. Am J Radiol 176:365–371

Mitchell MJ, Bielecki D, Bergman AG, Kursunoglu-Brahme S, Sartoris DJ, Resnick D (1995) Localization of specific joint causing hindfoot pain: value of injecting local anesthetics into individual joints during arthrography. Am J Radiol 164:1473–1476

Teng MM, Destonet JM, Gilula LA, Resnick D, Hembree JL, Oloff LM (1984) Ankle tenography: a key to unexplained symptomatology, part I. Normal tenographic anatomy. Radiology 151:575–580

Reinherz RP, Zawada SJ, Sheldon DP (1986) Tenography around the ankle and introduction of a new technique. J Foot Surg 25:357–363

Resnick D (1995) Diagnosis of bone and joint disorders. Saunders, Philadelphia

Schreibman KL, Gilula LA (1998) Ankle tenography: a therapeutic imaging modality. Radiol Clin North Am 36: 739–756

Sugimoto K, Samoto N, Takaoka T, Takakura Y, Tamai S (1998) Subtalar arthrography in acute injuries of the calcaneofibular ligament. J Bone Joint Surg [Br] 80-B: 785–790

Sugimoto K, Takakura Y, Samato N, Nakayama S, Tanaka Y (2002) Subtalar arthrography in recurrent instability of the ankle. Clin Orthop Relat Res 394:169–176

van Dijk CN, Molenaar AH, Cohen RH, Tol JL, Bossuyt PMM, Marti RK (1998) Value of arthrography after supination trauma of the ankle. Skeletal Radiol 27:256–261

Wybier M, Hamze B, Champsaur P, Parlier C (1997) Arthroscanner et tenoscanner de la cheville. Ann Radiol 40:92–98

3 Computed Tomography (CT) and CT Arthrography

R. W. WHITEHOUSE

CONTENTS

3.1 Introduction

Over the last two decades, sectional imaging has developed rapidly. Computed tomography (CT) and magnetic resonance (MR) imaging are now established methods of investigation of the foot and ankle, and both methods continue to develop so rapidly that descriptions of the current state of the art remain valid for only a few months. The clinical value of comparisons between techniques such as CT and MRI depends upon the condition being imaged, the model and age of the scanners used, the scanning protocol, and the experience and ability of the scanner operators and the radiologist. Whilst CT is 'loosing ground' to MRI for imaging the musculoskeletal system, it should not be forgotten that the methods are complementary. In addition, CT 'came first', is more widely available, cheaper, quicker and can be easier to perform well and interpret. CT remains more suitable than MRI in the assessment of acute trauma (e.g. intra-articular calcaneal fractures), whilst the advantages of MRI over CT for conditions such as tarsal coalition are small in terms of improved sensitivity and specificity. The addition of arthrography further increases the specificity and sensitivity of both MRI and CT for articular and some ligamentous lesions. There is a law of diminishing returns as these sensitivities and specificities creep ever closer to 100%, which also reduces the real difference between the two techniques. CT remains essential in the assessment of patients in whom MRI is contraindicated (e.g. due to intracranial aneurysm clips or cardiac pacemakers). CT therefore continues to have a role in the diagnosis and management of many pathologies of the foot and ankle. Having decided that CT is an appropriate investigation for an individual, the precise format of the examination will depend upon the suspected pathology and the equipment available. Whilst this chapter starts by describing the recent developments in CT scanners and the value of these to peripheral musculoskeletal imaging, the main aim is to outline those considerations that should optimise the images obtained whatever CT scanner is used.

3.2 Developments in CT

A CT image is a Cartesian co-ordinate map of normalised X-ray attenuation coefficients, generated by an electronically filtered, computerised back projection of X-ray transmission measurements in multiple

R.W. WHITEHOUSE, MD
Department of Clinical Radiology, Manchester Royal Infirmary, Oxford Road, Manchester, M13 9WL, UK

directions through a section of the object in question. This description is as true today as when Hounsfield first described the technique. Those areas where recent developments have been made include helical scanning, multislice acquisition and real-time CT 'fluoroscopy' (Dawson and Lees 2001). These developments have been made on the back of improving technology which includes slip-rings for power and data transmission to and from the gantry, higher heat-loading X-ray tubes, high-efficiency solid-state X-ray detectors, faster data transmission and processing abilities of the electronics.

3.2.1 Slip Rings

In order to acquire X-ray transmission data in all directions across a slice of the patient, the X-ray tube has to travel around the entire circumference of a circle around the slice. If the tube is supplied with power by cables, then these have to wrap around the circle as the tube moves. In order to unwrap the cables, the next slice is performed by rotating the tube in the opposite direction. This design requires more than 360° of tube rotation as initial acceleration and final deceleration distances are also required. Powerful motors and brakes are needed to cope with the inertia of this system (which may include the X-ray detectors and counterweights to balance the gantry), and a significant time delay is necessary between each slice acquisition to allow for these acceleration and deceleration phases. Replacing the cables with slip rings (large circumference electrically conducting rings) which encircle the X-ray tube path and transferring power from the rings to the X-ray tube via conducting brushes on the X-ray tube gantry allow the gantry to be continuously rotated in one direction. This has several advantages – rapid acceleration and deceleration of the gantry are no longer required, yet a faster rotation speed can be achieved, giving shorter scan acquisition times. The time delay between slices need be no longer than that required for table movement in the conventional acquisition mode, and the potential for acquiring continuously updated X-ray transmission data paves the way for both helical scanning and CT fluoroscopy.

3.2.2 X-ray Tubes

The development of slip rings resulted in a requirement for X-ray tubes to have both a higher heat capacity and a higher maximum tube current, as the mAs required for a single slice remained much the same while the time in which the slice was acquired was reduced. In addition, for helical scanning, continuous X-ray output for up to 60 s may be required. The disadvantage of these X-ray tubes is the increased ease with which high radiation doses can be given to patients during CT investigations. This disadvantage may be mitigated by the development of solid-state and multislice detectors.

3.2.3 X-ray Detectors

Xenon gas detectors, used in CT scanners for many years, have a conversion efficiency (X-rays to signal strength) of around 60%, which can diminish further if the detectors are not maintained. Solid-state crystal detectors may have conversion efficiencies of nearly 100%, resulting in a 40% reduction in the patient radiation dose for the equivalent scan appearances. The tendency for solid-state detectors to continue emitting light after the X-rays had terminated (afterglow) and other technical problems with respect to the size of the front face of the individual detectors and the interspace material between adjacent detectors have been largely overcome.

Although one of the earliest EMI CT head scanners acquired two slices at the same time with a pencil beam of X-rays passing to two adjacent detectors, the ease with which solid-state detectors can be stacked in parallel adjacent channels has facilitated the redevelopment of multislice scanners. These scanners can acquire several sections simultaneously, which can be separately processed to give large numbers of thin sections, or recombined to give fewer thicker sections with lower noise.

3.2.4 Helical CT (Spiral or Volume Scanning)

The requirement for a break in the X-ray emission whilst the table is moved to the next slice position was overcome by the development of helical scanning. Helical scanning is performed by moving the table continuously during the exposure, from the first slice location to the last. Thus, a helix of X-ray transmission data through the scan volume is acquired. To generate a CT image, the data from adjacent turns of the helix are interpolated to produce transmission data which are effectively from a single slice location. This process can be performed at any location within the helix (except the first and last 180° where there is no adjacent helix of data for interpolation). In this way overlapping slices can be produced without overlapping irradiation of the patient. The relationship between the X-ray fan beam collimation and the table movement per rotation of the gantry is called the pitch ratio. Extended or stretched pitch scans are performed with pitch ratios greater than 1. Such extended pitches can be used to trade off between greater scan volumes; shorter scan acquisition times and lower scan radiation doses. Stretching the pitch ratio to 1.25 has little effect on the image appearances, but pitch ratios greater than 1.5 produce images with effective slice thicknesses significantly greater than the nominal fan beam collimation thickness. By increasing the number of detector arrays ('multislice scanner') several interlaced helices can be acquired simultaneously (Fig. 3.1), with the table increment per gantry rotation increased proportionately.

The combination of multislice and helical scanning results in volume scan acquisition times which are 4 times faster than a single-slice helical scanner with the same gantry rotation speed and an order of magnitude faster than a non-spiral scanner. Multislice scanning reduces X-ray tube loading requirements as it acquires several slices simultaneously with the same tube loading as a single slice would require on a conventional scanner. The patient radiation dose is not directly reduced, however, and may be increased if greater volumes are scanned.

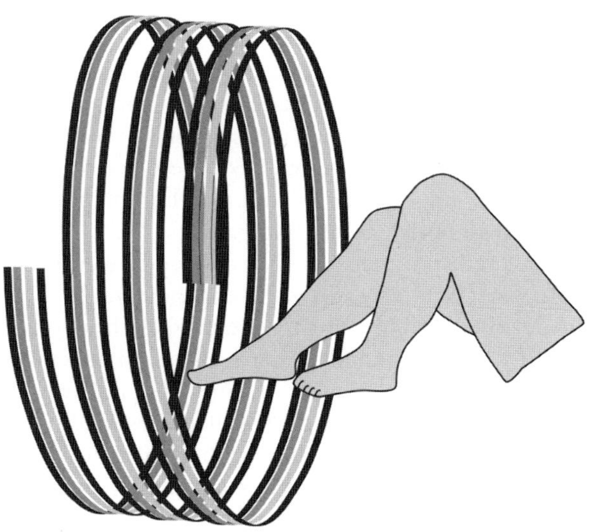

Fig. 3.1. Pictorial representation of the path followed by a single column of detectors for a four-beam multislice helical CT scan. The patient positioning illustrates a way of scanning a single foot in the coronal plane

3.2.5 CT 'Fluoroscopy'

In conventional CT, transmission data from a 360° gantry rotation are required to generate an image. This is because two opposing beam paths then exist for each ray across the imaging volume. This produces improved signal to noise, corrections for the effects of divergent X-ray beams along each ray and beam hardening effects. Images can also be produced using 270° or even 180° gantry rotation data sets. Such 'partial scan' images have acquisition times proportionately shorter than full rotation scans. This can be useful for reducing movement artefacts in selected patients. For a 0.5 s per rotation scanner, the effective scan acquisition time will be one-quarter of a second (250 ms). If the gantry continues to rotate and acquire data without table movement, continuously updated transmission data will be collected from which revised images can be generated. At any one time, image data of between 0 and 250 ms old will be available – i.e. data with an average age of 125 ms. With extremely rapid processors and appropriate reconstruction algorithms, further delay for image reconstruction can be minimised and a continuously updated CT image displayed in 'near real time' (Hsieh 1997). Such 'CT fluoroscopy' imaging can be used for CT-guided interventional procedures. As with all fluoroscopic procedures care should be taken to reduce the fluoroscopy time to the minimum necessary and to avoid operator irradiation – instruments designed to keep the operator's hands out of the CT section (Daly et al. 1998) and use of the lowest selectable tube current (50 mA is sufficient; Froelich et al. 1999) are advocated. To assist in maintaining short CT fluoroscopy exposure times, routine recording and auditing of fluoroscopy exposure times are advocated. An audible alarm after a preset exposure time may also assist in keeping exposures as short as possible. The use of a lead drape adjacent to the irradiated volume has been demonstrated to reduce operator exposure (Nawfel et al. 2000). High skin doses to patients and operators will occur if care is not taken.

3.2.6 Data Manipulation

The vast masses of image data acquired from a multislice spiral scanner produces problems of data storage and interpretation. It is no longer feasible to produce hardcopy images of every available section. With isometric voxels, reformatted images in any other image plane will have the same image quality as the acquisition images, potentially requiring even further hard copies.

Fast workstations, allowing rapid reformatting and display of examinations in the most appropriate plane for the pathology being demonstrated, are therefore necessary, with hard copy restricted to representative images. Other image reconstruction methods [curved planes, surface-rendered three-dimensional (3D) images, minimum or maximum intensity projections (Fig. 3.2)] can produce a bewildering array of visually stunning images, though demonstration of the clinical utility of these methods is currently limited.

The current state-of-the-art device has a multislice helical scanner with solid-state detectors, sub-second scan acquisition and image reconstruction times, CT fluoroscopy capability and a link to a powerful workstation with real-time image manipulation software.

3.2.7 Reformatted Images

As spiral multislice scanning produces overlapping sections and thinner slice collimation (less than 1 mm), in-plane and reformatted plane spatial resolutions are now potentially similar, even for CT images from small fields-of-view (Table 3.1). Volume acquisitions obtained in any plane can therefore be reformatted into other planes without a marked loss of image quality. For scanners not capable of such fine collimation, CT in the most appropriate plane for the expected pathology is still preferable if achievable.

As the best effective Z-axis resolution for a spiral scan acquisition is approximately half the X-ray beam collimation thickness, isometric voxels can consequently be achieved by selecting a combination of scan parameters such as those identified in Table 3.1. For non-helical scanners, overlapping transverse sections will provide better Z-axis resolution (e.g. 25 cm field-of-view, 1 mm slice collimation, 0.5 mm table increment between sections) but at twice the radiation dose to the patient.

Table 3.1. Effect of field-of-view, collimation and reconstruction interval on pixel and voxel sizes for CT images

Field of view	Pixel diameter on 512×512 matrix	Collimation/reconstruction interval required for isometric voxels (spiral mode)
12.5 cm	0.25 mm	0.5 mm/0.25 mm
25 cm	0.5 mm	1.0 mm/0.5 mm
50 cm	1.0 mm	2.0 mm/1.0 mm

3.3 Scan Image Quality

The amount of noise, beam-hardening and streak artefacts in a CT image are dependent upon the following factors:

- Collimation slice thickness
- Partial or full rotation dataset
- Mass and distribution of tissue in the scan plane
- Scan time/movement
- High density extraneous material (the contralateral limb, contrast medium spills, surgical metalwork)
- KVp and mAs
- Field-of-view
- Matrix size
- Reconstruction algorithm
- Post-processing image sharpening or softening filters
- Viewing window width and level settings

Most of these factors are amenable to selection or modification by the scanner operator and can markedly affect the quality of the final image. As Fig. 3.3 demonstrates, the relationships between image noise, mAs and patient size are non-linear, with a halving of patient size resulting in a quartering of image noise, whilst a fourfold increase in mAs is needed to halve the image noise. The figure also demonstrates that for small patients, the image noise is low at all mAs settings, and the absolute reduction in image noise achieved by quadrupling the mAs is small. For these reasons, only one foot or ankle should be scanned wherever possible, rather than both together (Fig. 3.1).

This reduces image noise, streak and beam-hardening artefacts caused by the contralateral limb. A lower mAs setting can then be used with a consequently reduced patient radiation dose, no tube loading limitations (cooling time, limited spiral length) and potentially increased tube life. If the pathology being imaged is osseous, the width of the usual viewing window renders noise imperceptible, and even when soft-tissue lesions are viewed on a narrow window, the noise is not intrusive.

Streak artefacts can be generated by high density material within the scan plane but outside the field-of-view of the scanner. Tabletops which contain

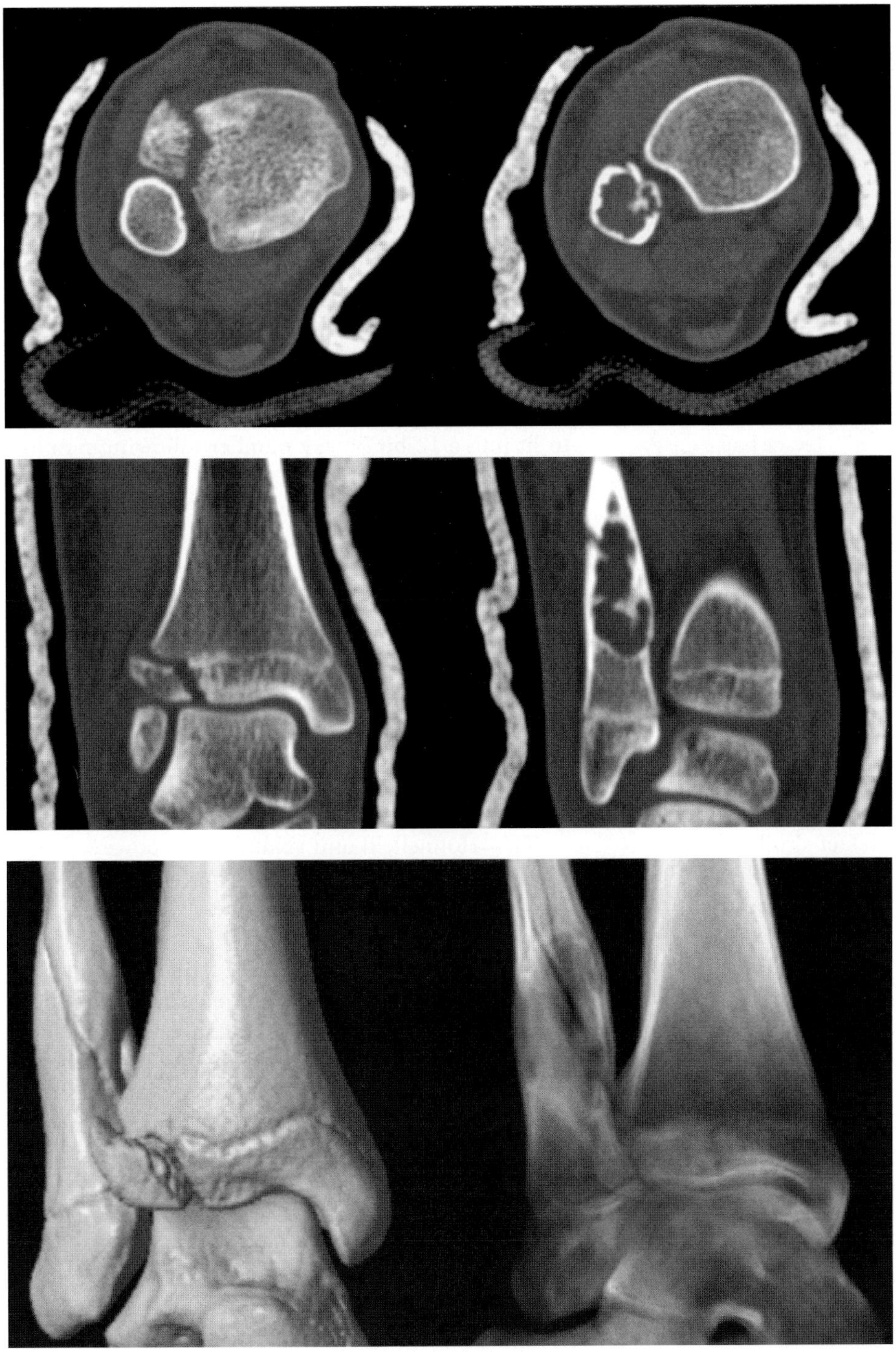

Fig. 3.2a–c. Examples of workstation manipulation of CT data sets. **a** Transverse CT images demonstrate a pathological fracture through a distal fibula non-ossifying fibroma, with further fracture through the tibia. **b** Coronal reformations. **c** Surface-rendered three-dimensional (3D) reconstruction and a thick block reformat segmented to the bone. (Images provided courtesy of Philips Medical Systems and Dr R.C. Berlin, MD, St. John's Hospital, Jackson, WY, USA)

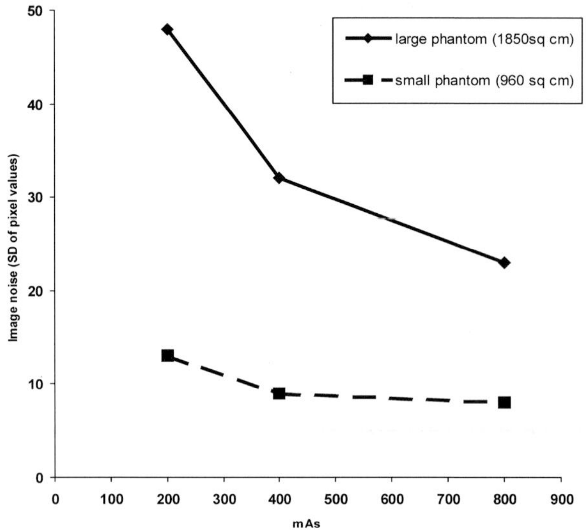

Fig. 3.3. Influence of size and mAs on image noise for a CT scanner. Sections were performed through water density phantoms with 10 mm slice collimation

edge grooves, tracks for the fixing of attachments or detachable mattresses can act as traps for spilt contrast media. Contrast droplets on the gantry window will also cause image artefacts. Scrupulous care to keep the tabletop and gantry clean is needed to remove these sources of artefact.

3.3.1 Internal Metalwork from Fixation Devices

The streak artefact generated from in-situ intramedullary rods is rarely excessive and does not prevent adequate assessment of the bone cortex, making CT of value in assessing fracture union in selected cases. More intrusive streak artefact is seen when the CT plane runs through locking screws in intramedullary rods, bone surface plates or fixation screws. Care in patient positioning (including decubitus positions where necessary), combined with gantry angulation in order to align the scan plane with the long axis of any screws present, will reduce the number of sections degraded by streak artefact from the screws to a minimum. In scanners with operator-selectable kVp, the use of the highest kVp setting will reduce streak artefact, as will the selection of a higher mAs (though the combination of increased kVp and mAs results in considerably greater tube loading and patient irradiation). Streak artefact also may appear visually less intrusive on volume-rendered (3D) images (Pretorius and Fishman 1999).

3.3.2 CT Number, Hounsfield Units, Window Width and Levels

The scale of numbers used to define the grey scale in CT images is artificially limited by data storage constraints. In the earliest days of CT, the number scale ran from –500 for air, through zero for water and up to +500 at the top of the scale. This allowed numerical values from –512 to +512 to be stored as a 10-bit binary number. This 'EMI number' scale was soon replaced by the CT number scale, still used now, where air has a value of –1000 and water has a value of zero. The top end of the scale is usually constrained to fit into a 12-bit binary number (allowing number values from –1024 to +3072 to be stored). The Hounsfield unit (HU) is the true value which the CT number should represent. Scanner drift, calibration error, artefact or other limitations may render this inaccurate, which is why measurements made from scan images are best called CT numbers.

The Hounsfield unit value for any material is defined by the following formula:

$$HU_s=1000\ (\mu_s-\mu_w/\mu_w)$$

where
HU_s=Hounsfield unit value for substance *s*
μ_s=linear attenuation coefficient for substance *s*
μ_w=linear attenuation coefficient for water

This formula relates the HU value to the linear attenuation coefficients of the material being measured and water. As the linear attenuation coefficients of all materials change with the X-ray beam energy, there are consequently only two fixed points on the Hounsfield scale. These are –1000, which is the HU value for no X-ray attenuation (i.e. a vacuum), and zero, which corresponds to the HU value for water (at the calibration pressure and temperature for the scanner). The HU scale is, in fact, open ended, with high atomic number, high-density materials having values way in excess of the upper end of the usual scale (even on 'extended scale' scanners) (Table 3.2).

As implied above, EMI units are converted into CT units by doubling them. In the early days of CT, it was usually stated that dense cortical bone had an EMI number of around 500 (i.e. the top of the scale), which became 1000 when the scale changed from EMI to CT numbers. However, the theoretical Hounsfield value for dense cortical bone calculated at an effective beam energy of 65 keV (equivalent to a scanner operating at around 120 kVp) is in the region of 1600 (Fig. 3.4). At

Table 3.2. Theoretical HU values for a variety of materials at 65 keV

Adipose tissue	-80
Water	0
Collagen	250
Dense cortical bone	1600
Aluminium	2300
Iron	34000
Iodine	141300
Lead	205000

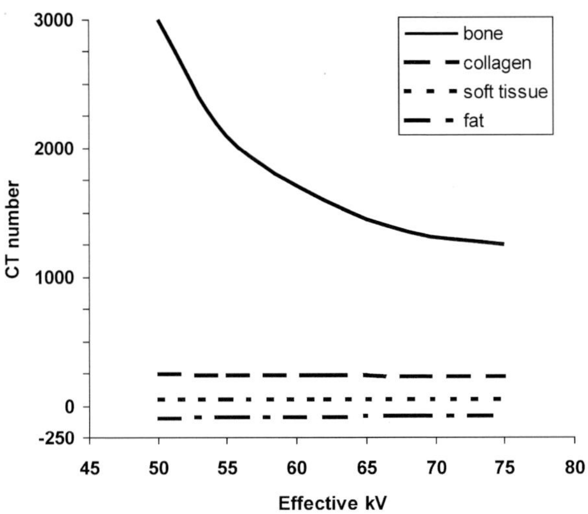

Fig. 3.4. Influence of scanner kVp on CT numbers for bone and soft tissues

lower energies (e.g. 55 keV – the approximate effective energy of a scanner operating at 80 kVp), the HU value for dense cortical bone is over 2000. Other high atomic number materials (contrast media, aluminium, and metal fixation devices) also show marked variation in HU value with beam energy. By contrast, the HU values of soft tissues, collagen and fat vary very little with effective beam energy as the linear attenuation coefficients for these materials closely follow those of water.

Consequently, in scanners which allow the operating voltage to be changed, the CT number for bone can be increased by using a low kVp (around 80 kVp). This increases the dependence of the CT number on the presence of bone or calcification and is particularly used for quantitative measurement of mineral density. A high kVp (usually around 140 kVp) can be selected to reduce the CT number of bone and metalwork, which has some effect in reducing streak artefacts.

For lower atomic number materials such as are present in soft tissues, the X-ray attenuation and consequent CT number are predominantly influenced by the electron density of the material, which is, in turn, closely related to the physical density of the material. Even the CT number of water is influenced by differences in temperature, and differences in density exist between water at room temperature and at body temperature. The presence of protein or high concentrations of salts will increase the CT number of body fluids. Measurement of the CT number of a region of interest in an image must therefore be considered only a guide to its composition. At an extreme not met in clinical practice but potentially relevant to research, the CT number of ice at 0°C (approximately –80 HU) is lower than that of fat (the CT number of which increases as it cools). Specimens scanned straight from the freezer may look quite different than expected (WHITEHOUSE et al. 1993).

The visual impression of the density of a region of interest is influenced by the window and level settings of the image, the calibration of the display and the densities in the surrounding part of the image. Particularly within bone, the surrounding high density of bone can give a lytic lesion the visual impression of a lower density than actually exists. Consequently, measurement rather than estimation of any region of interest is essential; recording an image in which the CT numbers of important regions of interest are measured is a useful addendum to the hard copy.

The window width and level are calibrated contrast and brightness settings for image display. All scanners have preset buttons allowing different window/level combinations to be instantly applied. These commonly have settings deemed appropriate for bone, lung, brain, etc., but typically the bone setting is aimed at an overview of trabecular bone, which may be inappropriate for subtle cortical bone lesions. The most appropriate window level for cortical bone will be influenced by the bone density and the effective scan energy, whilst the window width may need to be quite narrow to demonstrate subtle intracortical density changes.

Reviewing images on the console prior to printing hard copies is recommended to obtain the best image settings for individual patients and to avoid overlooking pathology not demonstrated at 'standard' settings.

3.4 CT of the Foot and Ankle

Most of the research literature on applying CT imaging to the distal lower extremity was published in the 1980s (MARTINEZ et al. 1985), as the technique became widely available and equipment improved. Descriptions of patient positioning, immobilisation methods and reformatting image data sets (including 3D reconstructions; ADLER et al. 1988) were all described, and much of what was said is still relevant to modern scanners. The detail in which the anatomy of the foot and ankle can be demonstrated and the clinical significance ascribed to its various structures have improved significantly.

3.4.1 Anatomy

The anatomy of the foot and ankle is complex, with detailed knowledge of the appearances in all imaging planes being necessary for adequate interpretation. A published comparison of the gross anatomy, CT images and line diagrams in all three orthogonal planes is available (SOLOMON et al. 1986), though the image quality is appropriate to the scanners of that time. Knowledge of anatomical structures not easily or consistently demonstrated on CT is still needed to assess the likelihood of their involvement by any pathology which is demonstrated. The anatomy of the region has been covered in other chapters. Selected CT images are included here for comparative purposes (Fig. 3.5).

For the clearest depiction of articular surfaces and fractures, images perpendicular to the plane of the articulation or fracture are usually best (*vide infra*), whilst for tendons and ligaments, an imaging plane perpendicular to the long axis of the structure is useful. Care in patient positioning to obtain direct coronal or even sagittal imaging planes may therefore be necessary (unless isometric voxels from thin-section spiral CT are available, allowing high-quality reformats).

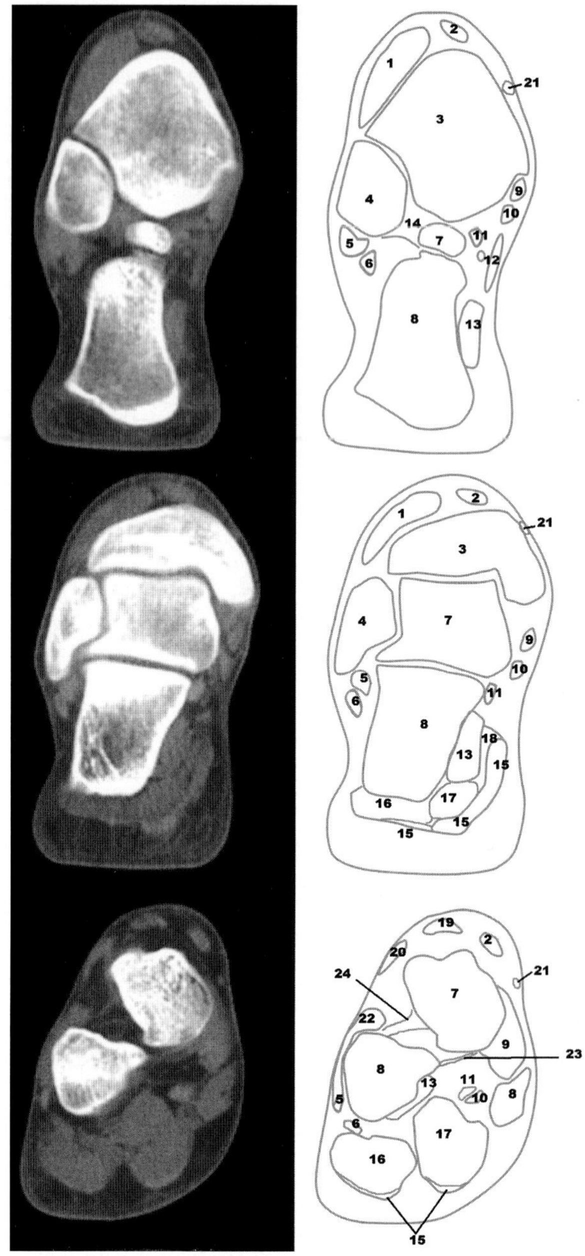

Fig. 3.5. Anatomy of the foot and ankle on selected coronal CT sections. Line drawings of each section identify structures as enumerated in Table 3.3

3.4.2 Immobilisation

Although CT of the foot and ankle is a rapid procedure, immobilisation is necessary to prevent movement artefacts, particularly in children. For adults, sandbags, velcro straps and sticking tape will usually suffice. In children, improved immobilisation can be achieved by the use of rubber-soled tennis shoes (without metal shoelace eyelets) which hold the foot steady and can themselves be firmly fixed to a plywood base attached to the scanner table (DONALDSON et al. 1987). Equipping the department with a full set of shoe sizes is inexpensive and useful if a large number of children of varying ages are likely to be scanned. Even better immobilisation is achieved routinely in trauma patients by the plaster of Paris cast or backslab they are usually fitted with. Scanning through a plaster cast does not significantly interfere with image quality, whilst the immobilisation achieved is usually excellent, such that a temporary cast is also worth considering for occasional patients inadequately immobilised by other methods.

Table 3.3. Anatomical structures in Fig. 3.6

1	Extensor digitorum longus and extensor hallucis longus musculotendinous region
2	Tibialis anterior tendon
3	Tibia
4	Fibula
5	Peroneus brevis
6	Peroneus longus
7	Talus
8	Calcaneus
9	Tibialis posterior tendon
10	Flexor digitorum longus tendon
11	Flexor hallucis longus tendon
12	Posterior tibial artery
13	Quadratus plantae muscle
14	Posterior talofibular ligament
15	Plantar aponeurosis
16	Abductor digiti minimi muscle
17	Flexor digitorum brevis muscle
18	Abductor hallucis muscle
19	Extensor hallucis longus tendon
20	Extensor digitorum longus tendons
21	Great saphenous vein
22	Extensor digitorum brevis muscle
23	Medial talocalcaneal ligament
24	Lateral talocalcaneal ligament

3.4.3 Patient Positioning

As described above, volume acquisitions obtained in any plane can be reformatted into other planes without a marked loss of image quality, though less beam-hardening artefact will be present if the initial acquisition plane is coronal. For scanners not capable of such fine collimation, CT scanning in the most appropriate plane for the expected pathology is still preferable. Care in positioning the patient on the scanner table and judicious use of gantry angulation are usually sufficient for both transverse and coronal plane scans. Lying the patient in a decubitus position with the relevant foot over the end of the table and a few additional supports can be used to achieve sagittal plane scans (Mann and Gilula 1989).

The true transverse and coronal planes of the foot are not aligned with the osseous structures of the foot. An improvement in the demonstration of the midfoot bones and articulations can be obtained by modifying the gantry angulation. Scan planes either parallel (for transverse oblique scans) or perpendicular (for coronal oblique scans) to the talus-first metatarsal axis as seen on a lateral scout view (Johnson and Timins 1998) more clearly demonstrate the bone cortices and articulations.

There are indications for scanning both feet or ankles, such as for the evaluation of bilateral tarsal coalitions or calcaneal fractures. It has been suggested that scanning both feet together in these situations allows direct comparison of the two sides on one image. In my experience the feet are almost never sufficiently accurately positioned to compare the two sides on the same image, but rather on adjacent images or even ones taken two frames apart. As the slice thickness is reduced, even more accurate positioning is needed to obtain anatomically identical levels on the two sides. The larger field-of-view required to encompass both feet also reduces the spatial resolution of the resultant images. This can be overcome by separately targetting image reconstruction to each side in turn. Scanning both feet together or each in turn is therefore going to be a decision based upon compromises between available scan time, machine wear and tear, required image quality (noise and beam-hardening artefact effects) and raw data reconstruction time (for retrospective targetting to each side in turn).

3.5 Indications

CT of the foot and ankle is particularly suited to the demonstration of complex bony anatomy such as the evaluation of bony morphological abnormalities, tarsal coalitions and fractures. Intra-articular calcaneal fractures in particular should be assessed by CT. Intraosseous tumours are well demonstrated; for example, the nidus of an osteoid osteoma, which can be overlooked on MR imaging, is characteristic and clearly demonstrated on CT. The presence of tumour matrix ossification or calcification is also clear on CT. In osteomyelitis, the presence and location of sequestra are revealed. With the addition of arthrography, talar dome osteochondral lesions are well demonstrated, whilst tenography allows the diagnosis of lateral collateral ligament disruption.

Soft-tissue pathology is less well demonstrated than with MRI, and intravenous contrast medium injection provides less satisfactory contrast enhancement than the equivalent MR examination, but valuable information on soft-tissue lesions is still obtainable from CT (for example size, extent, tumour calcification, enhancement, articular involvement). CT can be used to guide biopsy and aspiration procedures (Fig. 3.6).

The accurate 3D localisation of the bone anatomy with CT can be used to calculate the mechanical axes of long bones and the relationships of the joints. This can then be used in the preoperative planning of joint replacements. Tibofibular motion under applied loading can be measured on CT (Jend et al. 1985), as can talocrural and subtalar tilting (van Hellemondt et al. 1997), giving new insights into the pathological significance of these movements. CT retains a significant role in the identification and assessment of tarsal coalitions. The CT scanogram, usually used to identify the start and finish points for a CT investigation, can also be used for limb length measurements.

The limitations of CT are usually described in relationship to MRI, and consequently the poorer soft-tissue contrast of CT is top of the list. Where MRI is available and not itself contraindicated, it is the most appropriate modality for imaging soft-tissue lesions. The other limitations of CT in relation to MRI are the direct multiplanar capability of MRI and the use of ionising radiation with CT.

3.5.1 Trauma

In the acutely traumatised patient, speed and patient safety are important requirements for a satisfactory examination. This gives limited scope for scan technique modifications. As the primary aim of the examination is to determine the size and disposition of fracture fragments and joint alignments, the aim is to ensure adequate coverage of the injured region in a single helical acquisition with effective slice thickness appropriate to the size of the fracture fragments. For purely osseous detail, a low mAs is sufficient. A lateral scout view to determine appropriate start and end points for the acquisition should be routine. The smaller the collimation thickness, pitch and reconstruction interval, the better the quality of reformatted planar and 3D images, giving overlapping helical acquisition sections a small advantage over conventional contiguous transverse sections for fracture classification.

If helical scanning is not available, a mixed protocol of thicker sections to cover the extent of the fracture with thinner sections through the region of the articular surface depression can also be used. Three-dimensional surface reconstructions provide an easily interpreted overview of fracture fragment disposition, particularly useful in badly comminuted injuries (Pretorius and Fishman 1999).

For intra-articular fractures of the calcaneus, CT has now become essential as the classification and management are dependent upon features best demonstrated on CT (Fig. 3.7). The state of the posterior facet of the subtalar joint, the degree of comminution of the sustentaculum and the lateral wall of the

a 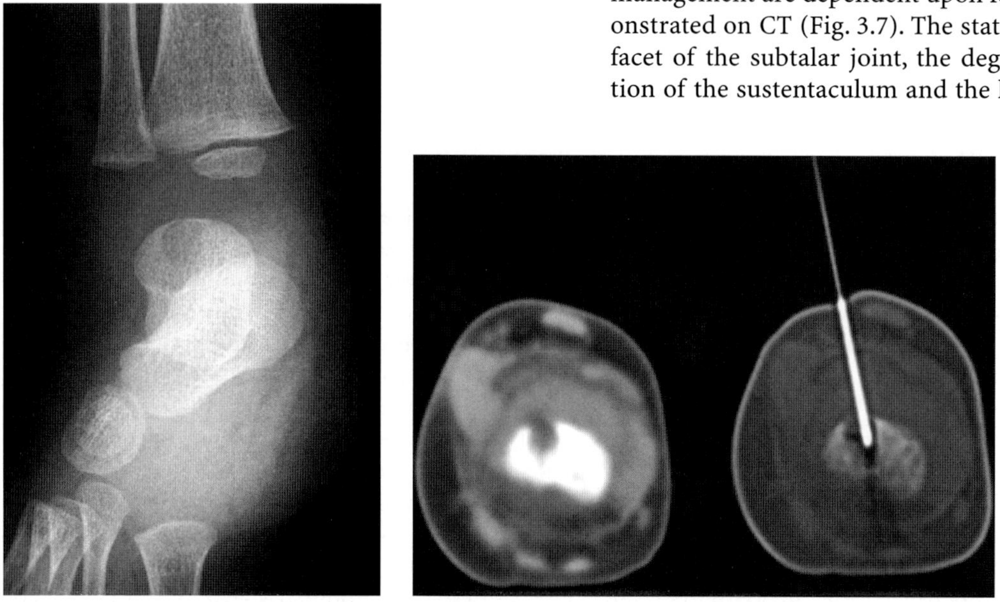 b

Fig. 3.6a. Plain film of the ankle demonstrating a subtle focal lytic area in the talus. **b** CT and CT-guided aspiration with a 20G spinal needle under general anaesthesia with the patient prone confirmed a Brodie's abscess

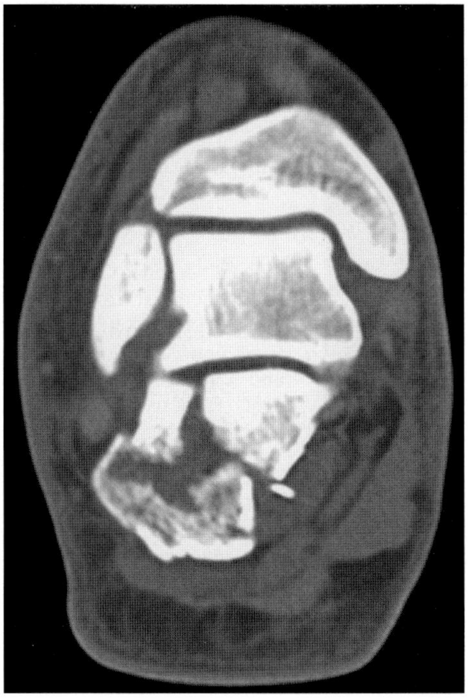

Fig. 3.7. Coronal 2 mm section through the hindfoot demonstrating a comminuted intra-articular fracture of the calcaneus

calcaneus, involvement of the calcaneocuboid joint and the overall shape of the heel are all of surgical importance and demonstrable with a combination of coronal and transverse CT scans (or reformations) through the hindfoot (Bearcroft 1998). A spiral acquisition in the transverse plane with 1-mm-thick collimation and a pitch of 1 mm allows the calcaneus to be covered in around 60 rotations, whilst coronal and sagittal reformations are of satisfactory quality. Direct coronal scanning requires more rotations, increased collimation thickness or pitch to cover the calcaneus and cuboid, but it is necessary if 1 mm collimation is not available.

A similar spiral protocol demonstrates comminution, fracture alignment and articular congruity of talar fractures (Wechsler et al. 1997).

3.5.2 Articular Cartilage

Thin-section CT (particularly multislice helical) combined with arthrography (see below) has been used as the gold standard for measuring articular cartilage thickness and volume in the knee. These techniques are equally applicable to the ankle.

These measurements are of increasing clinical importance as targetted treatments for osteoarthritis are being developed (Hangody et al. 1998). Many of these studies are aimed at validating MR methods of cartilage measurement rather than advocating the use of CT arthrography (Eckstein et al. 1997, 1998; Haubner et al. 1997). Nevertheless, CT arthrography currently remains more sensitive than non-arthrographic MR for subtle cartilage defects (Daenen et al. 1998), and the minimally invasive technique allows accurate measurement of capsular volume, fluid aspiration for laboratory studies and injection of therapeutic agents as required (Berquist 1997).

3.5.3 Tarsal Coalitions

Abnormal bridging by bone or fibrous tissue between two or more tarsal bones (tarsal coalition) is usually congenital in origin and causes foot pain and reduced movement, usually presenting in childhood or young adults. The most common forms are calcaneonavicular and talocalcaneal, accounting for approximately 90% of cases between them (Pachuda et al. 1990). Both transverse and coronal CT may be necessary to evaluate all the articulations adequately, though both talocalcaneal and calcaneonavicular coalitions are usually best seen on coronal scans (Fig. 3.8).

Coalitions are classified as complete (where bone bridges the articulation) or incomplete (fibrous or cartilaginous bridging). In the former, CT will readily demonstrate osseous continuity between the bones. In the latter, secondary features of joint space narrowing or irregularity, sclerosis and cyst formation of the articular 'subchondral' bone should be sought (Emery et al. 1998). Although differentiation of fibrous from osseous coalition is easier and more reliable on CT than MR imaging, currently, CT and MR scanning are approximately equivalent in diagnostic accuracy for detecting tarsal coalitions; both techniques also detected similar numbers of unrelated conditions accounting for the patients' symptoms where coalition was suspected but not present (Emery et al. 1998).

3.5.4 Soft Tissues

The imaging examination of soft-tissue masses and synovial diseases of the foot and ankle is best undertaken by MRI [with or without gadolinium diethylene tetra-amine penta-acetic acid (Gd-DTPA)

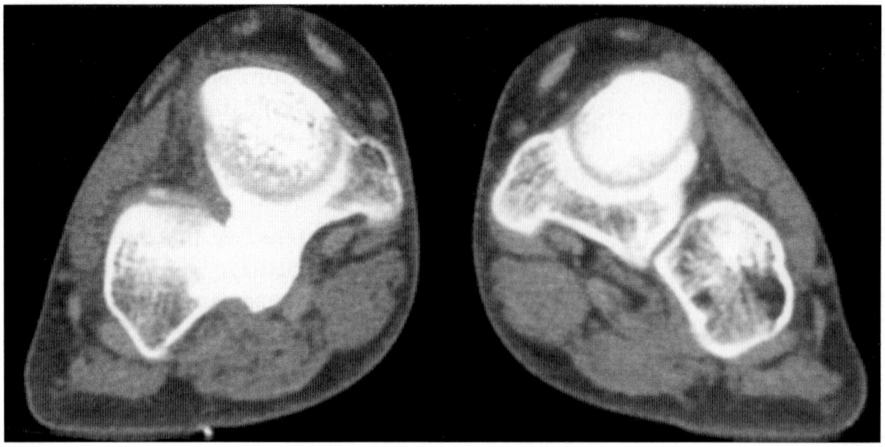

Fig. 3.8. Coronal CT of both feet demonstrating unilateral bone bridging (tarsal coalition) between the navicular and calcaneus (courtesy of Prof. H. Carty, Alder Hey Hospital, Liverpool, UK)

enhancement], augmented by radiographs and possibly specialist ultrasound (US) examination. CT has a limited role where these methods are contraindicated or unavailable, but some pathologies [e.g. fatty tumours such as lipoma arborescens, calcified lesions – synovial osteochondromatosis (Fig. 3.9), gouty tophi and dense lesions such as pigmented villonodular synovitis] may have characteristic appearances on CT (Chen et al. 1999; Lin et al. 1999). CT is unreliable for follow-up scanning of the resection site of soft-tissue sarcoma (Hudson et al. 1985).

Contrast enhancement can be used with volume rendering to demonstrate arterial and graft stenosis and obstructions after vascular surgery down to the popliteal vessels (Ishikawa et al. 1999) and other vascular lesions (Fig. 3.10). Similarly, soft-tissue enhancement in masses or the synovium can be demonstrated, but the timing is critical, with peak enhancement being later, less marked and more variable in onset than in the abdomen. CT scanner software which prescans at low mAs to detect the onset of enhancement and triggers the study at that point may be useful.

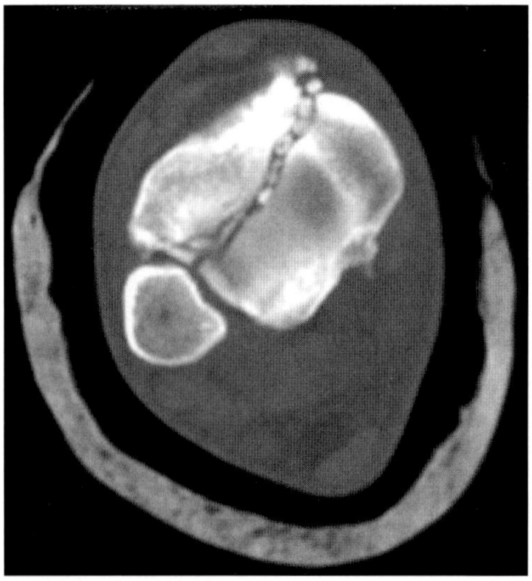

Fig. 3.9. Synovial osteochondromatosis – multiple, peripherally calcified lesions are present, which in this case have become trapped within a fracture of the plafond

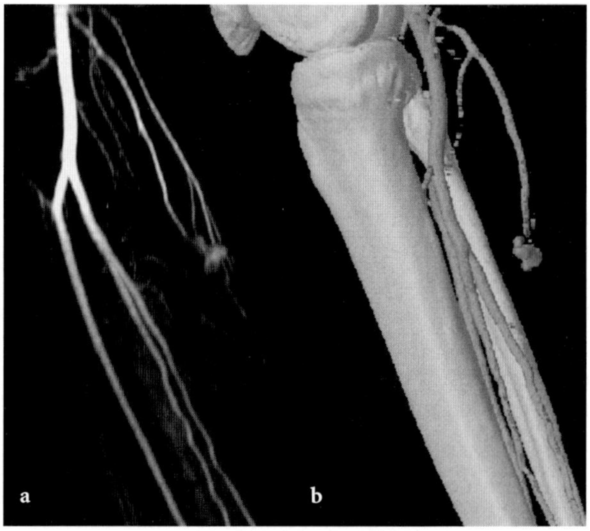

Fig. 3.10a. Maximum intensity projection from scans acquired during intravenous contrast infusion demonstrate the arterial vascular anatomy of the knee and proximal leg. Contrast extravasation from the distal muscular (sural) artery is noted. **b** 3D surface-rendered image from the same data as **a.** (Images provided courtesy of Philips Medical Systems and Dr R.C. Berlin, MD, St. John's Hospital, Jackson, WY, USA)

3.5.5 Tendons

The tendons of the foot and ankle are clearly depicted by CT. In cross-section, tendons appear as homogeneous, well circumscribed, rounded densities of higher attenuation than other soft tissues, usually having CT numbers in the range of 75 to 115 and thus being visible within their muscles of origin as well as when surrounded by fat in their more distal courses. Tendons are therefore best demonstrated with sections perpendicular to their courses (ROSENBERG et al. 1988). Fluid around the tendon can be identified on CT as a ring of lower attenuation surrounding the tendon (Fig. 3.11), though with less sensitivity to small quantities of fluid than MRI. Increased fluid around the flexor hallucis longus and flexor digitorum longus tendons can be normal findings due to communication of these tendon sheaths with the ankle joint in 10%–20% of people. Scar tissue around the tendon sheath appears as an indistinct soft-tissue density obscuring the surrounding fat. Tendinosis and tendon rupture can also be demonstrated on CT, with thickening and reduction in attenuation of the tendon being seen. Dislocation of tendons is easily identified by the demonstrated tendon position, peroneal tendon dislocation and bony abnormalities that may be associated (a shallow retromalleolar groove or fracture fragments encroaching on the tendon) being obvious on CT (ROSENBERG et al. 1986).

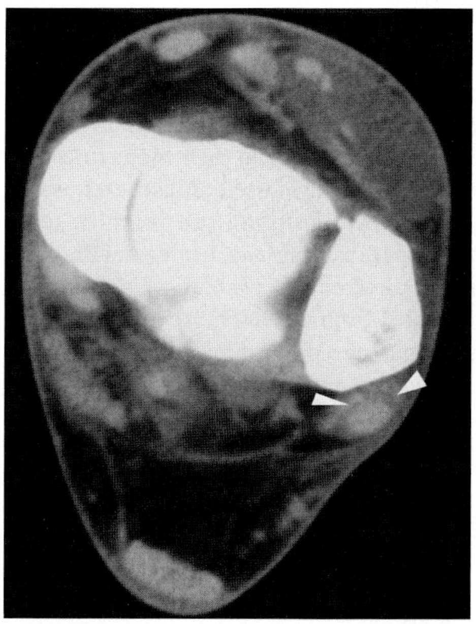

Fig. 3.11. Axial CT of the ankle demonstrating tenosynovitis (excess fluid) around the extensor digitorum longus tendons and longitudinal splitting of the peroneus brevis tendon (*arrowheads*)

Three-dimensional reformations from multiple thin sections can provide an exquisite demonstration of tendon and osseous anatomy (BELLON and HOROWITZ 1992). Thus, whilst CT can be used to demonstrate gross tendon pathology and associated osseous abnormality, MRI is more sensitive and more specific for the tendon lesion (CLARKE et al. 1997). Scar tissue, oedema, early tendon degeneration and small amounts of inflammatory fluid are difficult to differentiate on CT (CHEUNG et al. 1992).

3.6 Arthrography

CT arthrography can be performed as an adjunct to conventional ankle arthrography. With double-contrast arthrography, CT can be performed immediately after the conventional examination as only a small amount of iodinated contrast medium is injected (1–2 ml of 300 mg I/ml). If single contrast arthrography is performed with larger quantities of dense contrast, an interval of 2–3 h between the conventional technique and the CT examination allows the contrast medium density to dilute to a level appropriate for CT. If an immediate CT arthrogram is planned, appropriate reduction in the contrast medium concentration is needed, e.g. 150 mg I/ml non-ionic water-soluble contrast medium (Fig. 3.12).

Indications for CT arthrography are the demonstration of intra-articular loose bodies (TEHRANZADEH and GABRIELLE 1984), chondral lesions and osteochondral defects (DAVIES and CASSAR-PULLICINO 1989). CT arthrography can also be used for the evaluation of the ankle impingement syndrome (HAUGER et al. 1999).

3.6.1 Technique

Fluoroscopy screening is rarely needed for needle placement but confirms the correct location during injection of contrast medium. Local anaesthetic should not be necessary, though preparation of the skin with topical anaesthetic cream may be useful in children. Using an aseptic technique, a small gauge needle (23G) is introduced into the ankle joint from the midline, anteriorly, avoiding the dorsalis pedis artery (identified by palpation). Slight cephalad angulation of the needle

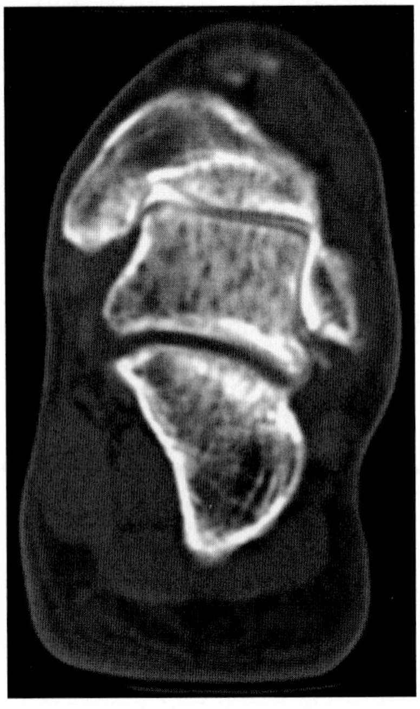

Fig. 3.12. Coronal ankle CT arthrogram with 3 ml of 150 mg/ml iodinated non-ionic contrast medium

to avoid the anterior lip of the tibia assists in accurate needle placement. A double contrast technique with 2 ml of contrast and 5 ml of air can be performed if a conventional arthrogram is also required. A single contrast technique with 2–5 ml of 150 mg I/ml contrast is satisfactory for a CT arthrogram and avoids the streak artefact that may occur at air/fluid interfaces. Lateral fluoroscopy during injection confirms correct needle location as contrast should flow rapidly away from the needle tip into the joint. A misplaced needle results in focal accumulation of contrast at the needle tip. After removing the needle, gentle manipulation ensures the contrast extends throughout all the joint capsular recesses. After a conventional arthrogram if required, coronal CT through the ankle is performed. Delayed post-arthrography scanning may be necessary if communication between the ankle joint and any nearby cyst or ganglion is suspected as there may be a 1–2 h delay before contrast appears within the cyst (Malghem et al. 1998).

3.7 CT-Guided Interventions

CT is being increasingly used to guide interventional procedures, recently encouraged by the development of CT fluoroscopy which enables more rapid and accurate placement of needles and interventional devices (Froelich et al. 1999; De Mey et al. 2000). As described above (Section 3.2.5), care needs to be taken to minimise operator and patient X-ray exposure during CT-guided biopsy. CT fluoroscopy times of around 10 s should suffice for most biopsy procedures (Goldberg et al. 2000). Limiting the fluoroscopy to identification of the needle tip rather than the entire needle will also reduce the operator and patient radiation dose (Silverman et al. 1999). The CT section thickness should be appropriate to the size of the lesion, otherwise partial volume averaging may include both the needle tip and the lesion in the same section, erroneously suggesting an accurate needle location. CT can be used to guide the biopsy of bone and soft-tissue lesions. Where primary malignancy is present, then the course of the biopsy track and the compartment(s) through which it passes may need excision with the tumour at the time of definitive surgery. Biopsy of such lesions must therefore only be performed after consultation and agreement of the approach with the surgeon who will carry out the definitive treatment. The accuracy of a CT-guided biopsy is increased if specimens are obtained for both cytology and pathology; an overall accuracy of around 80% should be acheived (Hodge 1999).

Percutaneous treatment of osteoid osteoma can also be performed with CT guidance. Again, a planned approach avoiding vascular structures is required, and a preliminary contrast-enhanced scan to identify the vessels clearly is valuable (Fig. 3.13). It is possible to treat osteoid osteomas by complete removal via CT-guided biopsy (Voto et al. 1990), but this may be difficult to achieve with biopsy needles unless a large bore needle is used and several passes are made through the lesion. More recently, techniques aimed at destroying the tumour with heat, either from a radiofrequency ablation probe or a laser-heated probe, both of which are available with fine probes for passage down a biopsy needle, have been used. In either case, to avoid complications, the lesion to be treated should be more than 1 cm from neurovascular or other critical structures. A preliminary biopsy for histological confirmation of the diagnosis is necessary as in one series 16% of lesions were not osteoid osteomas (Sans et al. 1999). Osteoid osteomas can cause severe pain when biopsied; although some series report the use of local anaesthesia, epidural or general anaesthesia may be necessary. Other CT-guided procedures described around the foot and ankle include steroid and local anaesthetic injection into the sinus tarsi for sinus

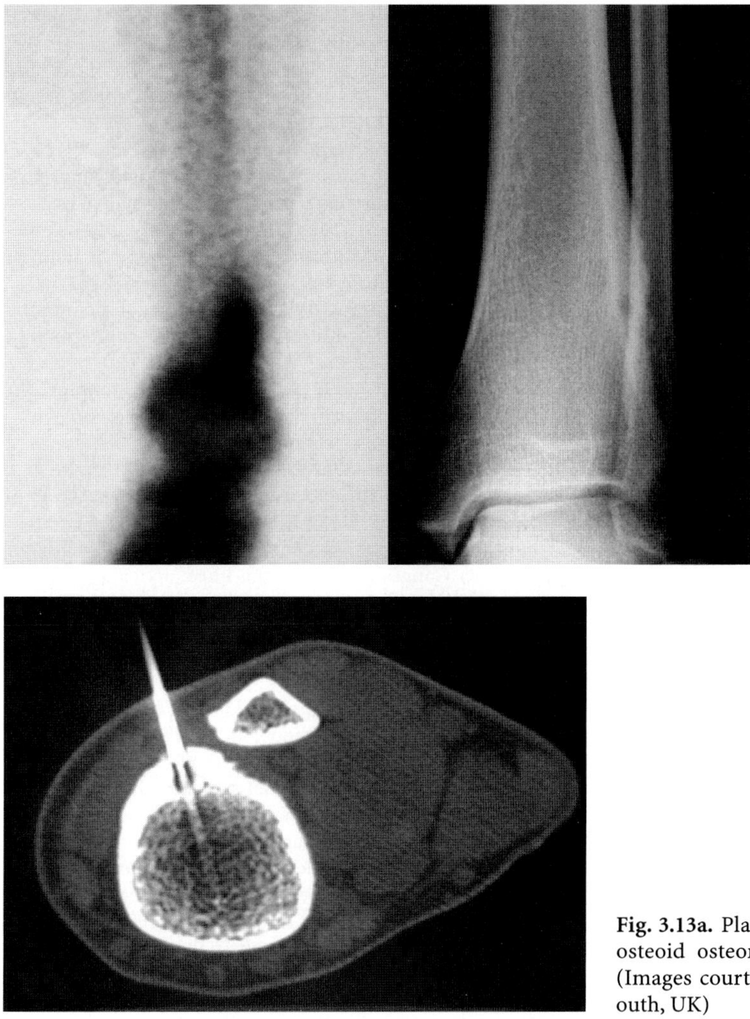

a

b

Fig. 3.13a. Plain film and isotope bone scan demonstrate an osteoid osteoma in the distal tibia. b CT-guided ablation. (Images courtesy of Dr P. Hughes, Derriford Hospital, Plymouth, UK)

tarsi syndrome (Ingham et al. 2001) and percutaneous drilling of osteochondral lesions of the talus and plafond (Shah et al. 2001).

Although the bulk of CT-guided interventional procedures are performed by radiologists in the Radiology Department, the development of mobile CT scanners has allowed the use of CT guidance for procedures performed in the operating theatre, allowing the orthopaedic surgeon to make greater use of CT guidance for minimally invasive procedures.

3.8 Conclusion

With appropriate attention to the technique, CT continues to play a role in the diagnosis and management of many conditions in and around the foot and ankle. Some pathologies will, however, only be adequately demonstrated using CT arthrography and a scanner capable of submillimetre resolution in the Y-axis.

References

Adler SJ, Vannier MW, Gilula LA, Knapp RH (1988) Three-Dimensional computed tomography of the foot: optimising the image. Comp Med Imag Graph 12:59–66

Bearcroft PWP (1998) The use of spiral computed tomography in musculoskeletal radiology of the lower limb: the calcaneus as an example. Eur J Radiol 28:30–38

Bellon RJ, Horowitz SM (1992) Three-dimensional computed tomography studies of the tendons of the foot and ankle. J Digital Imag 5:46–50

Berquist TH (1997) Imaging of articular pathology: MRI, CT, arthrography. Clin Anat 10:1–13

Chen CK, Yeh LR, Pan HB, Yang CF, Lu YC, Wang JS, Resnick D

(1999) Intra-articular gouty tophi of the knee: CT and MR imaging in 12 patients. Skeletal Radiol 28:75–80

Cheung Y, Rosenberg ZS, Magee T, Chinitz L (1992) Normal anatomy and pathologic conditions of ankle tendons: current imaging techniques. Radiographics 12:429–444

Clarke HD, Kitaoka HB, Berquist TH (1997) Imaging of tendon injuries about the ankle. Orthopedics 20:639–643

Daenen BR, Ferrara MA, Marcelis S, Dondelinger RF (1998) Evaluation of patellar cartilage surface lesions: comparison of CT arthrography and fat-suppressed FLASH 3D MR imaging. Eur Radiol 8:981–985

Daly B, Templeton PA, Krebs TL, Carroll K, Wong You Cheong JJ (1998) Evaluation of biopsy needles and prototypic needle guide devices for percutaneous biopsy with CT fluoroscopic guidance in simulated organ tissue. Radiology 209:850–855

Davies AM, Cassar-Pullicino VN (1989) Demonstration of osteochondritis dissecans of the talus by coronal computed tomographic arthrography. Br J Radiol 62:1050–1055

Dawson P, Lees WR (2001) Multi-slice technology in computed tomography. Clin Rad 56:302–309

De Mey J, Op de Beeck B, Meysman M, Noppen M, De Maeseneer M, Vanhoey M, Vincken W, Osteaux M (2000) Real time CT-fluoroscopy: diagnostic and therapeutic applications. Eur J Radiol 34:32–40

Donaldson JS, Poznanski AK, Nieves A (1987) CT of children's feet: an immobilisation technique. Am J Roentgenol 148: 169–170

Eckstein F, Adam C, Sittek H, Becker C, Milz S, Schulte E, Reiser M, Putz R (1997) Non-Invasive determination of cartilage thickness throughout joint surfaces using magnetic resonance imaging. J Biomech 30:285–289

Eckstein F, Schnier M, Haubner M, Priebsch J, Glaser C, Englmeier KH, Reiser M (1998) Accuracy of cartilage volume and thickness measurements with magnetic resonance imaging. Clin Orthop 352:137–148

Emery KH, Bisset GS 3rd, Johnson ND, Nunan PJ (1998) Tarsal coalition: a blinded comparison of MRI and CT. Pediatr Radiol 28:612–616

Froelich JJ, Ishaque N, Saar B, Regn J, Walthers EM, Mauermann F, Klose KJ (1999) Steuerung von perkutanen Biopsien mittels CT-Fluoroskopie. [Control of percutaneous biopsy with CT fluoroscopy.] Rofo Fortschr Geb Rontgenstr Neuen Bildgeb Verfahr 170:191–197

Goldberg SN, Keogan MT, Raptopoulos V (2000) Percutaneous CT-guided biopsy: improved confirmation of sampling site and needle positioning using a multistep technique at CT fluoroscopy. J Comput Assist Tomogr 24:264–266

Hangody L, Kish G, Karpati Z, Udvarhelyi I, Szigeti I, Bely M (1998) Mosaicplasty for the treatment of articular cartilage defects: application in clinical practice. Orthopedics 21:751–756

Haubner M, Eckstein F, Schnier M, Losch A, Sittek H, Becker C, Kolem H, Reiser M, Englmeier KH (1997) A non-invasive technique for 3-dimensional assessment of articular cartilage thickness based on MRI, part 2. Validation using CT arthrography. Magn Reson Imaging 15:805–813

Hauger O, Moinard M, Lasalarie JC, Chauveaux D, Diard F (1999) Anterolateral compartment of the ankle in the lateral impingement syndrome: appearance on CT arthrography. Am J Roentgenol 173:685–690

Hodge JC (1999) Percutaneous biopsy of the musculoskeletal system: a review of 77 cases. Can Assoc Radiol J 50: 121–125

Hsieh J (1997) Analysis of the temporal response of computed tomography fluoroscopy. Med Phys 24:665–675

Hudson TM, Schakel M, Springfield DS (1985) Limitations of computed tomography following excisional biopsy of soft tissue sarcomas. Skeletal Radiol 13:49–54

Ingham F, McAlinden P, Naraghi A, Padhiar N, Chan O (2001) CT guided injection of sinus tarsi in patients with sinus tarsi syndrome. UK Radiology Congress Abstracts, pp 60–61

Ishikawa M, Morimoto N, Sasajima T, Kubo Y (1999) Three-dimensional computed tomographic angiography in lower extremity revascularization. Surg Today 29:243–247

Jend H-H, Ney R, Heller M (1985) Evaluation of tibiofibular motion under load conditions by computed tomography. J Orthop Res 3:418–423

Johnson JE, Timins ME (1998) Optimal computed tomography imaging of the midfoot: an improved technique. Foot Ankle Int 19:825–829

Lin J, Jacobson JA, Jamadar DA, Ellis JH (1999) Pigmented villonodular synovitis and related lesions: the spectrum of imaging findings. AJR 172:191–197

Malghem J, Vande-berg BC, Lebon C, Lecouvet FE, Maldague BE (1998) Ganglion cysts of the knee: articular communication revealed by delayed radiography and CT after arthrography. AJR 170:1579–1583

Mann FA, Gilula LA (1989) Direct sagittal CT of the foot. Am J Roentgenol 153:886

Martinez S, Herzenberg JE, Apple JS (1985) Computed tomography of the hindfoot. Orthop Clin North Am 16:481–496

Nawfel RD, Judy PF, Silverman SG, Hooton S, Tuncali K, Adams DF (2000) Patient and personnel exposure during CT fluoroscopy-guided interventional procedures. Radiology 216: 180–184 (and comments pages 9–10)

Pachuda NM, Lasday SD, Jay RM (1990) Tarsal coalition: etiology, diagnosis and treatment. J Foot Surg 29:474–488

Pretorius ES, Fishman EK (1999) Volume-rendered three-dimensional spiral CT: musculoskeletal applications. Radiographics 19:1143–1160

Rosenberg ZS, Feldman F, Singson RD (1986) Peroneal tendon injuries: CT analysis. Radiology 161:743–748

Rosenberg ZS, Cheung Y, Jahss MH (1988) Computed tomography scan and magnetic resonance imaging of ankle tendons: an overview. Foot Ankle 8:297–307

Sans N, Morera-Maupome H, Galy-Fourcade D, Jarlaud T, Chiavassa H, Bonnevialle P, Giron J, Railhac JJ (1999) Resection percutanee sous controle tomodensitometrique de s osteomes osteoides. Suivi a moyen terme de 38 cas. [Percutaneous resection under computed tomography guidance of osteoid osteoma. Mid-term follow-up of 38 cases.] J Radiol 80:457–465

Shah FN, Naraghi A, McAlinden P, King JB, Chan O (2001) Percutaneous CT guided drilling of osteochondral lesions under local anaesthesia. UK Radiology Congress Abstracts, p 61

Silverman SG, Tuncali K, Adams DF, Nawfel RD, Zou KH, Judy PF (1999) CT fluoroscopy-guided abdominal interventions: techniques, results, and radiation exposure. Radiology 212: 673–681

Solomon MA, Gilula LA, Oloff LM, Oloff J, Compton T (1986) CT scanning of the foot and ankle. 1. Normal anatomy. Am J Roentgenol 146:1192–1203

Tehranzadeh J, Gabrielle OF (1984) Intra-articular calcified bodies: detection by computed arthrotomography. South Med J 77:703–710 van Hellemondt FJ, Louwerens JWK, Sijbrandij ES, van Gils APG (1997) Stress radiography and stress examination of the talocrural and subtalar joint on helical computed tomography. Foot Ankle Int 18:482–488

Voto SJ, Cook AJ, Weiner DS, Ewing JW, Arrington LE (1990) Treatment of osteoid osteoma by computed tomography guided excision in the pediatric patient. J Pediatr Orthop 10:510–513

Wechsler RJ, Schweitzer ME, Karasick D, Deely DM, Glaser JB (1997) Helical CT of talar fractures. Skeletal Radiol 26: 137–142

Whitehouse RW, Economou G, Adams JE (1993) The influence of temperature on Quantitative Computed Tomography: implications for mineral densitometry. J Comput Assist Tomogr 17:945–951

4 MRI

J. P. R. Jenkins

CONTENTS

4.1 Introduction

MR imaging is increasingly used in the investigation of the ankle and foot being particularly suited to the assessment of the bones and soft tissues. The complex anatomy of the ankle and foot can be daunting to the uninitiated. In this chapter the relevant technique and principles of MR imaging will be expounded followed by a review of the regional anatomy.

J. P. R. Jenkins, MBChB, FRCP, DMRD, FRCR
Department of Clinical Radiology, Manchester Royal Infirmary, Oxford Road, Manchester, M13 9WL, UK

4.2 Imaging Technique and Principles

Magnetic resonance (MR) imaging has a high soft-tissue contrast discrimination and resolution with the ability to image any plane, lending itself particularly to the demonstration of complex musculoskeletal anatomy. A major advantage of MR imaging in musculoskeletal imaging has been the deployment of fat saturation/suppression techniques, leading to improved confidence in the diagnosis, particularly when combined with contrast administration.

4.2.1 Patient Selection

Claustrophobia (approximately 5% of total MR imaging) is less of a problem in the assessment of the ankle and foot as positioning of the body part in the centre of the magnet in order to optimise the signal-to-noise ratio usually means the patient's head is at the edge or outside the magnet bore. If, however, the patient is still unable to undertake the examination because of claustrophobia, then sedation can be offered with intravenous diazepam (Diazemuls), titrated to the patient's response, with monitoring of the patient with a magnet-friendly pulse oximeter. The main side-effect with intravenous sedation is transient apnoea which can readily be treated by requesting the patient to take deep breaths. An open magnet system or a dedicated extremity MR imager can be used in patients with claustrophobia without the requirement for intravenous sedation (Peterfy et al. 1998). These magnet systems can also be used in very obese individuals who are unable to fit into a closed magnet bore. The downside of these magnet systems is that they tend to be of low field (less than 0.3 T) with subsequent lower signal-to-noise ratio and spatial resolution than more conventional magnet systems.

Patients in plaster casts (POP) can be imaged in the cast with no detriment to the image quality but may require a larger receiver coil to fit over the cast. Patients with a pacemaker in situ, intracranial aneurysmal clips, neurostimulators and some cochlear implants are contraindicated for MR imaging. Care is also required for individuals who have programmable intracranial ventricular shunts in situ as they are programmed by a small magnet, and placement within an MR system can alter the programme. Individuals who have had recent surgery are usually not a problem, even in those who have received prosthetic heart valves or undergone angioplasty, as long as the MR examination is delayed for 6–8 weeks to allow healing fibrosis. Although the heating of prosthetic implants was initially considered to be a problem in the early days of MR imaging, studies have shown the effects to be negligible and not a contraindication. Orthopaedic appliances (plates, screws, prosthetic implants, etc.) are usually made of non-ferromagnetic material (e.g. high-grade steel, cobalt-chromium, titanium or multiple alloys), but they do contain impurities (e.g. iron particles) which are paramagnetic, leading to susceptibility artefacts. External fixation devices are usually not paramagnetic, but if there is any doubt, these can be tested using a hand-held magnet. External fixation devices represent more of a problem as the patient may not be able to fit within a quadrature/phased-array receiver coil used (usually the neurovascular head coil), and this would require body coil imaging with subsequently reduced spatial resolution. Numerous safety aspects have been fully assessed, and the information is readily available in book form (Shellock and Kanal 1996) and on the world wide web (www. mrisafety.com).

Artefacts can be caused by metal in situ, but this usually produces a localised artefact. Usually, there are fewer artefacts with MR than CT. Following surgery, particularly with the use of a bone drill, tiny metallic fragments can be left in situ, probably from the drill hitting the bone or tissue retractor, although the image distortion is usually of no consequence. On MR the size of the area of signal void from the artefact is dependent on the size, shape and orientation of the metal object and the pulse sequences used. Least artefact is produced using T1-weighted and T2-weighted SE and STIR sequencing with the worse artefacts from GE scans.

4.2.2 Coil Selection

A quadrature or preferably a phased-array coil is required for uniform signal and high resolution imaging. Newly designed coils (with an open or chimney shape) offer space for the foot to be placed in the neutral position when imaging the ankle and hindfoot – important when assessing the Achilles tendon. The use of a flat surface coil whilst covering a small field of view may not be advantageous when imaging a tendon as it is important to demonstrate both its musculotendinous junction and distal insertion. Smaller coils can be used for assessment of the midfoot and forefoot (e.g. assessment for a Morton's neuroma). The operator parameters required for high spatial resolution imaging involve the smallest field of view necessary to cover the geographic area with thin slices countered by the need for good signal-to-noise images.

4.2.3 Patient Positioning

Patients are usually examined in the supine position with the foot in the neutral position, particularly for evaluating the Achilles tendon. The foot can be plantar flexed if the midfoot and forefoot are to be assessed to avoid inadvertent movement artefact. As the medial and lateral ankle tendons follow a curved course, they are susceptible to a magic angle effect (vide infra). This artefact can be minimised and the distal parts of the tendons more clearly delineated by imaging these tendons in an oblique transverse plane with the foot plantar flexed. The contralateral foot should be outside the field of view to prevent a wrap artefact, which is caused by the image of the contralateral foot being placed inside the other image.

4.2.4 Imaging Planes

Coronal, sagittal and transverse planes are routinely used in the assessment of the ankle and hindfoot (Tables 4.1, 4.2). The optimum imaging planes for assessment of the Achilles tendon is the sagittal plane aligned along the tendon to include the musculotendinous junction down to its distal insertion together with transverse images (Fig. 4.1) (Table 4.3). With reference to the midfoot and forefoot, transverse (long-axis views) and coronal (short-axis) views are usually obtained with additional sagittal sectioning if required (Table 4.4).

4.2.5 Pulse Sequences

The advance of digital radiofrequency pulses in the 1990s allowed faster imaging times with the constraint

Table 4.1. Routine imaging strategies for the ankle/hindfoot/midfoot (head coil) (ETL, echo train length; NEX, number of signal excitations)

Imaging plane Sequence	Sagittal T1-weighted FSE	Sagittal Intermediate-weighted FSE + fat suppression	Coronal T2-weighted FSE	Transverse T1-weighted FSE	Transverse Intermediate-weighted FSE + fat suppression
TR/TE	560/8.8	3200/12.3	4000/105	340/9.3	3000/9.3
ETL	2	10	12	2	10
Field of view (FOV) (cm)	20×20	20×20	20×15	16×12	16×12
Matrix	320×224	320×224	256×224	320×224	320×224
Slice thickness/gap (mm)	3/0.5	3/0.5	4/1	4/1	4/1
NEX	2	3	3	3	3
Acquisition time (min)	2.10	3.57	3.06	2.57	2.54

Table 4.2. Imaging strategies for the ankle/hindfoot/midfoot – ? soft-tissue mass/infection (head coil) (FOV, field of view)

Imaging plane Sequence	Sagittal T1-weighted FSE	Sagittal Intermediate-weighted FSE + fat suppression	Transverse T2-weighted FSE	Transverse T1-weighted FSE + fat suppression -/+ gadolinium-chelate	Coronal T2-weighted GE (optional)
TR/TE	560/8.8	3200/12.3	4000/105	600/15.4	450/20/20°[a]
ETL	2	10	12	2	–
FOV (cm)	20×20	20×20	16×12	16×12	20×15
Matrix	320×224	320×224	320×224	320×224	512×224
Slice thickness/gap (mm)	3/0.5	3/0.5	4/1	4/1	5
NEX	2	3	3	3	2
Acquisition time (min)	2.10	3.57	3.06	5.08	3.20

[a] 20°=flip angle

Table 4.3. Imaging strategies for the Achilles tendon (head coil)

Imaging plane Sequence	Sagittal T1-weighted FSE	Sagittal T2-weighted GE + fat suppression	Transverse T1-weighted FSE	Transverse Intermediate-weighted FSE + fat suppression
TR/TE	560/8.8	3200/12.3/20°	4000/105	3000/9.3
ETL	2	10	12	10
FOV (cm)	30×30	20×20	16×12	16×12
Matrix	320×224	320×224	320×224	320×224
Slice thickness/gap (mm)	3/0.5	3/0.5	6/2	6/2
NEX	2	3	3	3
Acquisition time (min)	2.40	7.18	3.27	3.23

Table 4.4. Imaging strategies for the midfoot/forefoot including ? Morton's neuroma (knee coil)

Imaging plane Sequence	Transverse (long axis) T1-weighted FSE	Transverse (long axis) Intermediate-weighted FSE + fat suppression	Coronal (short axis) T1-weighted FSE	Coronal (short axis) Intermediate-weighted FSE + fat suppression
TR/TE	550/15.6	3200/12.3/20°	340/16.4	3000/16
ETL	2	10	2	8
FOV (cm)	16×16	16×16	12×12	12×9
Matrix	320×224	320×224	320×224	256×256
Slice thickness/gap (mm)	3/1	3/1	3/1	3/1
NEX	3	3	3	3
Acquisition time (min)	3.14	3.15	3.56	3.42

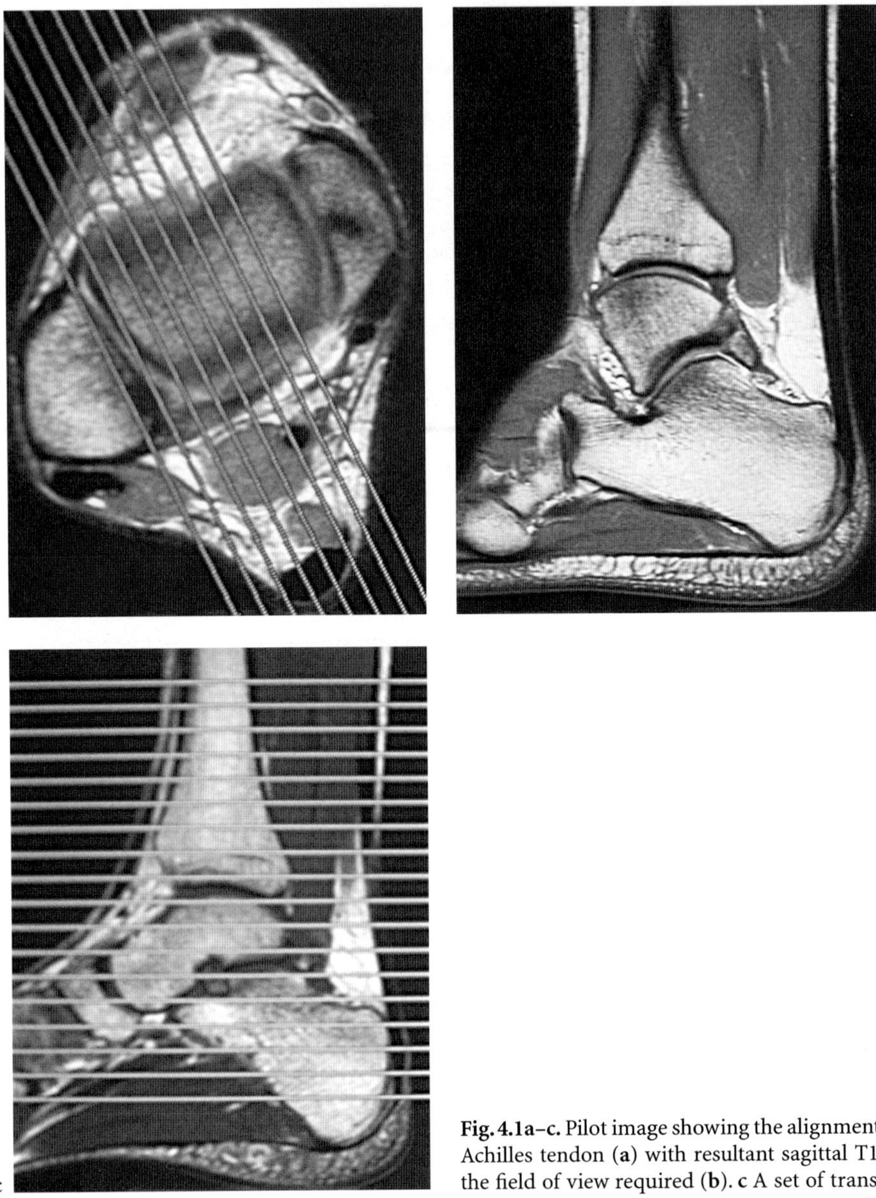

a b c

Fig. 4.1a–c. Pilot image showing the alignment for the sagittal sections through the Achilles tendon (**a**) with resultant sagittal T1-weighted SE image demonstrating the field of view required (**b**). **c** A set of transverse slices as prescribed from **b**

of slightly reduced contrast compared with conventional spin-echo imaging. The use of digital radiofrequency pulses allows multiple 180° refocusing pulses for spin-echo imaging providing turbo/fast spin-echo sequences with T1-weighting, intermediate/proton density and T2-weighting. The advent of fat suppression, particularly with spectral presaturation imaging, is of great benefit to MR imaging, aiding the detection of subtle soft-tissue and bone lesions, and enhancement following gadolinium -chelate.

Spectral presaturation imaging is frequency-specific (dependent on the fact that fat and water protons precess at slightly different frequencies) and can be applied as a preparatory pulse to conventional T_1-weighted and T_2-weighted spin-echo and gradient-echo sequences. A disadvantage of spectral presaturation imaging is that it may lead to inadvertent suppression of water protons within the image, particularly along curved regions that are off-centred, such as the ankle. This can lead to erroneous areas of high signal that can mimic pathology. Therefore, spectral presaturation requires good water-fat separation achieved in highly homogeneous magnet systems (usually 1 T or greater), whereas STIR, an alternative fat-suppressed pulse sequence, can be utilized with all magnet field strengths across a wide range of homogeneities. As the reduction in the fat signal is based on a frequency difference and not the relaxation time value, the spectral presaturation technique is more specific for the diagnosis of haemorrhage and can be used following gadolinium-chelate injection (intravenous or intra-articular). Fat suppression techniques are particularly useful in the demonstration of mass lesions, inflammation, infection and post-traumatic changes. They also provide for improved conspicuity of pathology compared with conventional T_1- and T_2-weighted sequences alone. The STIR sequence is used to advantage, however, in the presence of metal artefact.

Gradient-echo images, because of their susceptibility effects, are not used in the presence of metal or following surgery but are useful in demonstrating haemosiderin deposition which occurs under certain conditions (pigmented villonodular synovitis and rheumatoid arthritis). Fat-suppression sequences are relatively poor at demonstrating the signal void from haemosiderin deposition. Gradient-echo T2-weighted images with fat suppression are useful in the assessment of acute partial tear with haemorrhage in the Achilles tendon. Gradient-echo intermediate-weighting is also useful in the assessment of the articular cartilage of the talar and subtalar joint (Fig. 4.2).

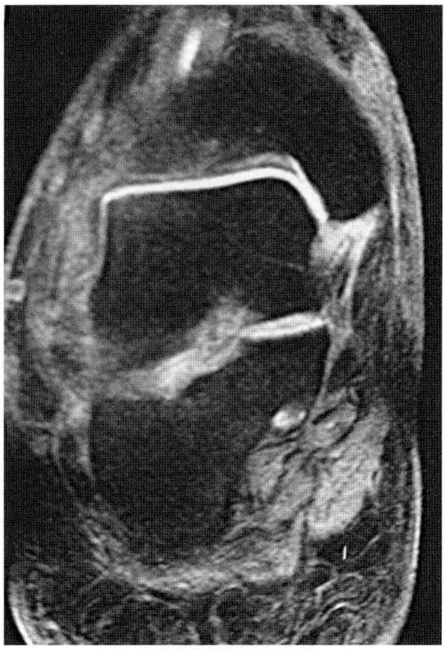

Fig. 4.2. A coronal intermediate-weighted fat-suppressed gradient-echo image through the talar dome and middle subtalar joint showing high signal contrast from articular cartilage

4.2.6 Contrast Administration

Intravenous injection of gadolinium chelate is used in suspected infection, synovitis or mass lesion to separate fluid/cyst from a solid soft-tissue mass/tumour. The usual concentration of contrast given is 0.1 mmol/kg body weight, which equates to 0.2 ml per kg body weight. The technique and anatomy for MR arthrography of the ankle are covered in the next chapter.

Table 4.5. Anatomical region selected by the clinical pathology suspected

Clinical diagnosis	Anatomical region
Focal/non-specific ankle pain	Ankle/hindfoot/midfoot
Trauma	
Tarsal coalition	
Infection/mass around ankle	
Achilles tendon pathology	Achilles tendon
Morton's neuroma	Forefoot
Infection/mass around foot	Midfoot & forefoot
Metatarsalgia	

4.2.7 Clinical Application

MR imaging is important in the problem-solving role of localised/diffuse pain of uncertain cause, in the diagnosis of clinically unsuspected bone contusion/bruising with micro-trabecular fracture, haemorrhage and oedema, and in the assessment of a soft-tissue mass/inflammation (Rosenberg et al. 2000). Imaging protocols are selected depending on the clinical diagnosis from four key anatomical areas – (1) ankle/hindfoot/midfoot, (2) Achilles tendon, (3) forefoot/toes, (4) entire foot (Table 4.5). One important aspect of MR imaging not to be underestimated is in the demonstration of normality with accuracy.

4.3 Anatomy

A clear understanding of anatomy and common anatomical variants is the key to the correct interpretation of MR images. The anatomy of the ankle and foot is complex and will be covered by a regional approach in the ankle to hindfoot, with a brief compartmental review of the midfoot and forefoot. The ankle and hindfoot can be divided into medial, lateral, anterior and posterior regions. The importance of understanding key anatomical areas such as the tarsal tunnel and sinus tarsi will be emphasised. For a full overview of the anatomy in the various imaging planes, reference should be made to published atlases (EL-KHOURY et al. 1995; STOLLER et al.1999).

It is important to have an understanding of the MR imaging appearance of normal anatomical structures. Cortical bone shows signal void on all sequences, with bone marrow having a lattice of low signal trabecular struts with intervening high signal fat. The appearance of bone marrow on MR imaging varies depending on the age of the individual studied, with the young and adolescent skeleton having areas of red marrow of low and intermediate signal on T1- and T2-weighted images, respectively (VALLEJO and JARAMILLO 2001). The appearance of patchy areas of red marrow can mimic pathology (Fig. 4.3). Articular (hyaline) cartilage is of intermediate signal, being well contrasted against low signal cortical bone and high signal synovial fluid on T2-weighted images. The ligaments of the ankle and foot appear of low signal, either as a uniform band or as alternating layers of low and intermediate signal.

Tendons demonstrate a homogeneous low signal on all sequences, except at their insertion where they can appear of intermediate signal (Fig. 4.4). Normal tendons can also show areas of increased signal due to the magic angle effect. This effect occurs when a structure courses at 55° to the main static magnetic field (Bo) and is seen on short TE (echo time) sequences (ERICKSON et al. 1991; HAYES and PARELLADA 1996). This artefact occurs with short TEs of 10–20 ms that are used in T1-weighted, intermediate/proton density-weighted and gradient-echo sequences. Depending on the orientation of the foot within the magnet, the medial and lateral tendons may be aligned to this angle along part of their length. However, the focal increased signal within the tendon from the magic angle effect remains low signal on T2-weighted images, allowing differentiation from pathology (tendinopathy and tears). A thin layer of fluid is normally seen around tendons and should not be interpreted as representing pathology (tenosynovitis). It should be noted that during fetal development the tendon invaginates its tendon sheath, forming a mesotendon which is located on

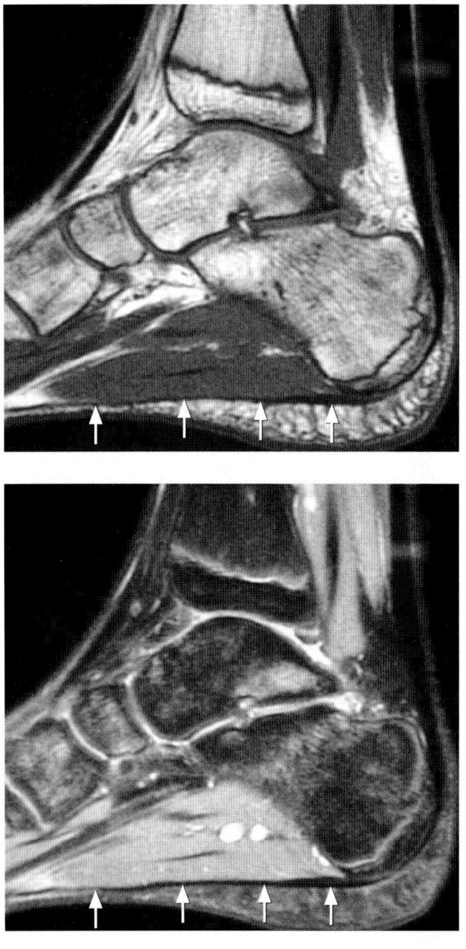

a

b

Fig. 4.3a,b. Sagittal T1-weighted SE (**a**) and intermediate-weighted FSE with fat suppression images (**b**) in a normal 13-year-old boy showing heterogeneity in marrow signals due to the presence of patchy red marrow. The normal plantar aponeurosis is shown (*arrows*)

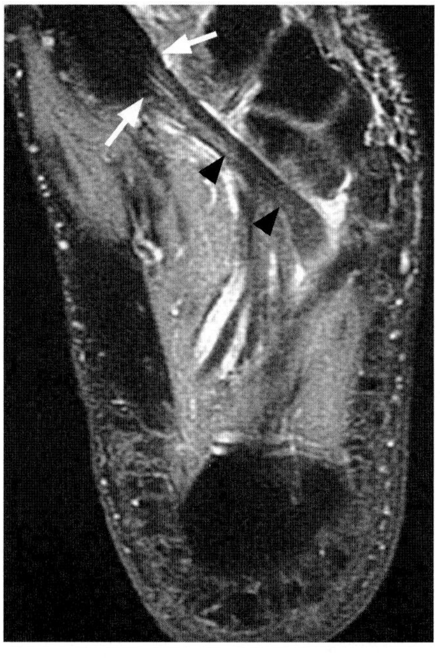

Fig. 4.4. Transverse intermediate-weighted FSE with fat-suppression image through the plantar surface of the foot showing the distal course (*arrowheads*) and insertion of the peroneus longus tendon onto the medial cuneiform and base of the first metatarsal (*arrows*). Note the fanning out of the tendon fibres at the sites of insertion with resultant increased signal

the nonfrictional surface of the tendon and allows passage of the blood supply to the tendon (Fig. 4.5).

Muscles are of uniform intermediate signal on all sequences and are useful as a reference tissue for comparing the signal intensity of lesions. The neurovascular bundles, small nerves and vessels, and retinacular structures are well visualised. Nerves are isointense or slightly hyperintense to muscle on T1- and T2-weighted images. Arteries, due to their fast blood flow, demonstrate a signal void within the lumen, whereas veins can appear high signal. Retinacula are thin structures that appear low signal on all sequences.

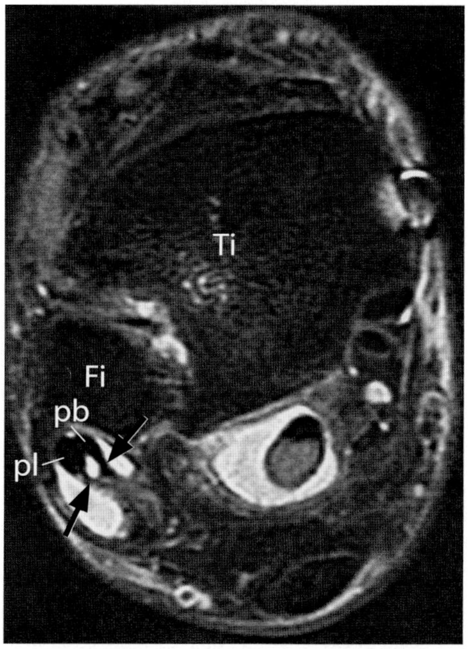

Fig. 4.5. Transverse intermediate-weighted FSE with fat-suppression image through the distal tibia (*Ti*) demonstrating excess fluid in the common peroneal tendon sheath (tenosynovitis) with resultant clear visualisation of the mesotendon structures (*arrow*) of both the brevis (*pb*) and longus (*pl*) tendons. Fi, fibula

4.3.1 Medial Aspect of Ankle

4.3.1.1 Tendons

There are three major tendons around the medial aspect of the ankle – tibialis posterior, flexor digitorum longus and flexor hallucis longus (a useful mnemonic which correctly ascribes the position of the tendons from medial to central is *Tom* (*t*ibialis posterior), *Dick* (flexor *d*igitorum longus) *And* (posterior tibial *a*rtery/neurovascular bundle) *Harry* (flexor *h*allucis longus) (Fig. 4.6). The largest, most medial and anterior tendon is tibialis posterior, which runs in the groove on the posterior part of the medial malleolus. The short axis diameter of the tibialis posterior tendon is normally twice the size of the adjacent medial tendons at the level of the medial malleolus. It is useful to compare the size of the tibialis posterior tendon with the other medial tendons as it commonly becomes thickened or thinned from tendinopathy. The tibialis posterior muscle has a complex origin from the posterior aspects of the upper tibia and fibula, and an intervening interosseous membrane in the deep posterior compartment. The tendon inserts onto the navicular, the three cuneiforms and the bases of the second to the fourth metatarsals. A sesamoid bone (os tibiale externum) occurs with a prevalence of 10%–16% within the distal tibialis posterior tendon (Schmidt and Freyschmidt 1993) (Fig. 4.7). A true accessory navicular refers to an osseous mass attached to the navicular by a synchondrosis, which can become painful from degenerative change (Lawson et al. 1984) (Fig. 4.8) and is associated with tibialis posterior tendon tears (Millar et al. 1995). Tibialis posterior assists in adduction, inversion and plantar flexion of the foot. The medial compartment

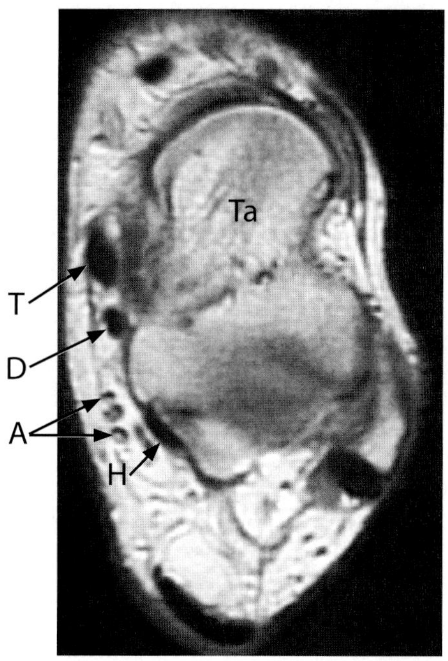

Fig. 4.6. Transverse T1-weighted SE image through the talus (*Ta*) showing the three medial tendons of tibialis posterior (*T*), flexor digitorum longus (*D*) and flexor hallucis longus (*H*). The posterior tibial neurovascular bundle (*A*) can be seen

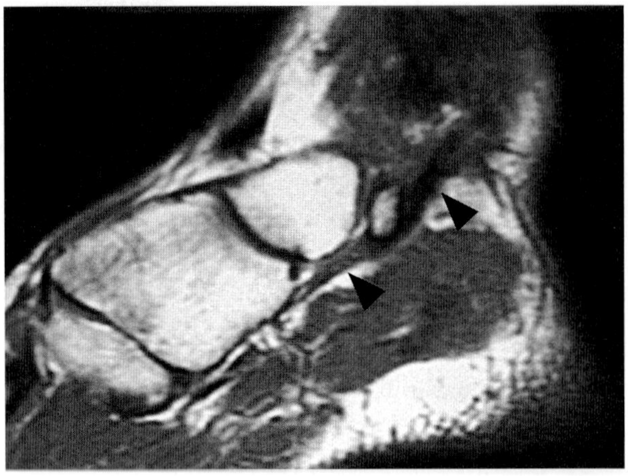

a

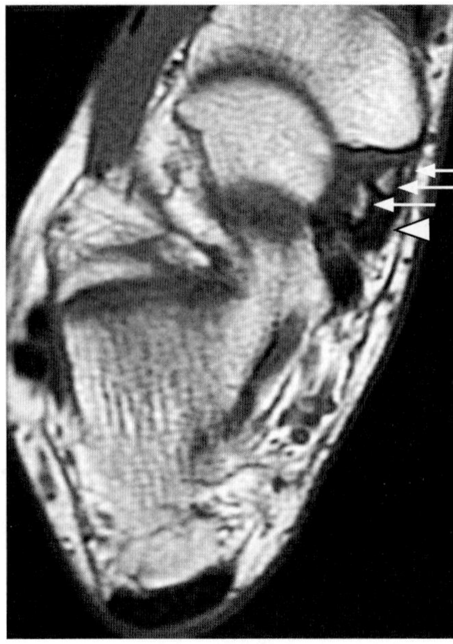

b

Fig. 4.7a,b. Accessory ossicles (os tibiale externum) (*arrow*) demonstrated in relation to the tibialis posterior tendon (*arrowheads*) close to its insertion onto the medial cuneiform (*Cm*) and navicular (*Na*) on sagittal and transverse T1-weighted SE images. Ta, talus; Ca, calcaneum

a b

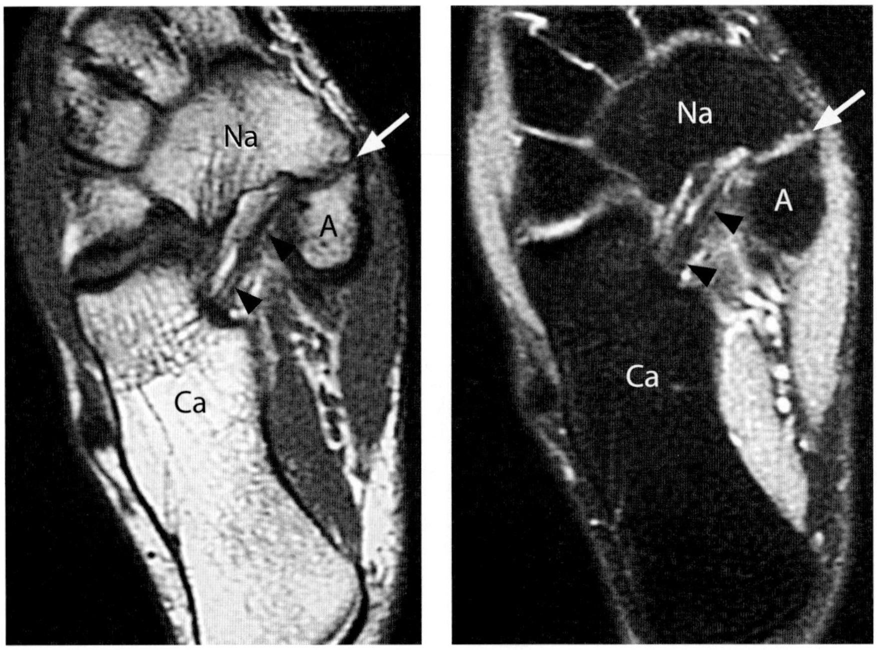

Fig. 4.8a,b. Accessory navicular (*A*) in a 23-year-old athlete showing degenerative change at the synchondrosis (*arrow*) on T1-weighted SE (**a**) and intermediate-weighted FSE with fat suppression (**b**). Part of the calcaneonavicular (spring) ligament is also shown (*arrowheads*)

musculature is innervated by branches from the tibial nerve and receives its blood supply from the posterior tibial artery.

The tibialis posterior tendon is of uniform low signal on all sequences, except at its insertion onto the navicular where it is normally heterogeneous and of intermediate signal (Schweitzer and Karasick 2000a). It is important to remember that the medial and lateral tendons do take an angled course around the ankle and are thus susceptible to magic angle effects. These effects can be offset to a degree by having the foot plantar flexed rather than in neutral position.

The flexor digitorum longus muscle originates from the posterior surface of the tibia, and its tendon inserts onto the plantar aspects of the bases of the distal phalanges of the second to the fifth digits. It acts as a flexor of the toes and supinator of the ankle.

Flexor hallucis longus is the closest to the midline of the other medial muscles and tendons, originating from the posterior mid-third aspect of the fibula and inserting onto the base of the distal phalanx of the great toe between the sesamoid bones. Fluid is commonly seen within the flexor hallucis longus tendon sheath in the presence of an effusion of the ankle joint as the tendon sheath communicates with the joint in approximately a fifth of normal individuals. A disproportionate amount of fluid within the tendon sheath relative to the joint is abnormal in keeping with tenosynovitis. It acts as a flexor of the great toe and ankle.

Anomalous muscles occur in relation to the medial tendons (Cheung and Rosenberg 2001) (Fig. 4.9). The flexor digitorum accessorius longus muscle has been reported in 2%–8% of dissected legs, being second in prevalence to the peroneus quartus muscle (vide infra). The flexor digitorum accessorius longus muscle has variable origins in the lower leg but is always posterior to the flexor hallucis longus muscle. It remains muscular within the tarsal tunnel and becomes tendinous as it exits the tarsal tunnel, where it is surrounded by quadratus plantae, and inserts into the tendon of flexor digitorum longus. Usually, the anomalous muscle remains asymptomatic but has been implicated as a cause of the tarsal tunnel syndrome as it abuts the posterior tibial nerve. Another accessory muscle in the medial compartment has been described, namely the peroneocalcaneus internus muscle. The latter is less frequent, found in 1% of individuals, and can be distinguished from the flexor digitorum accessorius longus muscle as it is separated from the posterior tibial neurovascular bundle by flexor hallucis longus. No symptoms have yet been reported due to the presence of a peroneocalcaneus internus muscle.

4.3.1.2 Ligaments

The medial (deltoid) ligament is a strong triangular group of fibres providing medial stability to the ankle, talus and subtalar joints. It lies deep to the medial flexor tendons and can be divided into three superficial and two deep components (Fig. 4.10). The superficial ligaments from posterior to anterior are the tibiotalar, tibiocalcaneal and tibionavicular ligaments. The superficial ligaments insert onto the navicular, spring ligament, sustentaculum tali and the medial tubercle of the talus. The anterior and posterior deep tibiotalar ligaments represent the deeper components. The superficial ligaments show a uniform low signal, with the deep components of the deltoid ligament complex usually demonstrating a striated pattern of light and dark bands (Fig.4.11).

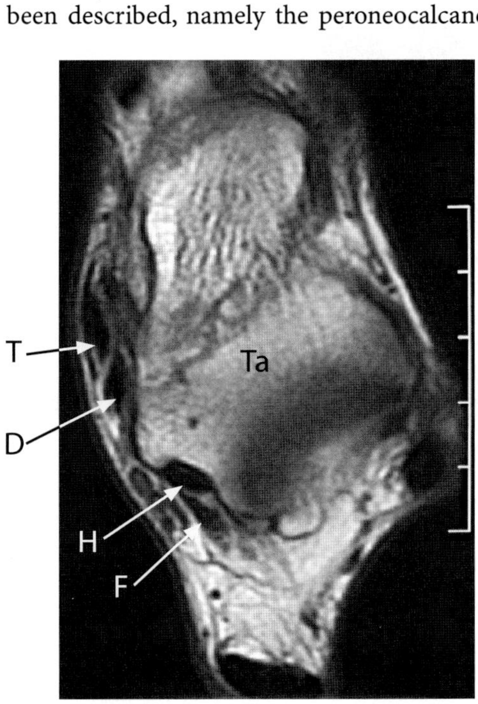

Fig. 4.9. Four medial structures are demonstrated on a transverse T1-weighted SE image at the level of the talus (*Ta*). There are the normal three tendons of tibialis posterior (*T*), flexor digitorum longus (*D*) and flexor hallucis longus (*H*), with an anomalous flexor digitorum accessorius longus muscle (*F*)

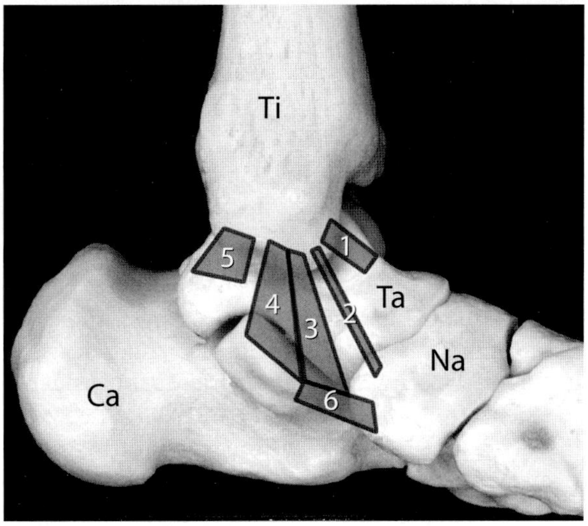

Fig. 4.10. Composite photograph showing the medial ankle ligaments: 1, anterior tibiotalar ligament; 2, tibionavicular ligament; 3, tibiospring ligament; 4, tibiocalcaneal ligament; 5, posterior tibiotalar ligament; 6, spring ligament. Ti, tibia; Ta, talus; Ca, calcaneum; Na, navicular

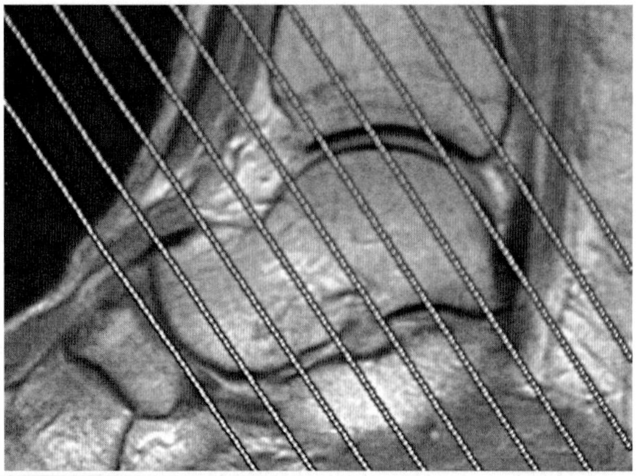

a

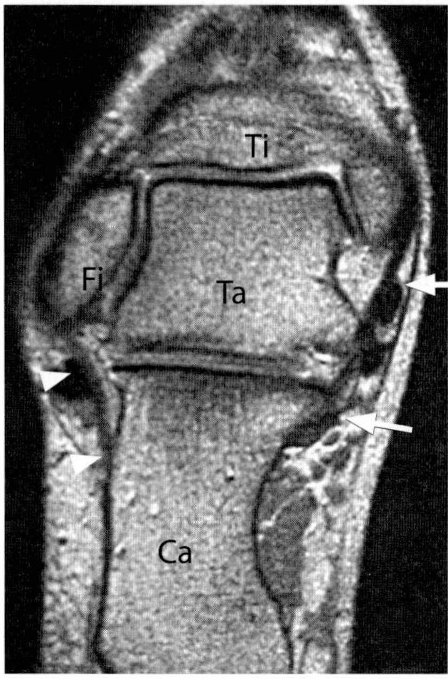

b

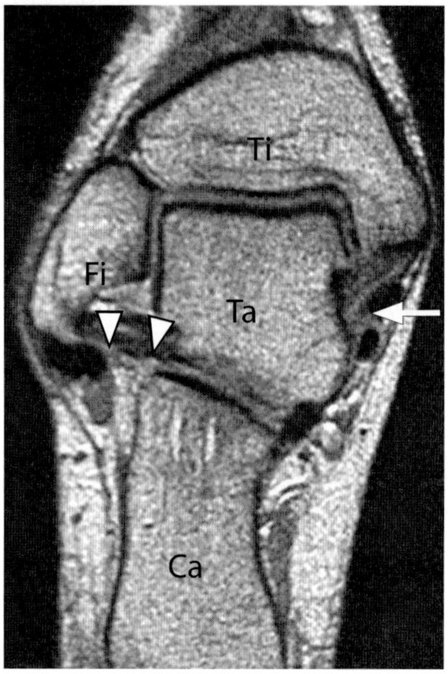

c

Fig. 4.11a–c. Pilot image (**a**) showing the alignment of the coronal-oblique T1-weighted images with **b** anterior to **c** demonstrating the superficial (*arrow* in **b**) and deep (*arrow* in **c**) medial ankle ligaments. The calcaneofibular ligament (*arrowheads* in **b**) and the posterior talofibular ligament (*arrowheads* in **c**) represent the lateral ligament complex. Same key as before

4.3.1.3
Tarsal Tunnel

The three medial tendons with the posterior tibial neurovascular bundle traverse in the tarsal tunnel and are isolated in their separate fibrous connective tissue tunnels. The proximal and distal boundaries of the tunnel are imprecise, but generally it is considered to extend from the level of the medial malleolus to the navicular (Fig. 4.12). The roof of the tarsal tunnel is formed by the flexor retinaculum, with the floor represented by the talus and calcaneum. The fibrous connective tissue (septa) which forms the separate tunnels connect the under-surface of the flexor retinaculum and medial malleolus. Some of the septa are attached to the neurovascular bundle, rendering it relatively immobile and therefore susceptible to traction injury or compression by an adjacent mass lesion. Either of these events may produce the sensory symptoms referred to a tarsal tunnel syndrome (an entrapment neuropathy).

4.3.2
Lateral Aspect of Ankle

4.3.2.1
Tendons

There are two peroneal tendons that traverse posterior to the lateral malleolus (see Fig. 4.5). The lateral malleolus can be concave, flat or convex. The peroneus brevis is the more anterior of the two tendons and traverses anterior to the peroneal tubercle, inserting onto

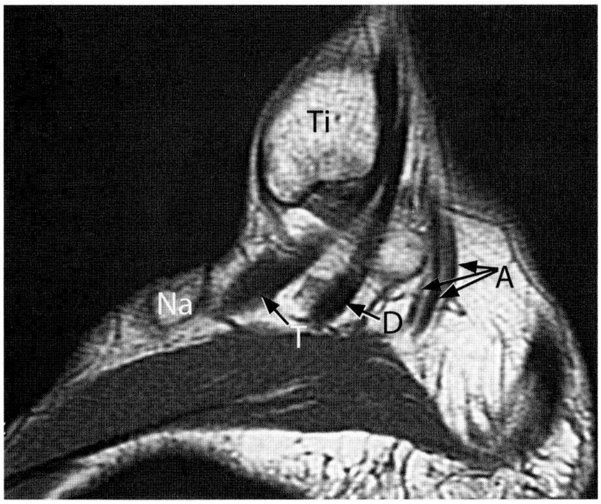

Fig. 4.12. Parasagittal T1-weighted SE image through the tarsal tunnel showing the position of the medial tendons of tibialis posterior (*T*) and flexor digitorum longus (*D*) being held in place by the fibrous septa. Key as before with A, posterior tibial neurovascular bundle

the base of the fifth metatarsal. It is frequently broader and flatter proximal to the tip of the lateral malleolus, compared with the peroneus longus tendon. It can be difficult to separate the two tendons at this level. Occasionally, the peroneus brevis is medial to the peroneus longus tendon. More distally, the tendons are more clearly demonstrated as two separate symmetrical entities (Fig. 4.13). The peroneus longus tendon passes posterior to the peroneal tubercle, when present, on the calcaneum, which acts as a pulley for the tendon as it courses distally beneath the cuboid to insert onto the base of the first metatarsal and medial cuneiform (see Fig. 4.4). The peroneus longus passes through a tunnel made by a groove in the plantar surface of the cuboid and long plantar ligament (see Fig. 4.33). In a fifth of individuals, there is a sesamoid bone (os peroneum) at the point of contact on the peroneus longus tendon and the cuboid. The two tendons have a common tendon sheath to the level of the distal tip of the lateral malleolus, but then diverge into separate sheaths. The peroneus brevis and longus muscles form the lateral compartment of the lower leg arising from the superolateral surface of the fibula. the peroneus longus muscle is superior and superficial to brevis. They are supplied by the peroneal artery (a branch of the posterior tibial artery) and innervated by the superficial peroneal nerve, also with a branch from the deep peroneal nerve to peroneus longus. They act as evertors of the foot and weak plantar flexors of the ankle.

The peroneus quartus is an anomalous muscle present in 10%–20% of normal individuals (Fig. 4.14). In the literature there is some confusion regarding its definition and even its name (otherwise known as peroneus quadratus) (Berquist 2000). The origin and insertion of this accessory muscle are variable, with insertion of the tendon onto the retrotrochlear eminence of the calcaneum in the majority, but it may

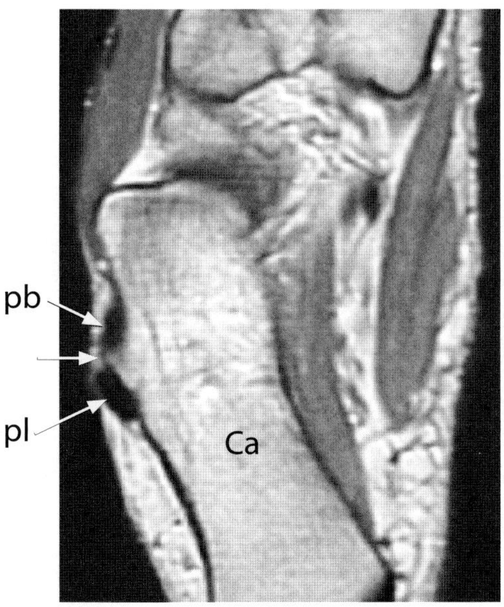

Fig. 4.13. Peroneal tubercle (*arrow*) separating the anterior peroneus brevis tendon (*pb*) from the more posterior peroneus longus tendon (*pl*) on a transverse T1-weighted SE image through the mid-calcaneum

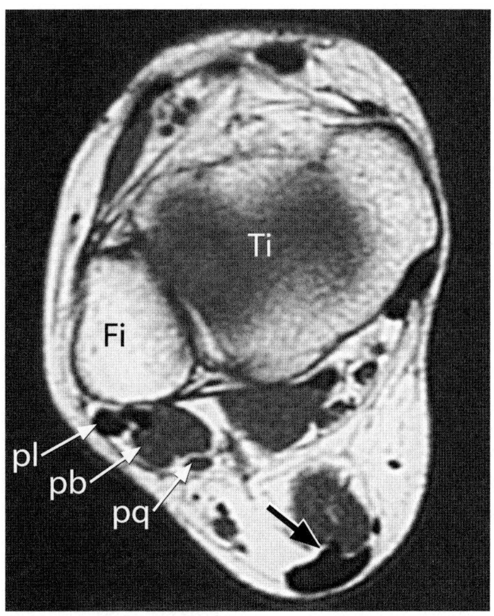

Fig. 4.14. Peroneus quartus (*pq*) on a transverse T1-weighted SE image at the level of the syndesmosis. Note the normal focal convexity (*arrowhead*) to the anterior margin of the Achilles tendon

also insert onto the inferior peroneal retinaculum (Cheung and Rosenberg 2001). The retrotrochlear eminence of the calcaneum is a constant protuberance posterior and proximal to the peroneal tubercle (trochlear process). The peroneal tubercle is an inconstant structure present in approximately 40% of individuals and, when present, separates the peroneus brevis and longus tendons (see Fig. 4.13). Although asymptomatic in the majority, if the peroneus quartus tendon is of sufficient size, its presence at the level of the lateral malleolus fills the peroneal tendon sheath and can predispose to tendinopathy of the peroneal brevis tendon. The anomalous tendon can also be used as an autologous graft for lateral ligament repair.

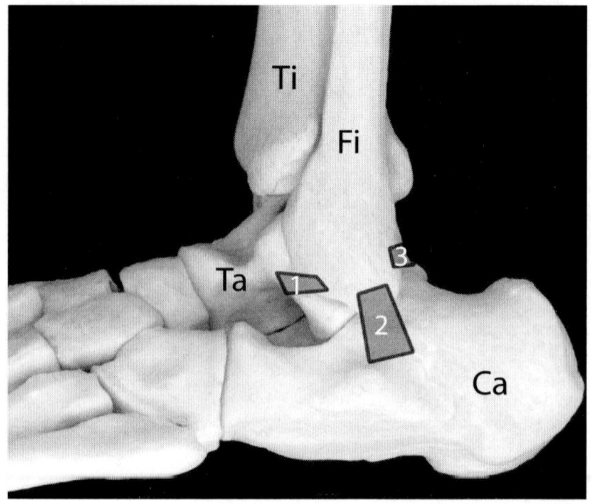

Fig. 4.16. Composite photograph showing the lateral ankle ligaments from the lateral aspect: 1, anterior talofibular ligament; 2, calcaneofibular ligament; 3, posterior talofibular ligament

4.3.2.2 Ligaments

The ligaments of the lateral ankle comprise the syndesmosis of the distal tibia and fibula and the lateral ligament complex (Fig. 4.15). The syndesmosis is composed of four components – anterior and posterior inferior tibiofibular ligaments, inferior transverse ligament (most inferior fibres of the posterior inferior tibiofibular ligament), and the interosseous membrane between the tibia and fibula. The lateral ligament complex is formed by three ligaments – anterior and posterior talofibular ligaments and a calcaneofibular ligament (Fig. 4.16). These ligament structures are best seen on transverse images with the ankle in the neutral position (Fig. 4.17). The calcaneofibular ligament is, however, not usually seen in its entirety on transverse sections with the ankle in the neutral position, but requires either oblique transverse imaging or the foot plantar flexed. Coronal imaging can also be used to show the entire ligament (see Fig. 4.11). The peroneal tendons are immediately superficial to the calcaneofibular ligament, which explains the arthrographic finding of contrast extending into the peroneal tendon sheath with lateral ligament injury. A useful landmark on transverse sections is the lateral malleolar fossa, a concavity on the inner margin of the distal fibula, which demarcates the level of the lateral ligament complex (Fig. 4.17). More proximally, the syndesmosis can be visualised where the inner margin of the fibula is flatter or convex (Fig. 4.18).

a

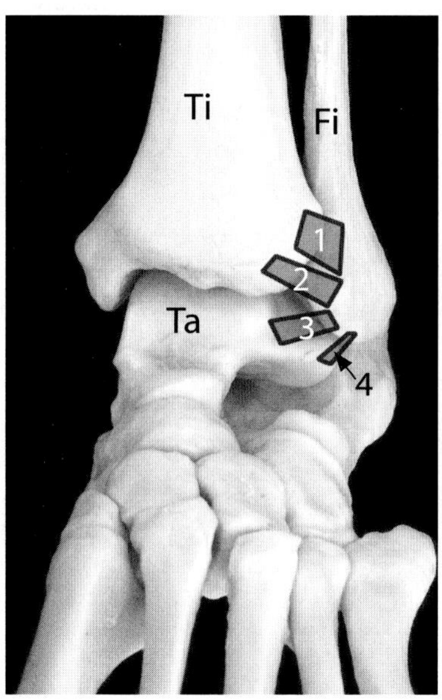

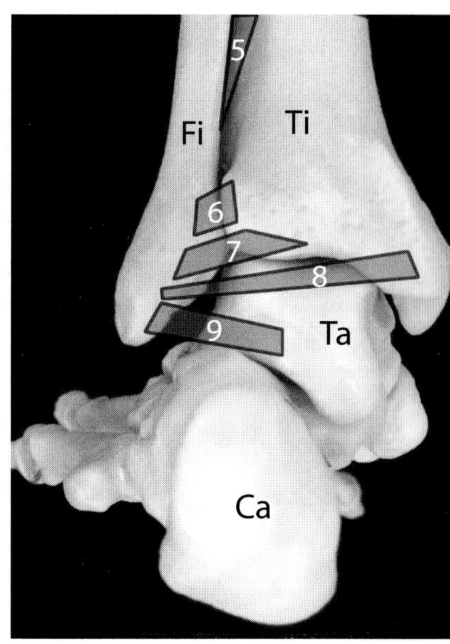

b

Fig. 4.15a,b. Composite photograph showing the lateral ankle ligaments and syndesmosis from anterior (**a**) and posterior (**b**) aspects: 1, anterior inferior tibiofibular ligament; 2, distal part of the anterior inferior tibiofibular ligament; 3, anterior talofibular ligament; 4, calcaneofibular ligament; 5, interosseous membrane; 6, posterior inferior tibiofibular ligament; 7, transverse inferior tibiofibular ligament; 8, posterior intermalleolar ligament; 9, posterior talofibular ligament

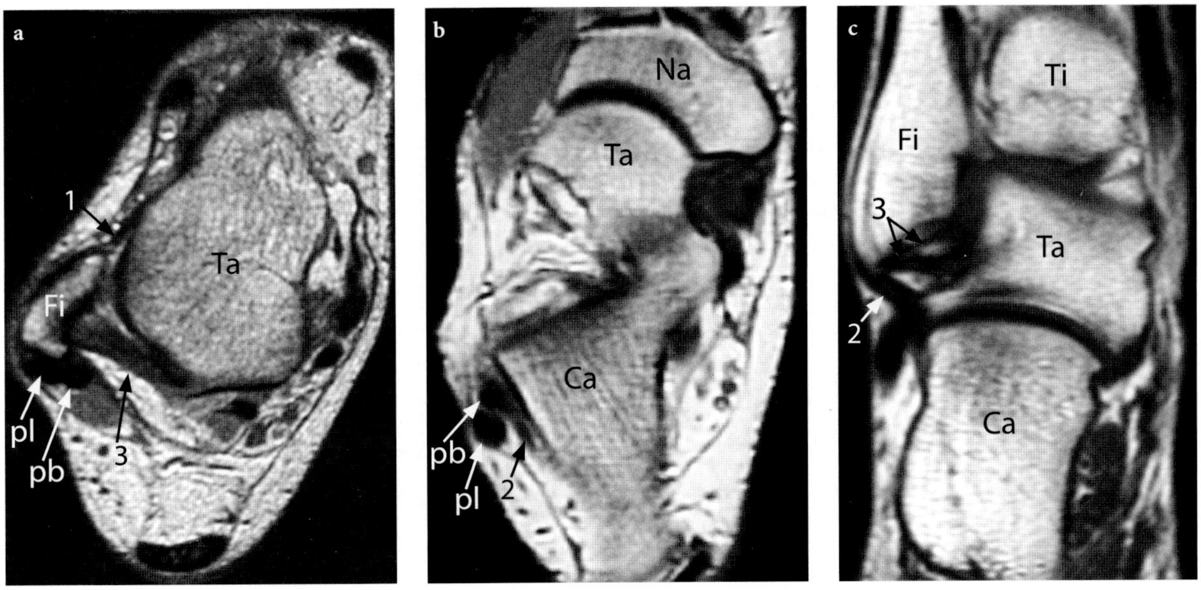

Fig. 4.17a–c. T1-weighted SE images showing the lateral ligament complex: **a** at the level of the lateral malleolus (*Fi*), anterior (*1*) and posterior (*3*) talofibular ligaments; **b** through the upper calcaneum showing the calcaneofibular ligament (*2*); and **c** coronal section demonstrating the calcaneofibular (*2*) and posterior (*3*) talofibular ligaments. Pl, peroneal longus tendon; pb, peroneal brevis muscle and tendon

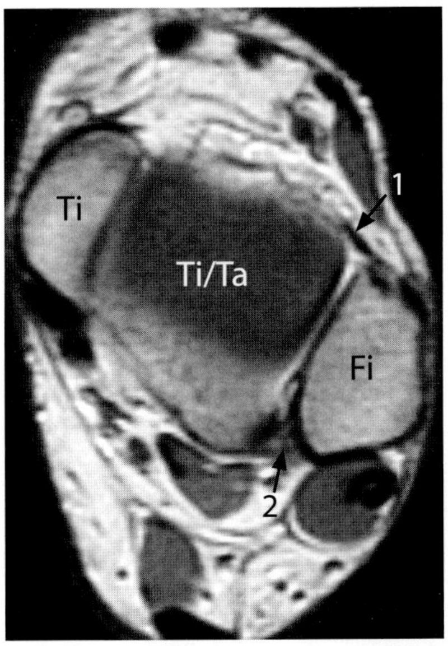

Fig. 4.18. T1-weighted SE image showing the syndesmosis with the anterior (*1*) and posterior (*2*) inferior tibiotalar ligaments. Ti/Ta, tibiotalar joint

The anterior and posterior inferior tibiofibular ligaments and the posterior talofibular ligament have a striated appearance, while the anterior talofibular and calcaneofibular ligaments are of uniform signal void. The anterior talofibular ligament is the weakest part of the lateral ligament complex and the one most commonly injured following an inversion injury. One pitfall to be aware of is the appearance of the posterior tibiofibular ligament on sagittal images as it is normally surrounded by joint fluid and can mimic a loose body in the posterior part of the tibiotalar joint (Fig. 4.19). There is also a posterior intermalleolar ligament which is present in 56% of cadaveric specimens, but reported in only a fifth of 97 clinical MR cases, being a normal variant lying between the posterior tibiofibular ligament and the posterior talofibular ligament (Bencardino and Rosenberg 2001) (see Fig. 4.15b).

4.3.3
Posterior Aspect of Ankle

4.3.3.1
Tendons

The main tendon in this position is the Achilles tendon which inserts onto the posterior part of the calcaneal tuberosity (see Fig. 4.1). The Achilles tendon is the largest and strongest tendon in the body, being about 15 cm in length. Anteriorly, the tendon receives muscle fibres from the soleus muscle almost to its distal insertion. The tendon fibres spiral through 90° with the medial fibres becoming more posterior. On transverse sections the anterior part of tendon is either concave or flat,

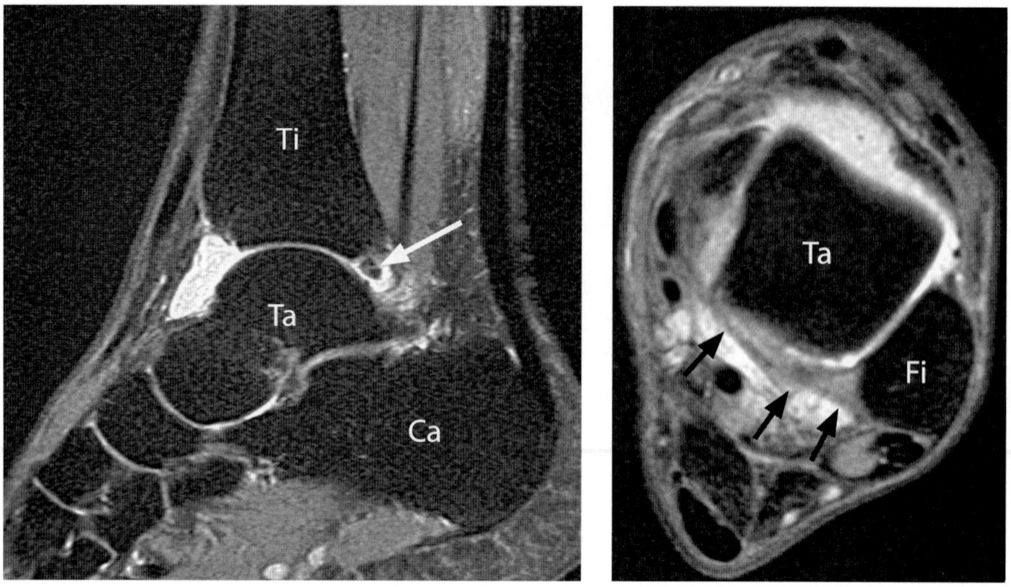

Fig. 4.19a,b. Posterior inferior tibiofibular ligament (*arrow*) mimicking a loose body within a tibiotalar joint effusion on sagittal (**a**) and transverse (**b**) intermediate-weighted FSE with fat suppression

measuring about 6–7 mm in anteroposterior diameter (Schweitzer and Karasick 2000b). There may be a focal anterior convexity to the tendon which spirals down the tendon from the lateral to the medial side due to soleus fibres merging with those of gastrocnemius (Figs. 4.14, 4.20). The tendon shows signal void on all sequences. Occasionally, there is a solitary vertical line of high signal in the mid-substance of the Achilles tendon which is thought to be the site of the junction of the soleus and gastrocnemius tendons, or possibly a vascular channel (Fig. 4.21, 4.24a).

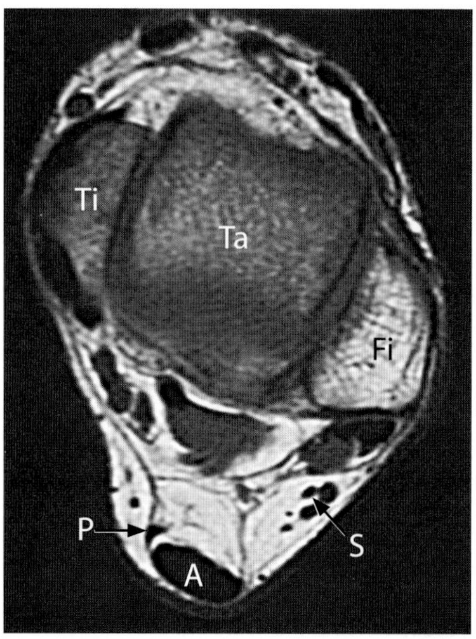

Fig. 4.20. Normal Achilles tendon showing a slight anterior bulging, and a prominent plantaris tendon (*P*) on its medial side on a transverse T1-weighted SE image. Ti, medial malleolus of the tibia; S, sural nerve adjacent to the lesser saphenous veins

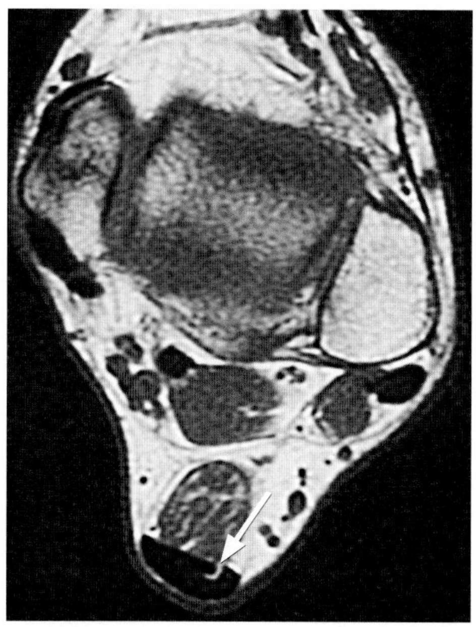

Fig. 4.21. Normal Achilles tendon showing a high signal from fat (*arrow*) at the junction of the soleus and gastrocnemius tendons, on a transverse T1-weighted SE image

The Achilles tendon is the only one in the human body without a tendon sheath, having a surrounding loose connective tissue termed the paratenon (or peritenon) (Fig. 4.22). The paratenon is present posterior, lateral and medial to the tendon, and can normally be identified as a thin linear area of intermediate signal posterior to the tendon on transverse sections (Bencardino and Rosenberg 2001) (Fig. 4.23). The presence of a paratenon allows free gliding of the Achilles tendon. It therefore does not develop a tenosynovitis, but the paratenon can become inflamed, producing a paratendinitis. There is normally a tiny amount of fluid within the retrocalcaneal bursa (anterior to the tendon) seen on fat-suppressed images. Posterior to the tendon lies a subcutaneous adventitial bursa (termed tendo Achilles bursa or retro-Achilles bursa) which is normally not visualised. These bursae can become inflamed, developing a bursitis which along with thickening of the adjacent distal Achilles tendon is known as Haglund's syndrome or 'pump-bump'. Its muscle components comprise the soleus and the medial and lateral muscle bellies of gastrocnemius, which are innervated by the tibial nerve with blood supply from the posterior tibial artery. They are the major plantar flexors of the foot. The sural nerve lies lateral to the Achilles tendon adjacent to the small saphenous vein in the subcutaneous space.

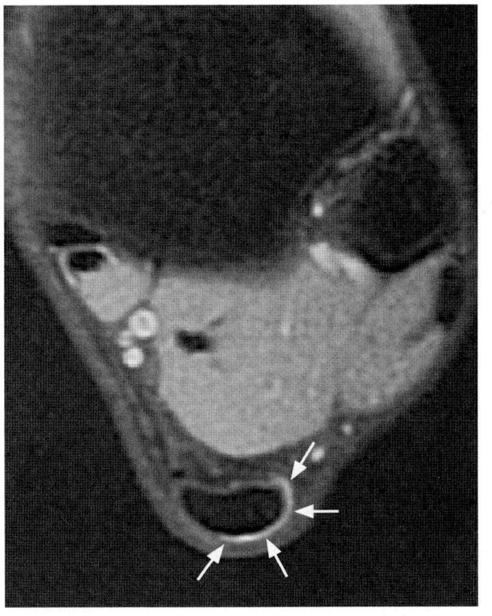

Fig. 4.23. Inflamed paratenon (*arrows*) on a transverse intermediate-weighted FSE with fat suppression image

In the majority (90%) of individuals (Daseler and Anson 1943), there is also a much smaller tendon (plantaris tendon) on the medial side of the Achilles tendon. The plantaris tendon is the longest tendon in the human body and has little functional significance, being a weak knee flexor with its muscle origin

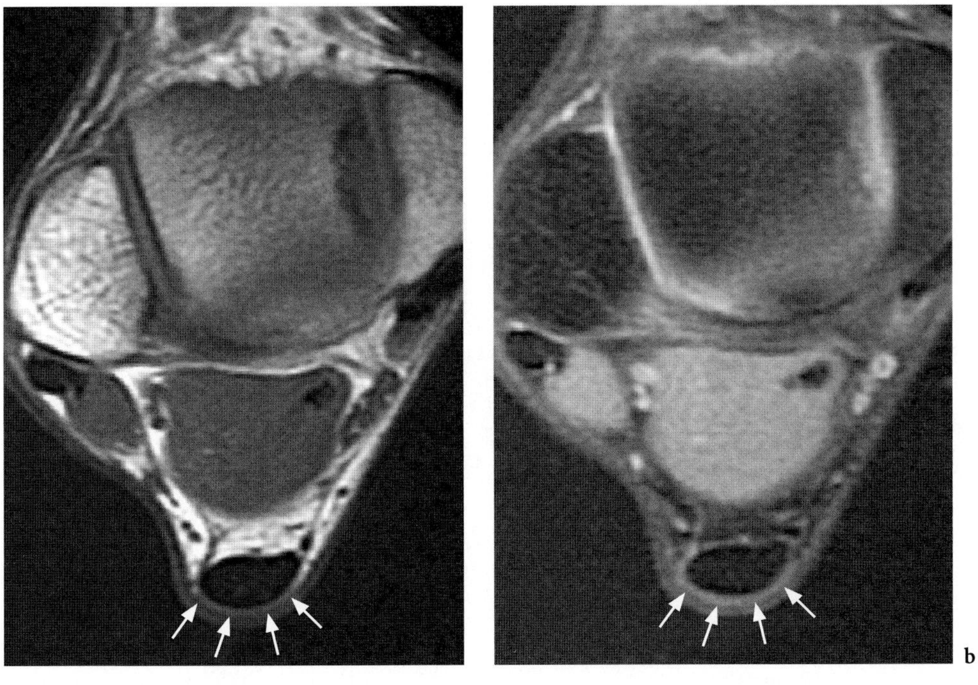

Fig. 4.22a,b. Normal paratenon (*arrows*) clearly visualised as intermediate signal on transverse T1-weighted (**a**) and intermediate-weighted FSE with fat suppression images (**b**)

from the posterior femur (see Fig. 4.20). The plantaris tendon inserts onto the calcaneum, Achilles tendon or flexor retinaculum, and can be used as an autologous graft for a lateral ligament reconstruction. It should not be mistaken for a partially torn Achilles tendon.

Anterior to the posterior tendons is a large triangular fat space termed Kager's triangle. An accessory soleus is an uncommon normal variant present in approximately 5% of cadaveric studies (Cheung and Rosenberg 2001) (Fig. 4.24). An accessory soleus muscle can fill Kager's fat space, mimicking a soft-tissue mass. Individuals with an accessory soleus muscle may complain of pain on exercise due to claudication as the accessory muscle has a tenuous blood supply. It inserts onto the medial part of the calcaneum or Achilles tendon.

Another normal variant is the os trigonum – a separate accessory bony ossicle which results from failure of fusion of the lateral tubercle of the posterior process of the talus to the body of the talus (Fig. 4.25). The os

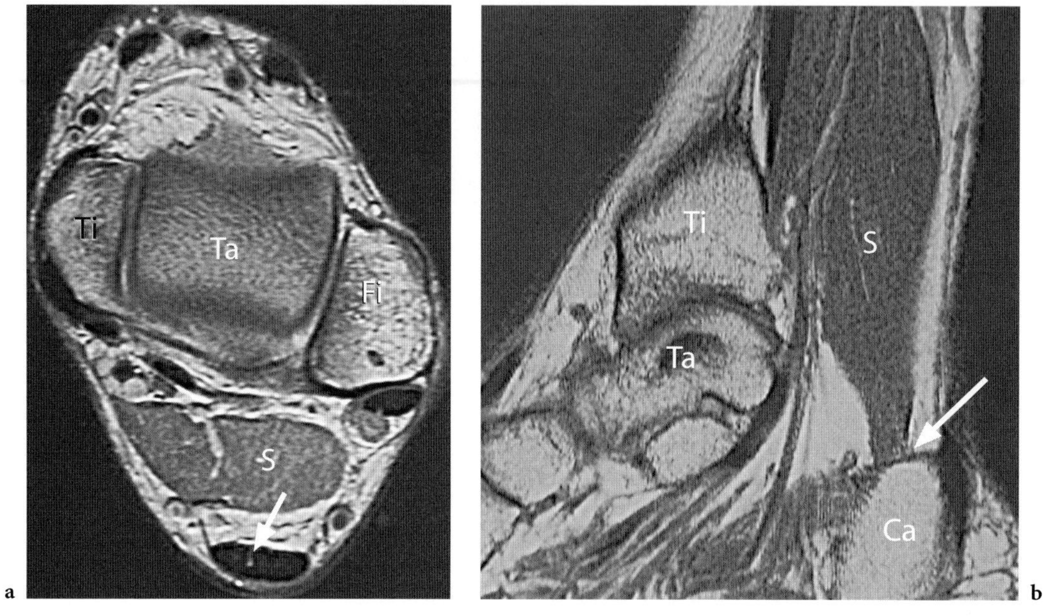

Fig. 4.24a,b. Accessory soleus muscle (*S*) on transverse (**a**) and parasagittal (**b**) T1-weighted SE images. Note the insertion site onto the medial side of the calcaneum (*arrow* in **b**), and the focal high signal in the central part of the normal Achilles tendon (*arrow* in **a**)

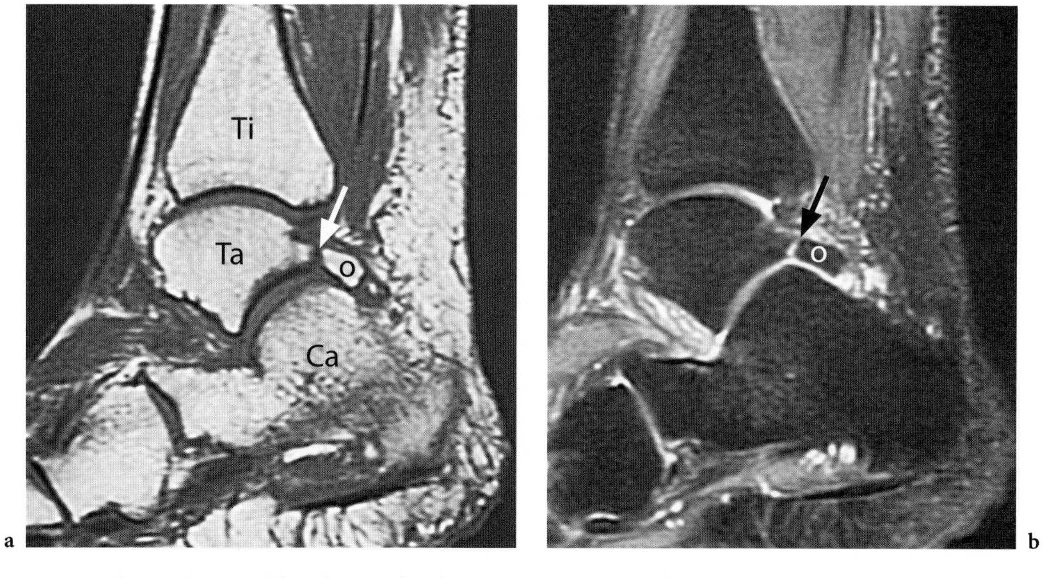

Fig. 4.25a,b. Os trigonum (*o*) with a synchondrosis (*arrow*) on sagittal intermediate-weighted FSE with fat-suppression images

trigonum is attached to the talus by a synchondrosis and is located lateral to the flexor hallucis longus tendon. It can be involved by an os trigonum syndrome (otherwise known as a posterior impingement syndrome) due to impingement of this ossicle with the adjacent flexor hallucis longus tendon upon plantar flexion. A prominent fused lateral talar tubercle is termed a Stieda process. Degenerative change can develop between the os trigonum/Stieda process and the adjacent calcaneum (Fig. 4.26).

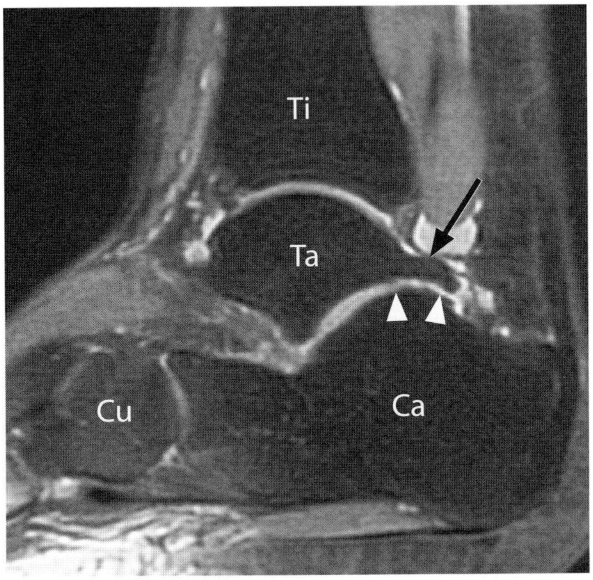

Fig. 4.26. Stieda process (*arrow*) with degenerative changes (*arrowheads*) in the adjacent joint on an intermediate-weighted FSE with fat-suppression images. Cu, cuboid

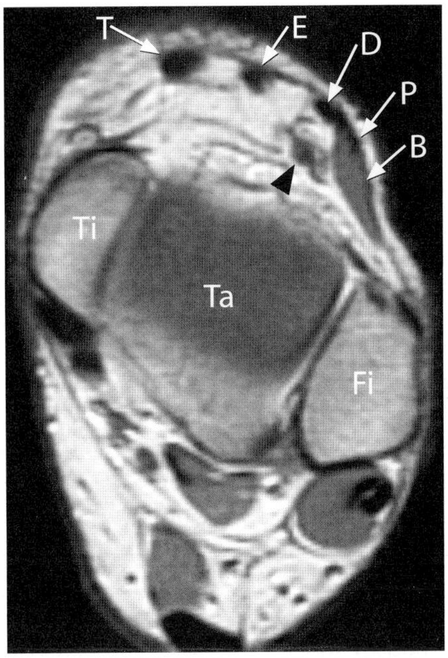

Fig. 4.27. Anterior aspect of the ankle on transverse T1-weighted SE image includes the tibialis anterior tendon (*T*), extensor hallucis longus tendon (*E*), extensor digitorum longus tendon (*D*), peroneus tertius tendon (*P*), extensor digitorum brevis muscle (*B*) and the anterior neurovascular bundle (*arrowhead*) of anterior tibial nerve and dorsalis pedis artery

4.3.4 Anterior Aspect of Ankle

4.3.4.1 Tendons

There are four tendons in the anterior/extensor compartment of the ankle (Fig. 4.27). From medial to lateral they are *t*ibialis anterior, *e*xtensor hallucis longus, extensor *d*igitorum longus (a helpful mnemonic is TED) and peroneus tertius. The tibialis anterior muscle originates from the proximal tibia, and its tendon inserts onto the medial cuneiform and the base of the first metatarsal (Fig. 4.28). It acts as a strong dorsiflexor and invertor of the foot. The extensor hallucis muscle lies deep to extensor digitorum longus and tibialis anterior, arising from the mid-

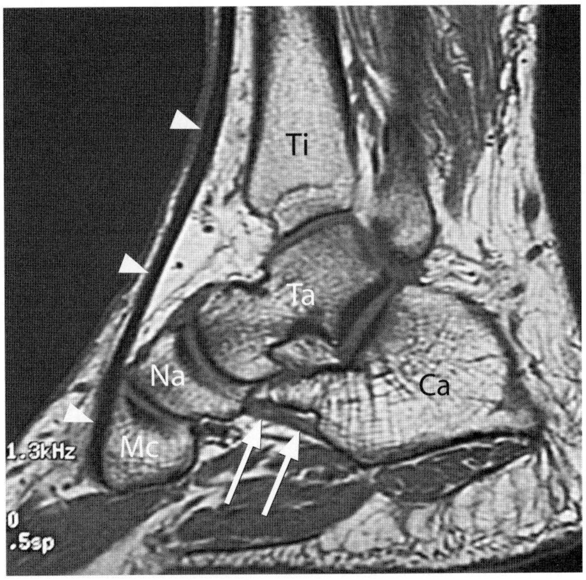

Fig. 4.28. Tibialis anterior tendon (*arrowheads*) and its insertion site onto the medial cuneiform on a parasagittal T1-weighted SE image. Note the spring ligament (arrowed). Mc, medial cuneiform

part of the fibula and adjacent interosseous ligament. Its tendon inserts onto the dorsal base of the distal phalanx of the great toe, and it acts as an extensor of the great toe, weak invertor and dorsiflexor of the foot. The extensor digitorum longus muscle arises from the lateral tibial condyle, anterior fibula and interosseous membrane. It has four tendon slips in a common sheath to insert onto the middle and distal phalanges of the second to the fifth ray. The peroneus tertius muscle is considered to be a portion of the extensor digitorum longus representing a fifth tendon (Williams et al, 1989). It arises from the distal anterior fibula, interosseous membrane and fascial membrane of peroneus brevis. Its tendon inserts onto the dorsal surface of the base of the fifth ray distal to the attachment of the peroneus brevis tendon. The muscle varies in size and may be absent. All four anterior tendons pass deep to the extensor retinacula, being innervated by the deep peroneal nerve and supplied by the anterior tibial artery. The dorsalis pedis artery and veins and deep peroneal nerve pass deep and parallel to the extensor hallucis longus muscle and tendon.

4.3.5 Foot

The foot can be divided anatomically into the hindfoot, midfoot and forefoot. Three longitudinal columns – medial, middle and lateral – have also been described. The medial column comprises the calcaneum, talus, navicular, medial and intermediate cuneiforms, and the first and second ray. The tibialis posterior tendon and the spring ligament act as supporting slings for the medial longitudinal arch. Loss of the medial longitudinal arch can occur with tibialis posterior tendinopathy.

4.3.5.1 Hindfoot

The soft-tissue anatomy of the hindfoot has already been covered above in the assessment of the medial, lateral and posterior compartments of the ankle. Some of the bony anatomy is covered as it relates to the various syndromes that occur around the ankle and foot, but for more detail the reader is directed elsewhere (Berquist 2000; Keats and Anderson 2001).

The hindfoot includes the talus and calcaneum and intervening subtalar joints, and surrounding soft tissues (Fig. 4.29). The posterior subtalar joint communicates with the tibiotalar joint in 10% of individuals. The anterior subtalar joint may communicate with the talonavicular or talocalcaneonavicular joint. The sinus tarsi (or tarsal sinus) is an anatomical space immediately anterior to the posterior subtalar joint between the inferior aspect of the talus (roof) and the superior aspect of the calcaneum (floor) (Fig. 4.30). The bony margins of the sinus are irregular. The space is cone-shaped with a narrow end medially posterior to the sustentaculum tali and inferior to the medial malleolus. Laterally, the sinus widens to below the lateral malleolus. It contains fat, ligamentous structures, a neurovascular bundle (branch of the posterior tibial artery) and an outpouching synovial bursa from the posterior subtalar joint. Nerve endings in the sinus provide proprioception for the hindfoot, with stability partly maintained by the interosseous ligament. The main ligament in the sinus is the talocalcaneal (or interosseous) ligament, which is composed of a single medial bundle with anterior and posterior bands laterally (Fig. 4.31). The anterior band of the ligament forms the cervical ligament. The lateral extensor retinaculum forms the most lateral portion of the sinus tarsi ligaments.

The MR anatomy of the sinus tarsi can be well demonstrated on sagittal and coronal imaging, the low signal ligaments contrasting against the surrounding higher signal from fat. Inflammation and

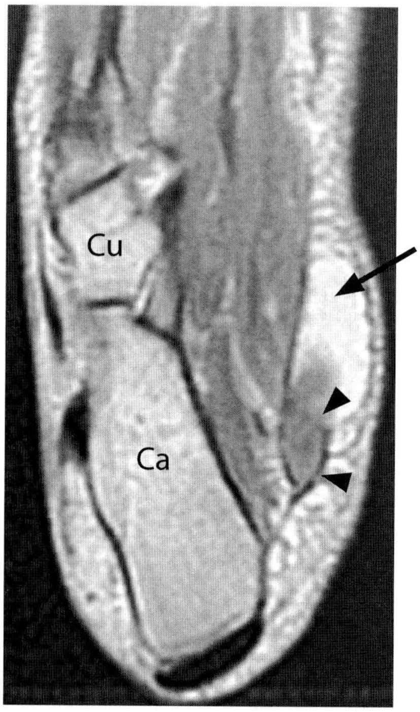

Fig. 4.29. Accessory abductor hallucis muscle (*arrowheads*) with an associated lipoma (*arrow*) on a transverse T1-weighted SE image. Cu, cuboid

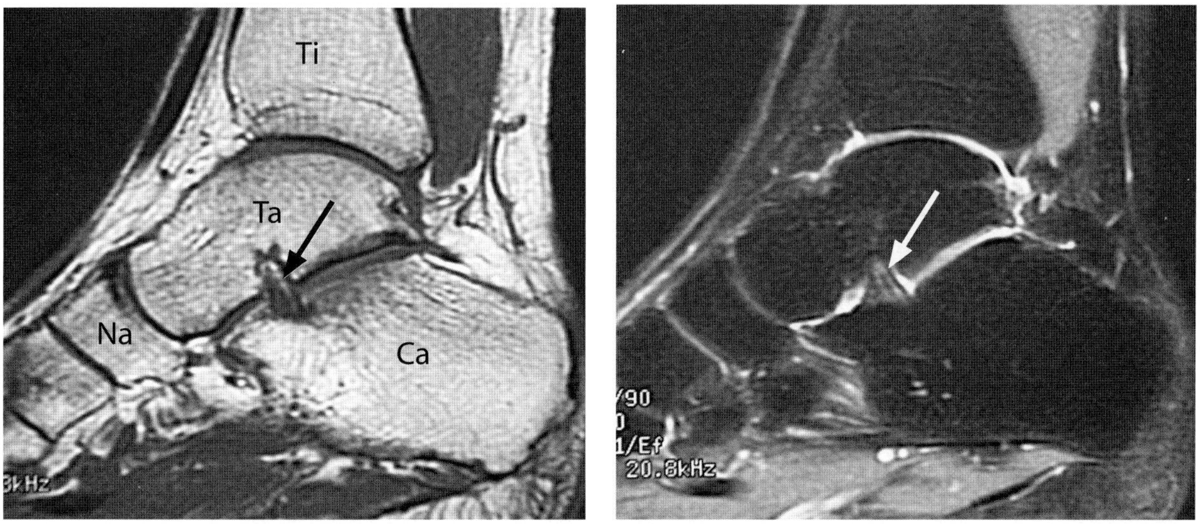

a b

Fig. 4.30a,b. Interosseous (talocalcaneal) ligament (*arrow*) within the medial aspect of the sinus tarsi on sagittal T1-weighted SE (**a**) and intermediate-weighted FSE with fat-suppression images (**b**)

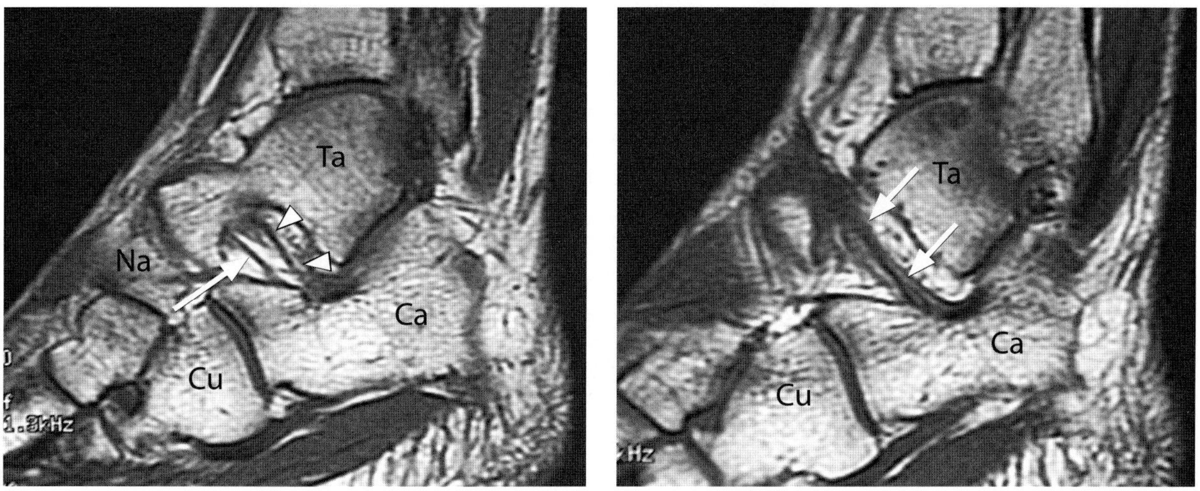

a b

Fig. 4.31a,b. Anterior (*arrow*) and posterior (*arrowheads*) bands of the talocalcaneal ligament (**a**) and lateral extensor retinaculum (**b**) (*arrow*) on parasagittal T1-weighted SE images: **b** more lateral than **a**, and both further lateral than Fig. 4.30

trauma can involve the sinus with loss of the ligaments and normal fat, producing a sinus tarsi syndrome with pain associated with hindfoot instability. It should be noted that MR imaging does not consistently identify the ligaments of the sinus tarsi even if intact, so the absence of the ligaments alone does not justify the diagnosis. It is important to look for any lateral ankle ligament damage and chronic tibialis posterior tendon tears, which are the associated features of a sinus tarsi syndrome.

The plantar fascia, otherwise termed plantar aponeurosis, is a thick, multilayered condensation of fibrous tissue comprised of three components (Theodorou et al. 2000) (Fig. 4.32). The larger central layer arises from the inferior part of the calcaneal tuberosity along the plantar surface of the flexor digitorum brevis and attaches distally to the plantar surface of the proximal phalanges and the skin. The central layer is cord-like, measuring 4 mm in normal thickness at the level of its attachment to the calcaneum (see Fig. 4.3). The medial and lateral portions of the aponeurosis are membrane sheets with the former being the fascia of abductor hallucis, and the latter arising from the lateral margin of the medial calcaneal tubercle close to the origin of the abductor digiti quinti (Kier 1994). The plantar fascia is easily

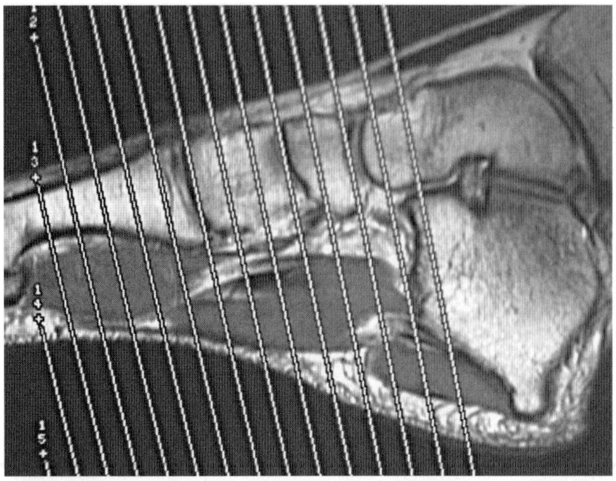

a

Fig. 4.32a–c. Pilot image (**a**) showing the alignment for short-axis (coronal-oblique) T1-weighted SE images (**b**, **c**); **b** is more proximal than **c**. Arrowheads, plantar aponeurosis; arrows, spring ligament; T, tibialis posterior tendon; DF, flexor digitorum longus tendon; H, flexor hallucis longus tendon; AbH, abductor hallucis muscle; Qp, quadratus plantae; Fb, flexor digitorum brevis muscle; Ab, abductor digiti minimi muscle; pl, peroneus longus tendon; pb, peroneus brevis tendon; B, extensor digitorum brevis muscle; DE, extensor digitorum longus tendon; E, extensor hallucis longus tendon; TA, tibialis anterior tendon; Mc, medial cuneiform; Ic, intermediate cuneiform; Lc, lateral cuneiform; Cu, cuboid; 5mt, base of fifth metatarsal

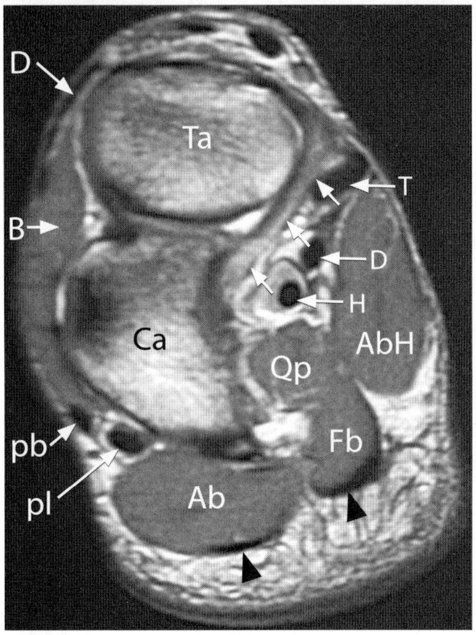

b

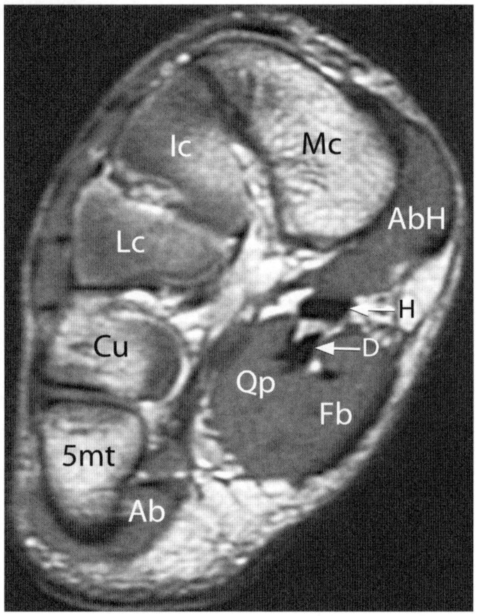

c

visualised on sagittal and coronal MR imaging, being of low signal on all sequences.

4.3.5.2
Midfoot

The midfoot compartment comprises the navicular, cuboid and three cuneiform bones, and is bounded proximally by the talonavicular and calcaneocuboid joints (Chopart's joint) and distally by the tarsometatarsal joints (Lisfranc's joint) (Fig. 4.33). The navicular lies on the medial aspect of the foot. It articulates with the talus proximally and with the three cuneiforms distally, occasionally with the cuboid. The cuboid is lateral to the navicular, articulating with the calcaneum proximally and with the fourth and fifth metatarsals distally. The medial side of the cuboid has a facet which articulates with the lateral cuneiform. There is a groove on the plantar surface of the cuboid for the peroneus longus tendon. The medial cuneiform is the largest of the cuneiforms, articulating with the intermediate cuneiform laterally and the first and second metatarsals distally. The intermediate cuneiform lies between the medial and lateral cuneiforms, articulating with both, and the second metatarsal distally. The lateral cuneiform lies between the intermediate cuneiform and cuboid articulating with both, and the second to the fourth metatarsals distally.

The spring (calcaneonavicular) ligament extends from the calcaneum to the tuberosity of the navicular on the plantar aspect (see Figs. 4.8, 4.28). It is a broad, thick band connecting the anterior margin of the sustentaculum tali to the plantar surface of the navicular.

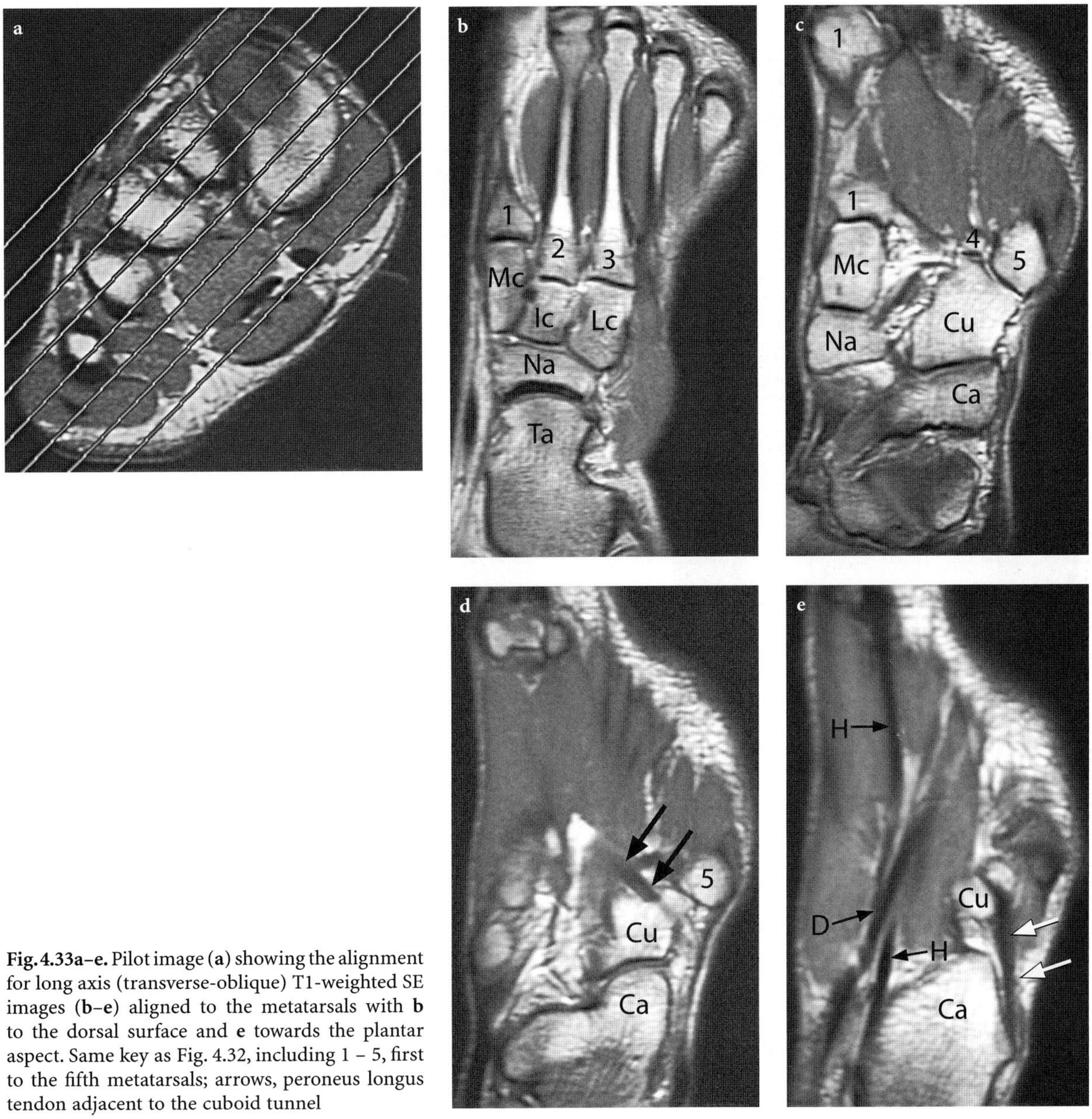

Fig. 4.33a–e. Pilot image (**a**) showing the alignment for long axis (transverse-oblique) T1-weighted SE images (**b–e**) aligned to the metatarsals with **b** to the dorsal surface and **e** towards the plantar aspect. Same key as Fig. 4.32, including 1 – 5, first to the fifth metatarsals; arrows, peroneus longus tendon adjacent to the cuboid tunnel

Both the spring ligament and the tibialis muscle and tendon maintain the medial longitudinal arch. Repair of the spring ligament is a major component of operative intervention in acquired flat foot deformity, but the value of imaging has yet to be established. There are short and long plantar ligaments which act to maintain the lateral longitudinal arch. The long plantar ligament is the longest ligament of the tarsus, extending from the plantar surface of the calcaneum and its anterior tubercle to the ridge and tuberosity of the cuboid, with superficial fibres extending to insert into the bases of the second to fourth/fifth metatarsals. The short plantar ligament is deeper, being closer to the bone than the long plantar ligament from which it is separated by fatty tissue. It is a strong, short, wide band (Fig. 4.34).

Although suspected midfoot pathology is an uncommon indication for MR imaging, this area is, however, usually included in MR imaging of the ankle and hindfoot. Unsuspected bone bruising/contusion/fracture and tarsal coalition (calcaneonavicular bar) can be identified (Fig. 4.35). For a full description of the soft-tissue compartmental anatomy of the midfoot, the reader is directed elsewhere (Farooki et al. 2001; Williams et al. 1989).

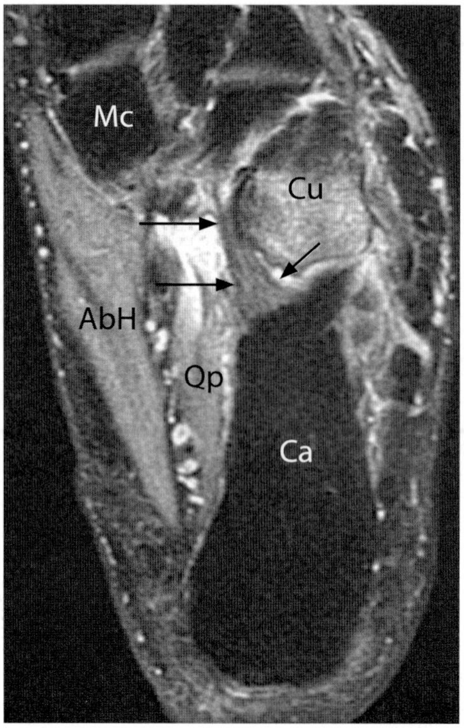

Fig. 4.34. Transverse intermediate-weighted FSE with fat-suppression image through the calcaneocuboid joint showing the short plantar ligament (*arrows*). Note there is marrow oedema within the cuboid due to bone contusion. Same key as Fig. 4.32

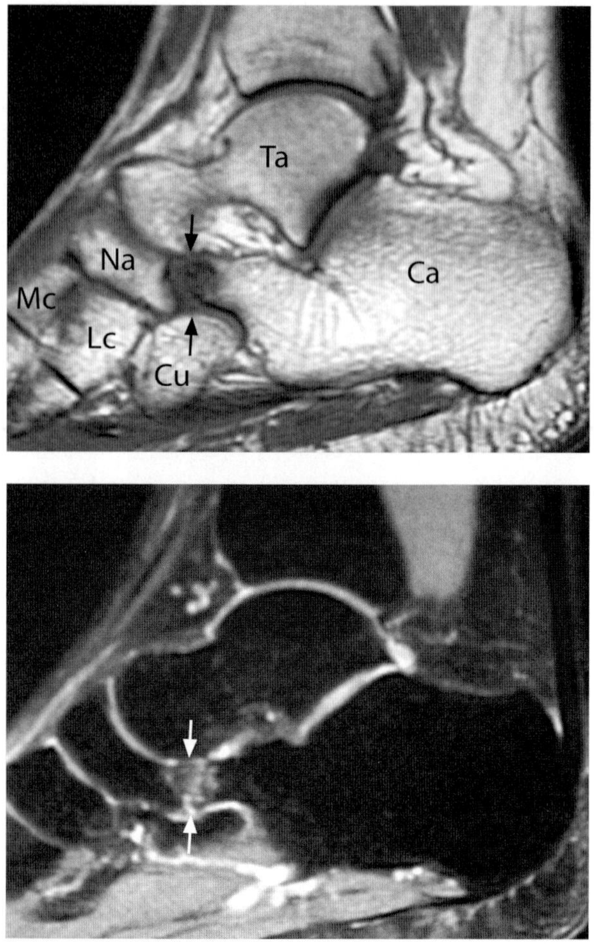

Fig. 4.35a,b. Calcaneonavicular coalition (*arrows*) with secondary degenerative changes at the synchondrosis on sagittal T1-weighted SE (**a**) and intermediate-weighted FSE with fat-suppression images (**b**)

4.3.5.3 Forefoot

This compartment includes the metatarsals and phalanges (Fig. 4.36). The digital nerves arise from the medial and lateral plantar nerves, being derivatives of the posterior tibial nerve. The digital nerves lie on the plantar surface of the deep transverse intermetatarsal ligaments and can become entrapped between the ligament and the plantar surface. The third digital nerve (in the third web space between the heads of the third and fourth metatarsals) is the largest of the digital nerves, being derived from branches of the medial and lateral plantar nerves, and is also, therefore, relatively fixed in position. The third digital nerve is susceptible to entrapment and compression and is the most common one to be involved by a Morton's neuroma.

For a full description of the compartmental anatomy of the forefoot, the reader is directed elsewhere (Kirsch and Erickson 1994; Williams et al. 1989).

4.4 Conclusion

MR imaging has an unrivalled ability in the assessment and detection of soft-tissue abnormalities and some bone lesions in the ankle and foot, and is being used more and more often. It is opening up new horizons in the diagnosis and treatment of various ankle and foot disorders. A clear understanding of the complex applied anatomy of the ankle and foot, together with a firm grasp of the normal appearances and variants as shown on MR, is vital to the correct interpretation of MR imaging and to an understanding of the various pathologies and syndromes to be expected.

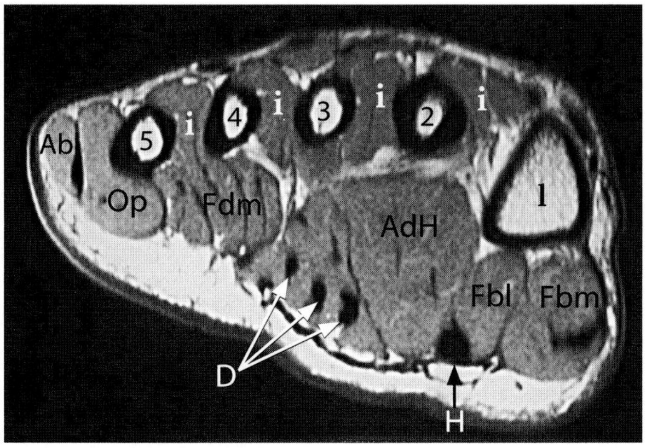

a

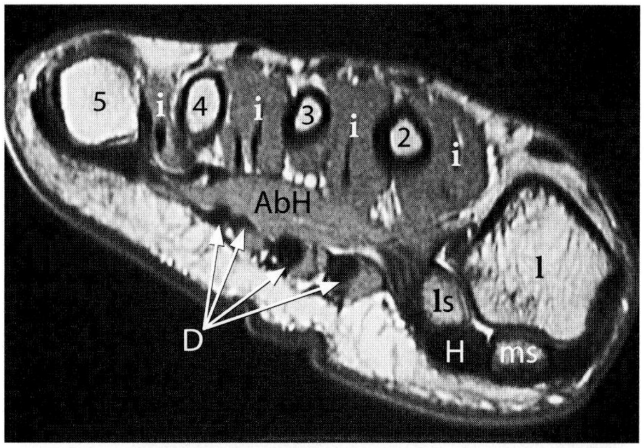

b

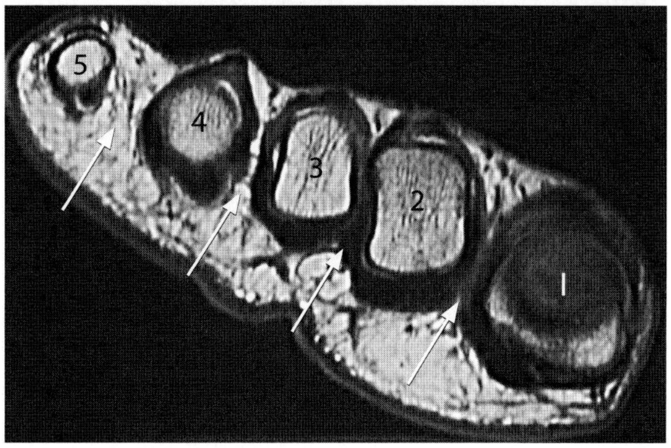

c

Fig. 4.36a–c. Short axis (coronal-oblique) T1-weighted SE images of the metatarsals: **a** at mid-shaft level; **b** through the first metatarsal head; **c** just distal in the web spaces. Same key as Fig. 4.33, including I, dorsal and plantar interosseous muscles; Ab, abductor digiti minimi muscle and tendon; Op, opponens digiti minimi muscle; Fdm, flexor digiti minimi muscle; AdH, adductor hallucis muscle; Fbl, lateral head of the flexor hallucis brevis muscle; Fbm, medial head of the flexor hallucis brevis muscle; ls, lateral sesamoid bone; ms, medial sesamoid bone; arrows in **c**, web spaces between the heads of the metatarsals

References

Bencardino JT, Rosenberg ZS (2001) Normal variants and pitfalls in MR imaging of the ankle and foot. In: Rosenberg ZS (ed) Update on the ankle and foot. MRI Clinics North Am 9:447–463

Berquist TH (2000) Anatomy, normal variants, and basic mechanics. In: Berquist TH (ed) Radiology of the foot and ankle, 2nd edn. Lippincott Williams & Wilkins, Philadelphia, pp 1–40

Campbell RSD, Grainger AJ (2001) Current concepts in imaging of tendinopathy. Clin Radiol 56:253–267

Cheung Y, Rosenberg ZS (2001) MR imaging of the accessory muscles around the ankle. In: Rosenberg ZS (ed) Update on the ankle and foot. MRI Clinics North Am 9:465–473

Daseler EH, Anson BJ (1943) The plantaris muscle. An anatomical study of 750 specimens. J Bone Joint Surg 25:822–827

Erickson SJ, Cox IH, Hyde JS, et al (1991) Effect of tendon orientation on MR imaging signal intensity: A manifestation of the «magic angle» phenomenon. Radiology 181:389–392

Farooki S, Sokoloff RM, Theodorou DJ, et al (2001) MR imaging of the midfoot. In: Rosenberg ZS (ed) Update on the ankle and foot. MRI Clinics North Am 9:419–434

Hayes CW, Parellada JA (1996) The magic angle effect in musculoskeletal MR imaging. Top Magn Reson Imaging 8: 51–56

Keats TE, Anderson MW (2001) Atlas of normal roentgen variants that may simulate disease, 7th edn. Mosby, St Louis

Kier R (1994) Magnetic resonance imaging of plantar fasciitis and other causes of heel pain. In: Beltran J (ed) The ankle and foot. MRI Clinics of NA 2:97–107

Kirsch MD, Erickson SJ (1994) Normal magnetic resonance imaging anatomy of the ankle and foot. In: Beltran J (ed) The ankle and foot. MRI Clinics North Am 2:1–21

Lawson JP, Ogden JA, Sella E, et al (1984) The painful accessory navicular. Skeletal Radiol 12:250–262

Millar TT, Staron RB, Feldman F, et al (1995) The symptomatic accessory tarsal navicular bone: assessment with MR imaging. Radiology 195:849–853

Peterfy CG, Roberts T, Genant HK (1998) Dedicated MR imaging. In: Mirowitz SA (ed) Special articles. MRI Clinics in North Am 6:849–870

Rosenberg ZS, Beltran J, Bencardino JT (2000) MR imaging of the ankle and foot. RadioGraphics 20:S153-S179

Schmidt H, Freyschmidt J (1993) In: Kohler/ Zimmer – Borderlands of normal and early pathologic findings in skeletal radiology, 4th edn. Thieme, Stuttgart, p818

Schweitzer ME, Karasick D (2000a) MR imaging of disorders of the posterior tibialis tendon. AJR 175:627–635

Schweitzer ME, Karasick D (2000b) MR imaging of disorders of the Achilles tendon. AJR 175:613–625

Shellock FG, Kanal E (1996) Magnetic resonance: bioeffects, safety, and patient management, 2nd edn. Lippincott-Raven, New York

Stoller DW, Ferkel RD, Beltran S (1999) The ankle and foot. In:

Stoller DW (ed) MRI, arthroscopy, and surgical anatomy of the joints. Lippincott-Raven, Philadelphia, pp 527–645

Theodorou DJ, Theodorou SJ, Kakitsubata Y, Lektrakul N, Gold GE, Roger B, Resnick D (2000) Plantar fasciitis and fascial rupture: MR imaging findings in 26 patients supplemented with anatomic data in cadavers. RadioGraphics 20:S181-S197

Vallejo JM, Jaramillo D (2001) Normal MR imaging anatomy of the ankle and foot in the pediatric population. In: Rosenberg ZS (ed) Update on the ankle and foot. MRI Clinics North Am 9:435–446

Williams PL, Warwick R, Dyson M, et al (eds) (1989) Gray's anatomy, 37th edn. Churchill Livingstone, London

5 MR Arthrography of the Ankle

J. W. HELGASON and V. P. CHANDNANI

CONTENTS

5.1 Introduction

Magnetic resonance (MR) imaging permits visualization of both osseous and soft tissues and is ideally suited to the evaluation of the musculoskeletal system. The major joints of the body, including the ankle, have been studied using MRI. The presence of joint fluid is widely known to improve the identification of intraarticular structures (YULISH et al. 1987). This is helpful in the acute setting, but joint fluid may be absent in chronic conditions. MR arthrography of the ankle employs contrast-enhanced joint fluid to facilitate discrimination between tissues within the ankle joint, simulating the 'arthrogram effect.' Primary signs, such as discontinuity of a ligament, and secondary signs, such as extravasation of contrast material, are both used in MR arthrography. This chapter describes the techniques and applications of MR arthrography of the ankle.

J. W. HELGASON, MD
Department of Radiology, Grant Medical Center, 111S. Grant Avenue, Columbus, OH 43215, USA
V. P. CHANDNANI, MD
Department of Radiology, Grant Medical Center, 111S. Grant Avenue, Columbus, OH 43215, USA

5.2 Indications

MR arthrography of the ankle has been studied and demonstrated to be useful in the evaluation of chronic ankle instability (CHANDNANI et al. 1994). After sustaining an ankle injury, patients whose careers depend upon maximum function and stability of the ankle, such as professional athletes or dancers, may be best evaluated with MR arthrography. Surgical intervention may be contemplated sooner in these patients. MR arthrography of the ankle aids in preoperative planning by improving the diagnostic accuracy regarding the extent of injury and allowing for the assessment of soft-tissue structures that may be used in surgical repair.

Lateral ligament injuries are not the only conditions which can be evaluated using MR arthrography. Recent investigators have found a wide spectrum of injuries that can occur in conjunction with ankle sprains or that may mimick the symptoms of lateral ligament tears. These include bone contusions, syndesmotic injuries, peroneal tendon tears and tendonopathy, fractures, osteochondral lesions, anterolateral impingement, sinus tarsi syndrome, osteoid osteoma, and intraarticular loose bodies (DIGIOVANNI et al. 2000; GERBER et al. 1998; HERTEL 2000; LEE and HOFBAUER 1999; PINAR et al. 1997). MR arthrography can be used to diagnose these conditions as well.

5.3 Technique

The enhancement of joint fluid can be accomplished either by intravenous administration or by direct intraarticular injection of contrast material. The former has been called indirect MR arthrography, and that designation will be used in this chapter. The latter technique will be referred to as direct MR arthrography. Most published studies have used direct MR arthrography.

5.3.1 Direct MR Arthrography

Joint access for direct MR arthrography is performed in the same manner as for conventional ankle arthrography. Marking the course of the dorsalis pedis artery can help prevent its puncture during the procedure. Any native effusion should be drained to reduce contrast dilution. The introduction of air bubbles should be avoided to prevent artifact mimicking intraarticular loose bodies. Contrast material is injected until slight resistance is felt by the examiner or patient. The injected volume generally ranges from 4 to 12 ml (Chandnani et al.1994; Trattnig et al. 1999).

The choice of gadolinium agent will depend on customary practice. Extensive research has been performed using gadopentetate dimeglumine. Theoretically, any of the commercially available chelates could be employed. The standard preparations of gadolinium agents for intravenous administration are of too high a concentration to be used in intraarticular injection. The optimal concentration for intraarticular use is 2 mmol/l (Engel 1990). This can be achieved by diluting stock preparation with normal saline in a 1:250 ratio (i.e. 1 ml gadopentetate dimeglumine in 250 ml normal saline). As MR arthrography has become more common, vendors are now marketing dilute gadolinium contrast agents for intraarticular use (Garcia 2000).

Joint puncture is often performed using fluoroscopic guidance. Confirmation of intraarticular placement of the needle requires injecting iodinated contrast material. Initial investigators using MR arthrography employed a minimal amount of iodinated contrast in order to limit potential contrast interactions and untoward magnetic effects of the iodinated contrast. This technique requires exchanging syringes during the procedure, risking the introduction of air bubbles or dislodging the needle from the joint. Brown et al. (2000) combined gadopentetate dimeglumine with iodinated contrast material with no ill effects. Iodinated contrast can be substituted as the diluent (i.e. 0.08 ml gadolinium chelate is diluted in 20 ml iodinated contrast). Using this method obviates the need for exchanging syringes.

While fluoroscopic guidance of joint puncture is most common, it is not the only technique used. Direct palpation using physical landmarks requires the most experience and skill. Ultrasound guidance (Fessell and van Holsbeeck 1999) and MR guidance (Trattnig et al. 1999) may be used to gain intraarticular access. Any of these techniques would eliminate the need for iodinated contrast.

5.3.2 Indirect MR Arthrography

Indirect MR arthrography is another means of enhancing the joint fluid. Gadolinium chelate is injected intravenously. The recommended dosage is 0.1 mmol/kg (Allmann et al. 1999; Vahlensieck et al. 1997). To ensure homogeneous enhancement of the joint fluid, the ankle is exercised through its range of motion for 5 to 15 min. Indirect MR arthrography has the advantage of being less invasive and less time consuming. It also does not involve the use of iodinated contrast. However, the joint capsule is not distended with indirect MR arthrography, which may limit the delineation of intraarticular structures.

5.3.3 Imaging

Imaging of the ankle is best carried out within 45 min after the intraarticular injection of contrast to maximize joint distention and joint fluid enhancement. If the indirect technique is used, then 5–15 min of exercise should precede imaging.

Images are obtained in the transverse, sagittal, and coronal planes. Images in the coronal oblique plane (Fig. 5.1) can also be acquired to improve visualization of the calcaneofibular ligament. T1-weighted sequences are used. Fat suppression is helpful in improving tissue contrast, which is especially important in indirect MR arthrography (Fig. 5.2). T2-weighted sequences may be obtained as desired and can provide additional

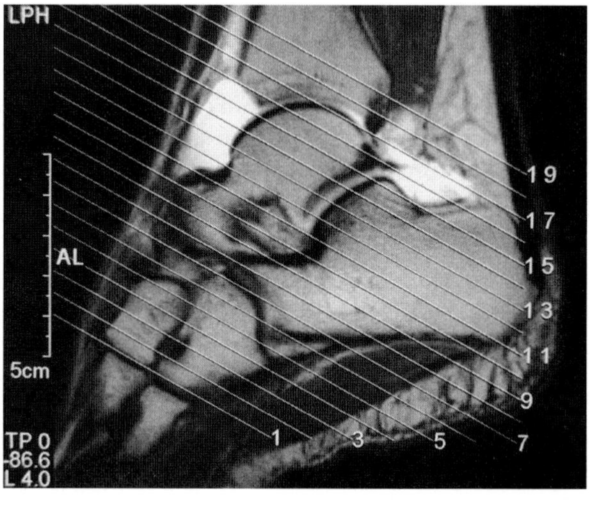

Fig. 5.1. Coronal oblique plane. Scout image shows the orientation of the coronal oblique plane used to maximize visualization of the calcaneofibular ligament

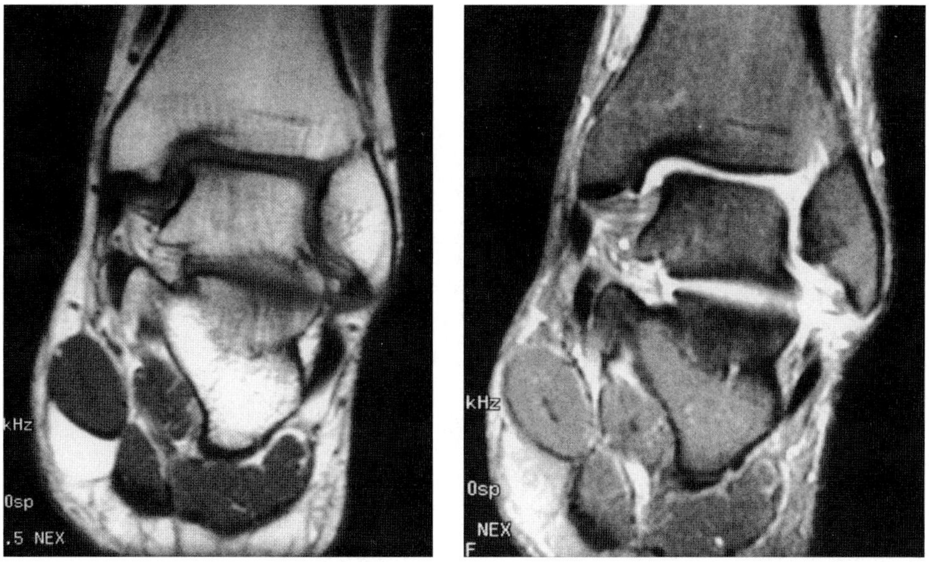

a b

Fig. 5.2a,b. Effects of fat saturation. **a** Coronal T1-weighted SE image from an indirect MR arthrogram. The joint fluid is of relatively low signal intensity compared with the bone marrow. **b** Same patient. After the application of fat saturation, there is marked improvement in contrast between joint fluid and other structures

information about the bone marrow and periarticular structures. A typical imaging protocol for a 1.5 T magnet is given in Table 5.1. Lower field-strength magnets can be used (Merhemic et al. 1999). For machines incapable of performing fat saturation, it may be necessary to substitute gradient-echo (GE) sequences for the T1-weighted fat-saturated sequences.

5.4 Complications

Complications associated with MR arthrography are rare. Intravenous adminstration of gadolinium-chelates is considered very safe, with a low incidence of adverse reactions (Runge 1999). In a survey of radiologists, Hugo et al. (1998) found that only 6 reported reactions occurred in over 13,000 MR arthrograms. These reactions were all minor and included pain, vasovagal reactions, and headaches. Animal studies have shown no serious effects within the joint (Hajek et al. 1990; Rahmouni et al. 1995).

5.5 Findings

5.5.1 Normal Findings

The ankle joint is formed by the distal tibia and fibula and the talus. Contrast material should be identified within this joint on MR arthrography. There may be communication of the tibiotalar joint with the flexor digitorum longus and flexor hallucis longus tendon sheaths and the subtalar joint in some individuals. Extravasation of contrast material beyond these boundaries is considered abnormal.

The lateral ligaments of the ankle are the anterior talofibular, calcaneofibular, and posterior talofibular

Table 5.1. Sample imaging protocol for direct MR arthrography of the ankle (1.5 T magnet)

Sequence	TR/TE	FOV	Matrix	Thickness/skip	NEX	Time
T1-weighted fat sat. coronal	464/18	14 cm	256×512	4 mm/1 mm	2	3:25
T1-weighted fat sat. transverse	392/13	14 cm	192×512	4 mm/1 mm	2	2:28
T1-weighted SE sagittal	535/18	16 cm	256×512	3 mm/1 mm	1	4:40
T2-weighted FSE transverse	3740/117	14 cm	192×512	4 mm/1 mm	2	2:43
T1-weighted SE coronal oblique	538/18	14 cm	256×512	4 mm/1 mm	2	3:58

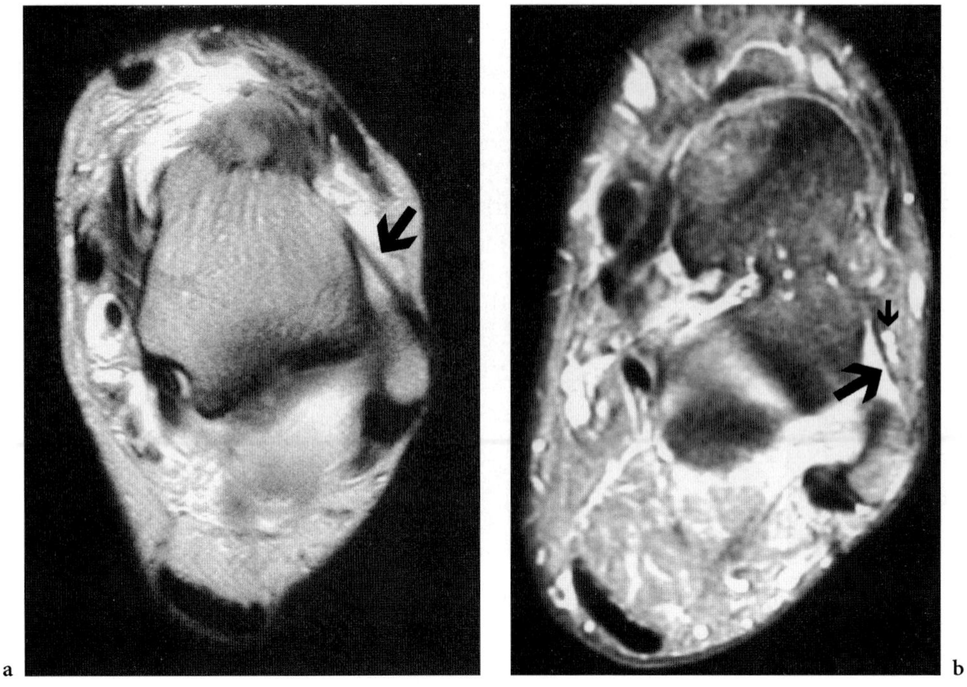

Fig. 5.3a,b. Normal anterior talofibular ligament (ATFL). **a** Transverse T2-weighted SE image from a direct MR arthrogram shows a normal anterior talofibular ligament (*arrow*). **b** Transverse T1-weighted fat-saturated image from an indirect MR arthrogram also shows a normal ATFL (*large arrow*). The high signal focus lateral to the ligament (*small arrow*) is an enhancing blood vessel

ligaments. These are the structures of primary concern in evaluating lateral instability. The anterior talofibular ligament (ATFL) can be seen as a band of low signal intensity spanning from the anterior margin of the lateral malleolus to the talus. It is best appreciated in the transverse plane (Fig. 5.3). The calcaneofibular ligament (CFL) is deep to the peroneal tendons, extending obliquely and inferiorly from the tip of the lateral malleolus to the lateral aspect of the calcaneus. It is best appreciated in the coronal or coronal oblique plane (Fig. 5.4). The posterior talofibular ligament (PTFL) attaches to the distal aspect of the fibula and the posterior aspect of the talus. It is typically thicker than the other two ligaments and is usually seen in both the transverse and coronal planes (Fig. 5.5).

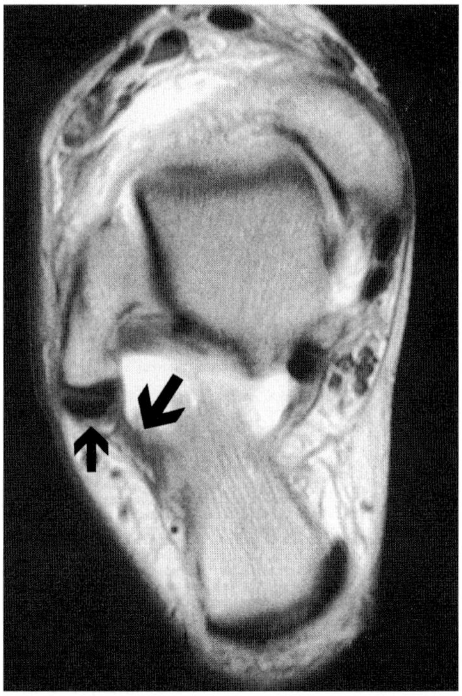

Fig. 5.4. Normal calcaneofibular ligament (CFL). T1-weighted SE coronal oblique image from a direct MR arthrogram demonstrates the normal calcaneofibular ligament (*large arrow*). The peroneal tendons (*small arrow*) are superficial to the CFL

5.5.2 Abnormal Findings

Tears of the lateral ligaments of the ankle can be diagnosed using primary signs. These are the absence or discontinuity of the ligament. Partial tears can be recognized as increased signal intensity or intravasation of contrast into the ligament, abnormal course of

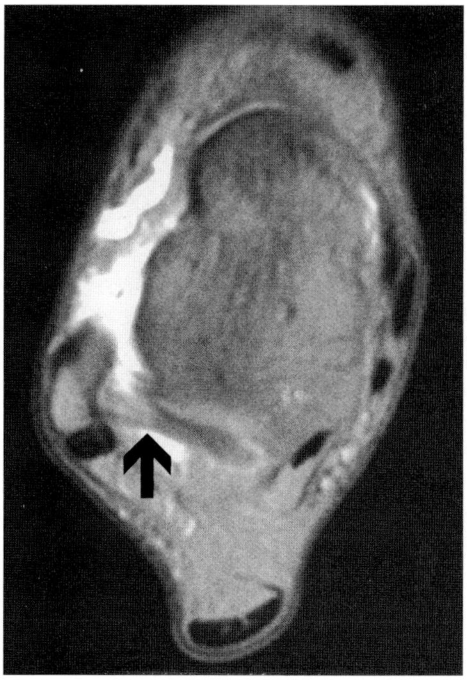

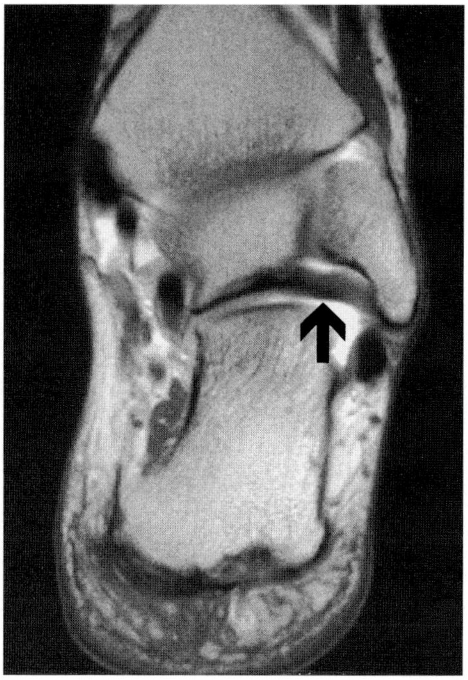

Fig. 5.5a,b. Normal posterior talofibular ligament. T1-weighted images from direct MR arthrograms are shown. In the transverse (**a**) and coronal (**b**) planes, the normal posterior talofibular ligament (*arrows*) is seen as a thick band

the ligament, or wavy, irregular contours of the ligament. Specific patterns of contrast extravasation can be used as secondary signs of lateral ligament tears. These are extravasation of contrast anterior and lateral to the anterior talofibular ligament in ATFL tear (Fig. 5.6), extravasation into the peroneal tendon sheath in CFL tear (Fig. 5.7), and extravasation into the soft tissues posterior to the posterior talofibular ligament in PTFL tear (Fig. 5.8). Injuries of the ATFL occur most frequently, either alone or along with CFL injury, and the PTFL is the least commonly injured ligament (Fallat et al. 1998).

Isolated tears of the deltoid ligaments are extremely rare. Tears of the distal tibiofibular syndesmosis are more common. Syndesmotic injuries are often associated with minimal swelling and may, therefore, be overlooked or underestimated. Syndesmotic sprains have been linked to prolonged disability (Gerber et al. 1998). The components of the syndesmotic ligamentous complex are best seen in the transverse plane cephalad to the ATFL (Fig. 5.9). Tears are identified as discontinuity of these ligaments (Fig. 5.10). Disruption of the interosseous ligament can be diagnosed by contrast extending cephalad into the interosseous space beyond the normal 1 cm synovial recess (Lee et al. 1998).

Osteochondral lesions are another frequent injury occurring with ankle sprains. MR arthrography can

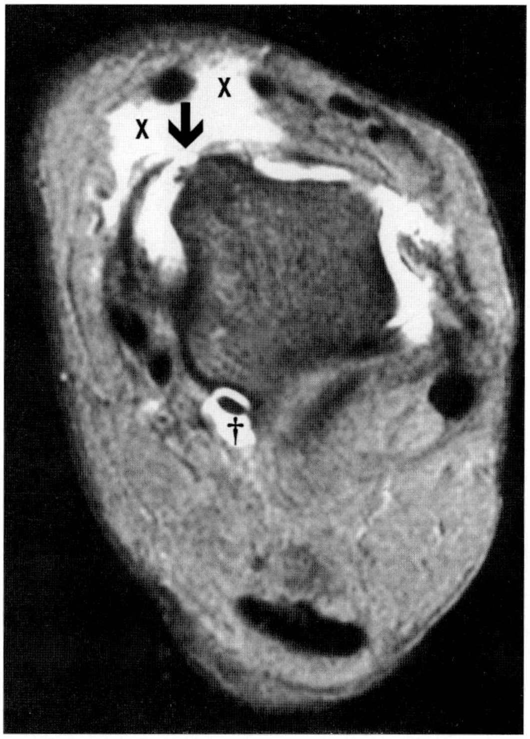

Fig. 5.6. ATFL tear. On this transverse T1-weighted fat-saturated image from a direct MR arthrogram, the anterior talofibular ligament is discontinuous (*arrow*), and there is extravasation of contrast material anteriorly (*X*). Contrast in the flexor hallucis longus tendon sheath (*dagger*) can be a normal finding

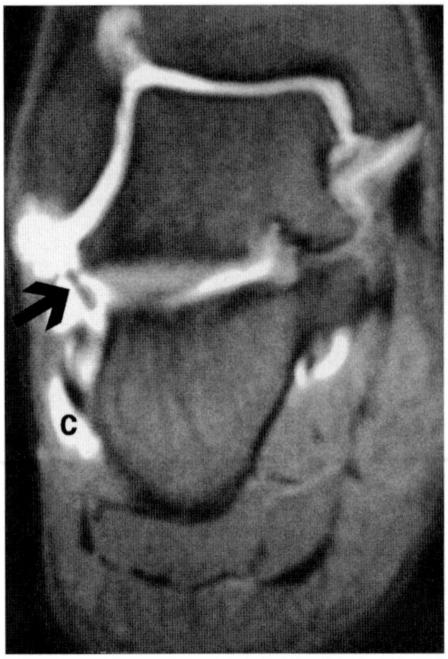

Fig. 5.7. CFL tear. Coronal T1-weighted fat-saturated image from a direct MR arthrogram shows discontinuity of the CFL. A small fragment of the ligament can be seen within the joint (*arrow*). The secondary sign of contrast material in the peroneal tendon sheath is present (*c*)

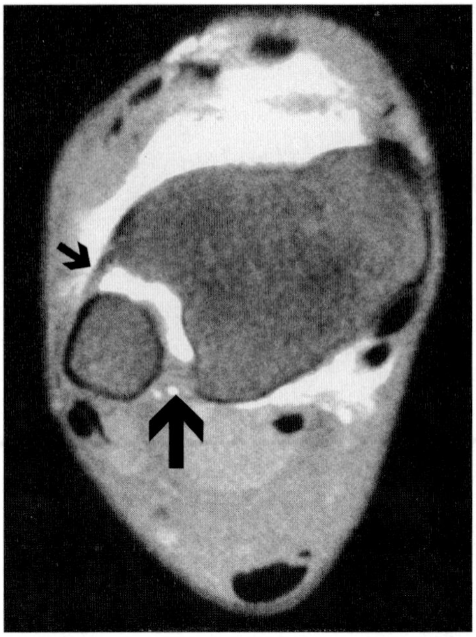

Fig. 5.9. Normal distal tibiofibular syndesmosis. The anterior (*small arrow*) and posterior (*large arrow*) tibiofibular ligaments are intact on this transverse T1-weighted fat-saturated image obtained after intraarticular contrast injection. Contrast can be present normally in the interosseous space, provided the contrast does not extend cephalad beyond the normal 1 cm recess

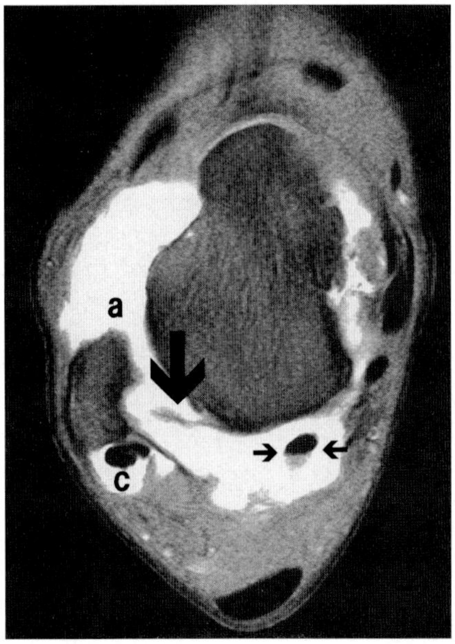

Fig. 5.8. PTFL tear. Transverse T1-weighted fat-saturated image from a direct MR arthrogram shows a torn posterior talofibular ligament (*large arrow*) with extravasation of contrast surrounding the flexor hallucis longus at its myotendinous junction (*small arrows*). This amount of fluid is much greater than expected with a normal communication. As is typical for tears of the PTFL, there is a tear of the ATFL, as evidenced by absence of the ligament (*a*), and a tear of the CFL, suggested by contrast in the peroneal tendon sheath (*c*)

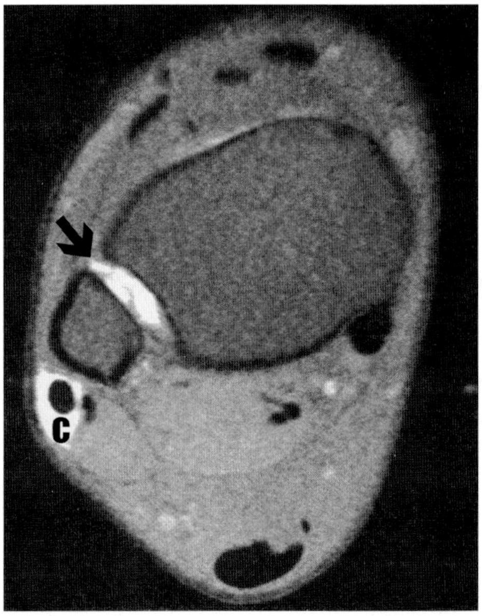

Fig. 5.10. Syndesmotic injury: direct MR arthrogram. Transverse T1-weighted fat-saturated image shows discontinuity of the ATFL (*arrow*). This tear has occurred in conjunction with a CFL tear. Contrast is present in the peroneal tendon sheath (*c*)

be used to diagnose and stage these defects accurately (Kramer et al. 1992). Using the classification system of Hepple et al. (1999), stage 1 is damage to the articular cartilage only. Stage 2a is cartilage injury with underlying fracture. In stage 2b, there is an underlying fracture but no adjacent bone marrow edema. Stage 3 involves a detached, but undisplaced fragment, and in stage 4, the fragment is displaced. Stage 5 is subchondral cyst formation. With MR arthrography, stages 1 and 2 can be identified as contrast intravasation into the articular cartilage. For stage 3, the contrast material will outline the fragment (Fig. 5.11). Contrast completely fills the fossa of the displaced fragment in stage 4 (Fig. 5.12).

Intraarticular loose bodies can occur as sequelae of osteochondral defects or other pathologic processes. Brossman et al. (1996) found MR athrography to be the most sensitive technique in detecting intraarticular loose bodies when compared with conventional MRI, CT, and CT arthrography. Loose bodies as small as 1 or 2 mm can be detected with MR arthrography (Steinbach and Schwartz 1998). It is important to distinguish air bubbles introduced during contrast administration from true loose bodies. Loose bodies will have signal characteristics of cartilage or bone. Air bubbles will produce magnetic susceptibility artifact, which will be compounded on gradient-echo images. Air bubbles will typically accumulate in non-dependent locations within the ankle joint.

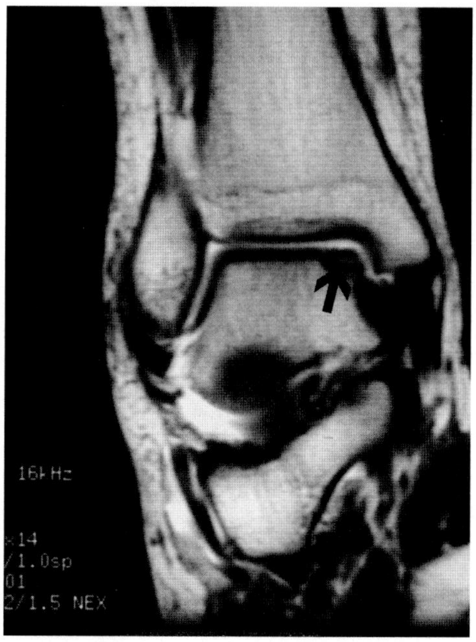

Fig. 5.11. Osteochondral defect, stage 3. Coronal T1-weighted SE image from a direct MR arthrogram shows contrast material outlining an unstable osteochondral fragment (*arrow*) in the medial talar dome. The fragment is not displaced

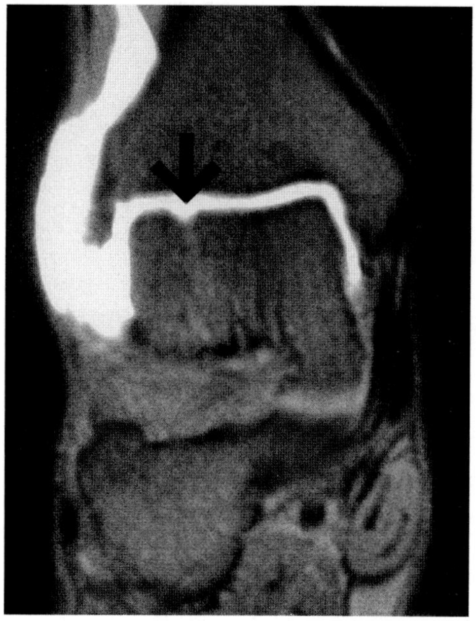

Fig. 5.12. Osteochondral defect, stage 4. Coronal T1-weighted fat-saturated image from a direct MR arthrogram shows a concavity in the medial talar dome (*arrow*). The osteochondral fragment is displaced, and contrast fills the fragment bed

The peroneus brevis tendon is often used in reconstruction of the lateral ligaments (Pisani 1998). Knowledge of its status is critical for surgical planning. Peroneal tendon abnormalities may be additional or alternative diagnoses in patients presenting with lateral ankle sprains (Fig. 5.13). Discontinuity of the tendon on sagittal images indicates a complete tear. Partial tears or longitudinal tears can also occur (Major et al. 2000). Tendonopathy is seen as increased signal within the tendon on T1-weighted sequences, typically accompanied by increased tendon girth.

Anterolateral impingement is a condition in which soft tissue becomes entrapped in the anterolateral gutter of the ankle. This material can be hypertrophied synovium, fibrotic scar, or part of the ATFL. A soft-tissue signal mass is seen in the anterolateral gutter on MRI (Jordan et al. 2000). Detection of this soft-tissue mass is improved when joint fluid is present, as in MR arthrography (Rubin et al. 1997).

5.6 Conclusion

Ankle injuries occur quite frequently and were the presenting injury in 23% of persons engaged in a regular exercise program (Gerber et al. 1998). Although many

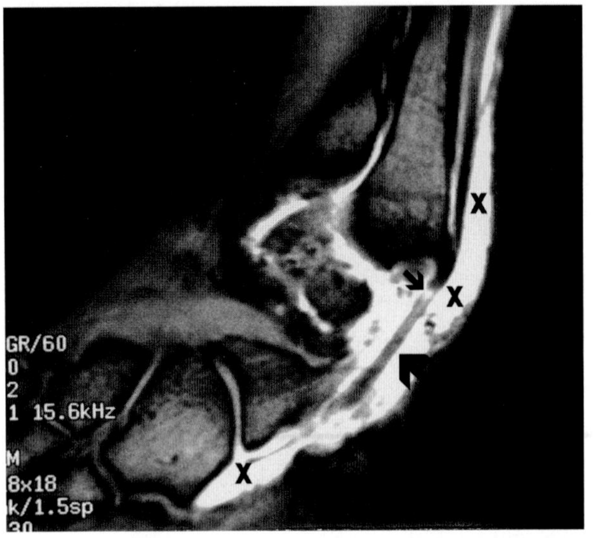

Fig. 5.13. Partial tear of the peroneus brevis tendon. Sagittal gradient-echo image from a direct MR arthrogram shows increased signal intensity in the peroneus brevis tendon (*large arrow*). There is focal intravasation of contrast into the tendon (*small arrow*). Massive contrast extravastion (*X*) can be seen in this patient with tears of all three lateral ligaments

patients go on to heal without incident, residual symptoms are being reported more and more commonly. Nearly 73% of patients in a general clinic-based population complained of residual symptoms 6–18 months after injury (Braun 1999). The recurrence rate can approach 75%, and chronic instability can occur in up to 20% (Yeung et al. 1994). Minimal or inadequate treatment has been found to lead to residual symptoms (Pijnenburg et al. 2000). The diagnostic goal is to identify those patients most at risk for instability so that an aggressive treatment regimen can be initiated (Macintyre and Joy 2000). This can be difficult given the great variation in clinical criteria establishing the severity of injuries and the treatment options (Lynch and Renström 1999). Biomechanical studies have shown a poor correlation between clinical stress tests and the extent of ligamentous disruption (Fujii et al. 2000). A more accurate method for evaluating the degree of ligamentous injury and the possibility of associated injuries is needed. MR arthrography of the ankle offers improved visibility of the intraarticular structures, thus leading to greater confidence in interpretation. It also provides for evaluation of the bone marrow and adjacent soft tissues. This is helpful in diagnosing alternative or associated injuries and assisting in preoperative planning.

MR arthrography is more invasive than conventional MRI. Indirect MR arthrography can be considered minimally invasive. However, recent patient surveys indicate that patients are willing to accept a more invasive test to achieve a more accurate diagnosis (Robbins et al. 2000).

Because of the additional procedures of needle placement and contrast administration, direct MR arthrography does result in a lengthier examination. The arthrographic portion of the exam can usually be completed within 15–30 min. Procedure times may shorten as examiners gain experience with the technique. More experience also leads to decreased fluoroscopy time. Alternatively, fluoroscopy can be avoided altogether if a nonionizing imaging modality is used for guiding needle placement.

The overall cost for MR athrography is higher than for conventional MRI. Over time, the cost of MRI can be expected to decline (Fletcher et al. 1999). Some investigators suggest that multiple patient doses of contrast can be acquired from a single vial of gadolinium-chelate, thus reducing expenditure on contrast agents (Kamishima et al. 2000). These reduced costs could be passed on to the public. While this practice is quite common with iodinated contrast media, manufacturers of gadolinium-chelates do recommend single-use only.

In summary, MR arthrography of the ankle is a useful technique in identifying patients at risk for developing chronic instability of the ankle. It accurately depicts the extent of injury and assists in the preoperative planning. MR arthrography can also be used to diagnose various other injuries associated with lateral ankle sprains.

References

Allmann K-H, Schäfer O, Hauer M et al (1999) Indirect MR arthrography of the unexercised glenohumeral joint in patients with rotator cuff tears. Invest Radiol 34:435–440

Braun BL (1999) Effects of ankle sprain in a genral clinic population 6 to 18 months after medical evaluation. Arch Fam Med 8:143–148

Brossman J, Priedler KW, Dänen B et al (1996) Imaging of osseous and cartilaginous intraarticular loose bodies in the knee: comparison of MR imaging and MR arthrography with CT and CT arthrography in cadavers. Radiology 200:509–517

Brown RR, Clarke DW, Daffner RH (2000) Is a mixture of gadolinium and iodinated contrast material safe during MR arthrography? AJR Am J Roentgenol 175:1087–1090

Chandnani VP, Harper MT, Ficke JR et al (1994) Chronic ankle instability: evaluation with MR arthrography, MR imaging, and stress radiography. Radiology 192:189–194

DiGiovanni BF, Fraga CJ, Cohen BE, Shereff MJ (2000) Associated injuries found in chronic lateral ankle instability. Foot Ankle Int 21:809–815

Engel A (1990) Magnetic resonance knee arthrography. Acta Orthop Scand 61:1–57

Fallat L, Grimm DJ, Saracco JA (1998) Sprained ankle syndrome: prevalence and analysis of 639 acute injuries. J Foot Ankle Surg 37:280–285

Fessell DP, van Holsbeeck M (1999) Foot and ankle sonography. Radiol Clin North Am 37:831–858

Fletcher J, Clark MD, Sutton FA, Wellings R, Garas K (1999) The cost of MRI: changes in costs 1989–1996. Br J Radiol 72:432–437

Fujii T, Luo Z-P, Kitaoka HB, An K-N (2000) The manual stress test may not be sufficient to differentiate ankle ligament injuries. Clin Biomech 15:619–623

Garcia J (2000) MR arthrography. J Radiol E 81:945–952

Gerber JP, Williams GN, Scoville CR, Arciero RA, Taylor DC (1998) Persistent disability associated with ankle sprains: a prospective examination of an athletic population. Foot Ankle Int 19:653–660

Hajek PC, Sartoris DJ, Gylys-Morin V et al (1990) The effect of intraarticular gadolinium-DTPA on synovial membrane and cartilage. Invest Radiol 25:179–183

Hepple S, Winson IG, Glew D (1999) Osteochondral lesions of the talus: a revised classification. Foot Ankle Int 20: 789–793

Hertel J (2000) Functional instability following lateral ankle sprain. Sports Med 29:361–371

Hugo PC, Newberg AH, Wetzner SM (1998) Complications of arthrography. Semin Musculoskelet Radiol 2:345–348

Jordan LK, Helms CA, Cooperman AE, Speer KP (2000) Magnetic resonance imaging findings in anterolateral impingement of the ankle. Skeletal Radiol 29:34–39

Kamishima T, Schweitzer ME, Awaya H, Abraham D (2000) Utilization of 'used' vials: cost-effective technique for MR arthrography. J Magn Reson Imaging 12:953–955

Kramer J, Stiglbauer R, Engel A, Prayer L, Imhof H (1992) MR contrast arthrography (MRA) in osteochondrosis dissecans. J Comput Assist Tomogr 16:254–260

Lee MS, Hofbauer MH (1999) Evaluation and management of lateral ankle injuries. Clin Podiatr Med Surg 16:659–678

Lee SH, Jacobsen J, Trudell D, Resnick D (1998) Ligaments of the ankle: normal anatomy with MR arthrography. J Comput Assist Tomogr 22:807–813

Lynch SA, Renström P (1999) Treatment of acute lateral ankle ligament rupture in the athlete. Sports Med 27:61–71

Macintyre J, Joy E (2000) Foot and ankle injuries in dance. Clin Sports Med 19:351–368

Major NM, Helms CA, Fritz RC, Speer KP (2000) The MR imaging appearance of longitudinal split tears of the peroneus brevis tendon. Foot Ankle Int 21:514–519

Merhemic Z, Breitenseher M, Trattnig S et al (1999) MRT des sprunggelenks. Radiologe 39:41–46

Pijnenburg ACM, Van Dijk CN, Bossyut PMM, Marti RK (2000) Treatment of ruptures of the lateral ankle ligaments: a meta-analysis. J Bone Joint Surg Am 82:761–773

Pinar H, Akseki D, Kovanlikaya I, Araç [a], Bozkurt M (1997) Bone bruises detected by magnetic resonance imaging following lateral ankle sprains. Knee Surg Sports Taumatol Arthrosc 5:113–117

Pisani G (1998) Reconstruction of chronic lateral ankle instability. In: Wülker N, Stephens M, Cracchiolo A (eds) An atlas of foot and ankle surgery. Mosby, St Louis, pp 277–282

Rahmouni A, Mathieu D, Chambon C, Dao T-H, Hernigou P, Vasile N (1995) Intraarticular tolerability and kinetics of gadolinium tetra-azacyclododecane tetraacetic acid. Acad Radiol 2:413–417

Robbins MI, Anzilotti KF, Katz LD, Lange RC (2000) Patient perception of magnetic resonance arthrography. Skeletal Radiol 29:265–269

Rubin DA, Tishkoff NW, Britton CA, Conti SF, Towers JD (1997) Anterolateral soft-tissue impingement in the ankle: diagnosis using MR imaging. AJR Am J Roentgenol 169: 829–835

Runge VM (1999) Safety of approved MR contrast media for intravenous injection. J Magn Reson Imaging 12:205–213

Steinbach LS, Schwartz M (1998) Elbow arthrography. Radiol Clin North Am 36:635–649

Trattnig S, Rand T, Breitenseher M, Ba-Ssalamah A, Schick S, Imhof H (1999) MR-arthrographie des sprunggelenkes. Radiologe 39:47–51

Vahlensieck M, Lang P, Sommer T, Genant H, Schild H (1997) Indirect MR arthrography: techniques and applications. Semin Ultrasound CT MR 18:302–306

Yeung MS, Chan K-M, So CH, Yuan WY (1994) An epidemiological survey on ankle sprain. Br J Sports Med 28: 112–116

Yulish BS, Montanez J, Goodfellow DB, Bryan PJ, Mulopulos GP, Modic MT (1987) Chondromalacia patellae: assessment with MR imaging. Radiology 164:763–766

6 Ultrasound Imaging of the Ankle

S. Bianchi, C. Martinoli, and J. Garcia

CONTENTS

6.1 Introduction

The recent development of high-resolution electronic transducers has increased the capability of ultrasound (US) to evaluate the normal structures of the musculoskeletal system as well as to detect and characterize subtle pathologic changes (Martinoli et al. 1999). US of the ankle has received increasing attention in recent years (Thermann et al. 1992; Cchem et al. 1993). Nowadays, it is considered an excellent modality for the assessment of a variety of ankle and foot diseases (Fessel et al. 1998; Fessel and van Holsbeeck 1999; Morvan et al. 2000) and can often replace MRI in the assessment of tendon disorders (Rockett et al. 1999).

The purpose of this chapter is to describe the technique of US examination and to present the normal US anatomy of the ankle.

S. Bianchi. MD
Division of Radiodiagnosis and Interventional Radiology, Hôpital Cantonal Universitaire, 24 rue Micheli-du-Crest, 1211, Geneva, Switzerland
J. Garcia, MD
Division of Radiodiagnosis and Interventional Radiology, Hôpital Cantonal Universitaire, 24 rue Micheli-du-Crest, 1211, Geneva, Switzerland
C. Martinoli. MD
Istituto di Radiologia, Università di Genova, Largo R Benzi 1, 16100, Genova, Italy

6.2 Standard US Examination

A detailed reference note from the clinician with the indication of the specific structures to be investigated and of the presumptive clinical diagnosis must be obtained. Focusing on a definite area of the joint not only reduces the time of examination but allows an in-depth, accurate assessment of the structures examined. US is inferior to other imaging techniques (MRI, CT) in the evaluation of intraarticular structures of the ankle. Since the clinician may ignore this limitation, knowledge of the presumptive clinical diagnosis is important to avoid useless examinations. On the other hand, compared with other modalities, US is efficient and economic in the assessment of superficial structures and can be considered the modality of choice in patients with paraarticular lesions.

We routinely obtain the patient's history and ask for a recent complete radiographic evaluation before starting the US examination. Taking the patient's history is helpful not only in focusing the examination but also in the interpretation of the US findings. The availability of standard radiographs can be essential for understanding troublesome US images related to disorders that can be obvious on plain films. Moreover, radiographs can show coincident bone lesions that can be detected by US.

Due to the superficial location of most ankle structures, high-frequency transducers working at 10–13 MHz are well suited for the assessment of the ankle region. Occasionally, in larger joints, a 5-MHz probe can help in depicting deeper structures such as the posterior joint space and the proximal portion of the flexor hallucis longus tendon. Although standard linear probes usually allow adequate evaluation of the region, taking into account the irregularity of the ankle surfaces, small transducers such as high-resolution intraoperative probes may be needed and often facilitate the study of perimalleolar areas. As an alternative, the employment of a stand-off pad can be helpful. Color and power Doppler are useful in the evaluation of vessels, assessment of the vascularity of paraarticular masses, and depicting synovial or tendon hyperemia. The use of extended field-of-view (EFW) provides a panoramic analysis of the region scanned. Utilization of this technique allows an optimal assessment of the Achilles tendon, which can be imaged from its origin from the triceps surae to its distal insertion onto the calcaneum. Moreover, EFW aids the interpretation of the US images by the referring physician.

US examination of the ankle is performed with the patient in the recumbent position. The ability to perform a dynamic examination is a particular advantage of US. Sonograms obtained with different degrees of flexion and extension of the ankle allow filling of the anterior and posterior synovial recesses and work well in the detection of small joint effusions. Ligaments and tendons can be examined at rest or during stress maneuvers or active muscle contraction. The stretching obtained with dynamic US helps in avoiding hypoechogenicity related to anisotropy and often adds additional information to the morphologic data. In the evaluation of intraarticular loose bodies, the displacement of fragments induced by movements of the joint is an important diagnostic criterion (Bianchi and Martinoli 1999). In the assessment of nerve tumor or entrapment neuropathies, US-guided pressure applied with the probe or with the examinor's finger can elicit the patient's symptoms and confirm the neurogenic nature of the lesion (US-guided Tinel's test).

If the normal US anatomy of the ankle is well known, contralateral examination is not essential and is not routinely performed. However, comparison with the opposite side can be helpful in selected cases such as patients with congenital anomalies or when the size of a pathological structure must be compared with the healthy contralateral one.

Standard US examination of the ankle starts with evaluation of the anterior aspect of the joint, followed by the medial, lateral, and posterior aspects.

6.2.1 Anterior Aspect

With the patient supine, the anterior aspect of the ankle is evaluated by axial, longitudinal, and oblique sonograms. In this region, US can image the anterior tendons and tendon retinacula, the anterior tibial vessels and the deep peroneal nerve, the distal end of the tibia, the anterior portion of the talus and its cartilage, as well as the anterior capsule and synovial recess (Figs. 6.1 and 6.2).

The anterior tendons include from medial to lateral: tibialis anterior (TA), extensor hallucis longus (EHL), and extensor digitorum longus (EDL). Axial sonograms are initially performed to show the different tendons in a single image and to assess their position. Tendons are identified on an anatomic basis, in relation to bone landmarks, and can be followed from the myotendinous junction to the foot region. Dynamic sonograms obtained during passive movements of the different toes can help the inexperienced examiner to distinguish the different tendons. Longitudinal sonograms are then obtained over each tendon for accurate evaluation of its structure. The development of high-frequency transducers has increased the ability to assess the internal tendon structure. Longitudinal sonograms show an internal network made up of many fine, tightly packed parallel echoes which resemble a fibrillar pattern. Such echoes are specular reflections of the US beam and become more clearly visible and better separated one from another as the transducer frequency increases (Martinoli et al. 1993). Tendon evaluation requires careful positioning of the probe. For each tendon, the transducer must be oriented perpendicular to its long axis in transverse scans and parallel to it in longitudinal sonograms. Even a slight obliquity of the angle of incidence of the US beam can result in an artifactual hypoechogenicity which may not only obscure textural details, but can even mimic tendinous disease.

Anterior ankle tendons, like the medial and lateral tendons, are surrounded by a synovial sheath and are held against the bone surface by the retinacula. The synovial sheath, composed of two thin membranes separated by a film of synovial fluid, facilitates tendon gliding. Under normal conditions, the synovial membrane cannot be detected by US. Retinacula are fibrous bands that insert onto the bone cortex and prevent dislocation of tendons during activation of muscles. They guarantee the correct direction of the tensile forces of the different tendons. The increased resolution of the newer electronic transducers allows demonstration of retinacula as thin hyperechoic bands overlying the tendons and inserting into the periosteum. The peculiar arrangement (Y shape) of the anterior retinaculum can be imaged by US. Dynamic longitudinal US, which shows smooth gliding of the tendons in normal subjects, is useful in the evaluation of peritendinitis or posttraumatic adhesions. In these conditions, passive movements of the ankle or toes induce displacements of the peritendineous tissue.

The anterior tibial vessels lie in a deep position, between the TA and EHL. The pulsatility of the artery allows its easy detection without the utilization of

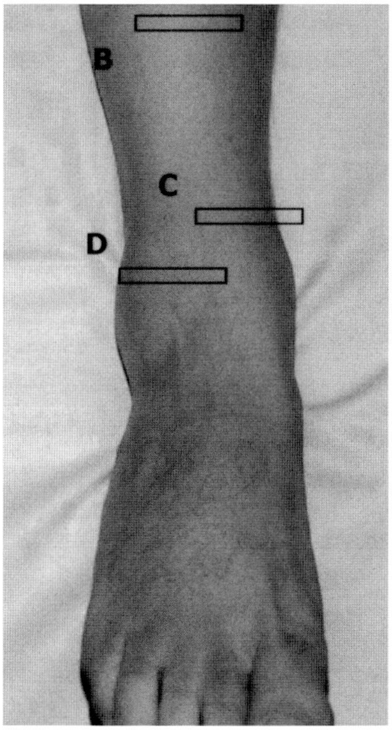

a

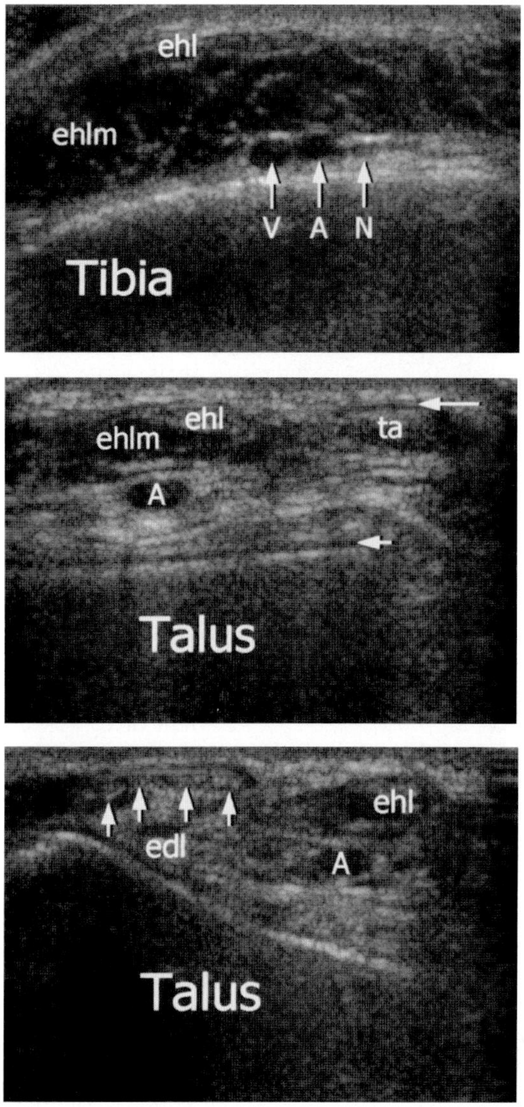

Fig. 6.1a–d. Anterior aspect. **a** Probe positioning for transverse examination. **b,c** Corresponding sonograms obtained from cranial to caudal. **b** Cranial sonogram. *ehlm*, extensor hallucis longus muscle; *ehl*, extensor hallucis longus tendon; *V*, anterior tibial vein; *A*, anterior tibial artery; *N*, deep peroneal nerve. **c** Distal sonogram (medial aspect). *ta*, tibialis anterior tendon; *short arrow*, cartilage of the talar dome; *long arrow*, retinaculum. **d** Distal sonogram (lateral aspect). *edl*, extensor digitorum longus tendons (*arrows*)

color Doppler. Arterial wall thickening as well as calcifications are easily assessed by US. The anterior veins are located adjacent to the artery. During their evaluation, attention must be paid to avoid excessive pressure with the probe, which can induce collapse of the veins.

Nerves present a particular appearance on US (Martinoli et al. 2000). Longitudinal sonograms demonstrate a fascicular aspect due to multiple, hypoechoic, parallel but discontinuous linear areas separated by hyperechoic bands. On transverse scans, the hypoechoic areas become rounded, embedded in a hyperechoic background. Histologic correlation demonstrated that the hypoechoic structures correspond to the fascicles and the hyperechoic background to the interfascicular epineurium. Due to its small size, only high-frequency probes can image the deep peroneal nerve. Since the nerve has a close relation with the anterior tibial artery, this acts as a useful landmark in its detection. The superficial peroneal nerve can also be imaged. Careful US scanning of the anterolateral face of the leg allows the demonstration, from cranial to distal, of its intramuscular and intrafascial portions. In the anterolateral region of the ankle, the nerve can be imaged in the subcutaneous adipose tissue where it splits into the terminal sensory branches.

Due to superimposition of different bones, the ankle joint cavity is poorly imaged by US. Anterior sagittal sonograms are obtained with the ankle in plantar flexion to allow evaluation of the articular surface of the talus. US shows from cranial to distal

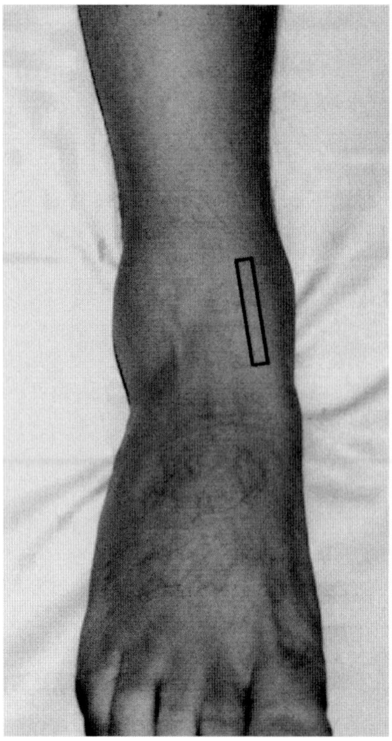

a

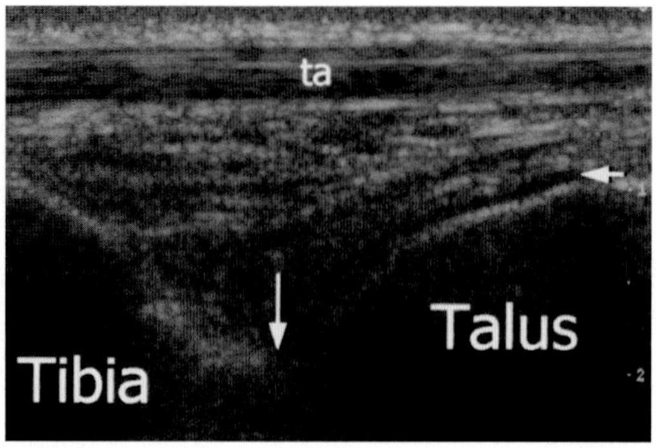

b

Fig. 6.2a,b. Anterior aspect. **a** Probe positioning for longitudinal examination of the tibialis anterior tendon. **b** Corresponding sonogram. *Long arrow*, ankle joint space; *short arrow*, cartilage of the talar dome; *ta*, tibialis anterior tendon

the distal epiphysis of the tibia, the anterior portion of dome, neck and head of the talus, and the dorsal surfaces of the tarsal bones. The anterior joint capsule can barely be distinguished from the paraarticular soft tissue. Under normal conditions, the anterior ankle synovial recess appears as a thin triangular anechoic structure located just anterior to the tibiotalar joint and posterior to the anterior fat pad (Jacobson et al. 1998). No echogenic material is depicted inside the recess. Since it is often difficult to clinically determine whether swelling of the ankles is due to arthritis or involvement of periarticular tissues, US evaluation of the anterior recess has practical value (Kellner et al. 1992). In a study comparing the ability of different techniques in revealing ankle effusions in cadaveric specimens, US was able to detect 2 ml of fluid in the anterior recess. However, care must be exercised in evaluating small amounts of fluid since US can also depict joint, bursal, and tendon sheath effusions in asymptomatic volunteers, thus implying that a detectable effusion does not necessarily indicate underlying abnormalities (Nazarian et al. 1995). A US diagnosis of pathological effusion must then be considered only if a large amount of fluid is demonstrated. In doubtful cases, correlation with clinical data and comparison with the controlateral side are helpful. When analysis of the synovial fluid is required for diagnostic or therapeutic purposes, US can assist joint puncture in accurately locating the joint space and allowing real-time correct positioning of the needle tip (Roy et al. 1999). Talocrural effusions are recognized as an increase of echo-free space between the bone and the joint capsule (Koski 1990).

6.2.2 Lateral Aspect

After examination of the anterior aspect, the patient is then asked to rotate the ankle internally to allow evaluation of its lateral aspect. Structures that can be imaged by US include the small saphenous vein and the sural nerve, the peroneal tendons and retinacula, the lateral ligaments, and the lateral aspect of the fibula, talus, and calcaneum (Figs. 6.3, 6.4, 6.5).

The small saphenous vein runs in the subcutaneous tissue of the lateral aspect of the ankle to reach the posterior aspect of the leg. Localization of the vein allows easy detection of the small sural nerve which lies close to it. Once the vein is detected, the sural nerve can be imaged on its medial aspect. The possibility to image the nerve with US has clinical applications since it can be injured during surgical stripping of the vein (Simonetti et al. 1999).

a b c d e f

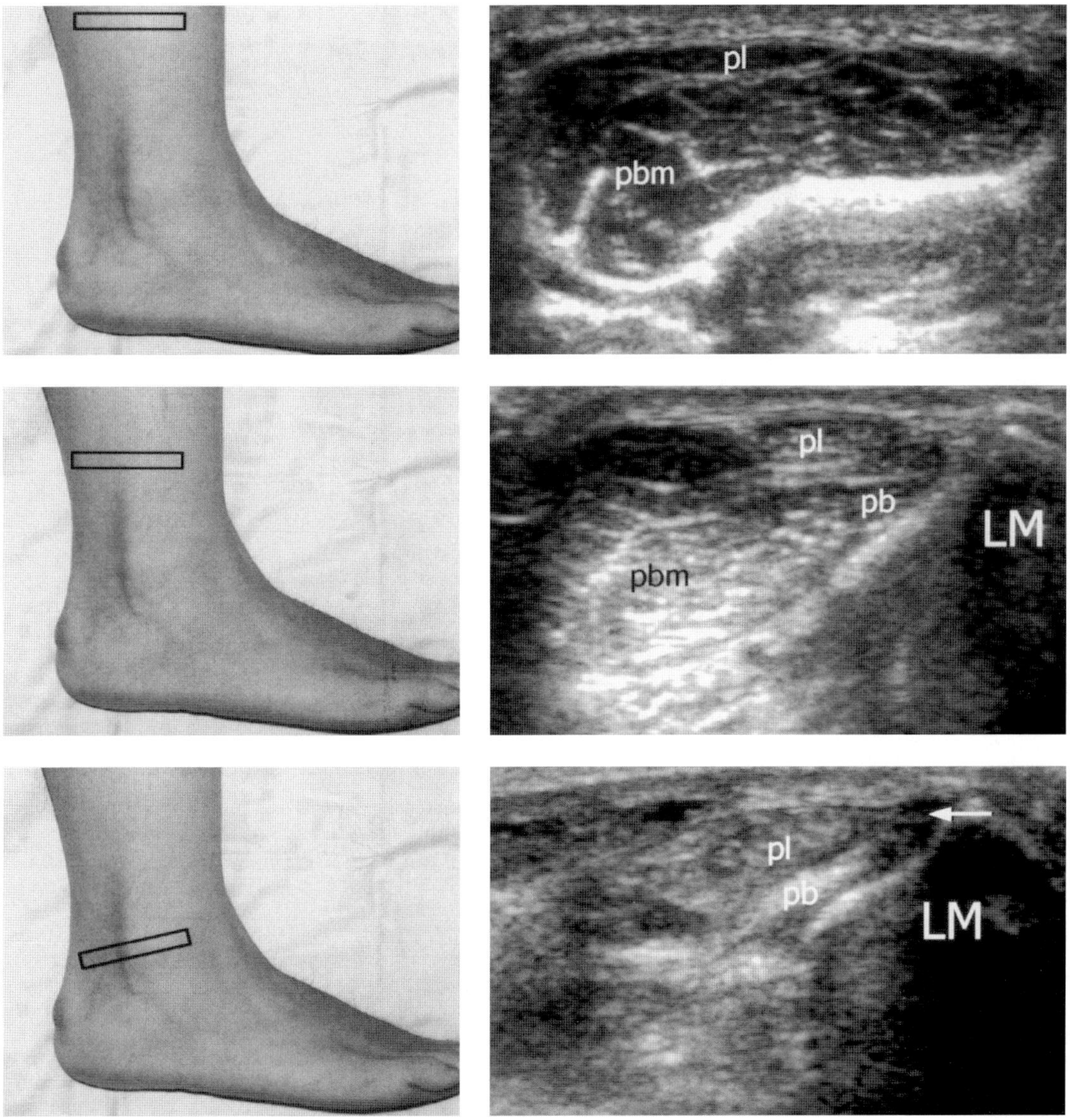

Fig. 6.3a–f. Lateral aspect. **a,c,e** Probe positioning for transverse examination of the supramalleolar region. **b,d,f** Corresponding sonograms obtained from cranial to caudal. *LM*, lateral malleolus; *pbm*, peroneus brevis muscle; *pb*, peroneus brevis tendon; *pl*, peroneus longus tendon; *arrow*, retinaculum

The peroneal tendons (PeT) include the peroneus longus (PL) and brevis (PB) tendons, which originate from the peroneal muscles and reflect under the lateral malleolus to insert onto the base of the first and fifth metatarsals, respectively. US allows accurate evaluation of both tendons in the supramalleolar, malleolar, and submalleolar regions. Because the tendons run obliquely, transverse sonograms perpendicular to their long axis are most useful to assess their location and internal structure. In the supramalleolar and submalleolar portions where the tendons are rectilinear, longitudinal sonograms are also obtained. In the supramalleolar region, PL lies lateral to the PB muscle. In the cranial part, it has a flattened appearance, while it becomes more oval in the caudal part. As the PB muscle approaches the external malleolus, the muscle fibers can be seen inserting in the curvilinear PB tendon, which is located anteromedial to the oval PL. In the malleolar region, the two tendons are closely retained against the lateral malleolus and are difficult to evaluate. In the inframalleolar region, both appear as oval structures that diverge and are separated by the peroneal tubercle of the calcaneum. PB passes superior to the tubercle, while PL is located inferior to it. The tendons present a common synovial sheath which splits

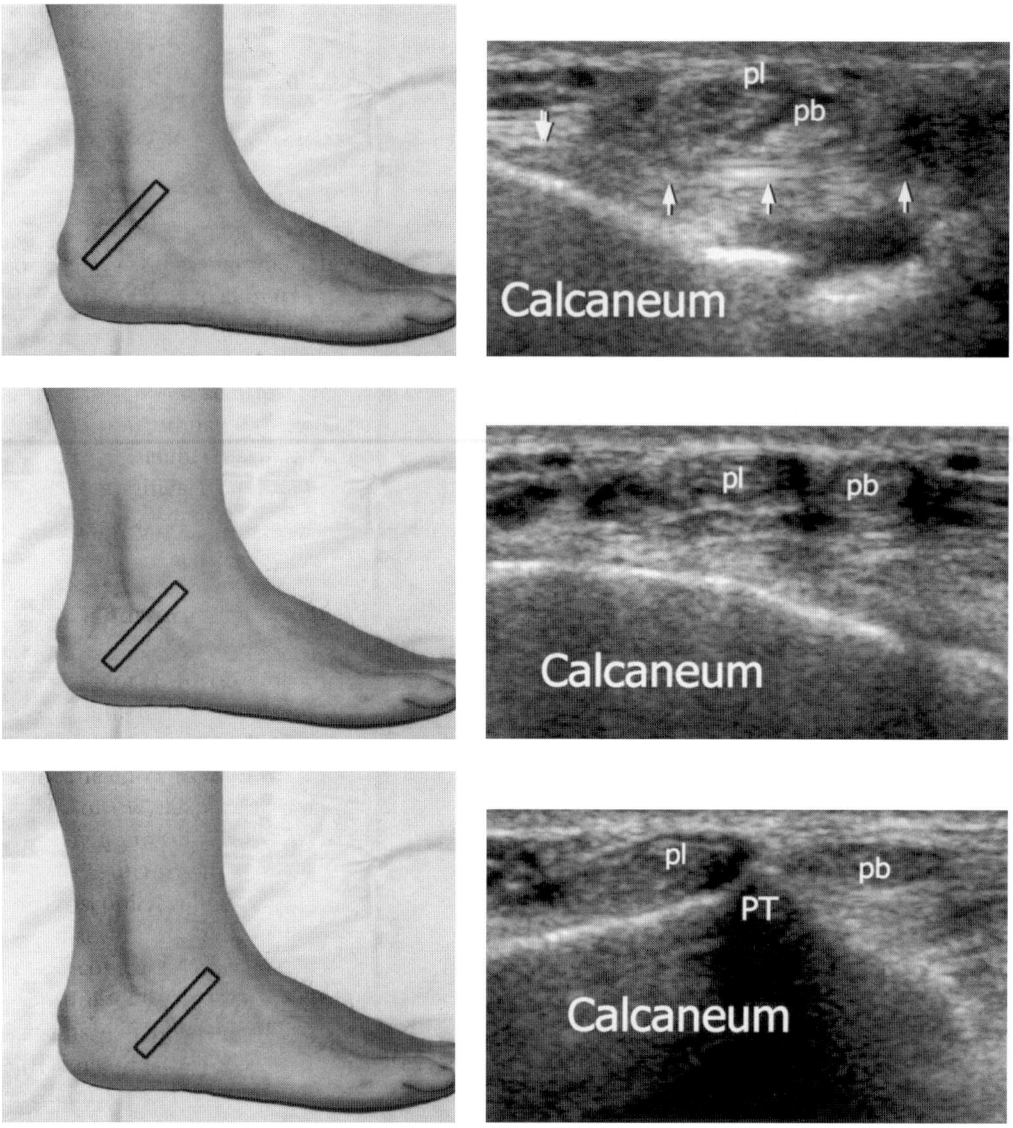

Fig. 6.4a–f. Lateral aspect. **a,c,e** Probe positioning for coronal oblique examination of the inframalleolar region. **b,d,f** Corresponding sonograms obtained from posterior to anterior. *PT*, peroneal tubercle; *pb*, peroneus brevis tendon; *pl*, peroneus longus tendon; *arrows*, peroneocalcaneal ligament

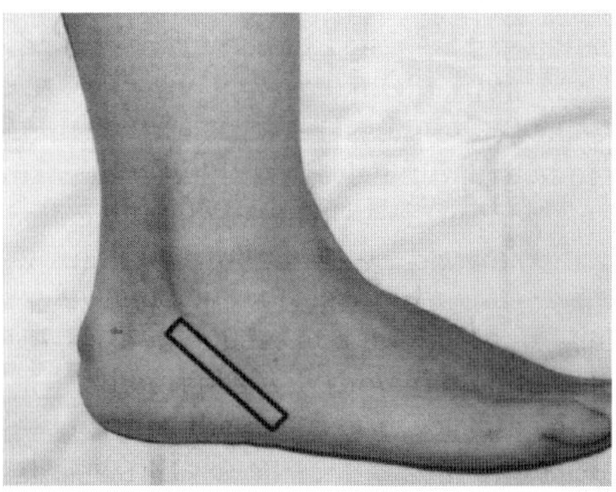

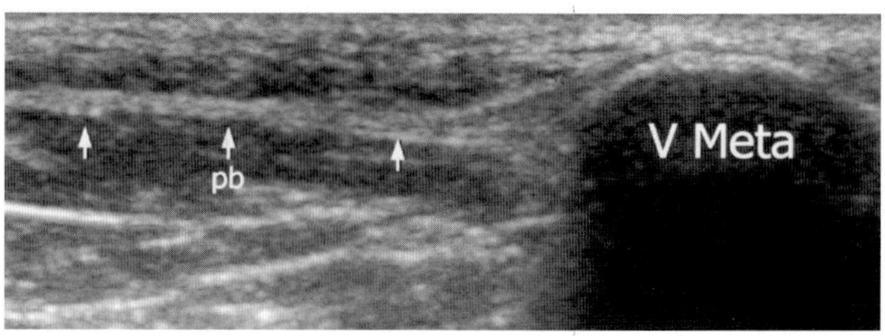

Fig. 6.5a,b. Lateral aspect. **a** Probe positioning for longitudinal examination of peroneus brevis tendon. **b** Corresponding sonogram; *V Meta*, base of fifth metatarsal; *pb*, peroneus brevis tendon (*arrows*)

distally to surround each tendon. Under normal conditions, the sheath and the small amount of internal synovial fluid cannot be detected with US. The superior retinaculum located in the malleolar region and the inferior retinaculum found at the level of the peroneal process can be demonstrated with US as thin laminar bands overlying the tendons and inserting onto the bone. The posterior face of the peroneal malleolus can be evaluated by US. Under normal conditions, a concave groove containing the PeT can be demonstrated. In patients presenting with anterior instability of the tendons, a flat or even a convex appearance, which can facilitate the dislocation, can be demonstrated. Dynamic sonograms of the ankle achieved in eversion can help in demonstrating intermittent PeT dislocation (Campbell et al. 1994; Magnano et al. 1998; Diaz et al. 1998).

The anterior talofibular (ATT) and calcaneofibular (CF) ligaments can be imaged by US on both longitudinal and axial sonograms. The possibility to image these ligaments is of clinical value since they are commonly injured in ankle sprains. Studies comparing US findings with anatomic data (Brasseur et al. 1994; Friedrich et al. 1993; Milz et al. 1996) show that US can accurately detect the ligaments and evaluate their thickness. As for tendon evaluation, care must be taken to accurately angle the transducer parallel to the ligament examined to avoid artifact hypoechogenicity. Sonograms obtained during joint stress tests (varus/valgus stress and anterior drawer maneuver) must be performed routinely as they increase the detection of tears and differentiate between complete and partial rupture (Campbell et al. 1994). The ATT ligament appears as a rectilinear hyperechoic band which joins the anterior aspect of the tip of the malleolus to the neck of the talus. The CF ligament has a similar echotexture but is more difficult to evaluate because of its curvilinear silhouette. The caudal part of the CF ligament can be imaged overlying the lateral face of the calcaneum, while the cranial portion is imaged deep to the peroneal tendons. Forced dorsiflexion of the foot straightens the ligament and allows better evaluation of it. Because of its deep location, the posterior talofibular ligament (PTT) cannot be assessed by US.

6.2.3 Medial Aspect

Axial sonograms of the internal aspect show from anterior to posterior and from medial to lateral the tibialis posterior (TP), flexor digitorum longus (FDL), and flexor hallucis longus (FHL) tendons (Figs. 6.6, 6.7, 6.8).

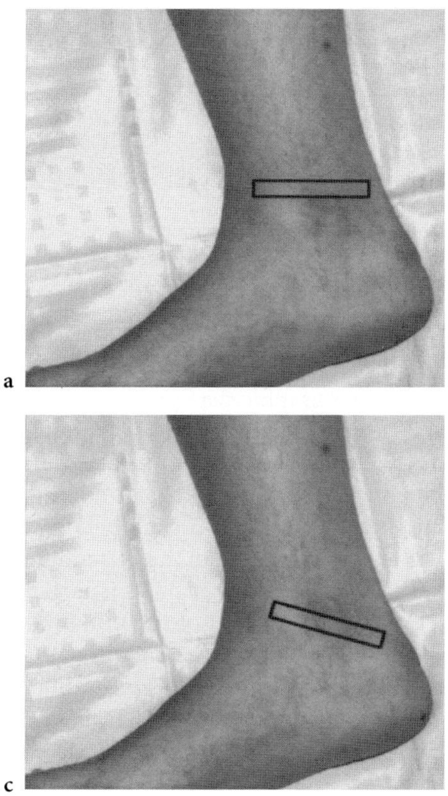

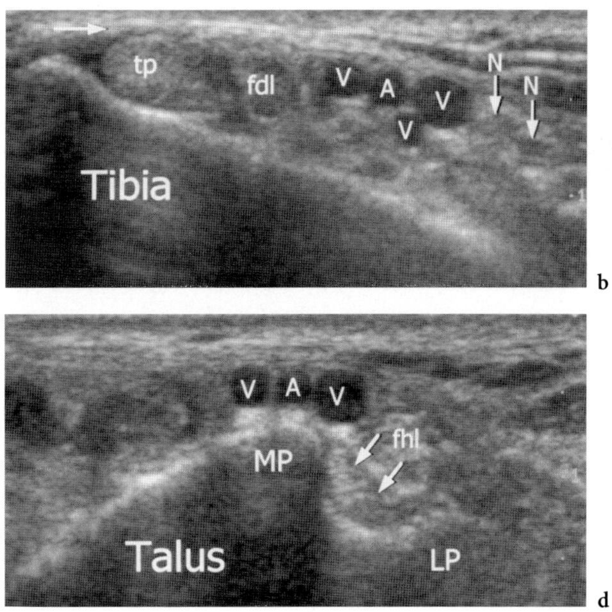

Fig. 6.6a–d. Medial aspect. **a,c** Probe positioning for transverse examination of the malleolar region. **b,d** Corresponding sonograms obtained from cranial to caudal. *tp*, tibialis posterior tendon; *fdl*, flexor digitorum longus tendon; *A*, posterior tibialis artery; *V*, posterior tibialis veins; *N*, medial and lateral branches of posterior tibialis nerve; *MP*, medial proces of the talus; *LP*, lateral process of the talus; *fhl*, flexor hallucis longus tendon (*arrows*)

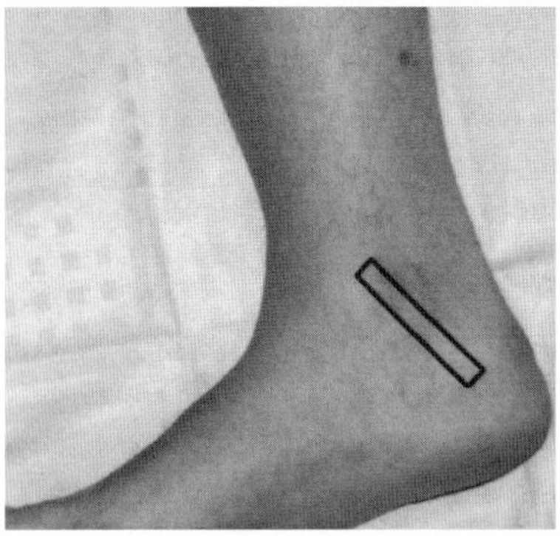
a

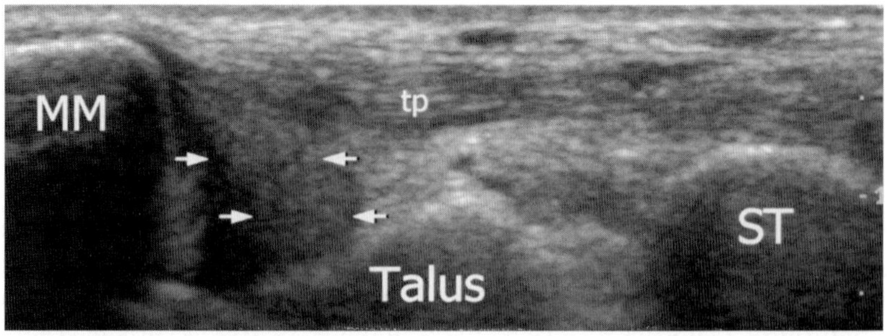

b

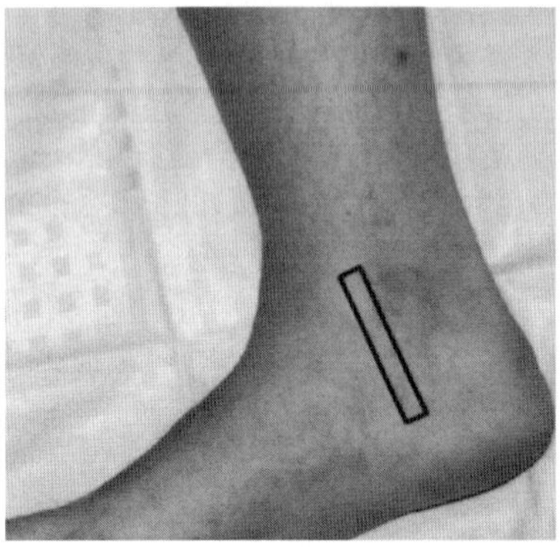
c

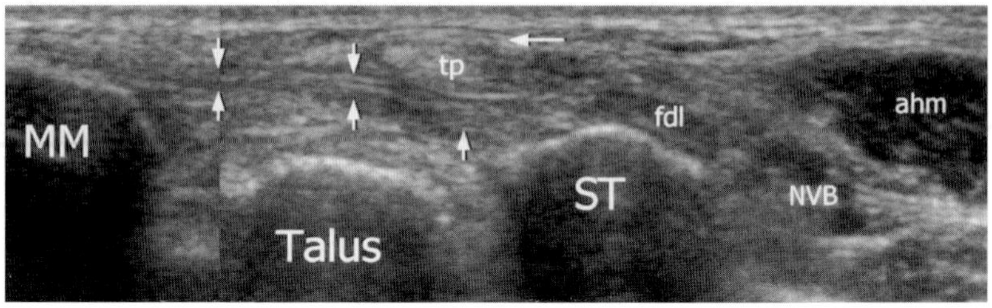

d

Fig. 6.7a–d. Medial aspect. **a,c** Probe positioning for coronal examination of the inframalleolar region. **b,d** Corresponding sonograms obtained from posterior to anterior. *MM*, medial malleolus; *ST*, substentaculum tali; *tp*, tibialis posterior tendon; *arrows* (**b**), deep component of the deltoid ligament; *fdl*, flexor digitorum longus tendon; *ahm*, adductor hallucis muscle; *NVB*, neurovascular bundle; *arrows* (**d**), superficial component of the deltoid ligament

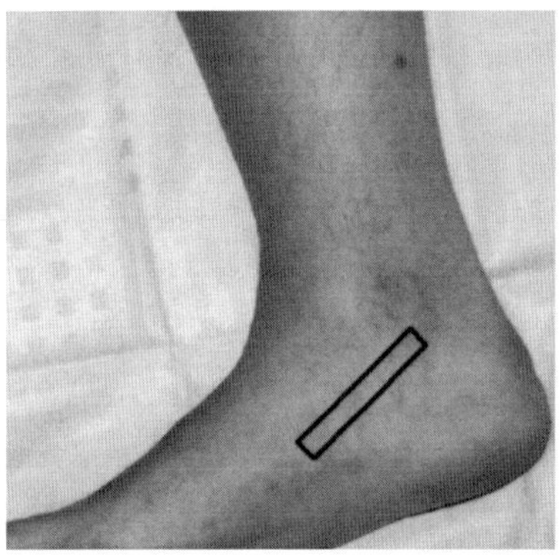
a

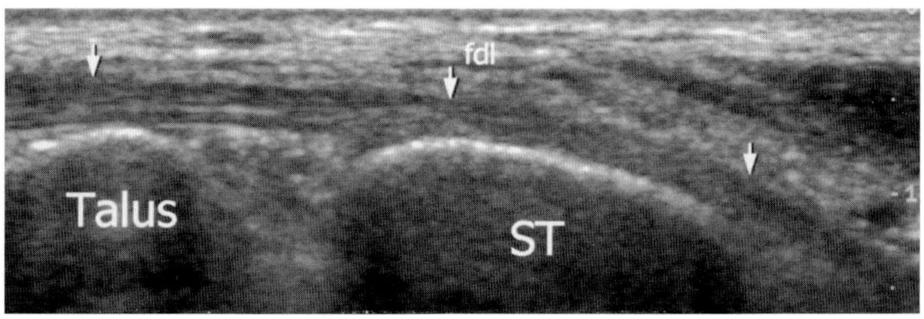

b

Fig. 6.8a,b. Medial aspect. **a** Probe positioning for longitudinal examination of flexor digitorum longus tendon. **b** Corresponding sonogram. *ST*, substentaculum tali; *fdl*, flexor digitorum longus tendon (*arrows*)

The TP tendon, the thickest and stronger internal tendon, appears as an oval hyperechoic structure (Hsu et al. 1997). It lies on the posterolateral aspect of the medial malleolus in a osteofibrous tunnel made by the bone surface and by a thick retinaculum. The tendon widens distally before its insertion on the tubercle of the scaphoid (principle insertion). The supplementary insertions (three cuneiforms and bases of 2nd–4th metatarsals) cannot be visualised with US. Occasionally, US can show a decreased echogenicity of the distal tendon. This may be related to the disparate orientation of collagen fibers in the different tendon portions which diverge to reach their insertions. Careful examination technique of the distal TP tendon and correlation with clinical data are essential for a correct interpretation of the sonographic data and can avoid an improper diagnosis of localized tendinosis. A small amount of fluid is commonly found in the distal sheath and must not be considered a pathological finding. The FDL is located just posterior and slightly lateral to the TP. Since it is always thinner than the TP tendon, its size can be used as a reference to evaluate a partial lesion of the TP. Coronal sonograms of the inframalleolar region show the tendon on the medial surface of the substentaculum tali. Because of its deep location, the FHL tendon is difficult to evaluate by US. Dynamic examination obtained during passive movements of the hallux enhance its detection. The supramalleolar portion is well depicted on sagittal sonograms obtained over the Achilles tendon. Both the muscle and the tendon can be visualized. The malleolar portion can be assessed only by axial oblique sonograms of the medial aspect. Careful examination technique is essential to display the two posterior processes of the talus (medial and lateral processes) delimiting a groove that contains the FHL. The distal portion can be evaluated by coronal and sagittal scans obtained on the sole of the foot. The differentiation between FHL and FDL is evident with dynamic examination.

The posterointernal neurovascular bundle (tibialis posterior artery, veins, and nerve) is found in a slightly lateral location with respect to the FDL tendon. The artery is differentiated from the adjacent veins by its pulsatility and on the basis of color Doppler findings. With the utilization of high-frequency transducers, the posterior tibialis nerve and its two terminal branches (medial and lateral) can be visualized. Occasionally, US can detect the thinner calcaneal sensory branch.

Both components of the ankle medial ligament (deltoid ligament) can be imaged by coronal sonograms. Due to its more pronounced obliquity, the posterior deep component appears as a hypoechoic thick structure connecting the medial malleolus to the medial surface of the talus. The most rectilinear superficial component is visible as a thinner hyperechoic structure linking the substentaculum tali with the medial malleolus. The anterior subtalar joint can be imaged in the coronal plane. Anatomic variations such as the talocalcaneal bone or fibrous collations can be diagnosed with US. In bone coalition, a continuous cortical hyperechoic line joining the two bones is evident, while fibrous collations can be suspected when marked irregularities of the joint boundaries are found. Bilateral examination can help in the evaluation of an unilateral coalition.

6.2.4 Posterior Aspect

Structures that can be imaged by US include the posterior aspect of the ankle and the Achilles tendon (AT). The patient is examined prone. Because of its superficial location, rectilinear appearance, and high frequency of ruptures, the study of the AT was one of the first applications of musculoskeletal US. Optimal stretching of the AT can be obtained by asking the patient to maintain the foot perpendicular to the leg. The tendon is examined by transverse and longitudinal images obtained from the myotendineous junction to the calcaneal insertion (Figs. 6.9 and 6.10). Longitudinal images show the AT as a fibrillar, homogeneous, hyperechoic structure which originates from

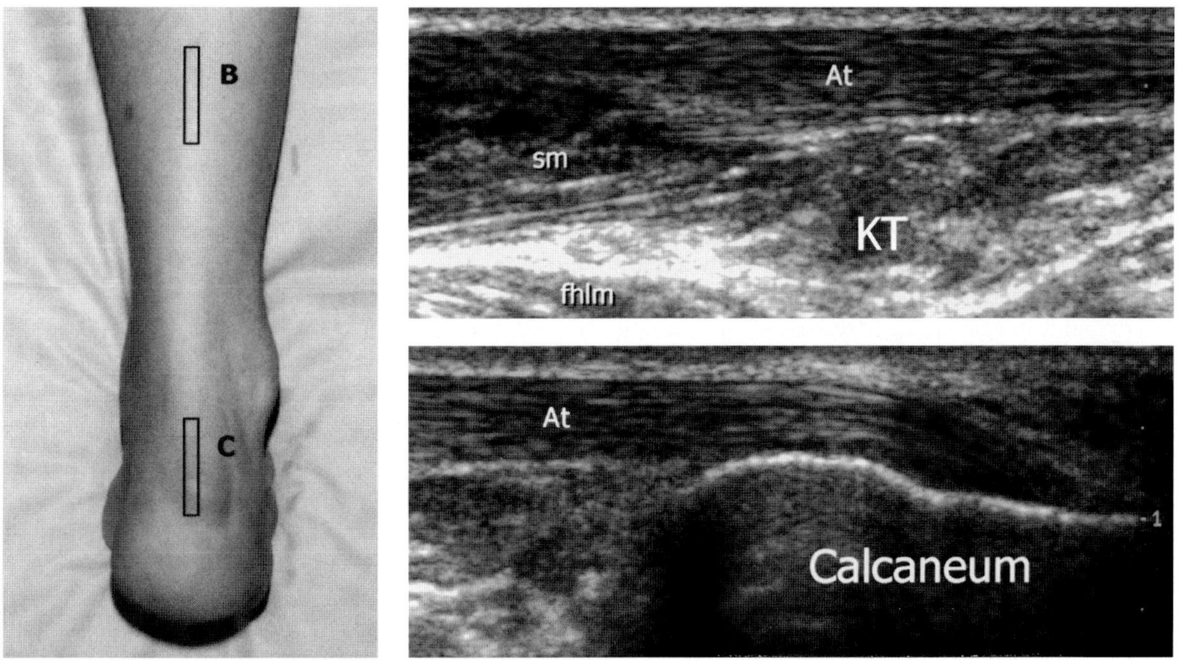

Fig. 6.9a–c. Posterior aspect. **a** Probe positioning for longitudinal examination of the Achilles tendon. **b,c** Corresponding sonograms obtained from cranial to caudal. *sm*, soleus muscle; *At*, Achilles tendon; *fhlm*, flexor hallucis longus muscle; *KT*, Kager's triangle

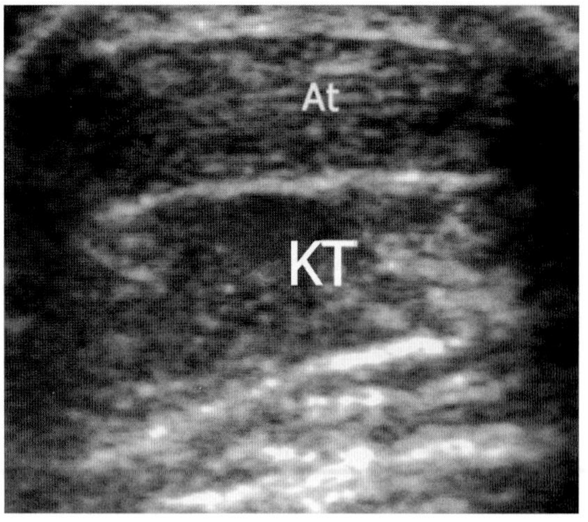

a

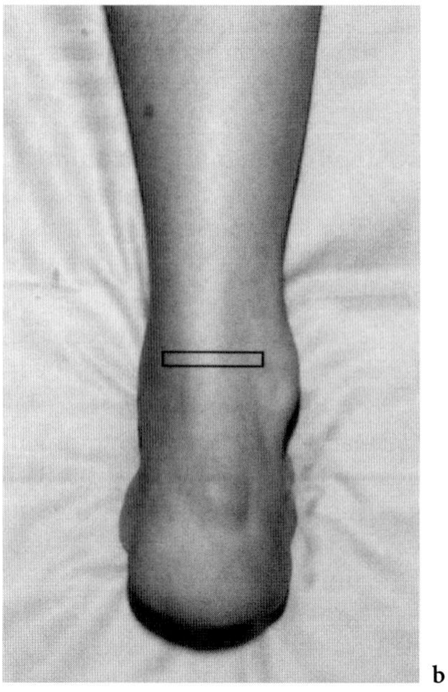

b

Fig. 6.10a,b. Posterior aspect. **a** Probe positioning for transverse examination of the Achilles tendon. **b** Corresponding sonogram. *KT*, Kager's triangle; *At*, Achilles tendon

the triceps surae muscle and inserts on the lower aspect of the posterior tuberosity of the calcaneum. Accurate examination of the proximal tendon reveals two components. The superficial component derives from the gastrocnemius muscle, while the deep one derives from the soleus muscle (Bertolotto et al. 1995). Axial sonograms are always performed since they yield accurate evaluation of the most peripheral area, which can be difficult to assess in longitudinal scans. The tendon has no synovial sheath but is surrounded by a layer of connective tissue, the paratenon, which appears as a regular hyperechoic line. The obliquity of the distal portion of AT can account for a hypoechoic appearance related to anisotropy that must not be interpreted as a focal tendinitis or tear. Changes in the angle of incidence of the US beam are necessary to evaluate this segment correctly. Longitudinal dynamic images obtained during passive flexion and extension of the foot show the smooth gliding of the tendon, and this works well in clinical practice to allow differentiation of partial and complete tears as well as to diagnose peritendinous adhesions.

The plantaris tendon can be identified in transverse images as a hyperechoic structure located at the medial aspect of the Achilles tendon. Identification of the tendon is useful before reconstructive surgery utilizing this tendon as an autologous transplant (Wening et al. 1996).

The normal retroachilles and retrocalcaneal bursae are rarely demonstrated as thin hypoechoic structures located, respectively, posterior to the TA and between it and the posterior tubercle of the calcaneum. Anterior to the AT, Kager's triangle appears as an adipose structure containing fibrous septa. An accessory soleus muscle can be found between the AT and the posterior aspect of the ankle (Palaniappan et al. 1999). US demonstrates it as a space-occupying lesion which presents with a normal muscle structure (Bianchi et al. 1995). The US diagnosis is obvious if this condition is kept in mind.

Deep to Kager's triangle, the myotendinous junction and supramalleolar portion of the flexor hallucis longus tendon as well as the posterior ankle recess can be demonstrated. In evaluating the deep posterior aspect of the ankle joint, care must be taken to adjust the focus of the US beam at the level of the tail of the talus. In larger ankles, a 5-MHz probe must be deployed. The posterior ankle recess fills with dorsal flexion of the ankle and is located between the posterior tibial malleolus and the talar queue but is hard to demonstrate in normal ankles. The posterior subtalar recess can be imaged only if distended by pathological effusion; it appears as an anechoic mass located between the talus and the calcaneum.

References

Bertolotto M, Perrone R, Martinoli C et al (1995) High resolution US anatomy of normal Achilles tendon. Br J Radiol 68:986–991

Bianchi S, Martinoli C (1999) Detection of loose bodies in joints. Radiol Clin North Am 37:679–90

Bianchi S, Abdelwahab IF, Oliveri M et al (1995) Sonographic diagnosis of accessory soleus muscle mimicking a soft tissue tumor. J Ultrasound Med 14:707–709

Brasseur JL, Luzzati A, Lazennec JY et al (1994) Ultrasono-anatomy of the ankle ligaments. Surg Radiol Anat 16:87–91

Campbell DG, Menz A, Isaacs J (1994) Dynamic ankle ultrasonography. A new imaging technique for acute ankle ligament injuries. Am J Sports Med 22:855–858

Chem RK, Beauregard G, Schmutz GR et al (1993) Ultrasonography of the ankle and the hindfoot. Can Assoc Radiol J 44:337–341

Diaz GC, van Holsbeeck M, Jacobson JA (1998) Longitudinal split of the peroneus longus and peroneus brevis tendons with disruption of the superior peroneal retinaculum. J Ultrasound Med 17:525–529

Fessell DP, van Holsbeeck MT (1999) Foot and ankle sonography. Radiol Clin North Am 37:831–858

Fessell DP, Vanderschueren GM, Jacobson JA et al (1998) US of the ankle: technique, anatomy, and diagnosis of pathologic conditions Radiographics 18:325–340

Friedrich JM, Schnarkowski P, Rubenacker S et al (1993) Ultrasonography of capsular morphology in normal and traumatic ankle joints. J Clin Ultrasound 21:179–187

Hsu TC, Wang CL, Wang TG et al (1997) Ultrasonographic examination of the posterior tibial tendon. Foot Ankle Int 18:34–38

Jacobson JA, Andresen R, Jaovisidha et al (1998) Detection of ankle effusions: comparison study in cadavers using radiography, sonography, and MR imaging. AJR 170: 1231–1238

Kellner H, Spathling S, Herzer P (1992) Ultrasound findings in Lofgren's syndrome: is ankle swelling caused by arthritis, tenosynovitis or periarthritis? J Rheumatol 19:38–41

Koski JM (1990) Ultrasonography of the metatarsophalangeal and talocrural joints. Clin Exp Rheumatol 8: 347–351

Magnano GM, Occhi M, Di Stadio M et al (1998) High-resolution US of non-traumatic recurrent dislocation of the peroneal tendons: a case report. Pediatr Radiol 28:476–477

Martinoli C, Derchi LE, Pastorino C et al (1993) Analysis of echotexture of tendons with US. Radiology 186:839

Martinoli C, Bianchi S, Derchi LE (1999) Ultrasound of tendon and nerves. Radiol Clin North Am 37:691–711

Martinoli C, Bianchi S, Gandolfo N et al (2000) US of nerve entrapments in osteofibrous tunnels of the upper and lower limbs. Radiographics 20 [Spec No]:S199–S217

Milz P, Milz S, Putz R et al (1996) 13 MHz high-frequency sonography of the lateral ankle joint ligaments and thetibiofibular syndesmosis in anatomic specimens J Ultrasound Med 15:277–284

Morvan G, Mathieu P, Busson J, Wybier M (2000) Ultrasonography of tendons and ligaments of foot and ankle. J Radiol 81:361–380

Nazarian LN, Rawool NM, Martin CE et al (1995) Synovial fluid in the hindfoot and ankle: detection of amount and distribution with US. Radiology 197:275–278

Palaniappan M, Rajesh A, Rickett A et al (1999) Accessory soleus muscle: a case report and review of the literature. Pediatr Radiol 29:610–612

Rockett MS (1999) The use of ultrasound in the foot and ankle. J Am Podiatr Med Assoc 89:331–338

Roy S, Dewitz A, Paul I (1999) Ultrasound-assisted ankle arthrocentesis. Am J Emerg Med 17:300–301

Simonetti S, Bianchi S, Martinoli C (1999) Neurophysiological and ultrasound findings in sural nerve lesions following stripping of the small saphenous vein. Muscle Nerve 22: 1724–1726

Thermann H, Hoffmann R, Zwipp H et al (1992) The use of ultrasonography in the foot and ankle. Foot Ankle 13:386–390

Wening JV, Katzer A, Phillips F et al (1996) Detection of the tendon of the musculus plantaris longus – diagnostic imaging and anatomic correlate. Unfallchirurgie 22:30–35

7 Intra-articular Injections of the Ankle and Foot

B. J. De Michaelis, S. L. Burrows, T. D. Berg, and G. Y. El-Khoury

CONTENTS

7.1 Introduction

Diagnostic injections of the foot are helpful in evaluating the cause of pain in patients who are candidates for arthrodesis, especially when pain management with medication has failed. The clinical diagnosis is often difficult in these cases, and imaging, including CT and MRI, may prove poor or misleading indicators of the pain source (Newberg 1998; Michell et al. 1995; Khoury et al. 1996). Surgical therapy is often altered by the results of such diagnostic injections (Newberg 1998; Lucas et al. 1997). Specifically, the decision of which and how many joints to fuse can be aided by these procedures (Chow and Brandser 1998). Pain relief from the diagnostic injection of an anesthetic correlates well with symptomatic relief from arthrodesis (Chow and Brandser 1998; Khoury et al. 1996).

B.J. De Michaelis, MD
Department of Radiology, University of Iowa Hospitals & Clinics, Iowa City, IA 52242, USA
S.L. Burrows, MD
Professor, Department of Radiology, University of Iowa Hospitals & Clinics, Iowa City, IA 52242, USA
T.D. Berg, MD
Department of Radiology, University of Iowa Hospitals & Clinics, Iowa City, IA 52242, USA
G.Y. El-Khoury, MD
Professor, Department of Radiology, University of Iowa Hospitals & Clinics, Iowa City, IA 52242, USA

Therapeutic administration of intra-articular corticosteroids is often beneficial in cases of inflammatory arthritis as well as osteoarthritis (Fig. 7.1).

Joint injection is generally contraindicated in cases of suspected joint sepsis. This is particularly true of corticosteroid administration (Newberg 1998). Intraarticular extension of a recent fracture also precludes steroid administration. Allergies to iodinated contrast and coagulopathy are relative contraindications. The reported risk of avascular necrosis due to the intra-administration of steroids is extremely low, and the causation not well substantiated; however, limiting the frequency and dosage of such treatment is prudent (Newberg 1998). Other potential complications include bleeding, allergic reaction to iodinated contrast agent, and joint sepsis. Post-injection pain is not infrequent and may relate to several factors. Joint distention causes discomfort at the time of injection and for

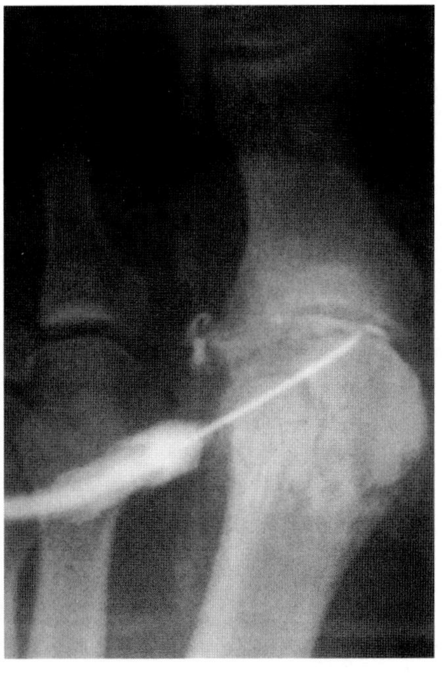

Fig. 7.1. Anteroposterior (AP) injection of 1st metatarsophalangeal (MTP) joint in a patient with osteoarthritis

a short time afterward. Contrast-induced chemical synovitis or steroid-induced (crystal) inflammatory flare may both be seen (NEWBERG 1998; HUGO et al. 1998).

7.2 Technique

In cases of diagnostic injections, fluoroscopic confirmation of intra-articular administration of the anesthetic or steroid is critical to the accuracy of the procedure. Spot films must be obtained for documentation. Obtaining spot films at different stages of the procedure (i.e., early in the procedure and upon completion) has been advocated and stresses the importance of this confirmation (NEWBERG 1998) (Fig. 7.2). Another critical aspect is documentation of any change in symptoms. The patient must be questioned before and after the procedure about the degree of symptomatic relief from the injection. Often, the patient is then examined by the referring clinician after the procedure. For patients with osteoarthritis or inflammatory arthritis involving specific joints, therapeutic injections may be performed for pain relief only.

The technique involved in joint injections begins with reviewing any prior imaging studies. The patient is then positioned to facilitate injection of the selected joint. The skin is marked, and any adjacent vascular structures are palpated to help prevent inadvertent vascular injury. Using sterile technique and local anesthetic, a needle is advanced under imaging guidance to the target. Often a 22-gauge needle is adequate for ankle and hindfoot injections; a 23- or 25-gauge needle may be required for small joints (i.e., intertarsal joints). Iodinated contrast is injected initially to confirm an intraarticular location. While air contrast may be useful to document the position in large joints, it is difficult to use in smaller joints. A small amount of iodinated contrast is typically used. The choice of administered medication should reflect the desired result. The anesthetic may be short-acting or long-acting. If successive joints are to be injected on the same day, then shorter-acting agents may be preferred. A longer-acting anesthetic is often used for single-joint injections and is often effective for several hours. This ensures a continued therapeutic effect if the patient goes on to be seen by the clinician after the procedure. The combination of anesthetic and steroid preparation is useful to immediately reduce the pain and allow the required time for the steroid to become effective. Various steroid preparations are marketed, and each has its respective merits (NEWBERG 1998). The steroid preparation we currently use most frequently is Celestone Soluspan (a combination of betamethasone sodium phosphate and betamethasone acetate). For the anesthetic, we use Bupivacaine 0.25% when a longer-acting agent is indicated, and preservative-free Lidocaine 1% as the

a b

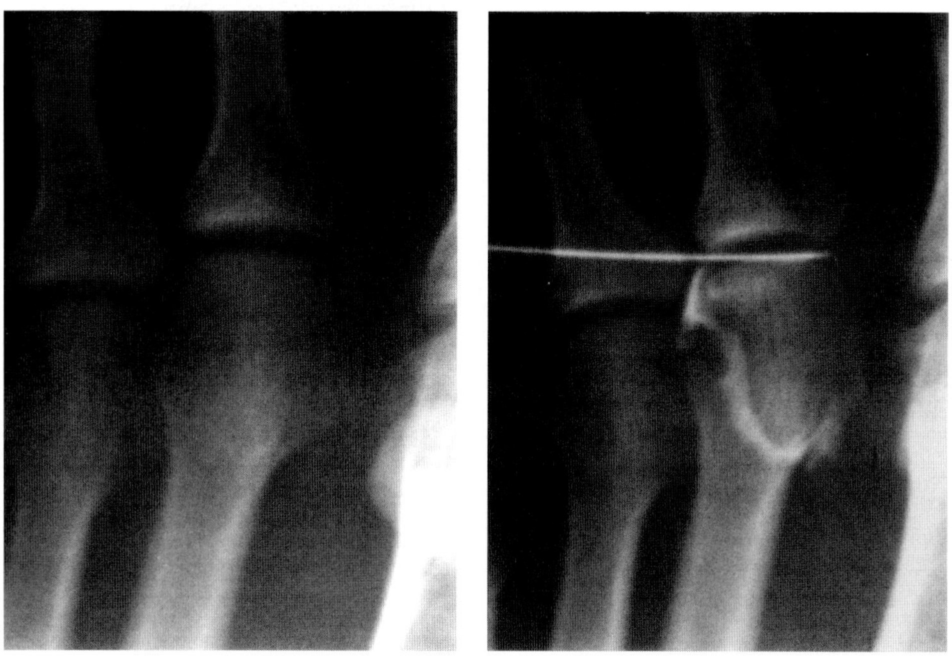

Fig. 7.2a,b. Pre-injection (**a**) and post-injection (**b**) spot films of 3rd MTP joint

shorter-acting agent. Care must be taken to ensure compatibility between the anesthetic and steroid preparation. The preservatives used in anesthetic preparations may cause precipitation of the steroid suspension.

Overall, the injection of anesthetic with or without steroid into joints of the foot and ankle provides useful diagnostic information and therapeutic relief (Chow and Brandser 1998). Osteoarthritis, both primary and secondary after trauma or inflammatory arthritis, is the most common cause of foot pain in this population. Occasionally, congenital abnormalities such as tarsal coalition or an accessory ossicle are the source of discomfort (Chow and Brandser 1998). Often, more than a single joint of the hindfoot or midfoot is injected during a single session. The patient is asked to rate the pain on a 1 (barely noticeable) to 10 (severest imaginable) scale, and the result is recorded. After each injection, the patient is ambulated, and maneuvers which ordinarily exacerbate the pain are attempted. The patient is asked to regrade the pain, and subsequent injections may be performed if symptoms persist. Often the response is fairly dramatic, and the patient must be encouraged to try to reproduce the symptoms. Communication between specific intertarsal joints is frequent and should be documented to acknowledge the treatment of more than one joint with a single injection.

7.2.1 Specific Joints

7.2.1.1 *Ankle*

There is a redundancy of the anterior and posterior portions of the ankle joint capsule. Access is obtained via an anterior approach. The patient is positioned supine with the knee slightly flexed, and the dorsalis pedis artery is palpated. The tibialis anterior (TA) and the extensor hallucis longus (EHL) tendons can be palpated by dorsiflexion of the foot and the great toe, respectively. The skin entry site is between the TA and EHL tendons. The patient is then placed in lateral decubitus, so that the dorsum of the foot is toward the radiologist. A 22-gauge needle is advanced under the anterior lip of the tibia and positioned in the joint under fluoroscopic guidance (Fig. 7.3). If difficulty is encountered, the foot can be plantar flexed to widen the anterior tibiotalar joint.

7.2.1.2 *Subtalar Joint*

The posterior subtalar joint is a frequent source of pain. Three approaches have been used to access this joint. We routinely use a *posterolateral* approach (Fig. 7.4a). The region of the lateral malleolus is prepared, and the needle is angled into the subtalar joint from a point just lateral to the Achilles tendon. With the lateral aspect of the foot facing the image intensifier, the posterolateral aspect of the joint can be accessed under direct visualisation. A fraction of a millilitre of contrast confirms the location in these smaller joints. Anesthetic is then administered. Other techniques have been described. The *anterolateral* approach (Fig. 7.4b) targets the anterior and lateral aspect of the posterior joint (at the crucial angle of Gisane) from a more direct lateral to medial needle orientation. The *posteromedial* approach begins posterior to the posterior tibial artery pulsation. The needle is oriented at an anterosuperior angle toward the posteromedial aspect of the joint (Ruhoy et al. 1998). Familiarity with these techniques and the underlying neurovascular and tendinous anatomy facilitates joint access in certain cases of advanced degenerative change or traumatic deformity. The subtalar joint may communicate with the ankle joint in 10% of cases (Chow and Brandser 1998).

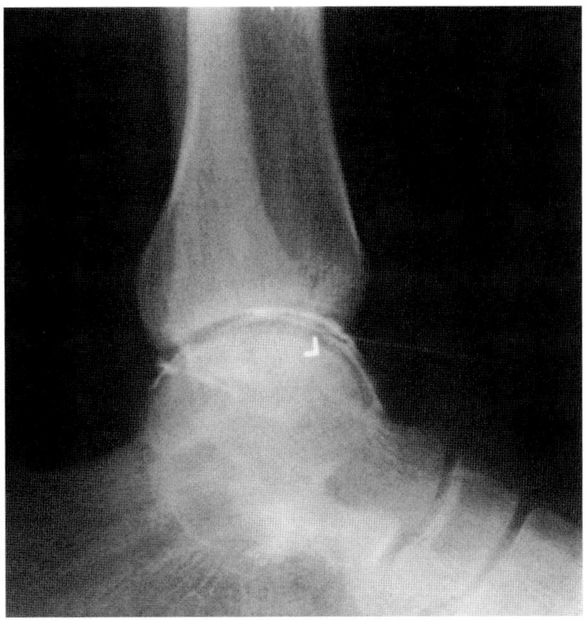

Fig. 7.3. Anterior approach for injection of left ankle joint

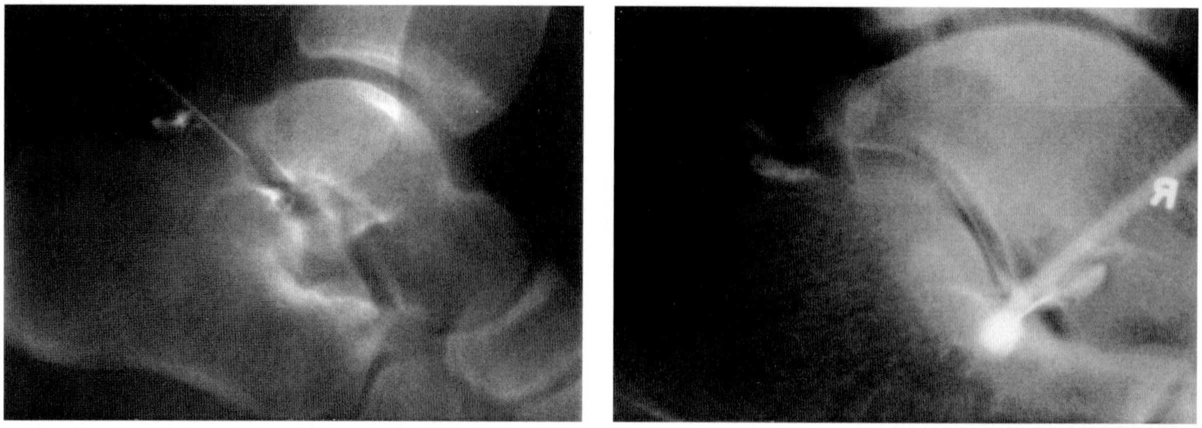

Fig. 7.4a,b. Subtalar joint injections from the posterior (a) and lateral (b) approaches

7.2.1.3 Talonavicular Joint

The talonavicular joint is easily injected from an anterior approach (i.e. through the dorsum of the foot)(Fig. 7.5). The foot is examined prior to sterile preparation. The foot is placed flat on the fluoroscopy table. The orientation of the joint is placed in line with the X-ray beam with dorsiflexion and maintained in this position by placing towels beneath the forefoot. If needed, the foot is placed with the medial side up and the needle advanced under direct fluoroscopic visualization. This joint routinely communicates with the middle subtalar joint and, for this reason, is also termed the talocalcaneonavicular joint (Chow and Brandser 1998; Pavlov 1979). This injection will therefore involve the middle talocalcaneal facet as well.

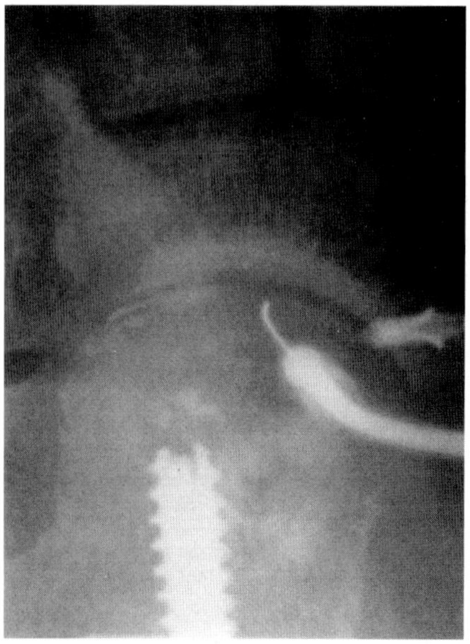

Fig. 7.5. AP view of talonavicular joint injection from anterior approach

7.2.1.4 Midfoot Joints

Midfoot joints can be injected through similar approaches with varying degrees of obliquity. Positioning is facilitated with the knee bent and internal/external rotation at the hip. The lateral oblique approach is used for the more lateral joints. Continuity between many of these joints should be considered when contemplating these injections. The naviculocuneiform joint communicates with the intercuneiforms, the lateral cuneocuboid, and the naviculocuboid joint when developed. The first tarsometarsal joint does not communicate with other joints. The second and third communicate with each other, as do the fourth and fifth (Chow and Brandser 1998; Resnick and Niwayama 1995) (Fig. 7.6).

7.2.1.5 Metatarsophalangeal Joints

Injection of the metatarsophalangeal (MTP) or interphalangeal joints requires distal angulation of the needle to pass beneath the dorsal lip of the phalangeal base. These joints can be accessed under fluoroscopic visualisation with the foot in a lateral position after marking the area in the anteroposterior position (Fig. 7.1).

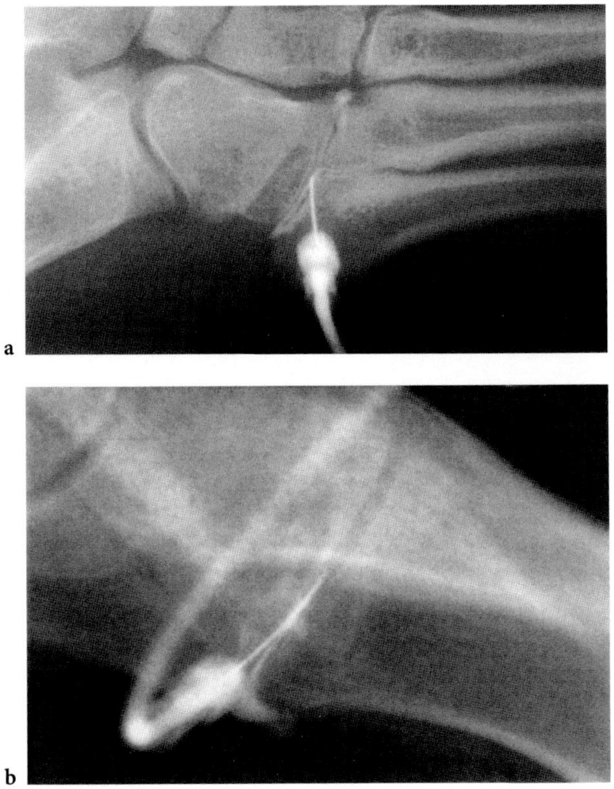

Fig. 7.6a,b. Demonstration of communication between 4th and 5th metatarsal joint (**a**) with lateral view of medial cuneiform 1st metatarsal injection (**b**)

7.2.1.6 Os Trigonum

In some patients who perform repetitive activities requiring pronounced plantar flexion, posterior ankle impingement (PAI) syndrome can develop. This syndrome is classically described in ballet dancers but can also be seen in individuals who are active in sports and those in non-sport-related activities (Bureau et al. 2000). With plantar flexion, there is compression of the posterior talus and the surrounding soft tissues between the posterior tibia and the calcaneous. This has been likened to a nut in a nutcracker (Hedrick and McBryde 1994). This compression of the posterior process of the talus and/or the ostrigonum can cause inflammation and pain. Also, there can be a fracture of the posterior process of the talus, with subsequent pseudoarthrosis mimicking an os trigonum. However, the flexor hallucis longus (FHL) and the posterior facet of the subtalar joint are in close proximity and may also cause pain in this region.

For both diagnostic and therapeutic purposes, the synchondrosis between the os trigonum and the talus can be injected with anesthetic and steroid to confirm the diagnosis of PAI syndrome and to provide therapeutic pain relief. A posteromedial approach is optimal (Hedrick and McBryde 1994), and contrast is injected to confirm the needle position and to assess for any joint communication.

References

Bureau NJ, Cardinal E, Hobdon R, Aubin B (2000) Posterior ankle impingement syndrome: MR imaging findings in seven patients. Radiology 215:497–503

Chow S, Brandser E (1998) Diagnostic and therapeutic foot and ankle injections. Semin Musculoskeletal Radiol 2: 421–431

Hedrick MR, McBryde AM (1994) Posterior ankle impingement. Foot Ankle 15:2–8

Hugo PC, Newberg AH, Newman JS, Wetzner SM (1998) Complications of arthrography. Semin Musculoskeletal Radiol 2:345–348

Khoury NJ, El-Khoury GY, Saltzman CL, Brandser EA (1996) Intra-articular foot and ankle injections to identify source of pain before arthrodesis. AJR 167:669–673

Lucas PE, Hurwitz SR, Kaplan PA, Dussault RG, Maurer EJ (1997) Fluoroscopically guided injections into the foot and ankle: localization of the source of pain as a guide to treatment – prospective study. Radiology 204:411–415

Mitchell MJ, Bielecki D, Bergman AG, Kursunoglu-Brahme S, Sartoris DJ, Resnick D (1995) Localization of specific joint causing hindfoot pain: value of injecting local anesthetics in to individual joints during arthrography. AJR 164:1473–1476

Newberg AH (1998) Anesthetic and corticosteroid joint injections: a primer. Semin Musculoskeletal Radiol 2: 415–420

Pavlov H (1979) Talo-calcaneonavicular arthrography. In: Freiburger RH, Kaye JJ, Spiller J (eds) Arthrography. Appleton-Century-Crofts, New York, pp 257–260

Resnick D, Niwayama G (1995) Anatomy of individual joints. In: Resnick D (ed) Diagnosis of bone and joint disorders. Saunders, Philadelphia, pp 762–764

Ruhoy MK, Newberg AH, Yodlowski ML, Mizel MS, Trepman E (1998) Subtalar joint arthrography. Semin Musculoskeletal Radiol 2:433–437

Clinical Problems

8 Congenital and Developmental Disorders

P. Renton

CONTENTS

P. Renton, FRCR
Consultant Radiologist, Royal National Orthopaedic Hospital, London W1W 5AQ, and University College London Hospitals, London WC1E 3BG, UK

8.1 Congenital Limb Deficiency

Limb deficiencies are usually sporadic but, if associated with other abnormalities, have an incidence in further pregnancies of up to 50% (Evans et al. 1991).

The incidence of limb deficiency is 1:2000 live births. Most syndromes with limb defects affect the upper limb; only a few affect both or just the lower limb (Table 8.1).

In 1989 an International Standard for the Nomenclature of Congenital Limb Deficiency was produced by the 'Kay' Committee of the International Organisation for Standardisation (ISO) in Geneva (Day 1991). The use of classical Greek terms, such as hemimelia, is to be avoided – the world no longer has the benefit of a classical education. The Standard therefore describes deficiencies as:

- *Transverse*, where the limb resembles an amputation, beyond which no skeletal development is seen, or
- *Longitudinal*, where there is absence or reduction of part of a limb along the long axis of the limb.

Total absence of the hemipelvis and distal elements is a *transverse* deficiency. These are described by naming (1) the segment at which the limb terminates and (2) describing the level with the segment beyond which no skeleton is seen, e.g. transverse tarsal total deficiency (Table 8.2).

If a *portion* of the hemipelvis is absent, the deficiency is *longitudinal*. Longitudinal defects may have skeletal elements distal to the deficiency. The deficient bones are named proximo-distally. Bones present and normal are not named.

Numbering of rays or digits in the foot starts on the tibial side (Fig. 8.1), e.g. longitudinal tibial total tarsus partial ray 1 total.

8.2 Proximal Femoral Deficiencies

Torode and Gillespie (1991) classify deficiencies into two groups. In group I the patients have a congenitally short femur, and the foot is (presumably) normal. In group II there may be a variable fibular deficiency, with a short fibula and valgus deformity at the ankle or, in severely affected cases, a deficient foot with absent rays (Fig. 8.2). Deficiency of bony elements may only become obvious during skeletal maturation.

8.3 Amniotic Band Syndrome (Streeter's Bands)

These bands apparently arise when the fetal limb penetrates a defect in the amniotic sac (Fig. 8.3).

Table 8.1. Syndromes presenting with lower limb deficiency (after Evans et al. 1991)

Aetiology	Syndrome	Lower limb deficiency
Single gene disorders:		
Autosomal dominant	EEC	Split hand/foot (ectrodactly)
	Adams Oliver	Transverse defect
	Split hand/foot	Split hand/foot
Autosomal recessive	Roberts	Longitudinal affecting whole limb
	Grebe	Hypoplastic radii, ulnae, tibiae
	Split hand/foot	Split hand/foot
X-linked recessive	Split hand/foot	Split hand/foot
Drugs	Alcohol	Longitudinal, all degrees
	Thalidomide	Longitudinal, all degrees
	Aminopterin	Hypoplasia (forearm), hypodactyly
	Varicella	Hypoplasia and hypodactyly
Infection associated with maternal diabetes	Caudal dysplasia	Hypoplasia of lower limb
	Femoral hypoplasia+unusual facies	Hypoplasia/absence of femur, fibula and humerus

Table 8.2. Designation of levels of transverse deficiencies of lower limb (after Day 1991)

Total	Pelvis[a]
Total	Thigh
Upper third	
Middle third	
Lower third	
Total	Leg
Upper third	
Middle third	
Lower third	
Total partial	Tarsal[b]
Total partial	Metatarsal[b]
Total partial	Phalangeal[b] (toe)

[a] Total absence of the hemipelvis (and all distal elements) is a transverse deficiency. If only a portion of the hemipelvis is absent, the deficiency is of the longitudinal type

[b] The skeletal elements marked are used as adjectives in describing transverse deficiencies, e.g. transverse tarsal total deficiency

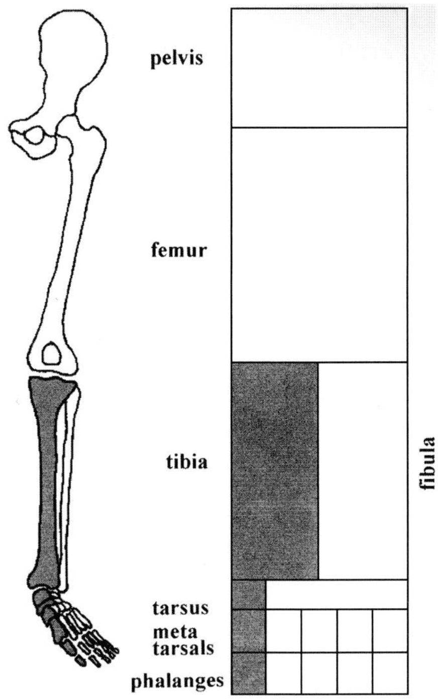

Fig. 8.1. Example of a longitudinal deficiency shown on the skeleton, together with Day's stylised representation (redrawn from DAY 1991)

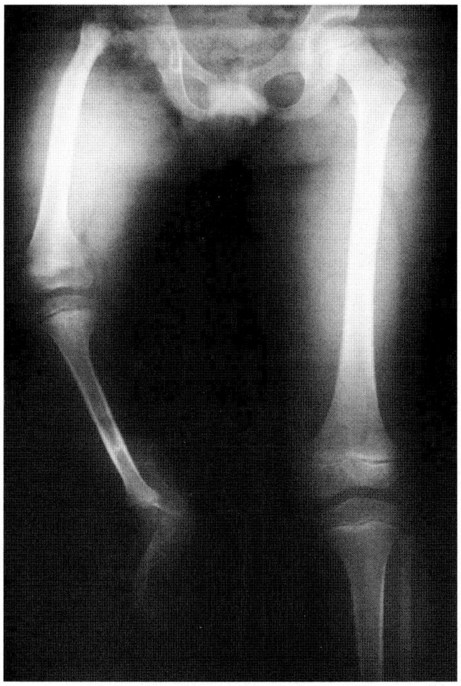

Fig. 8.2. Proximal femoral focal deficiency. There is congenital coxa vara. The proximal femur is hypoplastic. The femur as a whole is shortened, and the patella laterally subluxed. The tibia is also hypoplastic; the fibula exists only distally. The tarsus is defective; defects of the metatarsus and phalanges are noted

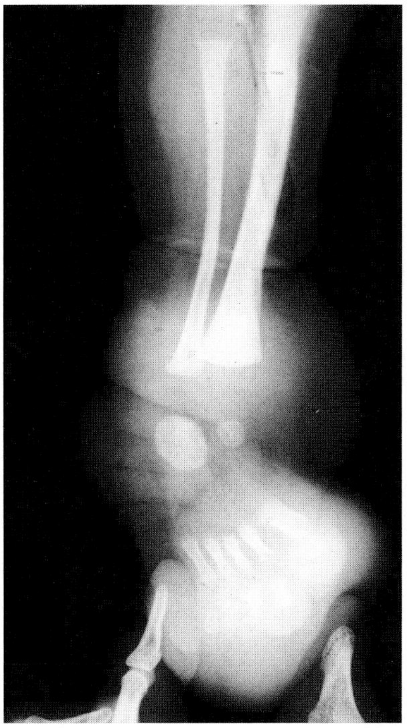

Fig. 8.3. Streeter's bands. Many bands of constriction are demonstrated in the soft tissues associated with intervening areas of soft-tissue thickening. Bone deformity is shown

The margins of the defect constrict the soft tissues and may amputate the underlying bone.

8.4 Foot Deformity in Children

In order to understand foot deformities in children, an appreciation of the normal anatomy is necessary. Besides the development of the skeletal tissue with growth, relationships between the bones of the foot change with age.

HOERR et al. (1962) list the time of appearance for the ossification centres in the foot for boys and girls (Fig. 8.4). The centres of ossification in individual bones may be central or eccentrically situated, but in the latter case, it is evident that as ossification proceeds, the *apparent* relationship between the bones of the foot alters. GAMBLE and YALE (1975) note that the talus seems to project beyond the calcaneus before 2 years of age because ossification is in its head rather than in the posterior part of the bone, while conversely there is more ossification in the posterior part of the calcaneus. Between 2 and 5 years of age, the posterior aspect of the talus ossifies, as does the

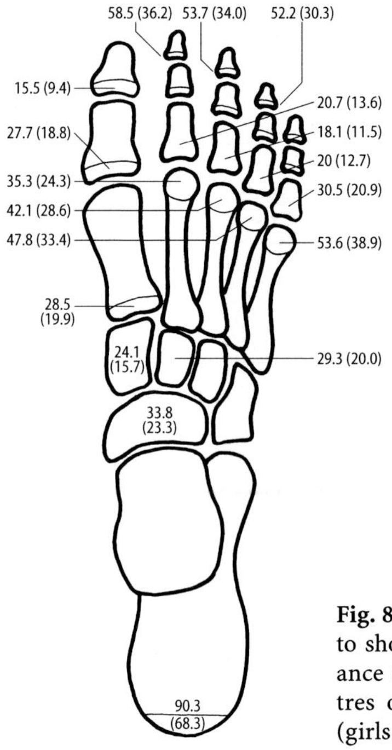

Fig. 8.4. Diagram of the foot to show the times of appearance (in months) of the centres of ossification for boys (girls in brackets)

8.4.1 Talipes Deformity

Talipes (from the Latin: *talus* ankle, *pes* foot) is defined as a congenital deformity of the foot, which is twisted out of shape or position (Fig. 8.5). *Talipes equinovarus* accounts for 75% of these (Gamble and Yale 1975).

8.4.1.1 Heel Valgus and Heel Varus

The normal heel, that is, the calcaneus, as seen from behind slants outwards by 5°–10° away from the midline. If the angle is increased above 10°, the heel is in *valgus*. Similarly, if the heel is adducted so that it points inward, it is in *varus*.

Freiberger et al. (1970) noted that when the heel is in valgus, on the AP radiograph the long axis of the talus lies *medial* to the first metatarsal but, when in varus, it lies *lateral* to the first metatarsal.

The lateral view radiograph then reflects these changes. In heel valgus, support is withdrawn from the anterior talus, which becomes disto-plantarflexed. The anterior part of the calcaneus, so that the apparent space between the two bones lessens.

In children, a line drawn through the long axis of the talus points to the head of the first metatarsal, and a line through the long axis of the calcaneus points to the head of the fourth metatarsal. The talocalcaneal angle between these two lines varies in normal children, gradually decreasing from infancy to 5 years of age. The lines of the metatarsal shafts are parallel in infants (Davis and Hatt 1955).

Altman (1968) examined 258 feet in the lateral plane in children aged from 6 months to 18 years and showed that the calcaneal pitch increased and the talar declination decreased up to 6 years of age. Templeton et al. (1965) examined 160 feet in the weight-bearing AP projection and showed a diminution of the calcaneotalar angle from 30°–50° to 20°–40° from 0 to 5 years of age, after which the angle stabilised. VanderWilde et al. (1988) examined the feet of 74 normal infants and children from 6 to 127 months of age and obtained measurements for 11 useful angles. They, too, showed how the angles change with age.

Measurements must always be assessed with caution. Not only do they change with age, but the angles measured alter with change in position of the foot and of the X-ray beam. If the foot is pronated, the talocalcaneal angle increases, while on the lateral view the calcaneal pitch decreases in pronation.

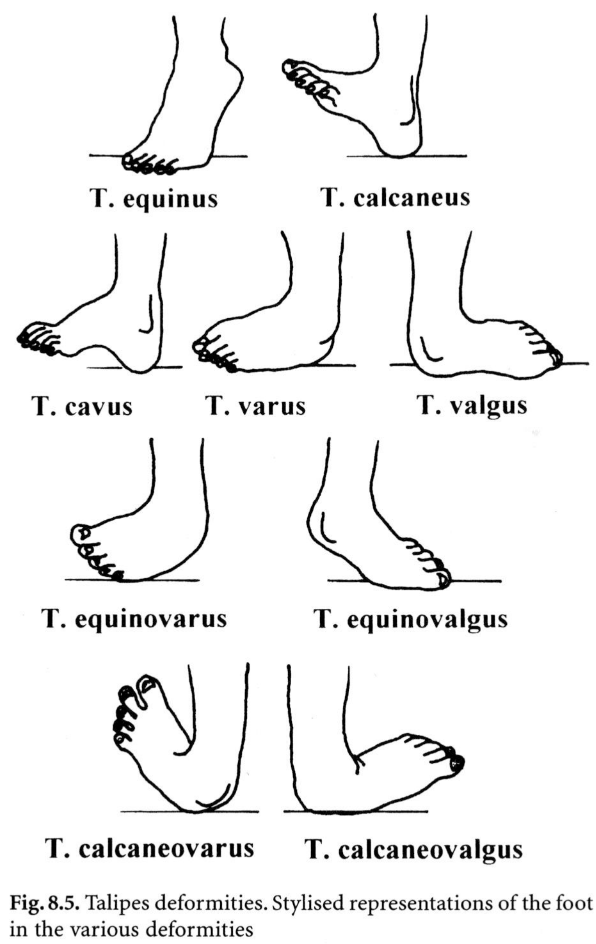

Fig. 8.5. Talipes deformities. Stylised representations of the foot in the various deformities

longitudinal arch flattens. In heel varus, the anterior calcaneus supports the talus, which cannot plantarflex. The long axes of the two bones become parallel.

8.4.1.2 Talipes Equinovarus (Clubfoot)

Congenital talipes equinovarus was first described by Hippocrates in 400 BC. The deformity occurs in 1.2:1000 live births in the United Kingdom, but is more common in Hawaiians (6.8:1000) and less common in Orientals (0.6:1000). If one child in a family is affected, the risk that a second will also be affected is 1 in 35 (Porter 1995). Clinically, the hindfoot is in equinus and varus; the forefoot is also in equinus and varus (Fixsen 1991).

Radiologically, on the AP view, the heel is in varus, and the forefoot is also adducted in varus (toward the midline). The talocalcaneal angle is narrowed, and the talus and calcaneus are parallel (Fig. 8.6). On the lateral view the calcaneus is in equinus. The forefoot is plantarflexed and in cavus. The forefoot is also adducted.

8.4.1.3 Talipes Equinus

Here, there is fixed plantar flexion of the calcaneus on the initial radiograph, giving an angle over 90° with the tibia.

8.4.1.4 Talipes Calcaneus

The calcaneus is abnormally dorsiflexed (the opposite of equinus); its anterior end elevates toward the vertical.

8.4.1.5 Talipes Cavus

Increased calcaneal pitch results in a high longitudinal arch of the foot (Fig. 8.7).

8.4.2 Metatarsus Adductus

This is seen either with heel valgus or normal heel alignment. The long axis of the talus is medial to the first metatarsal. The forefoot is in adduction and varus. On the lateral view the talus is disto-plantarflexed, but the calcaneus is *not* in equinus (Fig. 8.8).

8.4.3 Flat Foot

The heel is in valgus. The anterior talus is no longer supported by the calcaneus and is plantarflexed on the

a b c

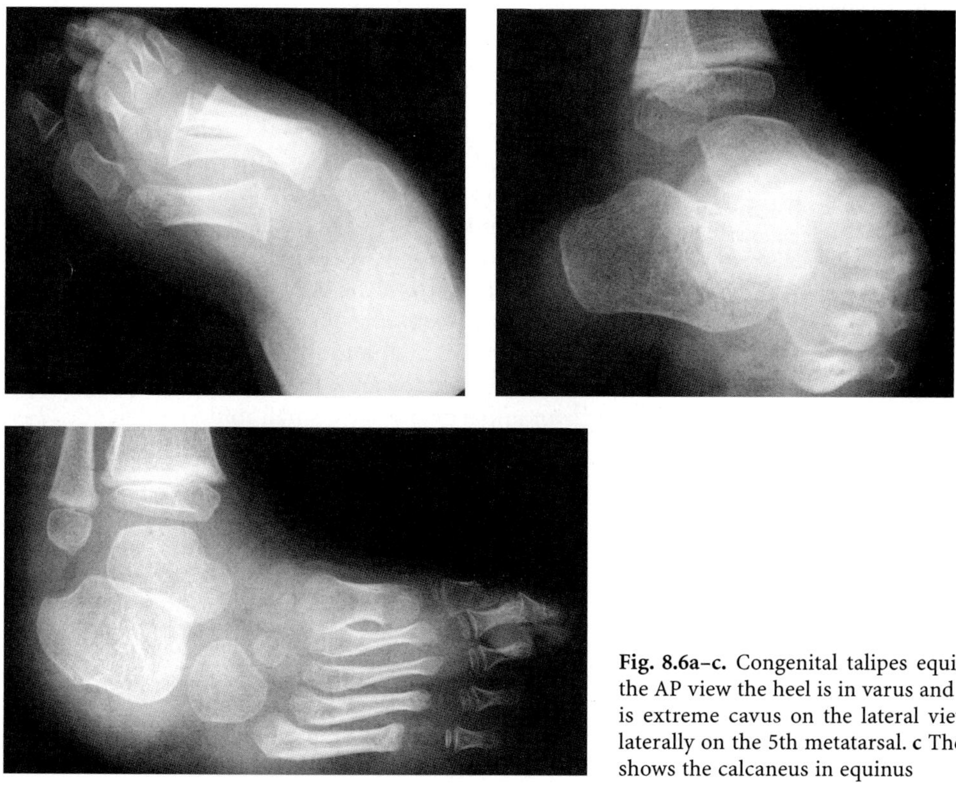

Fig. 8.6a–c. Congenital talipes equinovarus (clubfoot). **a** On the AP view the heel is in varus and the forefoot also. **b** There is extreme cavus on the lateral view. The foot bears weight laterally on the 5th metatarsal. **c** The oblique view of the foot shows the calcaneus in equinus

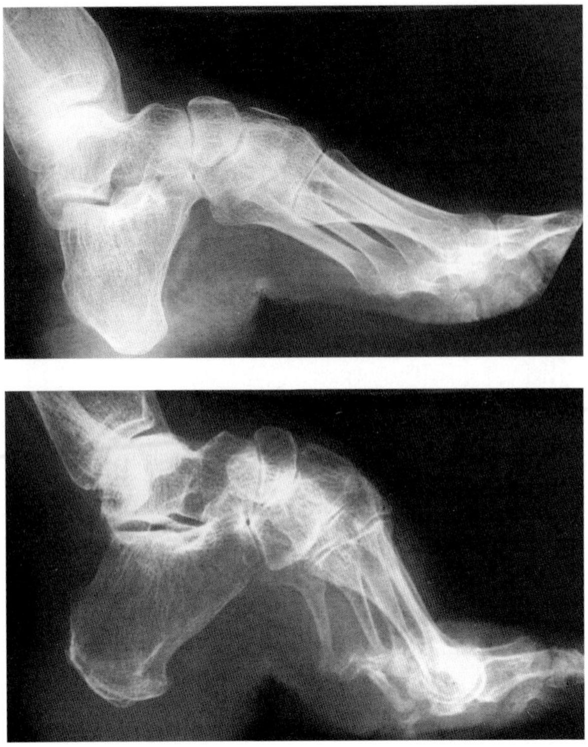

a

b

Fig. 8.7a. Pes cavus – an almost vertical orientation of the calcaneus. There is a soft-tissue deformity of the sole of the foot resulting from the pes cavus. b Chinese bound foot. The appearance is identical in this elderly woman from Liverpool. The soft-tissue deformity is again seen beneath the apex of the curve, but here there is also resorption of the metatarsals and phalanges, especially on the lateral aspect of the foot. The subtalar joints are remarkably well preserved in both cases. (By courtesy of Dr. Mary Cunningham, Fazakerley Hospital, Liverpool)

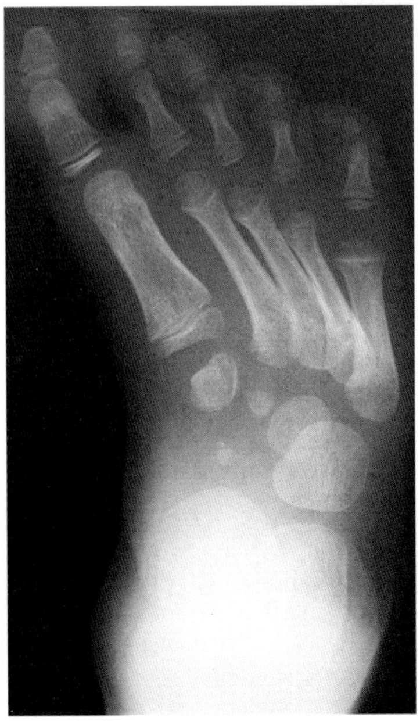

Fig. 8.8. Metatarsus adductus. All the metatarsals are adducted towards the midline

lateral view, in which the calcaneal pitch is plantigrade but not in equinus (Fig. 8.9). The long axis of the talus is no longer in alignment with the first metatarsal, but lies medial to it. The longitudinal arch is flattened.

8.4.4 Congenital Vertical Talus

On the AP view there is gross heel valgus. The long axis of the talus is very medial to the first metatarsal (Fig. 8.10). The forefoot is in valgus. The talocalcaneal angle is markedly increased.

The lateral view shows the heel in equinus (unlike flatfoot) with gross plantarflexion of the anterior calcaneus, giving a rocker-bottom foot. The talus is severely plantarflexed, with the navicular articulating with its neck. The dorsally displaced navicular and tibialis posterior tendon keep the distal talus plantarflexed.

8.5 Failure of Segmentation

8.5.1 Biphalangism

Failure of segmentation is a commonly seen phenomenon in the foot, usually affecting the distal interphalangeal joint of the fifth toe (Fig. 8.11). This innocent lesion occurs in around 35% of Europeans, but in 70% of Japanese. It is also more common in women. While symmetry is the rule, if only one foot is affected, it is usually the left (Venning 1960). The fourth toe is affected in <5%, the third in <2% and the second in <1% of Europeans.

The condition is seen in non-mineralised bone *in utero*, that is, from the very beginning of foot development. The middle phalanges are always smaller than the proximal and distal, and become progressively smaller towards the 5th; feet with biphalangism in particular have small middle phalanges 2–4. Venning believed that before a joint could form, a sufficiency of bone or cartilage had to be present to allow segmentation; if there was an insufficiency, the joint would not form.

8.5.2 Tarsal Coalition

Biphalangism perhaps helps us to understand the basic lesion in tarsal coalition, of which there are two major types.

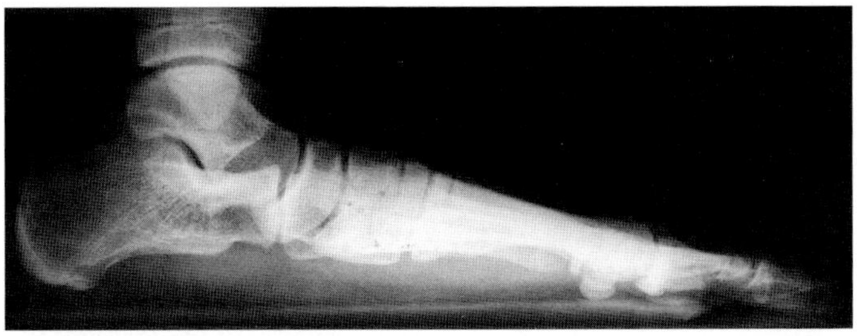

Fig. 8.9. Flat foot. Flattening of the longitudinal arch. The joint spaces are all well preserved

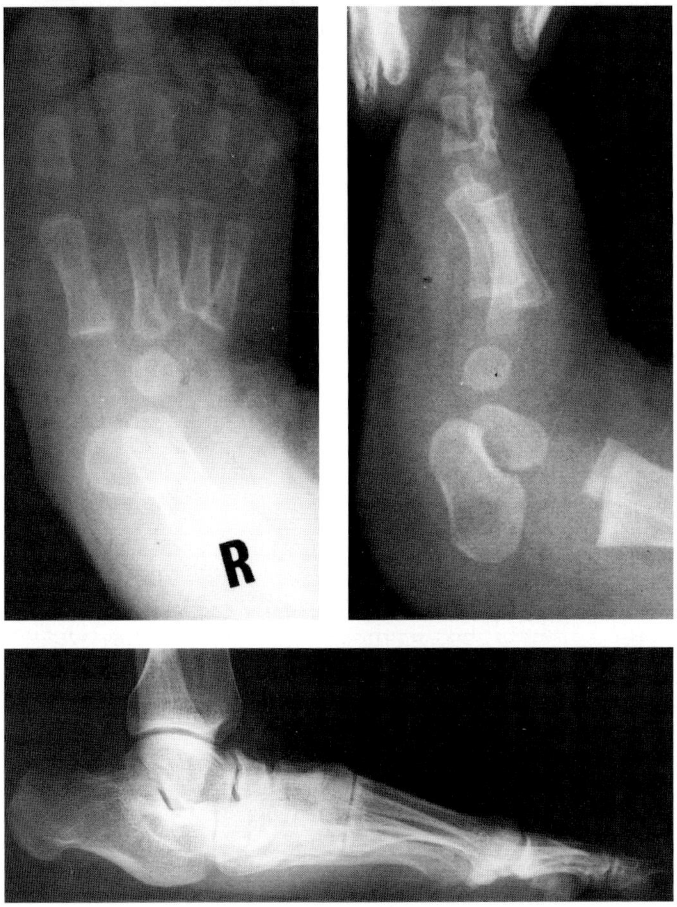

Fig. 8.10a–c. Congenital vertical talus. **a** The anterior view shows calcaneus valgus and metatarsus valgus. The long axis of the talus is very medial to the first metatarsal. **b** On the lateral view equinus of the calcaneus and vertical orientation of the talus are shown. The navicular has not yet ossified. **c** In this adult patient there is a rocker-bottom foot with vertical orientation of the talus. The navicular articulates with the anterior aspect of the talar dome and the neck. There is a flat longitudinal arch

Calcaneonavicular coalition was first described by CRUVEILHIER in 1829, and *talocalcaneal coalition* by ZUCKERKANDL in 1877. The first radiological description of calcaneonavicular coalition was by DWIGHT in 1907. SLOMANN (1926) demonstrated that coalition could be complete or incomplete (Fig. 8.12), so that a pseudarthrosis or cartilaginous coalition could be seen, sometimes with a contained *os secundarium calcis* – said to be present in 1% of the population and not to be confused with a fracture of the anterior process of the calcaneus. SLOMANN too recognised that the coalition was associated with a painful flat foot, as did HARRIS and BEATH (1948) who showed

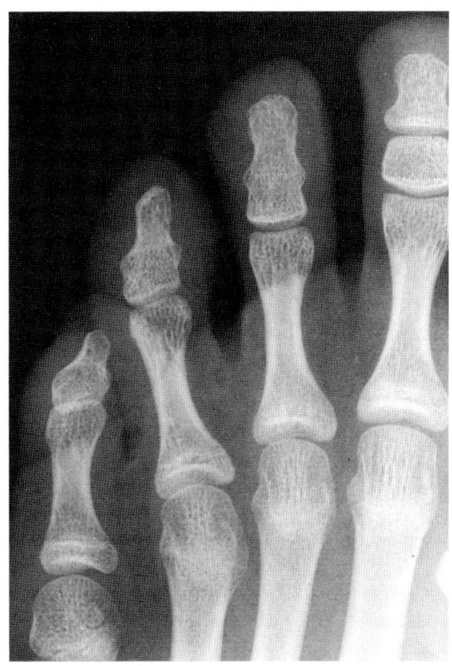

Fig. 8.11. Biphalangism is present at the third to fifth toes. Note the absence of segmentation of the distal interphalangeal joints

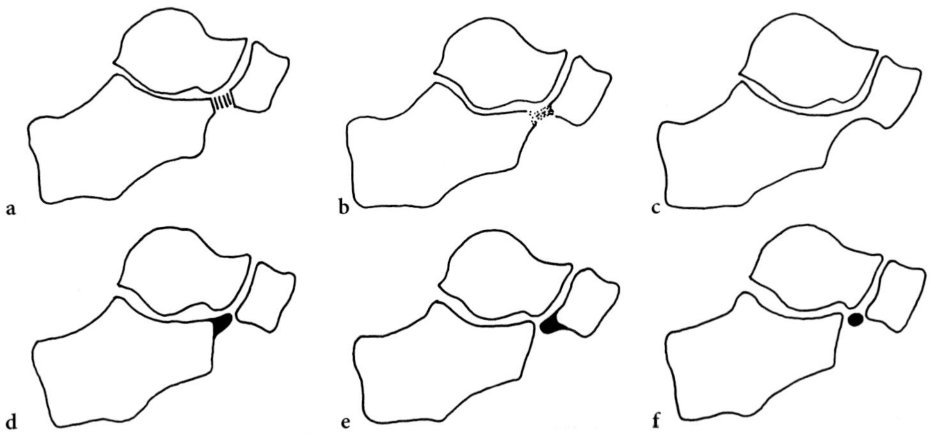

Fig. 8.12. Diagrammatic representation of the types of union: fibrous (*a*), cartilaginous (*b*), osseous (*c*), prominent process on the calcaneum (*d*), prominent process on the navicular (*e*) and separate calcaneonavicular ossicle (calcaneum secundarium) (*f*)

that coalition, occurring in 2% of male recruits into the Canadian army, was associated with the peroneal spastic flat foot syndrome (Table 8.3).

These two hindfoot coalitions are seen, as is biphalangism, *in utero* and so are likely to arise *ab initio* due to failure of segmentation of the cartilaginous primordium. The ossific nuclei for these two bones develop separately in the one piece of cartilage, and the initially cartilaginous bridge between the two allows some movement of the hindfoot. When the bridge becomes totally or partially ossified, however, the synostosis prevents hindfoot movement. Flattening of the longitudinal arch results in stretching of the peroneus longus tendon, which goes into painful spasm.

Talonavicular coalitions ossify at 3–5 years of age, calcaneonavicular at 8–12 years and talocalcaneal coalitions at 12–16 years, at which times they each become symptomatic (Jayakumar and Cowell 1977).

Signs of coalition may be primary or secondary.

Table 8.3. Incidence of causes of peroneal spastic flat foot in the literature (CNF, calcaneonavicular fusion; TCF, talocalcaneal fusion)

References	Cases	TCF	CNF	Both	Other	No bony lesion
Harris and Beath (1948)	17	12	3	0	–	2
Webster and Roberts (1951)	21	4	8	2	–	7
Jack (1954)	30	11	12	0	–	7
Chambers (1950)	17	12	3	–	2 (RA)	–
Harris (1965)	102	66	29	–	7	–

8.5.2.1 Primary Signs of Tarsal Coalition

Calcaneonavicular Coalition. Total or partial coalition is clearly seen on oblique radiographs of the foot (Fig. 8.13). There may be total bony union. With fibrous or cartilaginous union, enlargement of the opposing bony surfaces is seen, with their close approximation often at an irregular pseudarthrosis. Further imaging is not required.

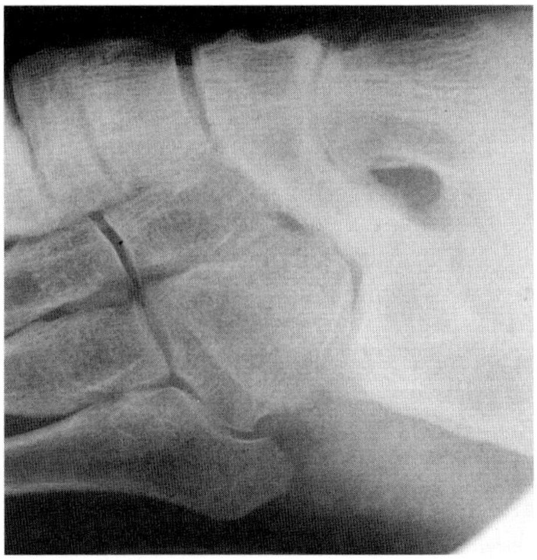

Fig. 8.13. Total calcaneo-navicular synostosis. The oblique view of the foot demonstrates this optimally. The anterior process of the calcaneus is much hypertrophied and fuses with the enlarged adjacent navicular

Talocalcaneal Coalition. The primary sign is the fusion of the subtalar joint, usually at the middle facet or sustentaculotalar articulation. This is demonstrated conventionally using the Harris, or ski-jump, view (Fig. 8.14a), in which the X-ray beam is angled down the joint, which is normally inclined at 30°–40° to the horizontal. However, this form of coalition is best demonstrated on CT scanning. With the foot plantigrade, the hindfeet are scanned axially. Total or partial coalition is clearly visualised, as are stress changes in the adjacent open joints (Fig. 8.14b). These stress changes are often seen as foci of increased uptake on the bone scan (Fig. 8.14c).

MR imaging of the hindfoot demonstrates the coalition, with marrow continuity across the joint (Fig. 8.14d). Emery et al. (1998) compared MRI and CT in the detection of tarsal coalition in 20 patients. CT was as effective as MRI in arriving at the diagnosis and is the more economical option, therefore representing better value for money.

Arthrography has been performed in the investigation of tarsal coalition. The posterior and mid-subtalar joint spaces may be injected directly, while the mid-joint space fills after talonavicular injection (Kaye et al. 1975). Failure to fill the sustentaculotalar joint space is seen with coalition.

8.5.2.2
Secondary Signs of Tarsal Coalition

Lateral weight-bearing plain radiographs demonstrate flattening of the longitudinal arch with non-visualisation of the subtalar joint spaces. In addition, a *talar beak* is seen. This bony prominence arises on the talar ridge, 3–6 mm posterior to the anterior talar articular surface, and is thus proximal to talonavicular osteophytes. The ridge and beak are located at the attachment of the talonavicular ligament. Restriction of movement in patients with coalition causes the navicular to impact on the talus, elevating the talonavicular ligament and periosteum, thus forming the beak (Fig. 8.15).

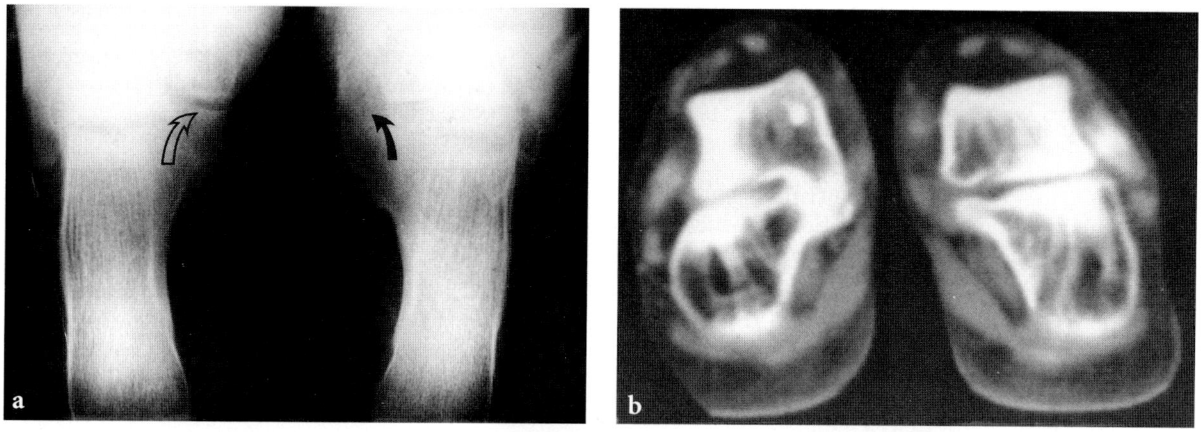

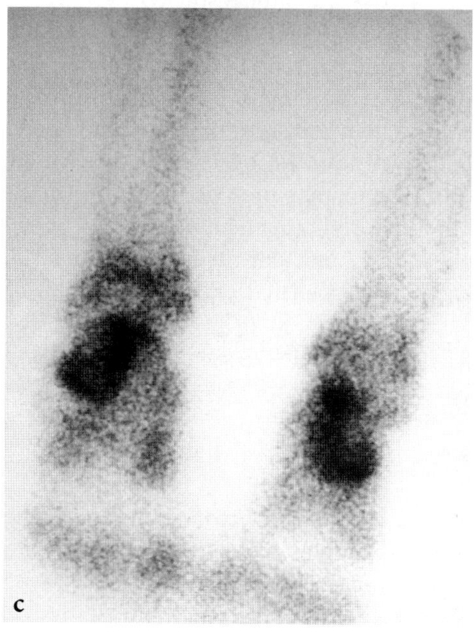

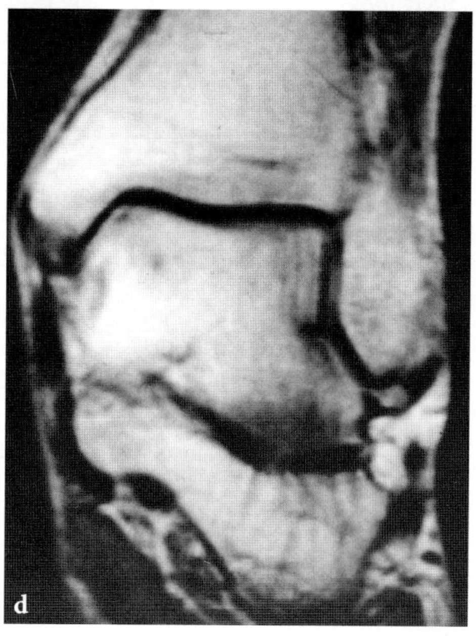

Fig. 8.14a–d. Talo-calcaneal coalition. **a** Axial (Harris) view showing unilateral coalition of the right middle facet (*solid arrow*). The left joint is normal (*open arrow*). **b** CT scan demonstrates fusion of the middle facet of the right subtalar joint. **c** This patient has bilateral talocalcaneal fusion. The bone scan shows a site of symmetrically increased uptake away from the fusion – a stress phenomenon. **d** Obliteration of the subtalar joint is seen on the MR image

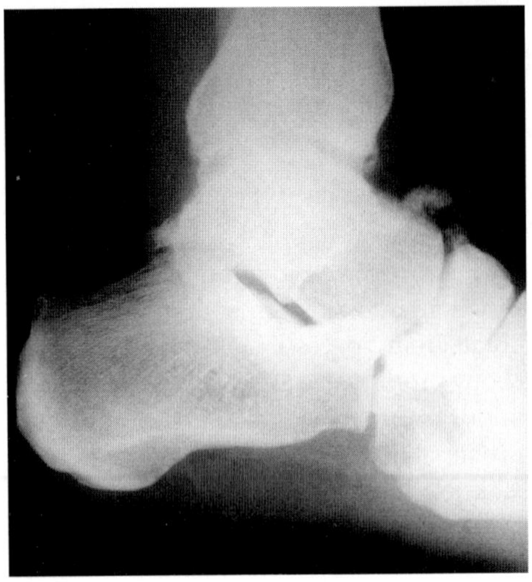

Fig. 8.15. Talar beak. This is an acquired talar beak in a professional football player and is an unusually well developed form of the lesion, occurring at the typical site proximal to the talonavicular articulation

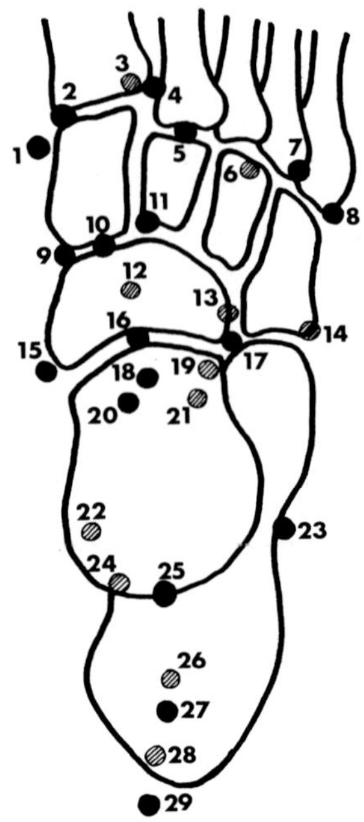

Fig. 8.16. Tarsal accessoria. Redrawn after TROLLE (1948) and O'RAHILLY (1953). TROLLE does not list nos. 12, 27 and 28, but does show an os tuberis calcanei (which could be similar to no. 28). *Black* = dorsal, *hatched* = more plantar. Os sesamoideum tibialis anterior (*1*), os cuneo-metatarsale I tibiale (*2*), os cuneo-metatarsale I plantare (*3*), os intermetatarsale I (*4*), os cuneo-metatarsale II dorsale (*5*), os unci (*6*), os intermetatarsale IV (*7*), os vesalianium (*8*), os paracuneiforme (*9*), os naviculocuneiforme I dorsale (*10*), os intercuneiforme (*11*), os sesamoideum tibialis posterior (according to TROLLE, this may be the same as no. 15) (*12*), os cuboideum secundarium (*13*), os peroneum (*14*), os tibiale (externum) (*15*), os talonaviculare dorsale (*16*), os calcaneus secundarius (*17*), os supertalare (*18*), os trochlare (*19*), os talotibiale dorsale (*20*), os in sinu tarsi (*21*), os sustentaculi proprium (*22*), calcaneus accessorius (*23*), os talocalcaneare (*24*), os trigonum (*25*), os aponeurosis plantaris (*26*), os supracalcaneum (*27*), os subcalcaneum (*28*) and os tendinis Achillis (*29*)

8.6 Accessory Bones in the Foot

Accessory centres of ossification are more commonly seen in the foot than in the hand. Some 50 have been described (HOERR et al. 1962), but only 20 occur with relative frequency. TROLLE (1948) listed 35 and O'RAHILLY (1953) 'about 30'. Figure 8.16 shows the best known ones.

The accessory bones have been defined as 'inconstant, independent, well-defined bones – in an otherwise normally developed foot – the existence of which is not due to a recent minor fracture or other pathological condition no matter whether these bones bear no, or a less, or more intimate relationship to the constant bones, or entirely replace them because of a division of the latter into several segments' (TROLLE 1948). They exist in the fetal foot in a cartilaginous state and develop *ab initio*, but are not seen radiologically until they begin to ossify. Their incidence increases radiologically with age, and the less common accessoria are seen more often when greater numbers of feet are examined. Only a few are commonly seen.

8.6.1 Os Tibiale Externum

The os tibiale externum is seen on the medial or internal aspect of the navicular (Fig. 8.17). It appears at around 10 years of age and accounts for 37% of tarsal accessory bones (SHANDS and WERTS 1953). The navicular may be protuberant medially in the absence of this ossicle. In the presence of the os tibiale externum as a separate bone, soft-tissue swelling is seen to overlie the medial bone protuberance on a plain X-ray. The pseudarthrosis between the navicular and the os tibiale externum may be the site of pain and degeneration, and then will show increased uptake on a radioisotope bone scan. An overlying bursitis may also be painful. The os may then be excised or fused by screw to the underlying navicular.

Occasionally, the navicular itself may be bifid, perhaps congenitally (KEATS 1996) or as a result of trauma.

8.6.2 Os Trigonum

The os trigonum is seen posterior to the talus, the posterior aspect of which may be round and smooth – the usual situation. Around 40% of feet X-rayed show a posterior process, while a separate ossicle

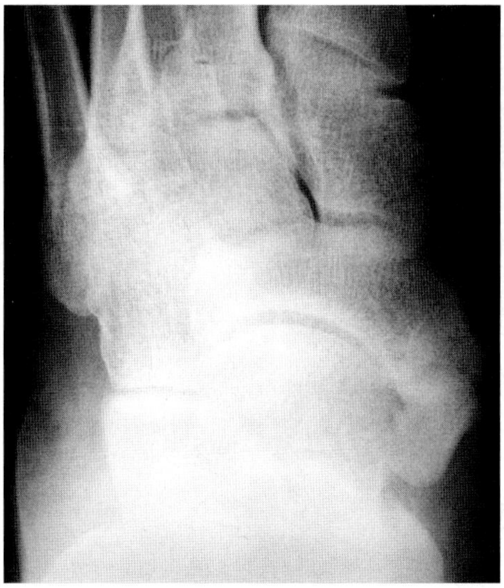
a

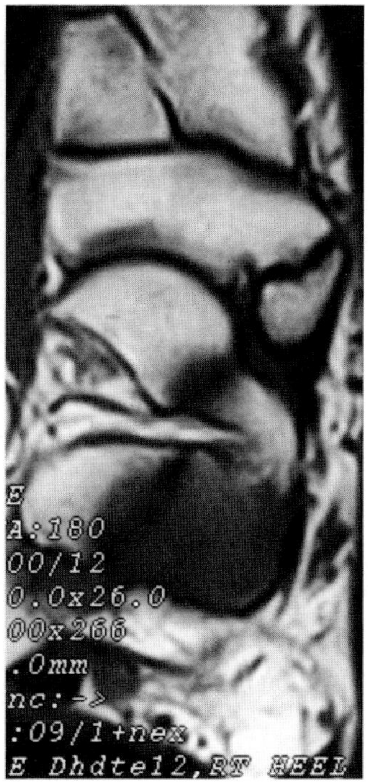
b

Fig. 8.17a,b. Os tibiale externum seen on plain radiography (**a**) and at MR imaging (**b**). The accessory ossicle lies medial to the navicular and enlarges it considerably. Degenerative change is occurring between the two bones

– the os trigonum – may be seen in 3%–15% of the population (Johnson et al. 1984) or in 30% of those with accessory bones (Shands and Werts 1953). This accessory bone is more commonly bilateral than unilateral (6:4).

This bone is of interest in that it was the first occasion in Europe in which an X-ray was used in a court of law, in Germany in 1897. A labourer, injured by an iron bar, complained of continual pain below the lateral malleolus. He was thought to be a malingerer, but a skiagraph showed him to have a 'fracture' of the talus. The labourer received an annuity of 30% but was later seen to be walking normally, and the clinician insisted that *both* feet be examined radiologically. The os trigonum was seen on both sides, and the labourer was forced to repay his annuity (Beck 1900).

Its position renders it liable to trauma in ballet dancers when it is trapped with the foot *en pointe* between the tibia and the calcaneus, and similarly in football players striking the ball.

Pain occurs, and local tenderness may be elicited by pinching the bone between thumb and forefinger anterior to the Achilles tendon. Plain radiographs show sclerosis, and a positive bone scan confirms the pathology (Fig. 8.18a,b). MR images may show local necrosis or inflammation, often with a mixed pattern of increase and decrease in signal (Fig. 8.18c). The radioisotope bone scan is positive at the abnormal os trigonum (Fig. 8.18d). Treatment is by excision.

8.6.3 Os Vesalianium

The os vesalianium is a small ossicle in a mature skeleton at the base of the 5th metatarsal which was first described by Vesalius in 1586 (Saunders and O'Malley 1950). When seen radiologically, it sits in a matching concave defect at the base of the 5th metatarsal (Fig. 8.19) (a similar ossicle exists at the base of the 5th metacarpal). This ossicle at the 5th metatarsal cannot be the local unfused apophysis, which has a different shape and alignment. It may, however, represent a detached and non-united basal tuberosity, but then should not be classified as an accessory ossicle (see definition above). There is thus some doubt as to whether this ossicle is a true accessory bone, but Thurston Holland came to believe in its existence as a rare entity (Holland 1928).

8.6.4 Os Peroneum

The os peroneum is seen in around 9% of feet (Trolle 1948). It lies in the peroneus longus tendon plantar to the calcaneocuboid joint and may be bipartite or multipartite – in which case it has probably been fractured. In such a case, in the acute state, the adjacent margins are not corticated (Fig. 8.20).

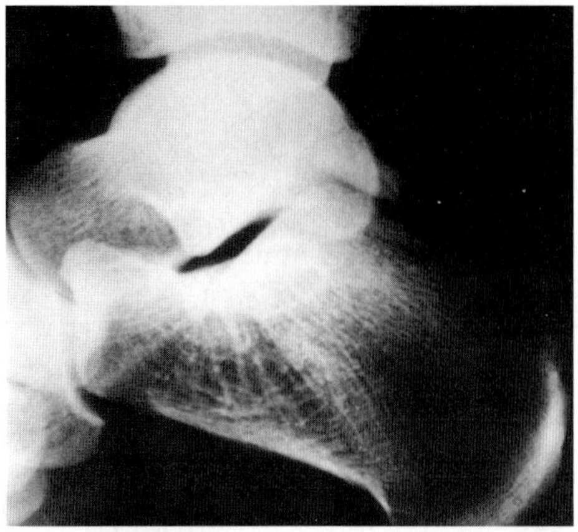
a

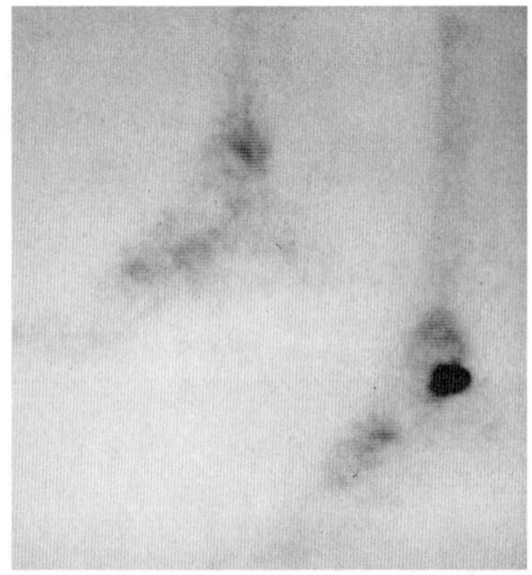
b

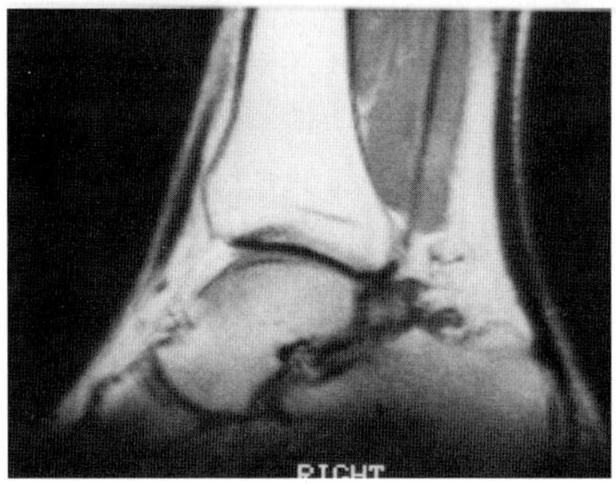
c

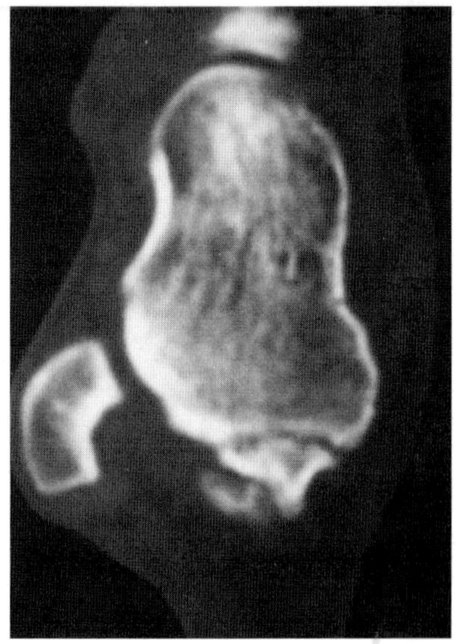
d

Fig. 8.18a–d. Avascular necrosis of the os trigonum. **a** The bone is irregular. **b** The radioisotope bone scan is strongly positive at the site of the os trigonum. **c** The MR sequence shows significant loss of marrow signal (T1-weighted), the result of intense mineralisation in the bone. **d** CT confirms the irregularity of the os trigonum and its rather irregular outline

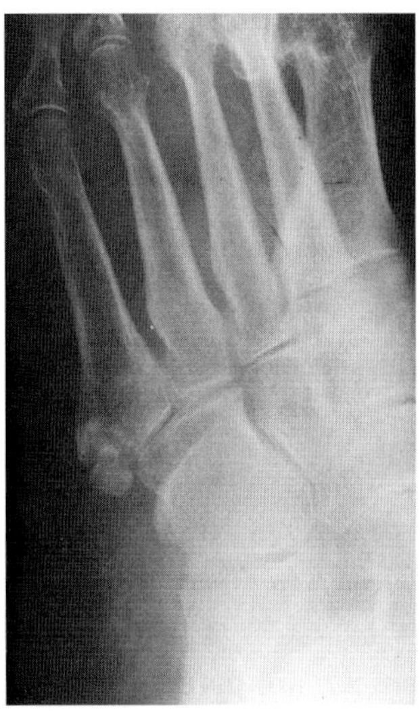

Fig. 8.19. Os vesalianium – a defect is present at the base of the 5th metatarsal within which sits a rounded ossicle. This cannot be the non-united apophysis, which has a completely different orientation, but may represent an unfused avulsion of the base of the 5th metatarsal

8.7 Sesamoids at the Metatarsal Heads

The medial sesamoid of the great toe is bipartite in up to 33% and the lateral, in up to 4%. Division is more common in women. A bipartite sesamoid is much larger than its counterpart, and its parts are well corticated all around. A fractured sesamoid is not corticated at its fracture line and is only slightly longer than its normal neighbours (Fig. 8.21). Fractures are mainly of the tibial sesamoids and usually occur in sportsmen. Burman and Lapidus (1921) give an excellent account of the sesamoids and their lesions, as does Helal (1988).

Sesamoids do occur at the other metatarsal heads, the next most common location being the 5th (Fig.8.22) (Bizarro 1921). A sesamoid at the plantar surface of the great toe interphalangeal joint is often associated with a local subungual exostosis, probably as a result of hyperextension of the local joint.

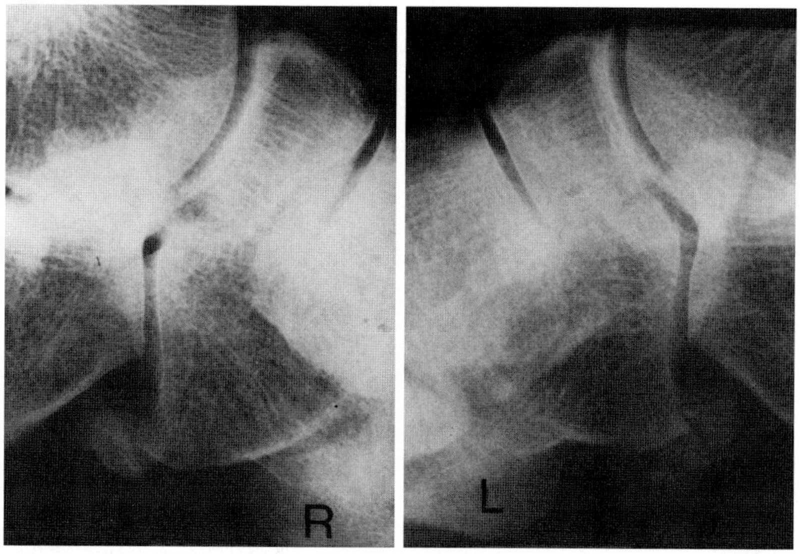

Fig. 8.20. Os peroneum. On the *right* the os peroneum is intact, while on the *left* it is fragmented and irregular following a fracture

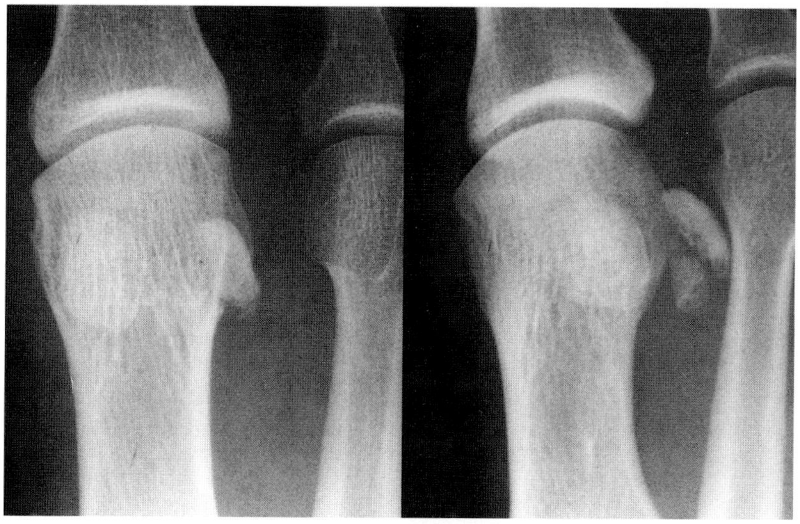

Fig. 8.21. Fracture of a sesamoid. The internal margins are irregular

a

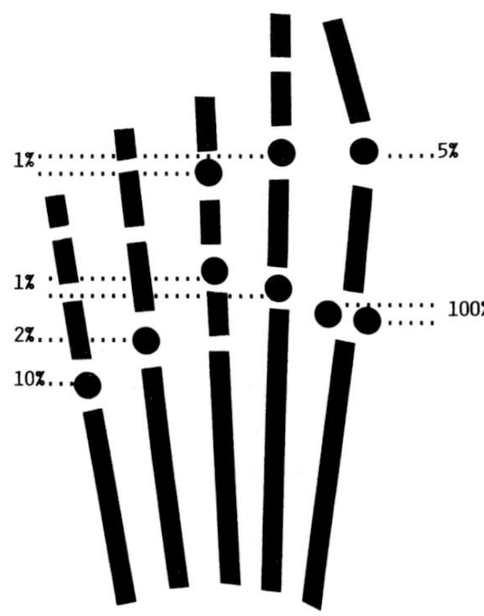

b

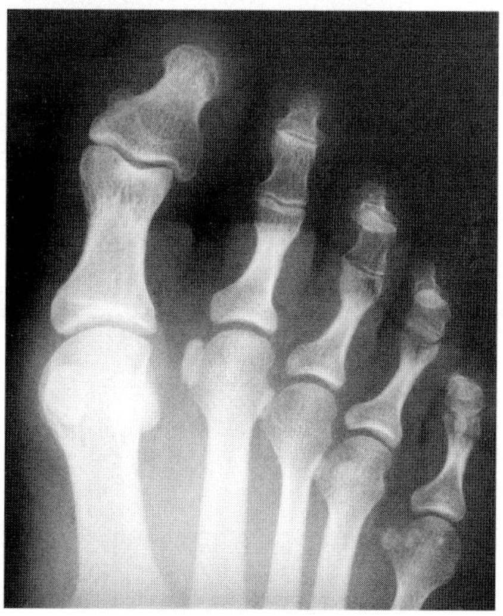

Fig. 8.22a. The percentages of foot sesamoid incidence in Bizarro's series. **b** Sesamoids are present at all the metatarsal heads, a very uncommon finding

Sesamoids may be seen in tendons or in joints related to synovium, in which case they may be involved in any local arthritic process – osteoarthritis, rheumatoid arthritis, infection or trauma. They may be eroded in ankylosing spondylitis or hyperparathyroidism. They are enlarged in acromegaly.

8.8 Short Fourth and Fifth Metatarsals

Bloom (1970) showed minor shortening of the 4th and 5th metacarpals and metatarsals in 8% of 1000 hands and feet examined in a casualty department. The degree of shortening was relatively minor, and in no case was less than half of the longest metacarpal or metatarsal.

Grosser forms of lateral metatarsal shortening are found in 70% of patients with pseudohypoparathyroidism and 97% of those with pseudopseudohypoparathyroidism (Poznanski 1984). Other causes include Turner's syndrome and juvenile chronic arthritis.

8.9 Pseudohypoparathyroidism

This is transmitted via a dominant gene, with a 2:1 female to male ratio. Patients are small and obese. They display symptoms of hypocalcaemia and soft-tissue calcifications, including cataracts. There may be mental retardation.

Radiologically, the 4th and 5th metatarsals are especially short. Cone-shaped epiphyses are present in the phalanges, which may be shortened due to premature growth plate fusion. Soft-tissue calcification and ossification are present (Fig. 8.23).

In the skull, vault thickening and basal ganglia calcification may be present.

8.10 Cone-Shaped Epiphyses

Cone-shaped epiphyses were originally described as part of a peripheral dysostosis in the hands by Brailsford in 1948. Such epiphyses have a cone shape with reciprocal change in the metaphyses, which may then have a basal flaring (Fig. 8.24). Premature growth plate fusion can then lead to brachyphalangy. This may be asymmetric, giving bending of involved rays. Similar changes occur in the metacarpus and metatarsus.

According to Giedion (1973), cone epiphyses are found in the toes in 26% of all normal girls and 8% of all normal boys, that is, as a minor variation in normal children, and should not indicate the presence of a peripheral dysostosis.

The 'severe type' of peripheral dysostosis described by Brailsford is associated with severe shortening and deformity, and may be seen in various syndromes (Table 8.4). In the hand, at any rate, some forms of cone-shaped epiphyses are diagnostic for some conditions, but these changes may not always be applicable in the foot.

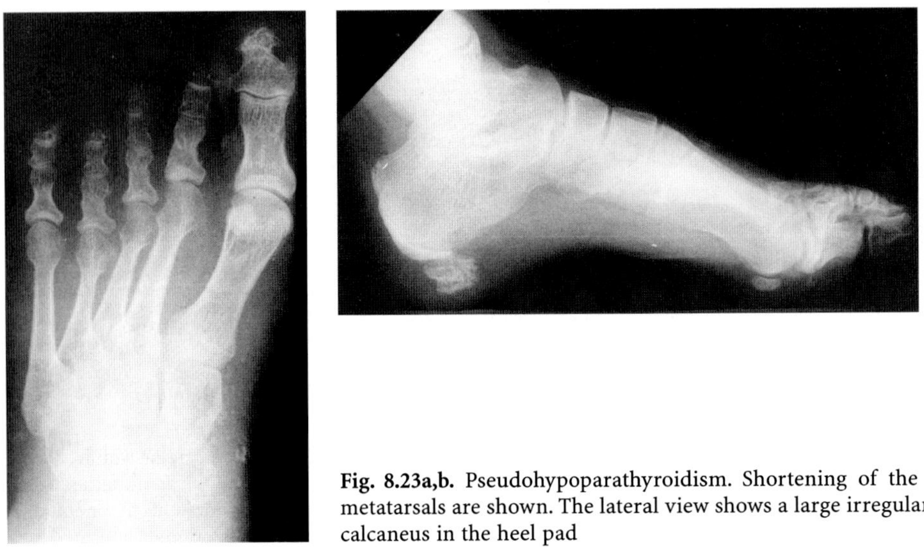

a b

Fig. 8.23a,b. Pseudohypoparathyroidism. Shortening of the third and especially fourth metatarsals are shown. The lateral view shows a large irregular ossicle situated beneath the calcaneus in the heel pad

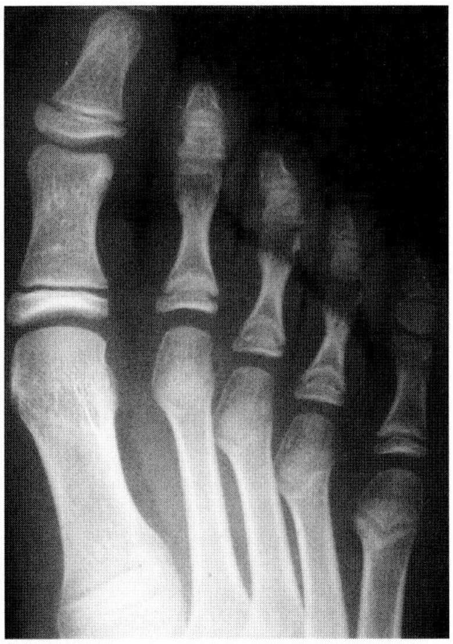

Fig. 8.24. Cone epiphyses. In this child minor cone epiphysis formation is demonstrated at the 2nd to 5th proximal phalanges. This is a normal variant in children, especially girls

Table 8.4. Cone-shaped epiphyses as a diagnostic indicator of generalised disorders (after GIEDION 1973)

Constitutional genetically determined disorders:
Asphyxiating thoracic dysplasia
Cleidocranial dysplasia
Dyschondrosteosis
Ellis-van Creveld syndrome
Hand-foot-uterus syndrome
Hereditary renal disease, retinitis pigmentosa and PD
Otopalatal digital syndrome
Peña's metaphyseal dysostosis
Pseudohypoparathyroidism
Pseudopseudohypoparathyroidism
Tricho-rhino-phalangeal syndrome
Acquired disorders:
Haemoglobin-S-dactylitis
Kashin-Beck's disease
Osteomyelitis variolosa

8.11 Terms Used in the Description of Congenital Anomalies

Syndactyly implies fusion of adjacent digits and may involve soft tissues and/or bone. In addition, there may be *polydactyly* - an increased number of digits; these may be pre- or post-axial. *Brachydactyly* means short phalanges (BELL 1931).

8.12 The Foot in Dysplasias

Much has been written on the *hand* in dysplasias. In particular, POZNANSKI (1984) attempted to diagnose the nature of the skeletal dysplasia by measuring metacarpal and phalangeal lengths. Each dysplasia was said to have a specific 'pattern profile'. Surprisingly little, however, has been written on dysplasias as they affect the foot in particular. The foot is more difficult to image than the hand, especially in children, and the phalanges are much shorter than those in the hand, which therefore lends itself better to the imaging and diagnostic process in dysplasias.

8.12.1 Chondrodysplasia Punctata (Chondrodystrophia Calcificans Congenita; Stippled Epiphyses)

This dysplasia exists in four forms, each with a different inheritance. Conradi's disease has an autosomal dominant inheritance. An X-linked dominant form is lethal in men. These two types have less severe rhizomelic shortening of the long bones than a severe recessive form and an autosomal dominant rhizomelic form of the disease. All forms show stippled or punctate calcification of cartilage.

In the foot, the hind foot in particular shows stippling, and the calcaneus has multiple ossification centres (Fig. 8.25a). Talipes equinovarus is seen. The metatarsals and phalanges may be shortened and broadened.

The calcifications eventually unite to form epiphyses which may be abnormal in form, some coming to resemble multiple epiphyseal dysplasia (see above) (Fig. 8.25b).

8.12.2 Stickler's Syndrome (Hereditary Arthro-ophthalmopathy)

Inheritance is autosomal dominant. The eye changes include retinal detachment, cataracts and glaucoma. Joints are painful. Epiphyses are irregular and show delayed ossification.

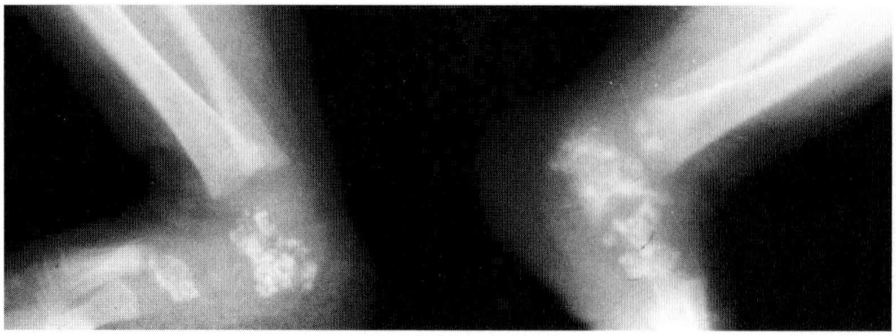

a

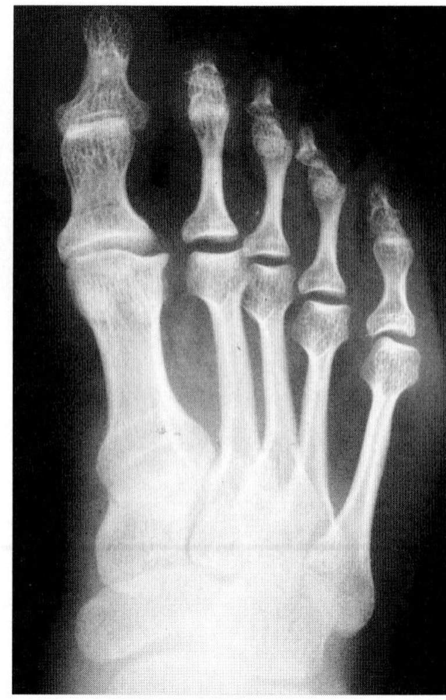

b

Fig. 8.25a,b. Dysplasia epiphysealis punctata; two cases at different levels of skeletal maturity. **a** This initial case is from a very young patient. There is very irregular ossification of the tarsal bones and, to a lesser extent, within the metatarsal cartilages. **b** An adult case showing the deformities at the metatarsal heads that are also seen at the femoral condyles, that is, distal concavity

In the feet the epiphyses show delayed ossification, and the metatarsals may be mildly shortened (Fig. 8.26).

8.12.3 Multiple Epiphyseal Dysplasia (Dysplasia Epiphysealis Multiplex)

This condition is inherited as an autosomal dominant with varying degrees of severity.

The major epiphyses at the shoulders, elbows, hips and knees are especially affected, being hypoplastic and irregular to varying degrees. The spine may also be affected; the vertebral bodies are flattened and irregular, giving a particular appearance, but involvement of the spine is not inevitable.

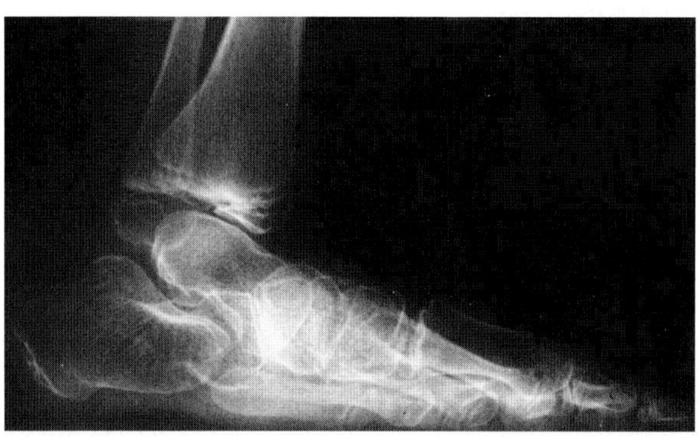

Fig. 8.26. Stickler's syndrome. Abnormal epiphyses are present at the ankle and at the calcaneus, which itself is abnormally shaped. Overall, the bones are demineralised

Shortening of the long bones and spine, if present, is moderate. The disease is of variable expression.

A talar tilt is seen (Fig. 8.27a). The tarsal bones are squared and irregular, and the metatarsals are short (Fig. 8.27b). The great toe metatarsals are broad, whilst the 2nd to 5th metatarsals have constricted necks. The phalanges too are short and broad. These severe changes are characteristic of the Fairbank type of the disease. Ribbing's disease is a milder form.

8.12.4 Achondrogenesis

There are two types of this disease, both with autosomal recessive inheritance. In both, death occurs *in utero* or shortly after birth. In type I the ribs are thinned and, more often, fractured. Bowing and shortening of the long bones are more severe in type I.

The feet are rarely commented upon (Fig. 8.28).

8.12.5 Thanatophoric Dysplasia

The mode of transmission is unknown. Death usually occurs shortly after birth. The enlarged skull vault has a clover leaf deformity, and the thorax is narrow. The long bones are short, broad and bowed; the metaphyses are flared. The acetabular roofs are horizontal, and the iliac blades vertically shortened.

The feet are not grossly abnormal (Fig. 8.29).

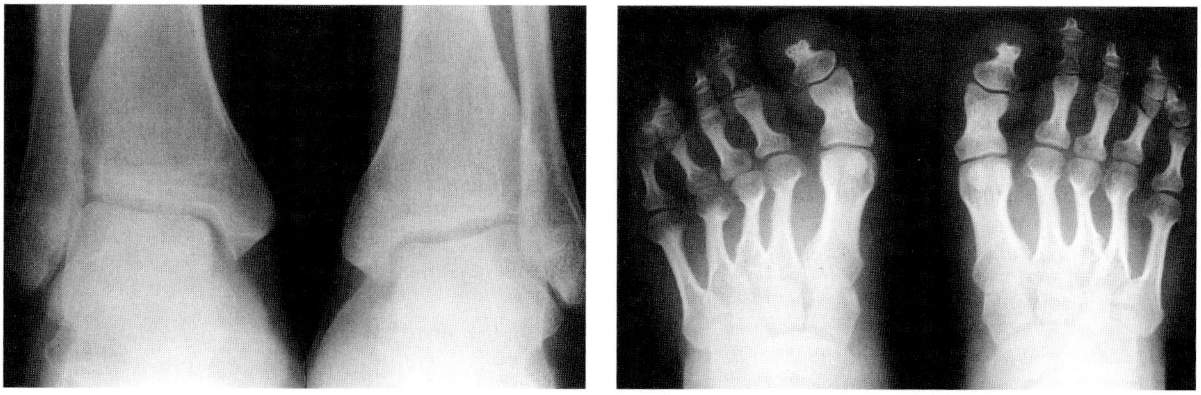

Fig. 8.27a,b. Dysplasia epiphysealis multiplex. **a** The ankle shows a mild talotibial slant. **b** In another patient there is conspicuous shortening of all the metatarsals, especially the 2nd to 5th. They are all roughly of the same length. There is minor deformity of the proximal phalanges of both great toes and of the distal phalanges also, but the second to fifth toes have a more normal modelling. The tarsal bones are angular and irregular in outline in this severe case

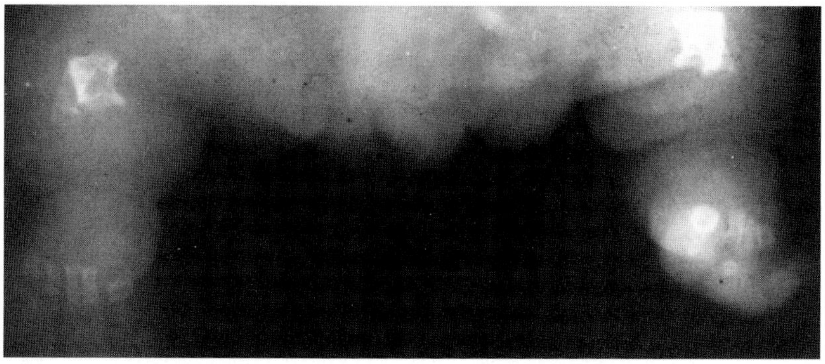

Fig. 8.28. Achondrogenesis type II. Short, broad metatarsals are seen with hypoplasia and non-mineralisation of some phalanges; the metaphyses are frayed and concave. There is gross shortening of the tibia and fibula

8.12.6 Chondroectodermal Dysplasia (Ellis-van Creveld Syndrome)

This has an autosomal recessive inheritance and presents with hypoplastic teeth, nails and hair, a ventricular septal defect or, less usually, atrial septal defect, and polydactyly. Hypoplasia of the proximal tibial epiphysis is characteristic, while at the ankle hypoplasia of the distal tibial epiphysis results in a tibio-talar slant.

Polydactyly is less common in the foot than in the hand and is post-axial (Fig. 8.30).

8.12.7 Short Rib-Polydactyly Syndrome

The Saldino-Noonan type has an autosomal recessive inheritance, but that for the Majewski type is unknown. In both types death occurs shortly after birth. The thorax is always narrow, and multiple cardiac and abdominal abnormalities are found.

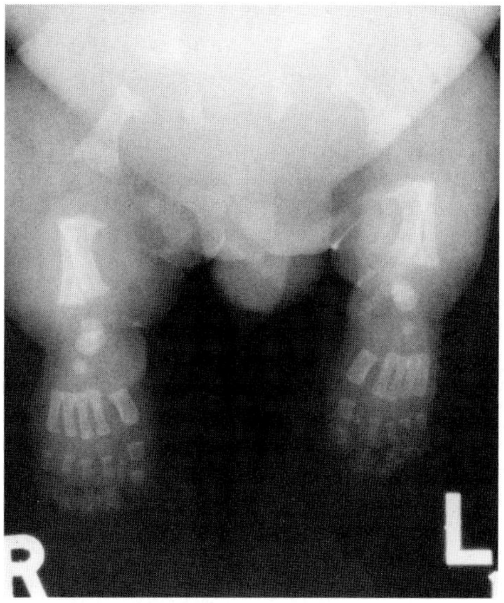

Fig. 8.29. Thanatophoric dwarfism. The tubular bones of the thigh and calf are short with broad, irregular metaphyses. The epiphyses at the knee have not yet ossified, though those of the ring epiphyses at the hind foot have. There is no marked abnormality of the bones in the foot. The great toes may show slight broadening of the metatarsals and phalanges

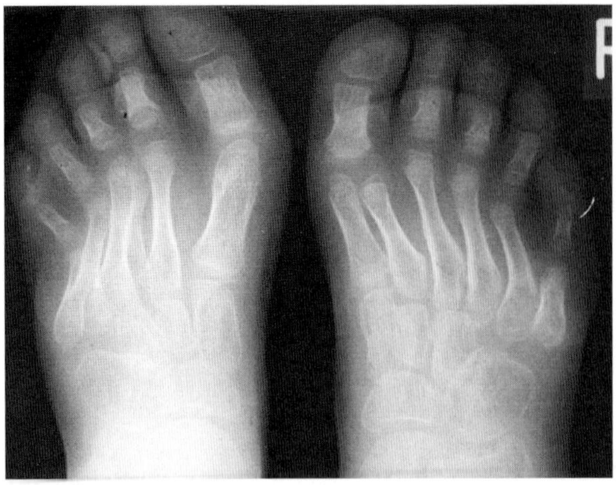

Fig. 8.30. Ellis-van Creveld syndrome. Both feet show six metatarsals, but only five phalanges. On the right there are two metatarsal shafts in the region of the great toe, which have the appearance of lateral metatarsals. This situation is not seen on the left, where there appears to be an extra lateral metatarsal, that is, the duplication may be both pre- and post-axial. There is also abnormal modelling of the metatarsals, the most lateral especially being hypoplastic. The distal phalanges, especially at the great toe, have a bullet shape

Radiologically, in the Majewski type, the pelvis is normal, and the polydactyly may be pre- or post-axial (Fig. 8.31), while the Saldino-Noonan type has a hypoplastic ilium and post-axial polydactyly. In both, the horizontally inclined ribs are extremely short.

8.12.8 Achondroplasia

This is the most common form of skeletal dysplasia associated with dwarfism. It is non-lethal. Those affected are of normal intelligence. Inheritance is autosomal dominant, though the majority of cases are spontaneous mutations. Homozygous cases, though less common than heterozygous, are more severely affected.

The changes in the foot are perhaps less dramatic than those in the hand (Fig. 8.32). The great toe metatarsal is broad, while the 3rd metatarsal is the longest. The 4th and 5th metatarsals are slightly shorter than the 3rd, but not grossly so. All the metatarsals seem relatively, but not severely, shortened. The phalanges do not appear grossly abnormal. No trident deformity is present.

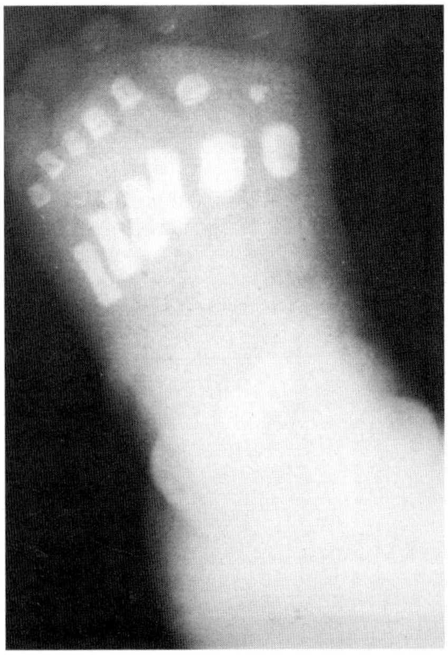

Fig. 8.31. Short rib-polydactyly syndrome – type Majewski. The polydactyly is associated with seven toes and seven metatarsals; the changes seem post-axial. The metatarsals are extremely short and broad. The proximal phalanges are hypoplastic, too, and the distal phalanges barely mineralised. In comparison, the polydactyly in chondroectodermal dysplasia is always a hexadactyly, and these children survive

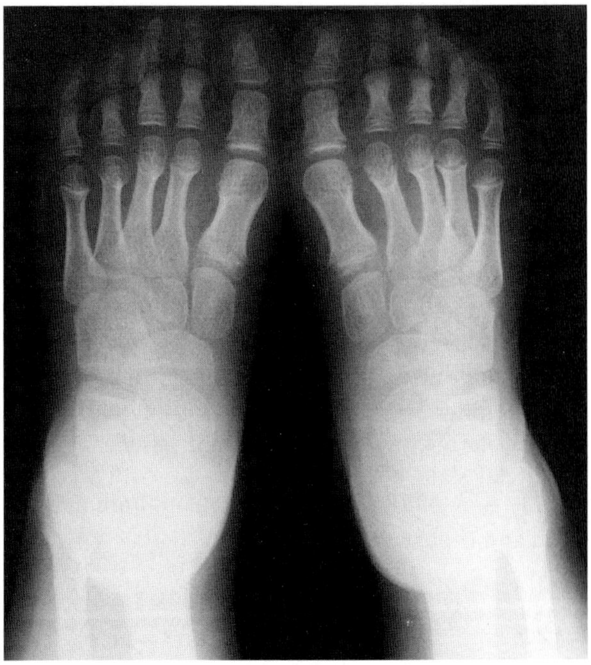

Fig. 8.32. Achondroplasia. Shortening of all the metatarsals is shown. The 3rd metatarsals seem to be the longest, which is not normally the case. The 4th and 5th, however, are slightly shorter. The proximal phalanges look fairly normal. The distal phalanx of the great toe has a bulbous basal epiphysis, while the epiphyses for the middle phalanges are not present. The cuboids seem markedly enlarged

8.12.9 Hypochondroplasia

This condition is inherited as an autosomal dominant. The skull is normal. The interpedicular distances narrow distally in the lumbar spine. The fibula is characteristically long.

The feet show cone-shaped epiphyses at the phalangeal bases (Fig. 8.33).

8.12.10 Metaphyseal Dysostosis

Multiple forms exist. As the name suggests, the metaphyses are abnormal with varying degrees of severity. They are broadened, fragmented and irregular, leading to shortening and deformity of the long bones in adult life.

8.12.10.1 Metaphyseal Dysostosis, Type Jansen

This is inherited as an autosomal dominant disorder. Patients have a short-limbed dwarfism. The skull is broad. There is hyperteliorism and nasofrontal hyperplasia.

Radiologically, the immature metaphysis is frayed, widened and cupped, rather like rickets, but the bony density is normal. Alignment anomalies are seen. There is subsequent shortening and curving of major tubular bones and, to a lesser extent, the tubular bones of the hands and feet (Fig. 8.34).

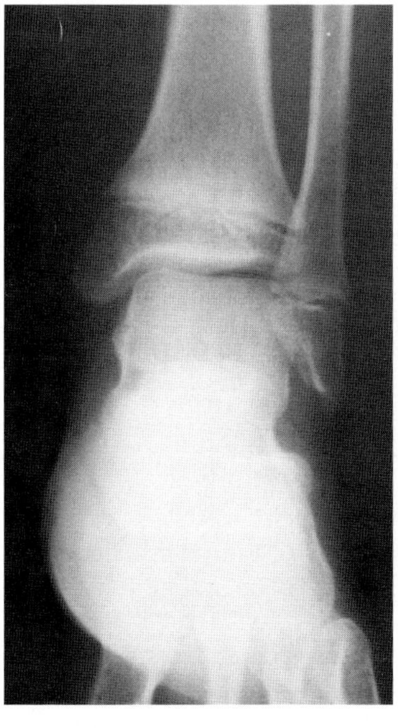

Fig. 8.33. Hypochondroplasia. The fibula is longer than the tibia. The medial malleolus is somewhat bulky

8.12.10.2 Metaphyseal Dysplasia, Type Schmid

This form is also inherited as an autosomal dominant disorder. The metaphyseal lesions are much less abnormal than in the Jansen type. Patients have

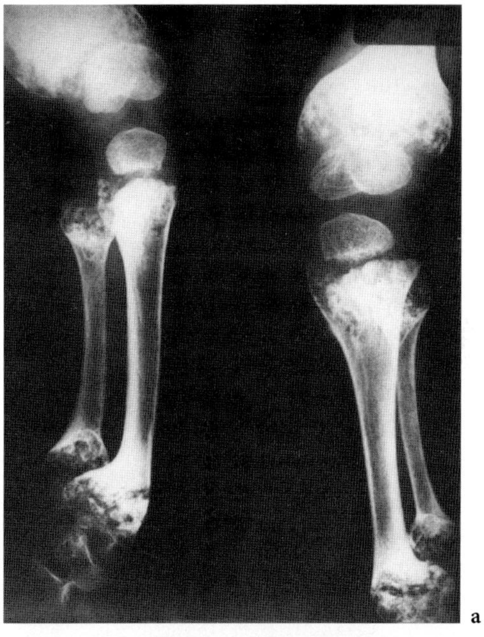

a

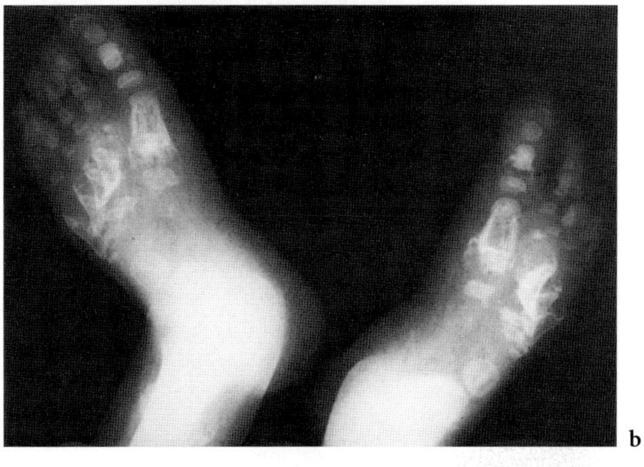

b

Fig. 8.34a,b. Metaphyseal dysostosis, type Jansen. **a** Severe deformity is demonstrated at the metaphyses around the knee and ankle, together with an overall deformity of alignment. The metaphyses are irregular and quite markedly sclerotic, as well as being expanded. **b** Irregularity of the tarsal bones is associated with sclerosis. Similarly, the metatarsals are hypoplastic, irregular and sclerotic, while the phalanges too are quite markedly disorganised, especially at the great toe a more normal physiognomy, although there is substantial short-limbed dwarfism.

Metaphyses are slightly flared and angular, but are well defined and sclerotic. Growth plates are widened to only a slight degree. Epiphyses show modelling abnormalities.

Tubular bones in the foot may show minor shortening.

8.12.11 Spondyloepiphyseal Dysplasia Congenita

The transmission is autosomal dominant. Change mainly affects the axial skeleton. The vertebral bodies flatten. A kyphoscoliosis develops, and the lumbar lordosis is exaggerated. The odontoid peg is hypoplastic. The long bones are short, and the metaphyses flared and irregular.

Changes in the feet are shown at the great toe with a distal metatarsal epiphysis (Fig. 8.35). The proximal phalanx is broad. There is minor modelling abnormality of the distal phalanges; they are short and broad.

8.12.12 Pseudoachondroplasia

This exists in autosomal dominant and recessive forms, which may be either mild or severe with major deformities.

The major tubular bones are short and bowed with flared metaphyses; the epiphyses are small and irregular.

In the feet, the tubular bones are short and broad, as they are in achondroplasia, while the tarsal bones are hypoplastic (Fig. 8.36).

The interpedicular distances are normal in the lumbar spine. In severe cases, major spinal deformity is seen.

8.12.13 The Mucopolysaccharidoses

8.12.13.1 MPS I-H (Hurler's Syndrome)

This is inherited as an autosomal recessive condition. It is apparent shortly after birth. There is mental retardation.

Radiologically, the skull shows macrocephaly, craniostenosis and a J-shaped sella. The ribs are paddle-shaped, widened anteriorly. Vertebral bodies have anterosuperior defects at the thoracolumbar junction. There is coxa valga and acetabular hypoplasia, and a tibiotalar slant in the ankle.

Skeletal retardation is present in the hands and feet. The metatarsals are demineralised and shortened, with pointed proximal ends. The phalanges are 'bullet-shaped', with pointed distal ends. Both metatarsals and phalanges are broadened (Fig. 8.37).

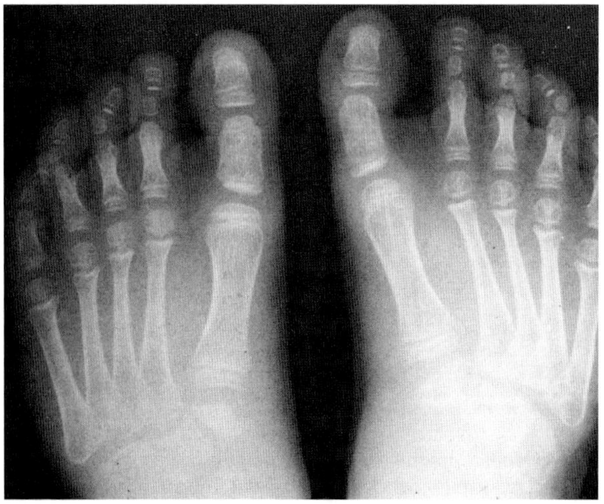

Fig. 8.35. Spondyloepiphyseal dysplasia congenita. The feet are minimally abnormal. The phalanges of the great toes in particular are short and broad. The epiphyses at the 1st metatarsal heads are an unusual feature, not occurring in the normal foot

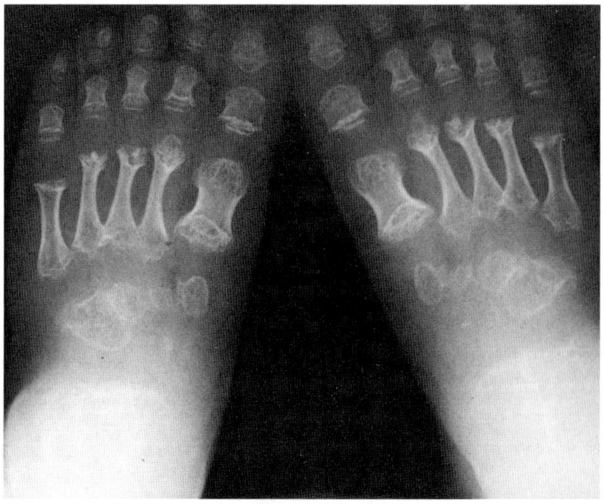

Fig. 8.36. Pseudoachondroplasia. The bones overall are demineralised. The tarsal bones are irregular and hypoplastic. The metatarsals are shortened and the metaphyses frayed. The phalanges are bullet-shaped; cone epiphyses are present

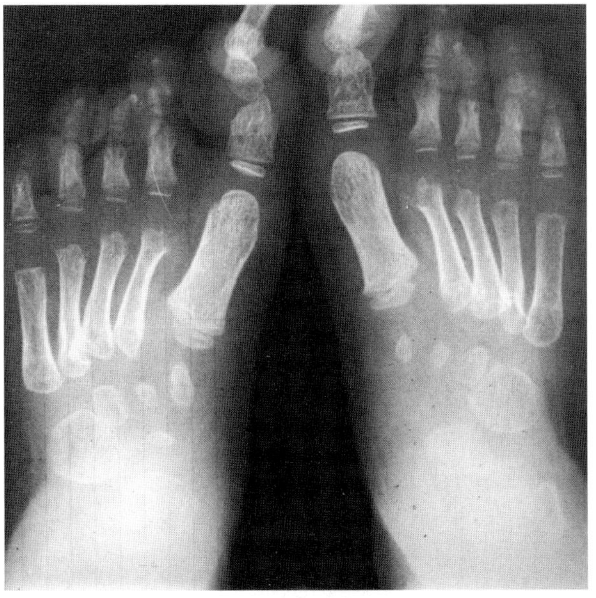

Fig. 8.37. MPS 1-H (Hurler's disease). Bullet-shaped phalanges are demonstrated. The epiphyses are irregular and angular. The metatarsals and phalanges are short and broad. Cupping of the distal metatarsal metaphyses is shown, and irregular epiphyses are included in them. The tarsal bones are extremely irregular. Overall, there is demineralisation

8.12.13.2
MPS IV (Morquio-Brailsford Syndrome)

Inherited as an autosomal recessive condition, this is a short spine dwarfism with no mental deficit.

In the spine central beaking of many vertebral bodies is present. Initially, the major epiphyses are fairly normal in appearance, but become progressively flattened, irregular and sclerotic.

A tibiotalar slant is seen. Metatarsals are short, broad and have pointed proximal ends. Phalanges are broadened (Fig. 8.38).

8.12.14
Skeletal Dysplasias with Anarchic Development of Bone

8.12.14.1
Dysplasia Epiphysealis Hemimelica (Trevor's Disease)

This is a rare condition of unknown genetic inheritance with a male preponderance (3:1).

There is progressive enlargement of an osteochondral exostosis on the epiphysis of one side of the body during growth, leading to progressive deformity of the involved joints. The lower limb is especially involved.

First described in 1926 in the French literature (Mouchet and Belot 1926) as *tarsomegalie*, ten cases were published by Trevor in 1950, who called the disease 'tarso-epiphyseal aclasis'. However, Fairbank pointed out that the lesion did not only affect the tarsus (Fairbank 1956). He coined the term 'dysplasia epiphysealis hemimelica'.

Changes in the feet are those of irregular exostoses on the articular surfaces, especially at the talar dome, and overgrowth of bone (Fig. 8.39).

8.12.14.2
Diaphyseal Aclasia (Multiple Exostoses)

This is inherited as an autosomal dominant, with a male preponderance.

The metaphyses are undertubulated, and exostoses form upon them, becoming progressively larger during adolescence (Fig. 8.40a). Growth anomalies result, especially at the distal radius and ulna, or tibia and fibula (Fig. 8.40b).

The exostoses cease to grow with the onset of skeletal maturity. Malignant change may supervene.

8.12.14.3
Enchondromatosis (Ollier's Disease)

There is no known mode of inheritance in this condition. Multiple, well-defined medullary carti-

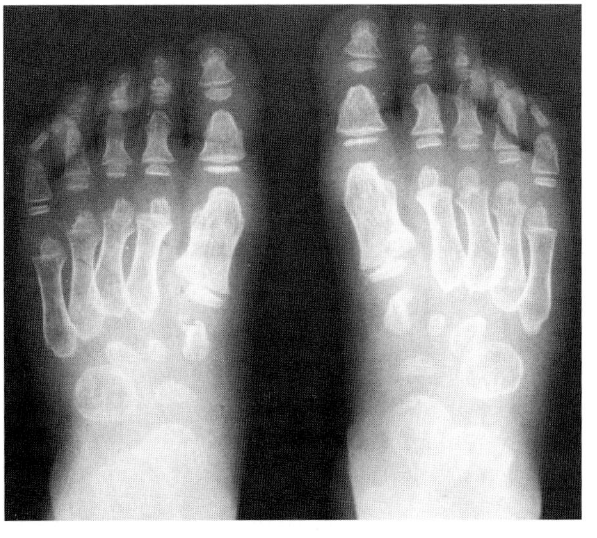

Fig. 8.38. MPS IV (Morquio-Brailsford disease). Here, the appearances are not as severe as those of MPS I-H, but the features are still those of a mucopolysaccharidosis. There is pointing of the metatarsal bases and irregularity of the tarsus. The phalanges are bullet-shaped

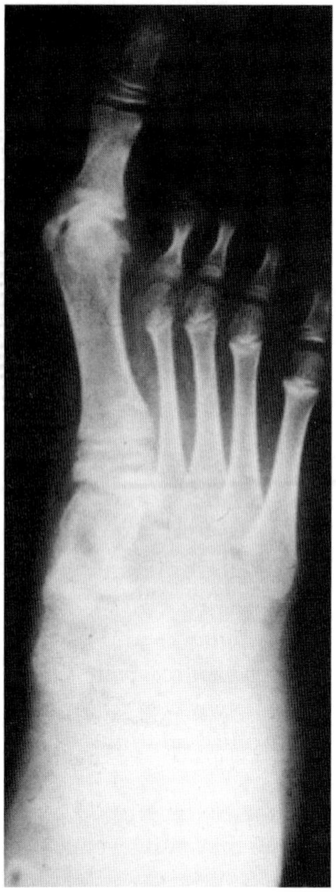

Fig. 8.39. Dysplasia epiphysealis hemimelica. The foot of this patient shows overgrowth of the great toe, especially involving the metatarsal, and there are ossicles present within the great toe metatarsophalangeal joint, as well as in the region of the first tarsometatarsal joint

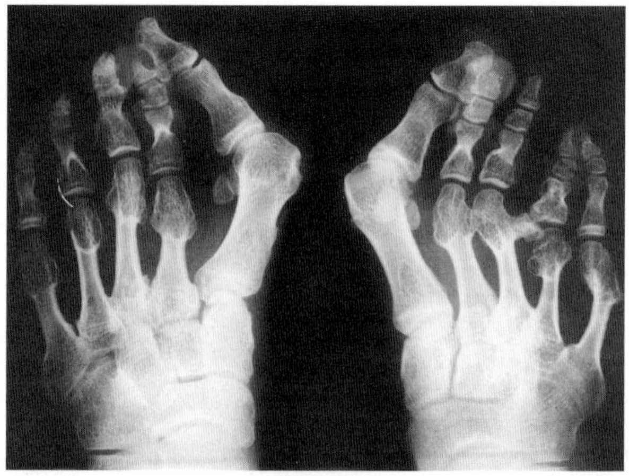

a

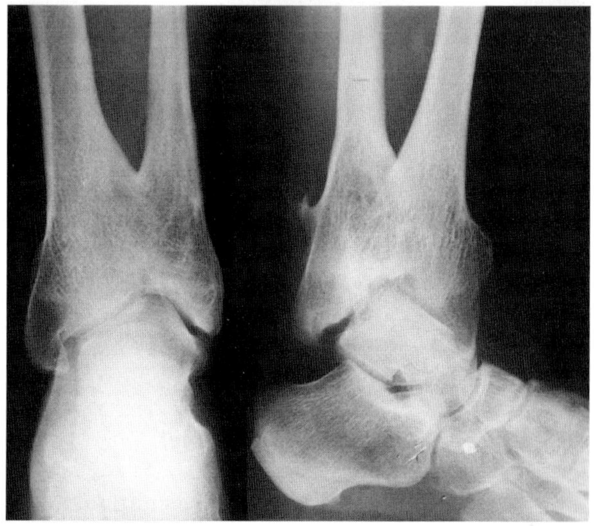

b

Fig. 8.40a,b. Diaphyseal aclasia. **a** The feet of this patient show quite marked shortening, especially of the metatarsals in association with exostoses. **b** In another case, expansion of the distal metaphyses is found in association with cross-fusion and growth arrest. A talotibial slant is seen. There are exostoses both anteriorly and posteriorly at the ankle joint

laginous tumours of varying size deform the tarsus, metatarsus and phalanges. Growth anomalies result (Fig. 8.41).

8.12.15 Dysplasias with Abnormality of Bone Density

8.12.15.1 Osteogenesis Imperfecta

Formerly divided into a severe recessive type and a less severe dominant type, osteogenesis imperfecta has been given a more modern classification (SILLENCE et al. 1979).

Four types exist, with numerous subtypes. Long bones may be 'thick' or 'thin', depending on the type of disease.

The bone changes in the feet reflect the type of disease seen elsewhere, with some bones being broad or cystic, and some thin or fragile (Fig. 8.42). Osteoporosis, fractures and deformity may also be present.

8.12.15.2 Osteopetrosis (Albers-Schönberg Disease)

This exists in several forms.

1. As a recessive, severe form (*congenita*);
2. As a milder dominant form (*tarda*);
3. As an intermediate recessive form;
4. Associated with renal tubular acidosis and diffuse cerebral calcification. This is linked to carbonic anhydrase-2 deficiency.

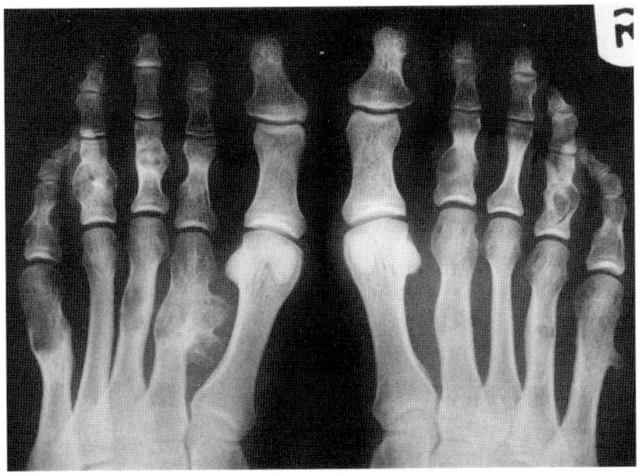

Fig. 8.41. Enchondromatosis (Ollier's disease). This is probably the most common benign tumour of the foot and hand. Multiple medullary lesions are shown, with thinning and displacement of the cortex. Some lesions are in the main lucent, while others show mineralisation. Abnormal modelling is quite marked in the small bones of the hand and foot

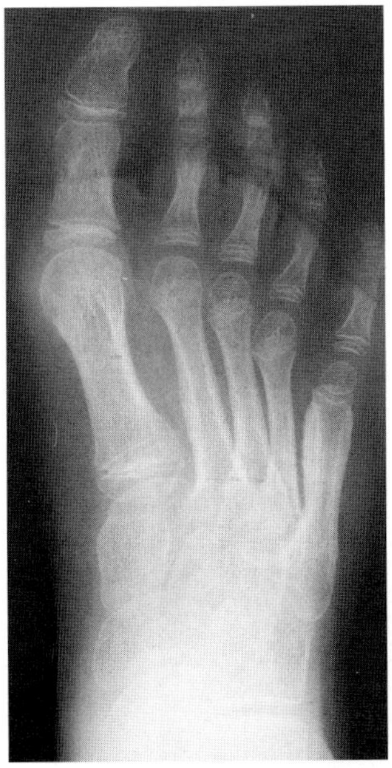

Fig. 8.42. Osteogenesis imperfecta. Overall there is osteoporosis. Prominent periosteal reactions are noted, especially on the 2nd and 5th metatarsals – the result of trauma and perhaps subperiosteal haemorrhage

Sclerosis may be uniform (Fig. 8.43A), or the intermittent nature of the disease may result in bands of normal and abnormal bone – a 'bone within a bone' appearance (Fig. 8.43b). Sclerosis and undertubulation may be barely perceptible in the dominant or tarda variety. Fracture may occur *in utero* in severely affected cases, or later in life in the tarda form.

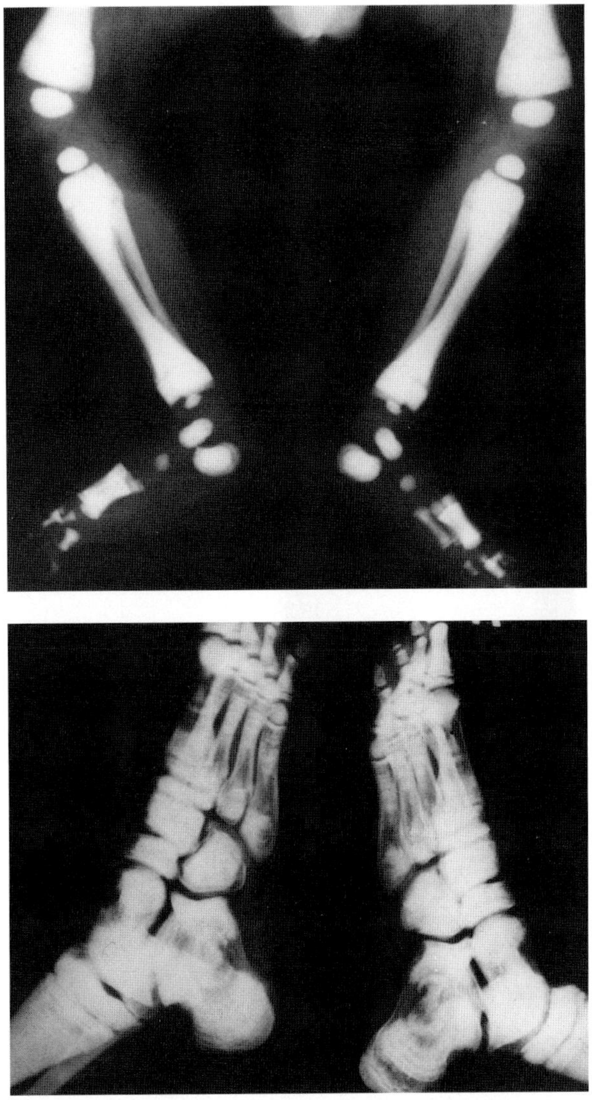

a

b

Fig. 8.43a,b. Osteopetrosis. **a** Erlenmeyer flask-like changes are shown at the distal femoral metaphyses, as well as the proximal and distal tibial metaphyses. There is quite marked bone sclerosis, but a 'bone-within-a-bone' appearance is still discernible. **b** There is an extensive 'bone-within-a-bone' appearance and undertubulation

8.12.15.3 Melorheostosis

This sclerosing bone dysplasia is usually found in a single limb or side of the body. The spine is infrequently affected.

Sclerotic new bone is laid down along the cortices of tubular bones, often in continuity around joints (Fig. 8.44). This change has been likened to flowing candle wax. Soft-tissue ossification occurs around

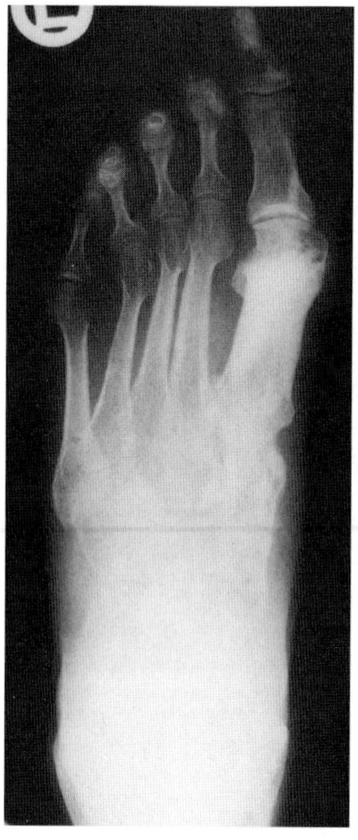

Fig. 8.44. Melorheostosis. Partial sclerosis is shown of the great toe metatarsal, which is overgrown, and linear sclerosis at the base of the adjacent proximal phalanx. The medial cuneiform and navicular are also partially affected. The change lies in the distribution of the L5 sclerotome

affected joints in about 25% of cases. The affected areas of bone are overgrown, and overgrowth may be associated with soft-tissue haemangiomas and enlarged superficial blood vessels.

The lesions were shown by Murray and McCredie (1979) to lie in the distribution of sclerotomes, that is, the nervous innervation of bone.

Other sclerosing bone dysplasias include osteopathia striata and osteopoikilosis.

8.12.15.4 Osteopoikilosis

Numerous, dense focal areas of osteosclerosis resembling bone islands are seen around joints (Fig. 8.45). The diaphyseal areas are spared. The lesions do not alter under long-term observation (unlike metastatic lesions, which may initially have a similar appearance).

8.12.15.5 Osteopathia Striata

Rather than being round, the sclerotic lesions are linear and extend to the joint (Fig. 8.46). Again, the changes are asymptomatic.

Some patients show a mixture of both linear and nodular density.

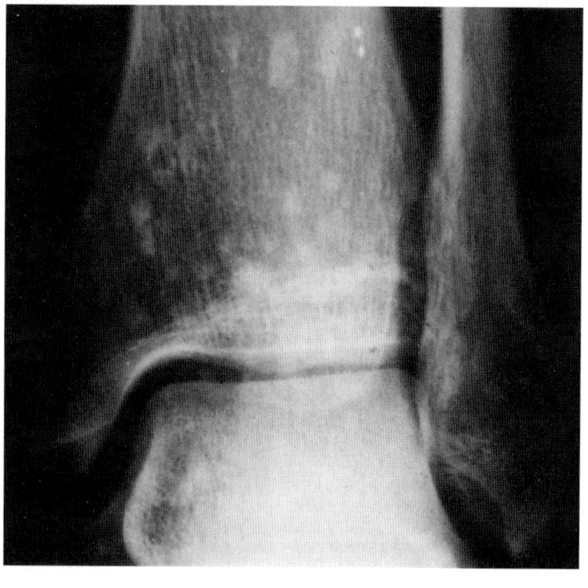

Fig. 8.45. Osteopoikilosis. Multiple, well-defined, focal areas of bone sclerosis, resembling bone islands, are shown around the ankle joint

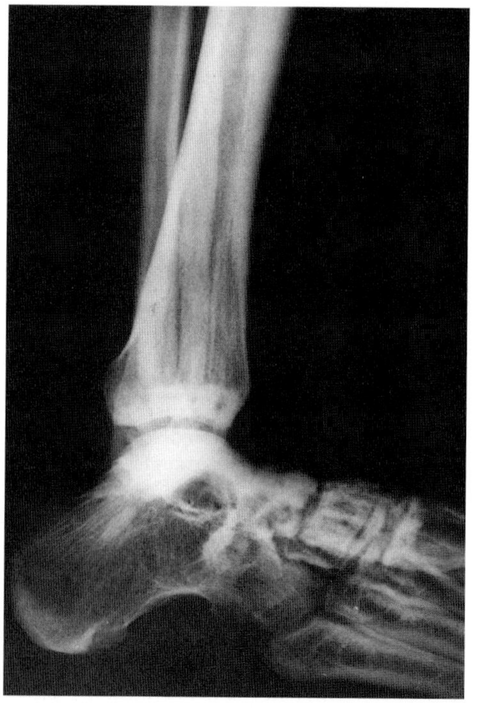

Fig. 8.46. Osteopathia striata. Linear streaks of increased density extend to the ankle joint and are also seen in the tarsus

8.12.15.6
Metaphyseal Dysplasia (Pyle's Disease)

This is inherited as an autosomal recessive disorder. The face is unremarkable.

Radiologically, the skull shows slight thickening of the vault and mild sclerosis of the base. However, there is marked thickening of the ribs, clavicles and ischiopubic bone. The tubular bones show marked diametaphyseal flaring with an extreme form of an Erlenmeyer flask appearance.

Phalanges and metatarsals show undertubulation and a lack of diaphyseal constriction (Fig. 8.47).

8.12.15.7
Diaphyseal Dysplasia (Camurati-Engelmann Disease)

Inherited as an autosomal recessive disorder, the face is grossly abnormal with hyperostosis of the facial bones (leontiasis ossea). This leads to foraminal stenosis, raised intracranial pressure and premature death.

Radiologically, the skull and mandible show gross sclerosis and expansion. The long bones show undertubulation at the diaphyses with osteopenia and cortical thinning.

Tarsal bones show irregular ossification. Metatarsals show undertubulation and expansion and are occasionally fused (Spranger et al. 1974). The phalanges are expanded (Fig. 8.48).

8.12.16
Miscellaneous Congenital Disorders

8.12.16.1
Cleidocranial Dysplasia

Inherited in the main as an autosomal dominant, some 30% are spontaneous mutations.

Failure of midline fusion occurs at the symphysis pubis and symphysis mentis. The clavicles are hypoplastic, and Wormian bones are typically found in the skull.

In the feet, acro-osteolysis is seen, and cone epiphyses (Fig. 8.49).

8.12.16.2
Acrocephalosyndactyly Type I (Apert's Syndrome)

This disease has an autosomal dominant inheritance. Craniostenosis results in a short head with a vertical, tall forehead. The maxilla is hypoplastic and the nasal bridge depressed.

The feet show soft-tissue syndactyly of some or all toes, which are grossly deformed and hypoplastic (Fig. 8.50).

Initially, the lateral toes are deficient in phalanges. Subsequently, cross-fusion develops across the tarsal and metatarsal joints. The metatarsals also cross-fuse. The phalanges of the great toe are hypoplastic, especially the proximal, which is laterally displaced.

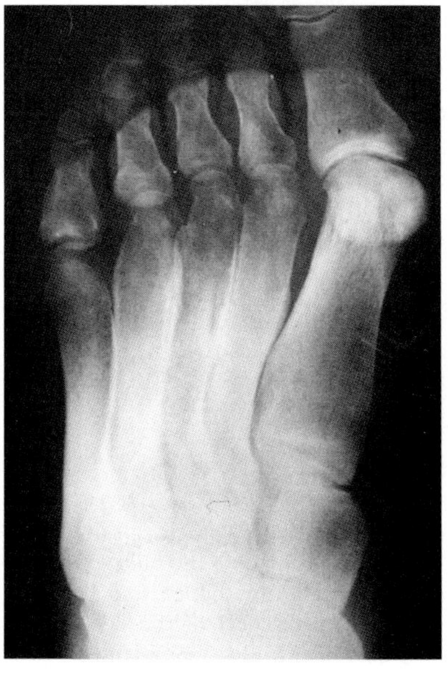

Fig. 8.47. Metaphyseal dysplasia (Pyle's disease). Diametaphyseal broadening of the metatarsals with cortical thinning and generalised osteopenia

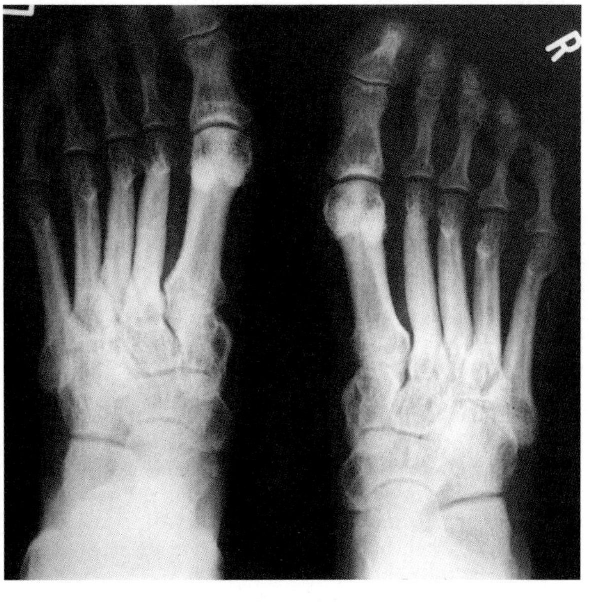

Fig. 8.48. Diaphyseal dysplasia (Camurati-Engelmann's disease). Diametaphyseal thickening in this case with sclerosis of bone and obliteration of the medullary cavities of the metatarsals

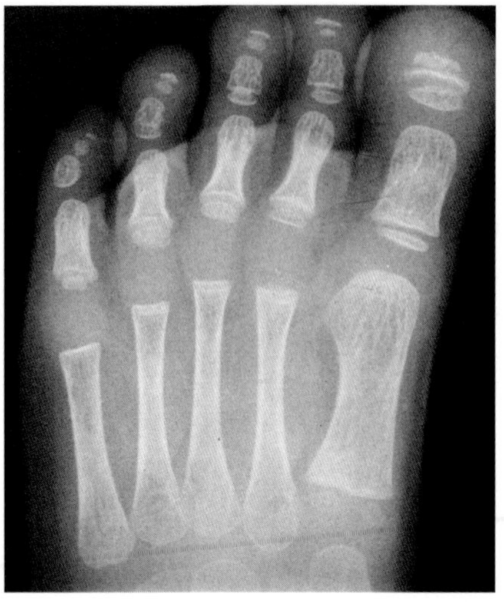

Fig. 8.49. Cleidocranial dysostosis. There is quite marked acro-osteolysis with associated pseudoclubbing of the soft tissues. The epiphysis for the base of the great toe metatarsal is bifid. The middle phalanges show abnormal basal epiphyses. That for the third toe seems to be a fusing cone epiphysis, while the epiphyses for the fourth toe and former fifth toe have not segmented at all. The distal metaphyses of the metatarsals have a slightly abnormal shape, being concave distally

8.12.16.3 Larsen's Syndrome

This syndrome is characterised by multiple dislocations at major joints. There is a flat face, a depressed nasal bridge and often a cleft palate. Cervical spine malformations are common.

Changes in the feet include vertical talus, navicular dislocation and a bifid calcaneus (Fig. 8.51).

8.12.16.4 Arthrogryposis Congenita Multiplex

The disease is recognised shortly after birth. The muscles are hypoplastic. Contractures develop around joints, especially in the lower limbs, leading to flexion deformities, especially at the hips and knees. Because movements are limited, bone hypoplasia results.

Most cases are sporadic mutations, but a few are described as X-linked recessive.

Radiologically, bilateral club foot and vertical talus are seen (Fig. 8.52). Tarsal and, more frequently, carpal coalition may be present.

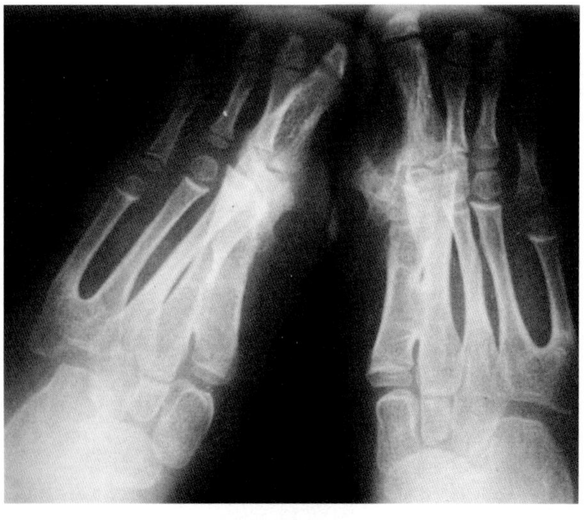

Fig. 8.50. Apert's syndrome. There is not only soft-tissue fusion, but also bony cross-fusion bilaterally. The metatarsals seem elongated and thinned. The phalanges also show abnormal modelling. The proximal phalanges of the second toes in particular seem overgrown and of abnormal bone texture. There do not appear to be any distal phalanges, and the middle phalanges are hypoplastic in association with soft-tissue fusion. The epiphyses of the metatarsophalangeal joints are abnormal in shape, and the right third toe shows failure of segmentation of the epiphyses at the metatarsophalangeal joint

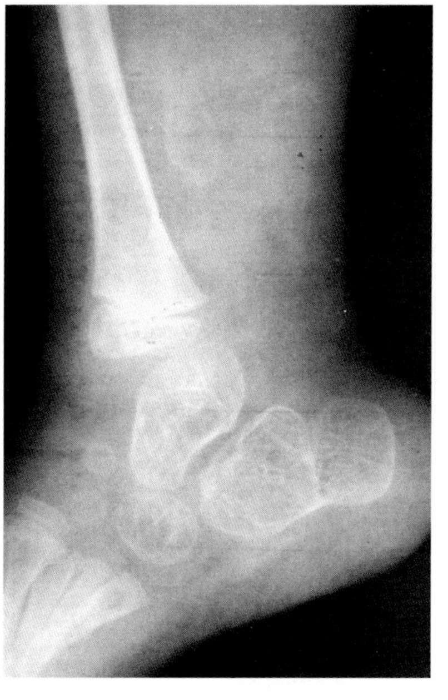

Fig. 8.51. Larsen's syndrome. An abnormal calcaneum is shown with an extra ossification centre on the point of fusing with the main centre. The talus is misshapen and tends to a vertical alignment. The anterior aspect of the distal tibial epiphysis is bulbous. The navicular no longer articulates with the talus and is also misshapen

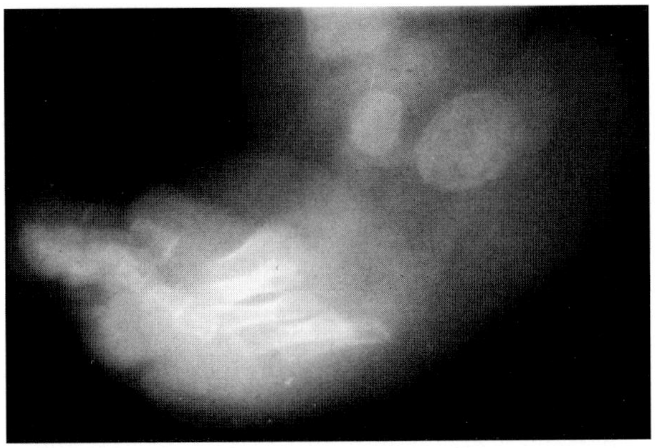

Fig. 8.52. Arthrogryposis multiplex congenita, presenting with club foot and vertical talus

8.12.16.5
Rubenstein-Taybi Syndrome

Patients have short stature and mental retardation. There are minor modelling abnormalities of the phalanges of the second to fourth toes, which show hypoplasia. The hallux in particular has abnormal phalanges, which are markedly broad and short (Fig. 8.53). Cervical spondylolisthesis is also seen.

8.12.16.6
Marfan's Syndrome

This is inherited as an autosomal dominant condition. Patients are tall and thin, with disproportionate elongation of tubular bones, which are gracile. Long fingers (arachnodactyly) are the classic finding upon which the diagnosis is made by the metacarpal index. The feet have a similar long, narrow appearance.

Radiologically, the metatarsals and phalanges are seen to be elongated and thinned (Fig. 8.54). Bone maturation is normal. Pes planus and a vertically orientated talus are described (Wynne-Davis et al. 1985).

8.12.16.7
Fibrodysplasia Ossificans Progressiva

In this rare and eventually fatal condition, progressive ossification of the voluntary musculature takes place, especially over the rib cage. Skeletal anomalies include cervical vertebral fusion and enlargement of the femoral and mandibular condylar necks.

In this condition the thumb (75%) and great toe (50%) are unusual in shape (Fig. 8.55).

8.12.17
Focal Foot Hypertrophy

8.12.17.1
Fibrous Dysplasia

This occurs in monostotic and polyostotic forms, the latter often with a preponderantly unilateral distribution. The McCune-Albright syndrome is associated with skin pigmentation and precocious puberty.

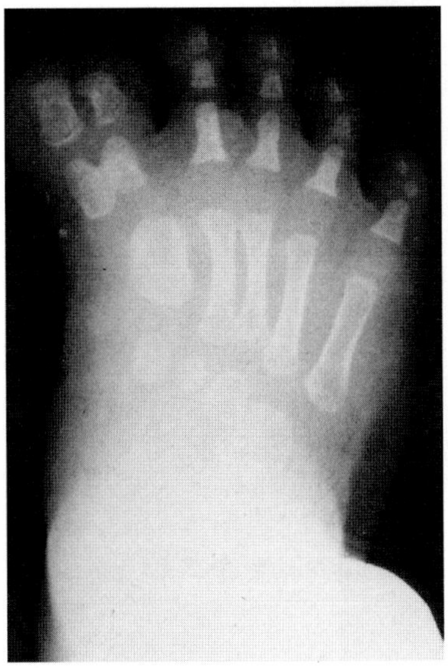

Fig. 8.53. Rubinstein-Taybi syndrome. Pre-axial polydactyly with broadening and shortening of the great toe metatarsal is associated with fusion of the proximal phalanges. There is slight broadening of all the phalanges

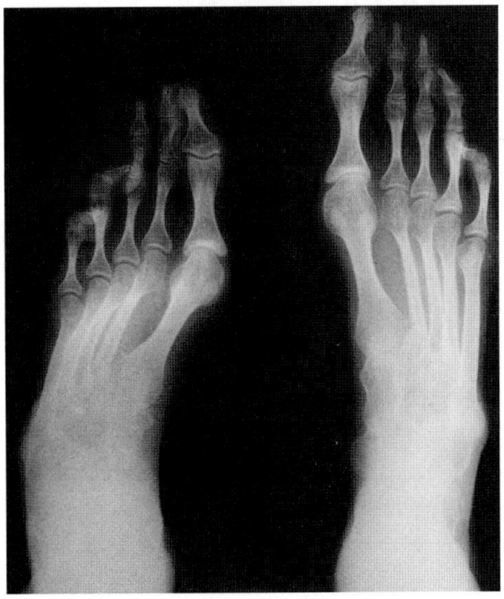

Fig. 8.54. Marfan's syndrome. The tubular bones are long and thin. There also seems to be early acro-osteolysis of the distal phalanges

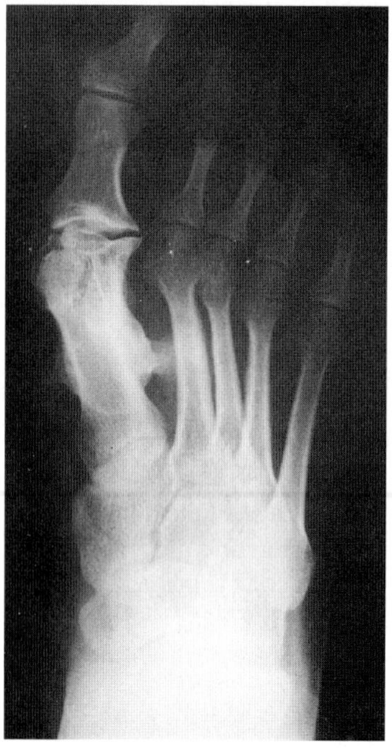

Fig. 8.55. Fibrodysplasia ossificans progressiva. Overgrowth of the great toe is demonstrated, with exostosis formation and a disorganised metatarsophalangeal joint

The affected bone is focally or generally enlarged. Well-defined lesions cause endosteal scalloping. Bone lesions may be lucent or cystic, sclerotic, or ground-glass, or all in combination (Fig. 8.56). Longitudinal overgrowth results.

8.12.17.2
Neurofibromatosis (von Recklinghausen's Disease)

This is inherited as an autosomal dominant. Type I affects the periphery of the body, and type II the central nervous system.

Skeletal overgrowth occurs in 30% of cases and is associated with soft-tissue enlargement. Plexiform neurofibromas often supply the overgrown part. There is associated blood vessel overgrowth, naevus formation and lymphatic hyperplasia.

Soft-tissue neurofibromas erode the adjacent bony structures (Fig. 8.57).

8.12.17.3
Macrodystrophia Lipomatosa (Neural Fibrolipoma)

In this rare disease, a fatty mass invades and infiltrates a nerve, which subsequently atrophies. In one-third of cases, the bone and soft tissues supplied by the nerve hypertrophy (as in neurofibromatosis), but unlike neurofibromatosis, the nerve is atrophied.

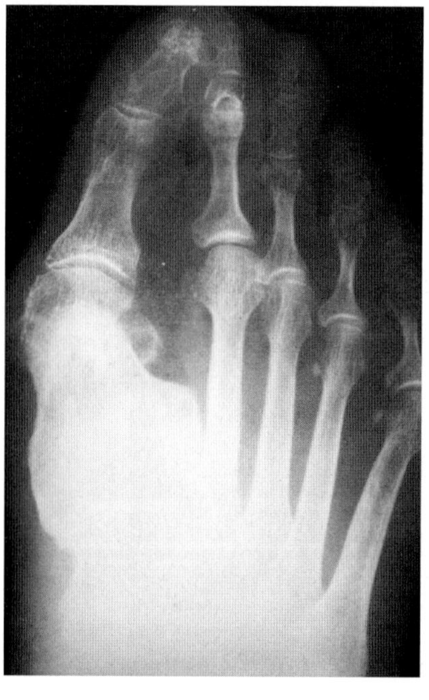

Fig. 8.56. Fibrous dysplasia. There is quite marked expansion of the great toe metatarsal. The abnormal bone shows a ground-glass texture. The abnormality is confined to this bone

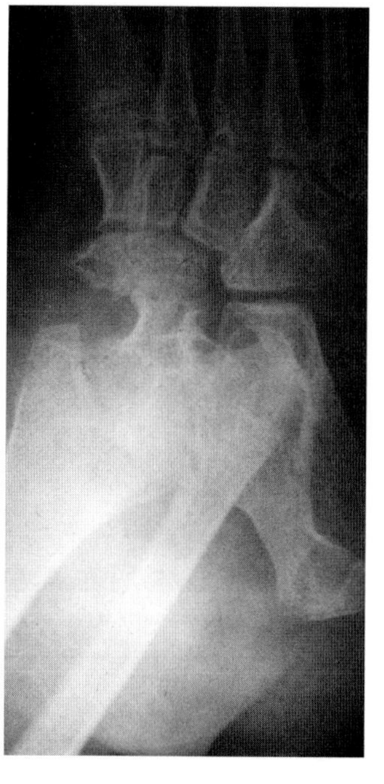

Fig. 8.57. Neurofibromatosis. The bones are demineralised and show overtubulation. Large soft-tissue masses are demonstrated, causing well-demarcated erosions of the underlying bone

The plain radiographs show major enlargement of one or more rays. The soft-tissue masses contain fatty lucency. The involved bones show major expansion; the marked hypertrophy of bone around joints resembles severe degenerative change (Fig. 8.58).

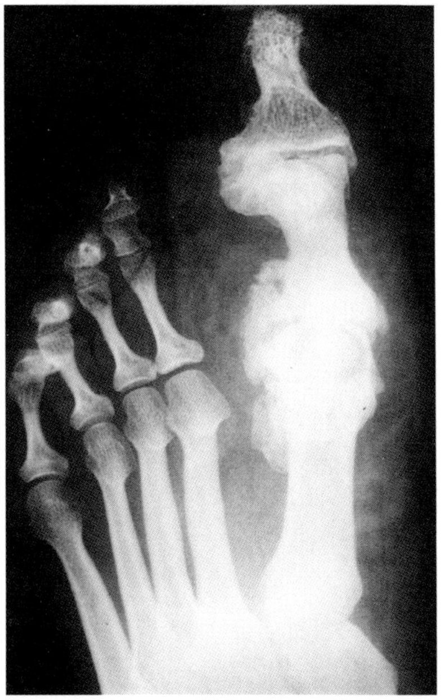

Fig. 8.58. Macrodystrophia lipomatosa. There is gross soft-tissue thickening which contains numerous fatty lucencies. The bones are overgrown, and the joints look degenerate, with large exostoses arising around the joints

References

Altman MI (1968) Sagittal plane angles of the talus and calcaneus in the developing foot. J Am Podiat Assoc 58: 463–470

Beck C (1900) Fractures, with an Appendix on the Practical Use of the Röntgen Rays. Saunders, Philadelphia

Bell J (1931) On brachydactyly and symphalangism. Cambridge University Press, Cambridge, pp 1–31 (The treasury of human inheritance, vol 1)

Bizarro AH (1921) On the sesamoid and supernumerary bones of the limbs. J Anat (Cambr) 55:56–268

Bloom RA (1970) The metacarpal sign. Br J Radiol 43: 133–135

Brailsford JF (1948) The radiology of bones and joints. Churchill Livingstone, Edinburgh

Burman MS, Lapidus PW (1921) Functional disturbances caused by the inconstant bones and sesamoids of the foot. Arch Surg 22:936–975

Chambers CH (1950) Congenital anomalies of the tarsal navicular with particular reference to calcaneo-navicular coalition. Br J Radiol 23:580–586

Cruveilhier J (1829) Anatomie pathologique du corps humain. Baillière, Paris

Davis LA, Hatt WS (1955) Congenital abnormalities of the feet. Radiology 64:818–825

Day HJB (1991) The ISO/ISPO classification of congenital limb deficiency. Prosthet Orthot Int 15:67–69

Dwight T (1907) Variations of the bones of the hands and feet. Lippincott, Philadelphia

Emery KH, Bisset GS III, Johnson ND, Nunan PJ (1998) Tarsal coalition: a blinded comparison of MRI and CT. Pediatr Radiol 28:612–616

Evans DGR, Thakker Y, Donnai D (1991) Heredity and dysmorphic syndromes in ngenital limb deficiencies. Prosthet Orthot Int 15:70–77

Fairbank TJ (1956) Dysplasia epiphysialis hemimelica (Tarso-epiphyseal aclasis). J Bone Joint Surg (Br) 38:237–257

Fixen JA (1991) The foot in childhood. In: Klenerman L (ed) The foot and its disorders, 3rd edn. Blackwell Scientific, Oxford

Freiberger RH, Hersh A, Harrison MO (1970) Roentgen examination of the deformed foot. J Bone Joint Surg (Am) 70: 341–353

Gamble FO, Yale I (1975) Clinical foot roentgenology, 2nd edn. Krieger, New York

Giedion A (1973) Acrodysplasias: cone-shaped epiphyses, peripheral dysostosis, Thiemann's disease and acrodysostosis. Prog Pediatr Radiol 4:325–345

Harris RI (1965) Retrospect: peroneal spastic flat foot (rigid valgus foot). J Bone Joint Surg Am 47:1657-1667

Harris RI, Beath T (1948) Aetiology of peroneal spastic flat foot. J Bone Joint Surg (Br) 30:624–634

Helal B (1988) The accessory ossicles and sesamoids. In: Helal B, Wilson D (eds) The foot, vol 1. Churchill Livingstone, Edinburgh, pp 567–580

Hoerr NL, Pyle SI, Francis CC (1962) Radiographic atlas of skeletal development of the foot and ankle. Thomas, Springfield, Ill

Holland CT (1928) The accessory bones of the foot. In: Fairbank HAT (ed) The Robert Jones birthday volume. Oxford University Press, Oxford

Jack EA (1954) Bone anomalies in the tarsus in relation to 'peroneal spastic flat foot'. J Bone Joint Surg Br 36: 530–542

Jayakumar S, Cowell HR (1977) Rigid flat foot. Clin Orthop 122:77–84

Johnson RP, Collier BD, Carrera GF (1984) The os trigonum syndrome: use of bone scan in the diagnosis. J Trauma 24: 761–764

Kaye JJ, Ghelman B, Schneider R (1975) Talocalcaneonavicular joint arthrography for sustentacular-talar tarsal coalitions. Radiology 115:730–731

Keats TE (1996) Atlas of normal roentgen variants that may simulate disease, 6th edn. Mosby Year Book, Chicago

Mouchet A, Belot J (1926) La tarsomegalie. J Radiol Electrol 10:289

Murray RO, McCredie J (1979) Melorheostosis and the sclerotomes: a radiological correlation. Skeletal Radiol 4:55–71

O'Rahilly R (1953) A survey of carpal and tarsal anomalies. J Bone Joint Surg (Am) 35:626–642

Porter RW (1995) Clubfoot: congenital talipes equinovarus. J R Coll Surg Edinb 40:66–71

Poznanski A (1984) The hand in radiologic diagnosis. Saunders, Philadelphia

Saunders JBdeC, O'Malley CD (1950) Vesalius: the illustrations from his works. World Publishing, Cleveland, Ohio

Shands AR, Werts IJ (1953) Foot problems in children. Surg Clin North Am 33:1543–1566

Sillence DO, Senn A, Danks DM (1979) Genetic heterogeneity in osteogenesis imperfecta. J Med Genet 16:101–116

Slomann H (1926) On the demonstration and analysis of calcaneo-navicular coalition by roentgen examination. Acta Radiol 5:304–312

Spranger JW, Langer LO, Wiedemann H-R (1974) Bone dysplasias. Saunders, Philadelphia

Templeton AW, McAlister WH, Zim ID (1965) Standardization of terminology and evaluation of osseous relationships in congenitally abnormal feet. Am J Roentgenol 93:374–381

Torode IP, Gillespie R (1991) The classification and treatment of proximal femoral deficiencies. Prosthet Orthot Int 15: 117–126

Trevor D (1950) Tarso-epiphysial aclasis. A congenital error of epiphyseal development. J Bone Joint Surg (Br) 32:204–213

Trolle D (1948) Accessory bone of the human foot (translated by E Aagensen). Munksgaard, Copenhagen

VanderWilde R, Staheli LT, Chew DE, Malagon V (1988) Measurements on radiographs of the foot in normal infants and children. J Bone Joint Surg [Am] 70:407–415

Venning P (1960) Variation of the digital skeleton of the foot. Clin Orthop 16:26–40

Webster FS, Roberts WM (1951) Tarsal anomalies and peroneal flat foot. JAMA 146:1099–1104

Wynne-Davies R, Hall CM, Apley AG (1985) Atlas of skeletal dysplasias. Churchill Livingstone, Edinburgh

Zuckerkandl E (1877) Über einen Fall von Synostose zwischen Talus und Calcaneus. Allg Wein Med Zeitung 22:293

9 Bone Trauma

P. N. M. Tyrrell and V. N. Cassar-Pullicino

CONTENTS

9.1 Introduction

Injury to the ankle and foot can be extremely debilitating for the patient and can greatly interfere with mobility. Bone injuries of the ankle can be very subtle and easily overlooked, due in part to the large number of bones tightly packed together with multiple overlap. Careful scrutiny of radiographs together with the use of extra or alternative views can help in the detection of subtle injury. Computed tomography (CT) is particularly valuable in those instances where the radiograph is normal but a high index of suspicion prevails. CT also has a particular role to play in the evaluation of calcaneal fractures.

P. N. M. Tyrrell, MD; V. N. Cassar-Pullicino, LRCP, MRCS, MD, DMRD, FRCR
Department of Diagnostic Imaging, The Robert Jones and Agnes Hunt Orthopaedic and District Hospital, Oswestry, Shropshire SY10 7AG, UK

9.2 Indications for Radiography in Suspected Injury

Trauma to the ankle is a very common injury presenting to the Accident and Emergency (A+E) Department. In the past an ankle radiographic series was found to be the second most commonly requested musculoskeletal examination in the A+E Department (after a cervical spine series), with more than 90% of such injuries being radiographed (Stiell et al. 1992). The yield of clinically significant fractures (those requiring plaster immobilisation or reduction) is less than 15% (Stiell et al. 1993). In an attempt to reduce the number of negative investigations following injury, Stiell introduced a number of clinical criteria, known as the Ottawa Ankle Rules, to determine the need for radiographs of the ankle (Stiell et al. 1994). These criteria included point tenderness over the posterior edge of either the medial or the lateral malleolus (including the distal 6 cm of the tibia and fibula) and inability to bear weight immediately after the injury or for four consecutive steps in the Emergency Department. Later studies demonstrated that application of the Ottawa Ankle Rules can adequately screen for ankle fractures (Verma et al. 1997).

Although patients may present with symptoms and signs suggestive of an ankle injury, careful perusal of the radiograph at the base of the fifth metatarsal may reveal a clinically unsuspected injury. There are a number of accessory ossicles in relation to the ankle and especially the foot, and these should not be confused with avulsion injuries. An accessory ossicle can usually be identified by its characteristic location and well corticated margin (Fig. 9.1). By comparison, an avulsed fragment will have an irregular margin, and the point from which it was avulsed may be identifiable.

In the absence of bone injury, soft-tissue swelling and tenderness are often indicative of significant soft-tissue injury. Such injuries are often referred to as ankle sprains. Since soft-tissue injuries about the ankle are almost always treated conservatively,

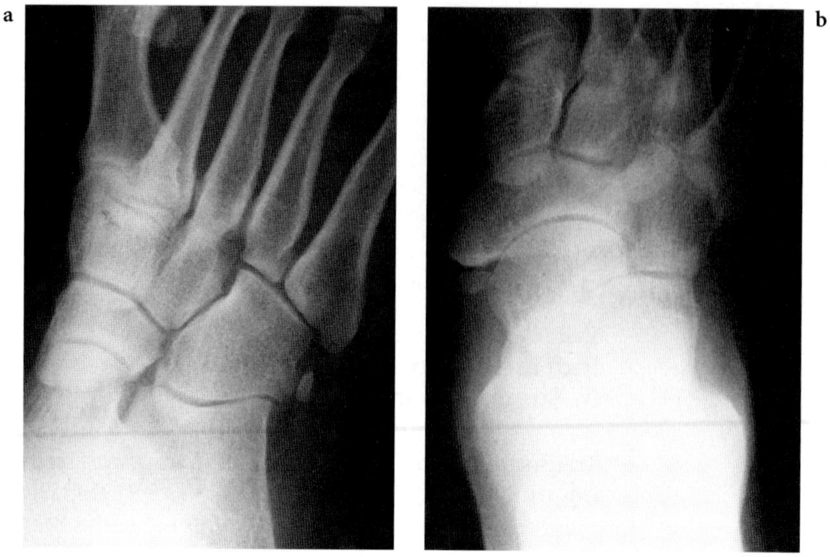

Fig. 9.1. a Oblique view of the foot demonstrating an accessory ossicle – the os vesalianum. **b** Oblique view of mid-foot demonstrating an accessory ossicle – the os tibiale externum

provided the conventional radiograph is negative for bone injury, it is unusual for patients to proceed to further imaging investigation in the form of CT or magnetic resonance imaging (MRI). However, in those centres where ultrasound is readily available, if tendon or ligamentous injury is suspected, transonic examination may often be carried out. Soft-tissue injuries are dealt with in more detail in the relevant chapter.

9.3 The Ankle

There are a number of classification systems used in respect of fractures (together with associated ligamentous injuries) at the ankle. The pattern of injury depends on the position of the foot at the time of injury and the direction, magnitude and rate of application of the loading forces. Although forces acting on the ankle may essentially be occurring in one direction and hence result in a single type of injury, such as avulsion of a bone fragment from a particular part of the joint, often the injuries are rather more complex, involving a combination of movements. The classification systems commonly employed at the ankle are those of Lauge-Hansen (1954), Danis (1949) and Weber (1972), the latter two being modified in the AO system. Lauge-Hansen (1950, 1954) highlighted the influence that the position of the foot has on the injury pattern and correlated this position with the direction of the deforming forces. In his system of classification, the position of the foot (pronation or supination) at the time of injury is described first, and the direction of the deforming force (abduction, adduction, eversion and inversion) is described second. Lauge-Hansen found that injuries occurred in a sequential manner.

The Lauge-Hansen classification of injuries is rather complex. However, one advantage of this system is that a particular mechanism of injury is associated with a sequence of injuries which if recognised, can allow one to deduce and assume their presence, even if they are not actually visualised/identified on the radiograph.

The Danis (1949) classification was modified by Weber (1972) (and more recently modified by the AO group). It is based on the level of the fracture of the fibula relative to the syndesmosis and the horizontal portion of the tibiotalar joint. While this system is simpler than the Lauge-Hansen classification, initially it ignored the medial malleolar injuries that were thought to be biomechanically important. Weber's classification has three types of fracture – A, B and C (Fig. 9.2). The more proximal the fracture of the fibula, the greater the risk of injury to the syndesmosis and tibiofibular ligaments and the more likely that the ankle mortice will be unstable. Some authors have advocated the expansion of this classification to incorporate medial injuries, and this would almost certainly increase the complexity of the classification (Harper 1992). This is essentially what the AO modification has done.

Henderson (1932) produced a classification system based on radiographic findings that separated injuries into three groups: (1) isolated fractures of the medial, lateral, posterior or anterior malleolus,

a

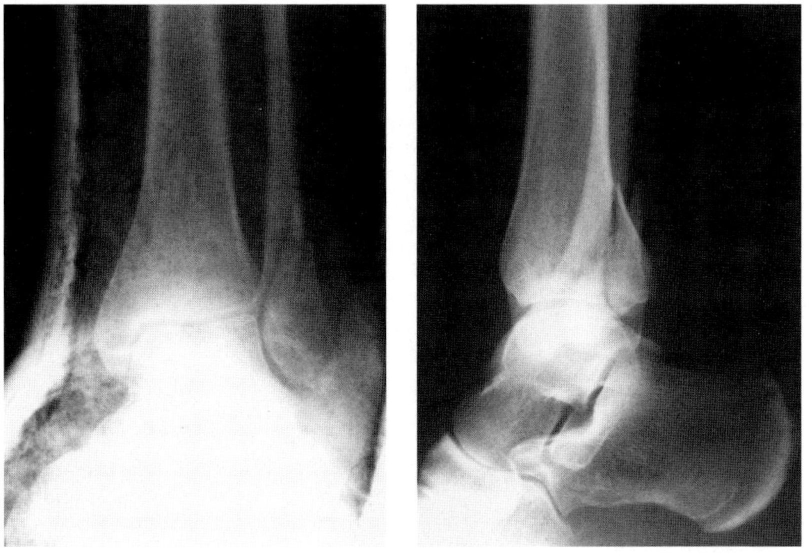

b

Fig. 9.2. a Anteroposterior view of the ankle demonstrating a fracture of the distal fibula commencing at the level of the tibiotalar joint space and extending proximally: a Weber type B injury. b Lateral view of the ankle shows the fibular fracture and also a fracture of the posterior malleolus of the tibia

(2) bi-malleolar and (3) tri-malleolar fractures. This is a simple descriptive classification that is sometimes used.

Vertical loading drives the talus into the distal tibia. The position of the foot and the rate of loading affect the injury pattern, which can range from isolated fractures of the anterior or posterior lip of the tibia to complex intra-articular fractures of the distal tibia (pilon fracture). The term pilon was first used by Destot in 1911. He compared this explosive injury of the talus impacting against the tibia to that of a hammer striking a nail. This fracture involves the tibial plafond of the ankle joint (Fig. 9.3). The injury is associated with high energy, as in falling from a height, and with a large compressive force, significant comminuted disruption of the articular surface, and extensive soft-tissue injury (Ayeni 1988; Mainwaring et al. 1988; Ruwe et al. 1993).

Isolated avulsion type fractures at the ankle can occur. Fractures of the medial malleolus may be transverse or oblique. Transverse fractures are the result of tensile forces mediated by the deltoid ligament and may involve the anterior colliculus alone or both the anterior and the posterior colliculi. Oblique fractures usually extend upwards and inwards from the corner of the plafond. These are due to angular forces generated by movement of the talus against the medial malleolus. Fractures of the medial malleolus distal to the corner formed in the ankle mortice within the plafond are more stable than those arising within the plafond, due to the buttressing effect afforded by the medial malleolus. An isolated fracture of the posterior colliculus due to avulsion by the deep portion of the deltoid ligament has been described by Bonnin (1970) and Pankovich and Shivaram (1979). The fragment extends superiorly and posteriorly and is relatively undisplaced due to the overlying tibialis posterior tendon. It may be seen as a long, thin fragment of cortical bone projected just lateral to the cortical contour of the malleolus. It can be difficult to visualise on an anteroposterior radiograph and may be better seen on an external oblique projection.

Classification systems are often employed to facilitate comparisons between different treatment/management regimens. In practical terms, what the orthopaedic surgeon wants to know from the radiograph is: what structures are fractured, the degree of separation, displacement or malalignment, and whether the injury is stable or unstable. Instability is confirmed if abnormal movement or displacement occurs under normal loading. The answer to these questions largely determines whether conservative or surgical management is required. The appropriate management employed will then hopefully minimise the risk of post-traumatic complications.

Inversion or adduction of the ankle places tension on the lateral collateral ligament, resulting either in ligamentous rupture or a transverse fracture of the distal fibula inferior to the level of the tibial plafond. The most common fracture of the lateral malleolus is an oblique or spiral fracture extending from the anteroinferior margin upwards and backwards to the posterior margin of the shaft of the distal fibula (Fig. 9.2). Fractures may also occur within the distal mid-shaft or proximal shaft of the fibula. Ankle injuries created by external rotation of the foot can be associated with a fracture of the proximal shaft of the fibula, as described

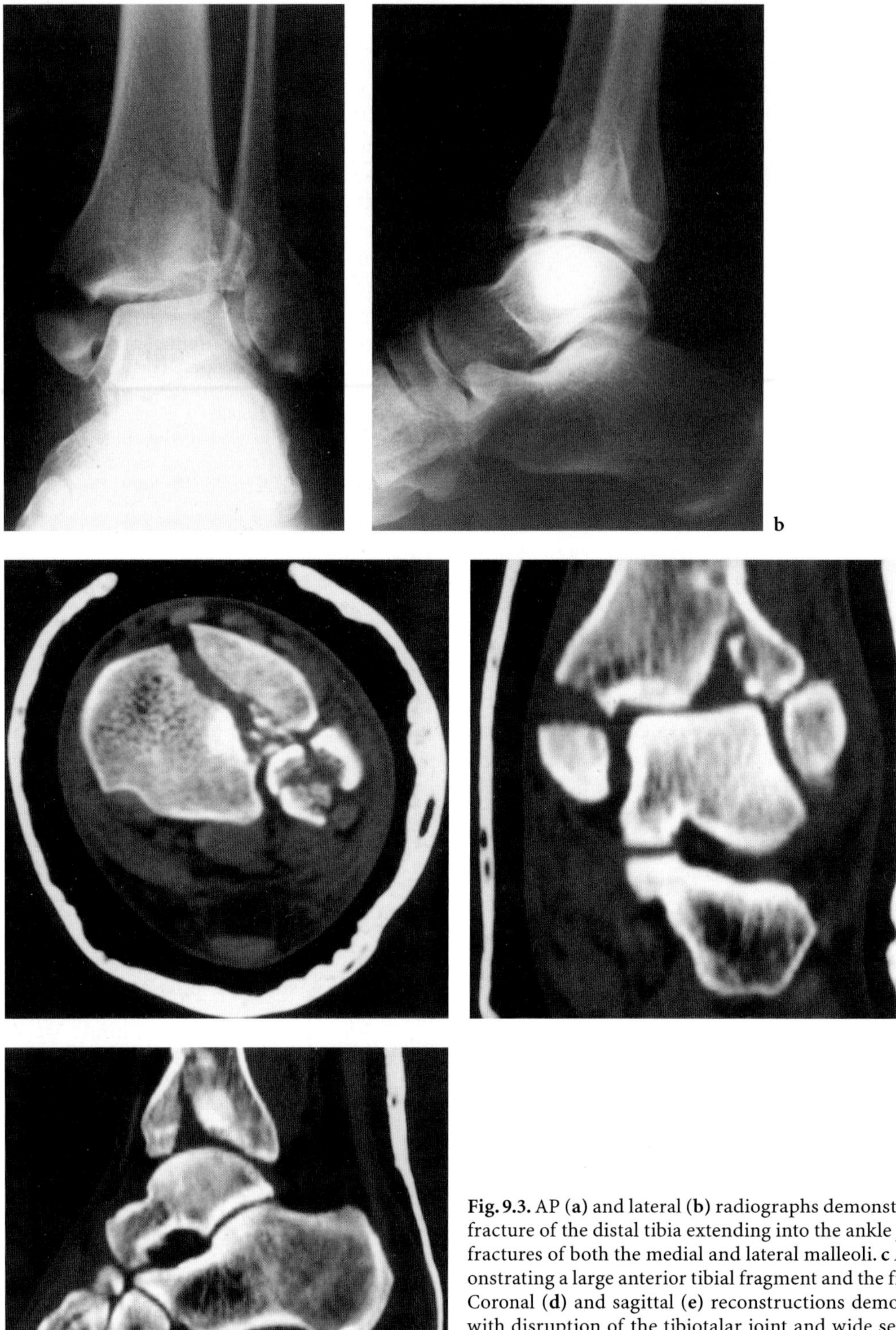

Fig. 9.3. AP (**a**) and lateral (**b**) radiographs demonstrating a comminuted fracture of the distal tibia extending into the ankle joint, associated with fractures of both the medial and lateral malleoli. **c** Axial CT image demonstrating a large anterior tibial fragment and the fractured distal fibula. Coronal (**d**) and sagittal (**e**) reconstructions demonstrate the fractures with disruption of the tibiotalar joint and wide separation of the anterior fragment from the parent bone

by MAISONNEUVE (1840). This fracture is easily overlooked since patients rarely complain of pain in the region when there are more painful ankle injuries. A Maisonneuve fracture should be suspected and full-length views of the tibia and fibula obtained when ankle radiographs demonstrate an apparent isolated fracture of the posterior lip of the tibia, widening of the medial or lateral clear space, an isolated displaced fracture of the medial malleolus, or when tenderness can be elicited clinically over the syndesmosis or anteromedial aspect of the joint capsule in the absence of obvious underlying injury (ROGERS 1992).

Avulsion fractures can occur from the distal tip of the lateral or medial malleolus due to pull of the lateral or medial collateral ligaments. These fractures need to be differentiated from the secondary centres of ossification. An isolated small avulsion fracture of the posterolateral aspect of the lateral malleolus may be associated with dislocation of the peroneal tendons due to the retinaculum which binds down the tendons being avulsed. The fracture flake consists of a small bone fragment 1–2 mm in width but 1–2 cm in length. It lies parallel to the lateral or posterolateral aspect of the lateral malleolus and is best seen on AP or an internal oblique projection. The injury is not uncommon in skiers and occurs when the peroneal muscles are tensed and the ankle dorsiflexed. Surgical treatment is required to repair the retinaculum, and the bone fragment is either excised or reattached. A similar small avulsion injury has been identified just proximal and medial to the medial malleolus, associated with rupture of the tibialis posterior tendon. This is associated with either a transverse fracture of the medial malleolus or bi-malleolar fractures of the pronation-external rotation variety with the fibular fracture located proximal to the joint line.

Avulsion fracture of the anterior tubercle of the tibia is the result of tension within the anteroinferior tibiofibular ligament and is known as the Tillaux fracture (CANCELMO 1962; PROTAS and KORNBLATT 1981). This is due to external rotation of the foot. The Wagstaffe-Le Fort fracture is an avulsion fracture at the fibular attachment of the anterior tibiofibular ligament. Fractures of the posterior malleolus or posterior lip of the tibia occur as a result of avulsion at the site of attachment of the posterior tibiofibular ligament. These may be small and flake-like or larger and involve some portion of the posterior joint surface of the tibia. The latter are due to vertical compression of the talus against the tibia. The fracture line is vertically oriented in the coronal plane. Fragments consisting of more than 25% of the articular surface may require surgical fixation. These fractures often occur as part of the tri-malleolar fracture. Dorsiflexion of the foot may result in fractures of the anterior lip of the tibia. Their size determines the need for surgical reduction. If large, they may be associated with a fracture dislocation.

In bi-malleolar fractures, the path of the fracture on one side is often transverse because of tensile forces, while the other fracture is spiral or oblique. Tri-malleolar fractures involve the posterior lip of the tibia in addition to the malleoli. Usually, these are fracture dislocations. Most are due to external rotation of the foot and, therefore, are laterally and posteriorly displaced. The lateral collateral ligament remains intact, as does the posterior tibiofibular ligament.

9.4 The Talus

Half of the injuries to the talus consist of fractures, 50% of which are avulsions while the rest are vertical or oblique fractures traversing the neck or body in the coronal plane. Some 25% of all injuries are fracture dislocations, with fracture of the neck being associated with either subtalar or posterior dislocation of the body. Another 20% are other forms of dislocation without fracture, and the remaining 5% consist of other fractures including compression fractures of the talus.

Avulsion or chip-type fractures occur at the superior aspect of the neck and head of the talus and also at the lateral, medial and posterior aspect of the body. The most common avulsion fracture involves the anterosuperior aspect of the neck at the point of attachment of the capsule (Fig. 9.4). This fracture needs to be differentiated from an os supratalare. A fracture from the lateral aspect of the body of the talus involves the lateral process that projects laterally beneath the tip of the lateral malleolus. An avulsion fracture may occur at the attachment of the deltoid ligament medially, and fractures of the posterior talar surface may occur in extreme plantar flexion. This injury is to be differentiated from the accessory ossicle, the os trigonum.

Vertical fractures usually occur as a result of a force from below driving the neck of the talus upward against the anterior lip of the tibia (Fig. 9.5). These are not infrequently seen in road traffic accidents, when the sole of the foot is jammed against the brake pedal. They can be associated with dislocation if the forces were strong enough. The mechanism of injury is continuation of the dorsiflexion force that pro-

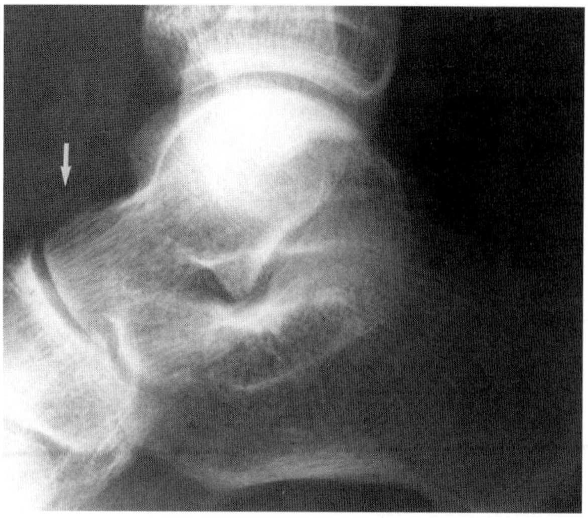

Fig. 9.4. Lateral view of the ankle. Note the avulsion fracture from the neck of the talus (*arrow*)

duced the fracture of the neck, resulting in rupture of ligamentous structures that bind the talus to the tibia and calcaneum.

Hawkins (1970) proposed a classification of talar fractures: type I – non-displaced fracture of the neck of the talus without subluxation or dislocation; type II – displaced fracture of the talar neck with subluxation/dislocation of the subtalar joint (the ankle joint remains aligned); and type III – displaced fracture of the talar neck with complete dislocation at the ankle and subtalar joints. Despite posteromedial displacement of the body with most type II injuries, the posterior tibial neurovascular bundle is usually spared. However, in type III injuries with posteromedial displacement of the body, the neurovascular structures are definitively at risk. Fractures of the neck of the talus can be associated with calcaneal (10%) (Lorentzen et al. 1977) and malleolar fractures (19%–28%) (Canale and Kelly 1978; Lorentzen et al. 1977).

Fractures of the body of the talus may involve compression fractures of the talar dome often following a fall from a height. Only the superior articular surface of the talus may be involved with disruption of the tibiotalar joint, or the entire body of the talus may fracture with involvement of both the tibiotalar and the subtalar joints. Post-traumatic complications of osteonecrosis and degenerative arthritis can be minimised by anatomical reduction with or without internal fixation. The blood supply of the talus is tenuous, and a vertical fracture of the neck is associated with a risk of avascular necrosis (AVN) of the proximal fragment (Fig. 9.5) (Haliburton et al. 1958; Kelly and Sullivan 1963). The risk of disruption of the blood supply and subsequent AVN increases progressively with each type of talar fracture.

9.5 The Calcaneum

This is the most frequently fractured bone of the tarsus. Approximately 25% of fractures are extra-articular, sparing the subtalar joint, consisting of

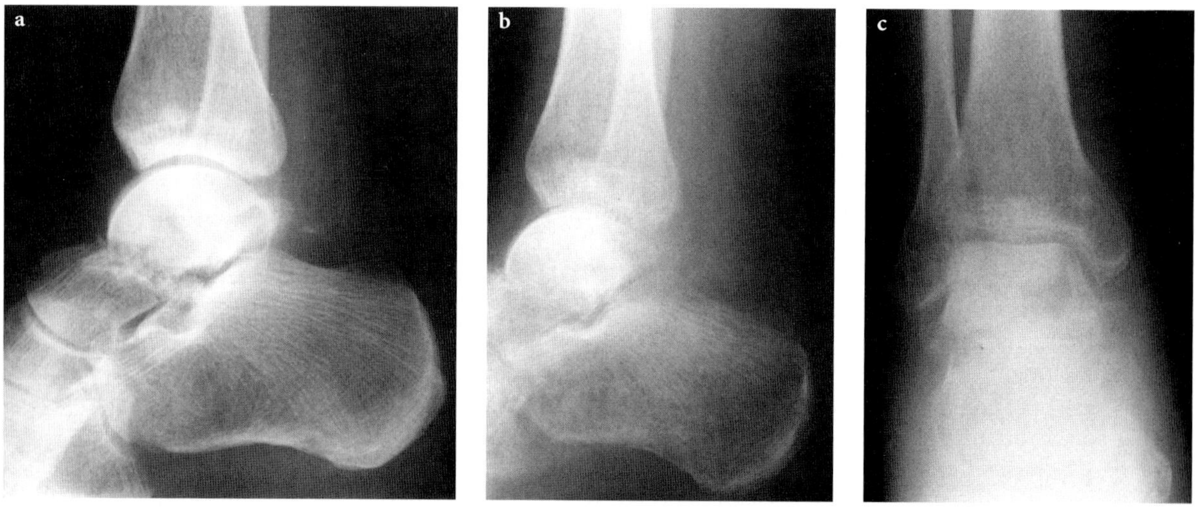

Fig. 9.5. **a** Lateral radiograph of the ankle demonstrating a fracture through the neck of the talus. **b** Lateral radiograph 10 weeks post-injury. There is a generalised osteopenia. The relative sclerosis of the talar dome indicates the presence of avascular necrosis. **c** Note the typical geographical distribution of avascular necrosis as seen on the AP view

avulsion of the various processes. The remaining 75% are intra-articular, involving the subtalar joint and body of the calcaneum. These are invariably due to compression forces such as landing on the feet following a fall from a height. Fractures of the calcaneum are associated with proximal fractures of the tibia and spine in 10%–12% of cases. Normally, a dorsiplantar projection, a lateral and an axial calcaneal view will allow identification of most fractures. Oblique projections may be needed for further clarification (ISHERWOOD 1961).

Non-compressive/Avulsive-Type Fractures. These involve the anterior process, the sustentaculum tali, the superior portion of the tuberosity and the medial or lateral surface of the tuberosity (Fig. 9.6). These fractures spare the subtalar joint. Vertical fractures of the tuberosity may occasionally spare the subtalar joint, extending obliquely from the medial to the lateral surfaces of the bone.

A fracture involving the anterior process of the calcaneum needs to be differentiated from an accessory ossicle, which can occur adjacent to the anterosuperior tip of the calcaneum, known as the os calcaneus secondarius.

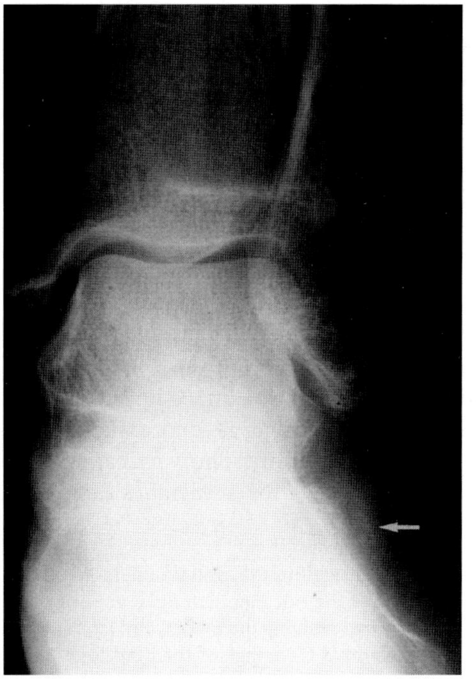

Fig. 9.6. AP view of the ankle. An avulsion fracture from the lateral calcaneum is visible (*arrow*)

Compressive Fractures. Böhler's tuber joint angle is seen on lateral projections (Fig. 9.7). It is the complement of the angle formed by two lines: one drawn between the highest part of the anterior process and the highest part of the posterior articular surface, and one drawn between the same point on the posterior articular surface and the most superior point of the tuberosity. The angle normally measures between 25° and 40° and is usually similar bilaterally.

The lateral process of the talus is wedge-shaped on lateral projection with its apex directed to the 'crucial angle' as originally described by Gissane (HARTY 1973). Axial compressive forces impact the talus into the calcaneum, disrupting the subtalar joint and distorting this anatomical angle. The force results in an oblique fracture extending from the apex of the angle, separating the body of the calcaneum. Simultaneously, a vertical split is created within the posterior facet, producing a lateral fragment which is usually larger and contains one-half to two-thirds of the posterior facet. There is often comminution and depression of the posterior facet from the lateral cortex. The lateral cortex is seen as a thin fragment of cortical bone. The smaller remainder of the facet is attached to a medial fragment containing the sustentaculum tali. Additional forces depress the lateral fragment, containing the majority of the posterior facet, into the body of the calcaneum.

ESSEX-LOPRESTI (1952) has defined two princi-

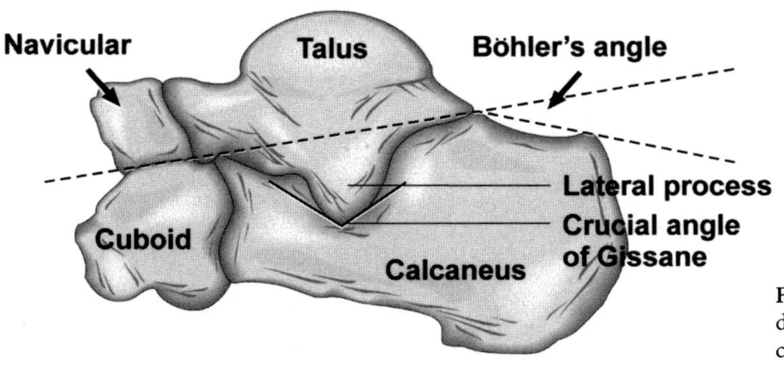

Fig. 9.7. Lateral line diagram of the hind foot demonstrating Böhler's angle and the talocalcaneal relationship

pal types of depressed fracture of the calcaneum. In one, the principal fragment of the posterior facet contains the upper portion of the tuberosity. Due to its appearance on the lateral projection, this fragment is designated the 'tongue' type. In the second, more common form, the principal fragment containing the posterior facet is separated from the tuberosity by a vertical fracture line just posterior to the posterior facet. This type is referred to as the 'central lateral' compression type, where central lateral refers to the principal fragment containing the posterior facet, which is laterally situated and depressed into the central portion of the calcaneum. Usually, the lateral fragment is depressed downwards and displaced laterally. The vertical split of the posterior facet allows for a variable degree of compression of the medial and lateral fragments.

A limited degree of information about these injuries can be obtained from conventional radiographs, including the particularly important radiographic sign of reduction of Böhler's angle to less than 25°. A significantly greater amount of information, facilitating a better assessment of the degree and nature of the injury, is obtained by CT (Guyer et al. 1985; Heger et al. 1985; Hindman et al. 1986; Rosenberg et al. 1987) (Figs. 9.8–9.10). Coronal images give a particularly good assessment of the degree of depression of the posterior facet, the size and number of fragments, the degree of fragment displacement and calcaneal widening. Sagittal reconstructions will also facilitate three-plane evaluation of the injury. In CT of fractures of the calcaneum, not infrequently the peroneal ten-

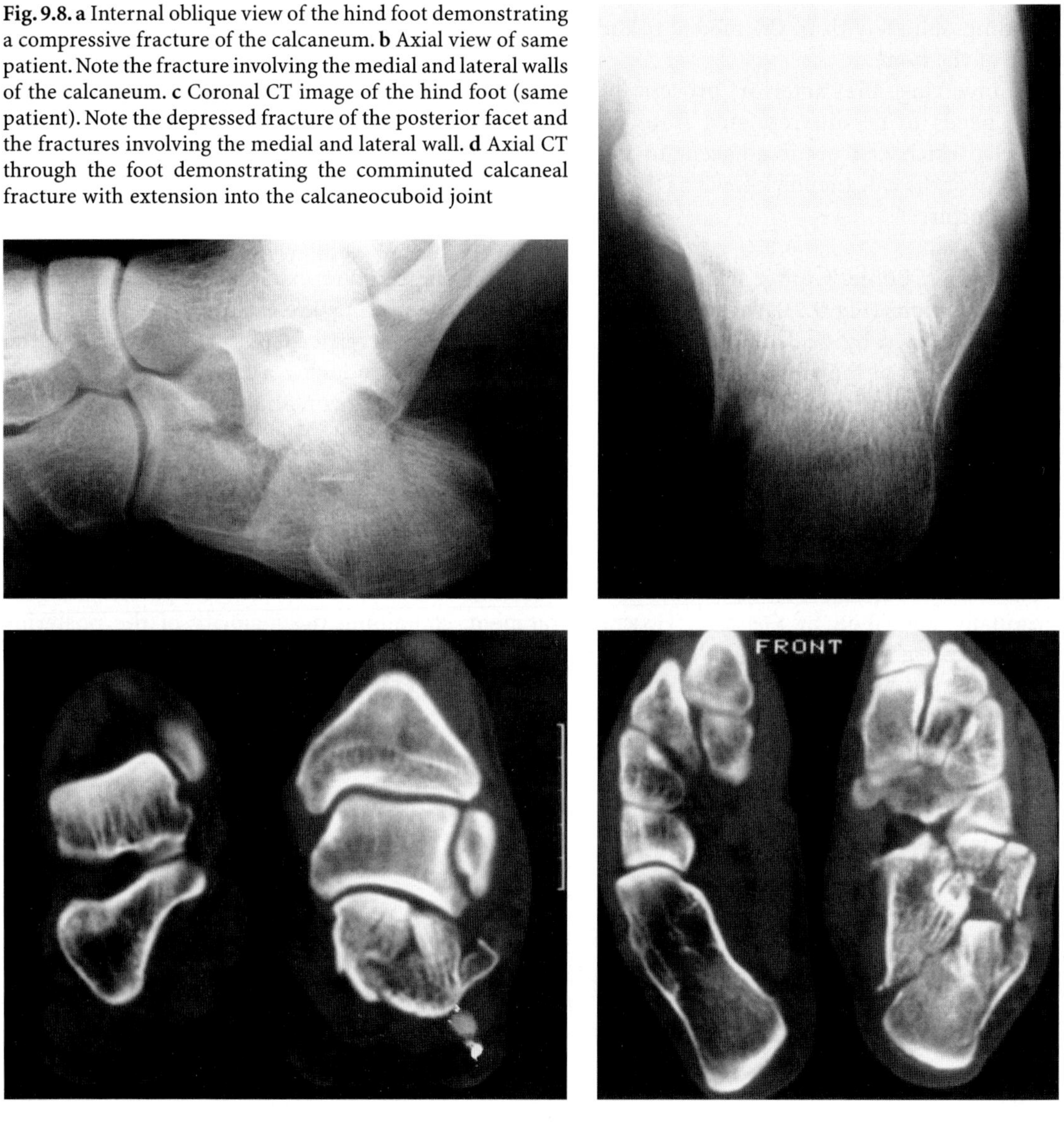

Fig. 9.8. a Internal oblique view of the hind foot demonstrating a compressive fracture of the calcaneum. **b** Axial view of same patient. Note the fracture involving the medial and lateral walls of the calcaneum. **c** Coronal CT image of the hind foot (same patient). Note the depressed fracture of the posterior facet and the fractures involving the medial and lateral wall. **d** Axial CT through the foot demonstrating the comminuted calcaneal fracture with extension into the calcaneocuboid joint

a b c d

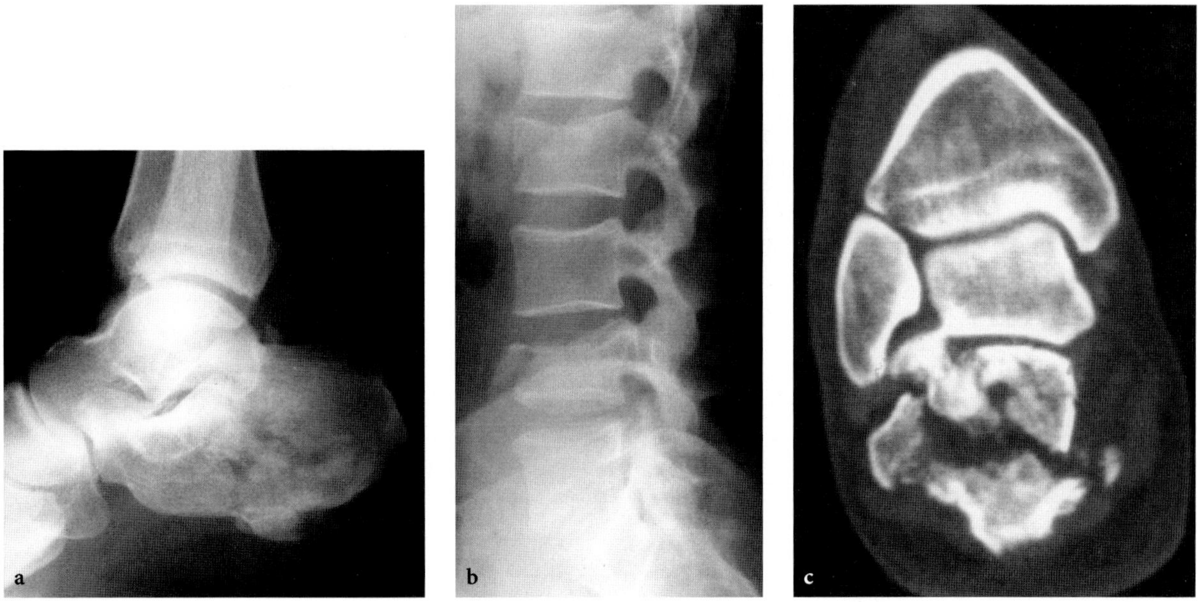

Fig. 9.9. a Lateral radiograph demonstrating a compressive fracture of the calcaneum with extension into the subtalar joint. **b** Coronal CT image demonstrates the pattern of the fracture. **c** Lateral lumbar spine of same patient, demonstrating fractures of the bodies of L2 and L4 sustained during the same injury (fall from a height)

dons may either be dislocated or impinged between the bone fragments and the inferiormost aspect of the fibula. CT is also particularly good in the follow-up evaluation of these fractures and particularly in the assessment of post-traumatic arthritis, a common complication following these injuries.

9.6 The Navicular Bone

Fractures of the navicular bone are uncommon. Fractures of the body of the navicular bone occur either in the horizontal or more commonly the vertical plane. They may be associated with dislocation, particularly the vertical fracture. The vertical fracture will only be visualised on the anteroposterior projection. When associated with dislocation, there is usually medial dislocation of the medial fragment. If a horizontally orientated fracture is associated with dislocation, there is usually dorsal dislocation of the dorsal fragment.

Avulsion fractures are more commonly seen in relation to the navicular bone. The most common of these is from the dorsal aspect of the bone, in the region of the talonavicular joint. This fracture should not be confused with an accessory ossicle, the os supranaviculare. An accessory ossicle can usually be readily differentiated from a fracture fragment by its smooth, well corticated margin. Another site of an avulsion fracture is in relation to the navicular tuberosity. This is the site of attachment of the tibialis posterior tendon. The fracture occurs during abduction of the foot. This fracture is not to be confused with the accessory navicular bone (Fig. 9.11). This is often a moderately large sized ossicle, attached to the body of the navicular by a synchondrosis. With abduction injuries of the foot, although an actual fracture may not occur, there may be some disruption of the synchondrosis, and this is manifest by slight widening of the synchondrosis. The ossicle itself is differentiated from an acute fracture by its well corticated margin. Occasionally, small ossicles may be seen just proximal to the navicular tuberosity. These lie in the substance of the posterior tibial tendon and are known as the os tibiale externum.

9.7 The Cuboid and Cuneiform Bones

An avulsion fracture from the lateral aspect of the cuboid bone can occur with adduction injuries (Fig. 9.12). This small bone fragment should also not be confused with accessory ossicles along the lateral aspect of the foot, namely the os peroneum and the os vesalianum. Compression fractures of

a b c d e f

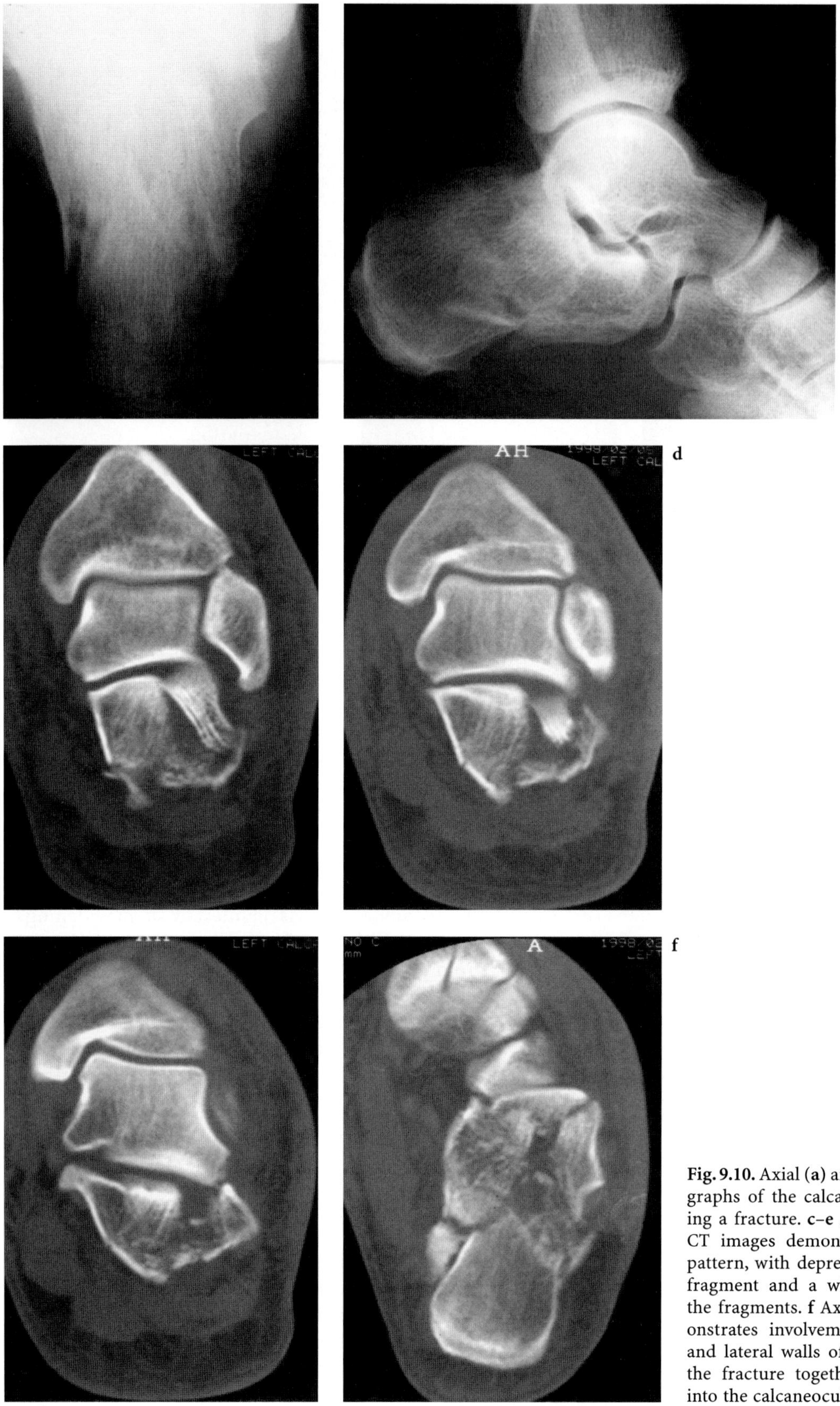

Fig. 9.10. Axial (**a**) and lateral (**b**) radiographs of the calcaneum demonstrating a fracture. **c–e** A series of coronal CT images demonstrate the fracture pattern, with depression of the lateral fragment and a wide space between the fragments. **f** Axial CT image demonstrates involvement of the medial and lateral walls of the calcaneum in the fracture together with extension into the calcaneocuboid joint

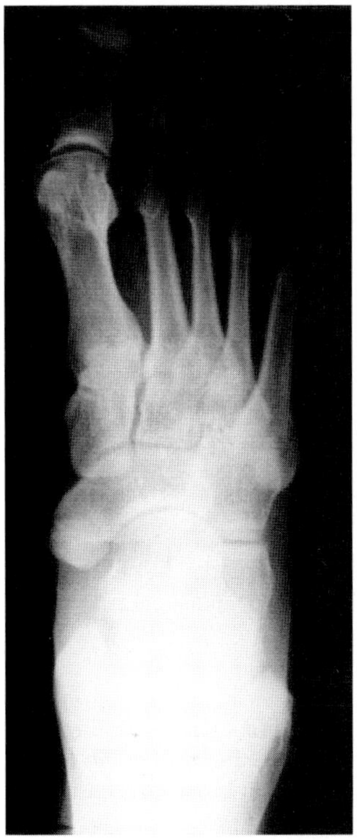

a

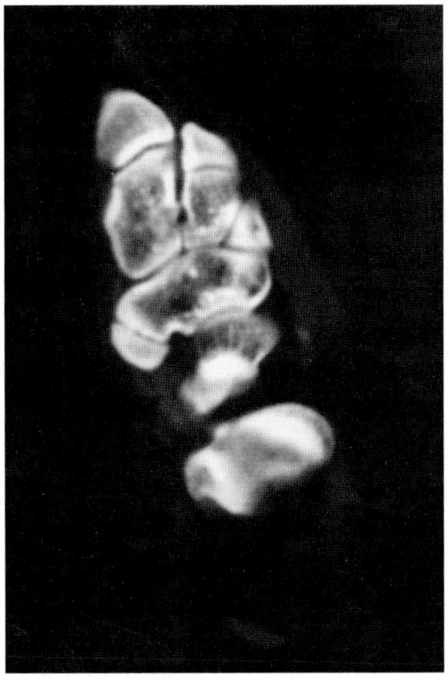

b

Fig. 9.11. a AP view of the foot demonstrating an accessory navicular ossicle. **b** Axial CT image demonstrating the synchondrosis of the accessory navicular with the parent bone

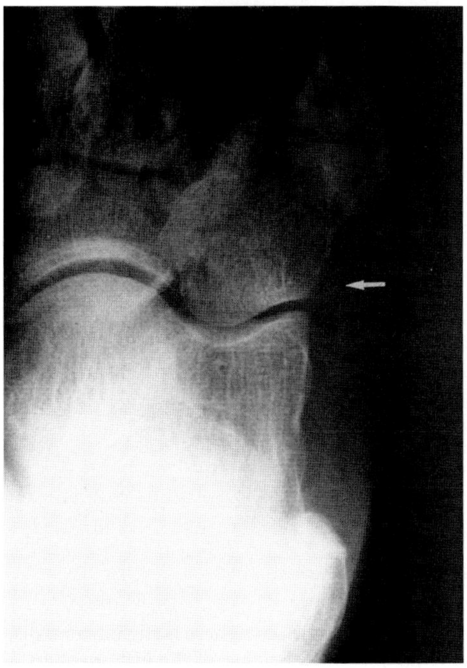

Fig. 9.12. Radiograph of the mid-foot demonstrating an avulsion fracture from the lateral aspect of the cuboid bone (*arrow*)

the cuboid bone or anterior process of the calcaneum may be associated with fracture of the tuberosity of the navicular bone.

Isolated fractures of the cuneiform bones are extremely unusual. If such a fracture is identified, the possibility of tarsometatarsal dislocation (Lisfranc) should be strongly suspected (Fig. 9.13). In this instance, further radiographic views or alternatively a CT scan should be obtained.

9.8 The Metatarsals

Fractures at the base of the fifth metatarsal are not uncommon (Dameron 1975; Torg et al. 1984). These tend to be transverse fractures. There are two distinct types, both of which are due to inversion of the foot. One is an avulsion fracture from the tip of the tuberosity (Figs. 9.14, 9.15), and the other a transverse fracture of the proximal shaft located approximately 1.5–2 cm distal to the tip of the tuberosity, just distal to the tarsometatarsal joint. This fracture is commonly known as the Jones's fracture, originally described by Sir Robert Jones in 1902. The avulsion fracture from the proximalmost tip of the fifth metatarsal occurs at the site of insertion of the pero-

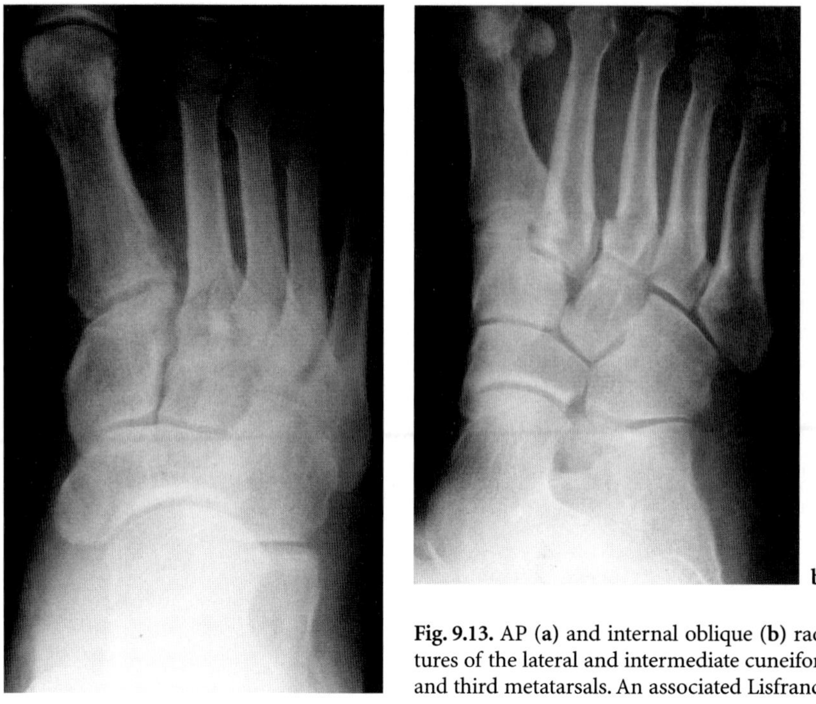

a b

Fig. 9.13. AP (**a**) and internal oblique (**b**) radiographs of the foot demonstrating fractures of the lateral and intermediate cuneiform bones and also the bases of the second and third metatarsals. An associated Lisfranc dislocation should be strongly suspected

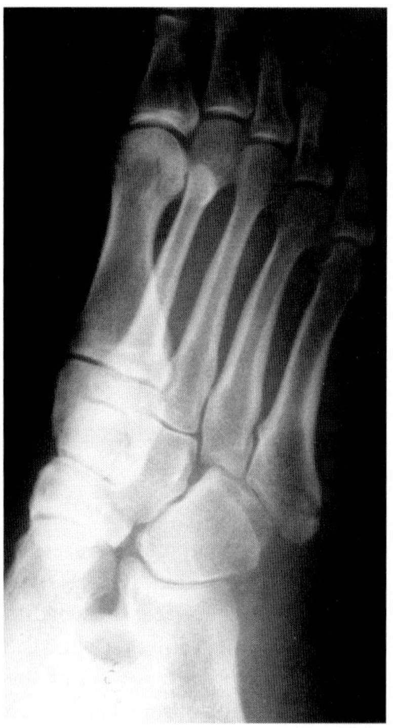

Fig. 9.14. AP internal oblique view of the foot. There is a transverse fracture of the base of the fifth metatarsal which extends into the calcaneocuboid joint. There is also widening of the calcaneocuboid joint space

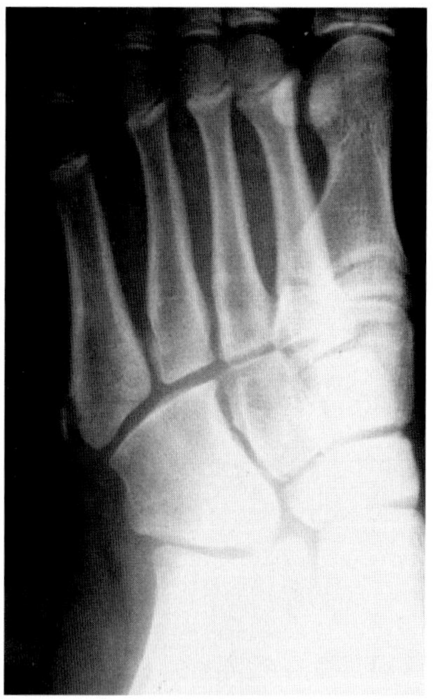

Fig. 9.15. AP oblique view of the foot. There is slight lateral displacement of the apophysis at the base of the fifth metatarsal. There is also an undisplaced transverse fracture at the base of the metatarsal

neus brevis tendon. Both of these fractures should be differentiated from the presence of a normally occurring apophysis just lateral to the base of the metatarsal (Fig. 9.15). The differentiating feature is that the apophysis lies in a longitudinal orientation, and the radiographic space between it and the parent bone is directed longitudinally. Both of the aforementioned fractures are transverse. On occasion, both a transverse and a longitudinal lucency can be identified, this simply representing a transverse fracture in the presence of an unfused apophysis.

Fractures of the metatarsal shafts can occur often due to a heavy load falling on the foot. The metatarsal shafts are common sites of stress fractures.

Freiberg's disease is avascular necrosis of the head of a metatarsal, usually the second, and should not be confused with an acute fracture (Helal and Gibb 1987). There is often a modelling anomaly, with slight flattening of the metatarsal head. There may be a cortical infraction, but there is usually altered density of the bone, and the combined radiological features allow differentiation from an acute injury.

9.9 Stress Fractures

A stress fracture occurs as a result of repetitive abnormal stress on physiologically normal bone. This is to be differentiated from an insufficiency fracture which occurs as a result of a normal stress on abnormal bone, usually due to metabolic bone disease. There are multiple characteristic sites of these fractures in the bones of the foot (Eisele and Sammarco 1993). The most common is the 'March' fracture, occurring in the mid-shafts of one or more metatarsals, an injury commonly found in soldiers. These fractures present with pain, but the fracture may not be visible on initial radiography. Repeat radiographs 3–4 weeks later usually show evidence of a fracture. Even if a discrete fracture line is not observed, there may be a very subtle periosteal reaction consistent with the injury. Radionuclide bone scan is diagnostic when the radiograph is negative. Stress fractures of the navicular bone are not uncommon, but such fractures can occur in almost any bone in the foot (Meurman 1981) including the sesamoids (Van Hal et al. 1982).

Common sites of insufficiency fractures in the foot include the calcaneum (Figs. 9.16, 9.17) and the navicular bone. The presence of pain in a patient whose radiographs demonstrate osteoporosis should raise a strong suspicion of an underlying insufficiency fracture. Again, a radionuclide bone scan at this time may well be positive when the radiograph does not demonstrate any sign of fracture.

9.10 Dislocation

9.10.1 Dislocation of the Talus

Subluxation or dislocation of the talus can occur either with or without a talar fracture. Three joints may be involved – the talotibial, the subtalar and the talonavicular. Total talar dislocation involves all three joints. This is usually an open injury. Characteristically, the talus is found to lie transversely in front of the lateral malleolus.

The pure form of subtalar dislocation of the foot involves dislocation at the subtalar and talonavicular joints (Fig. 9.18). Most commonly, the dislocation is medial, with the calcaneum and the navicular bone displaced medially, and the head of the talus lying dorsolaterally. Less commonly, the subtalar dislocation occurs laterally, with the calcaneum, navicular and forefoot lying lateral relative to the talus. The diagnosis is best made on anteroposterior radio-

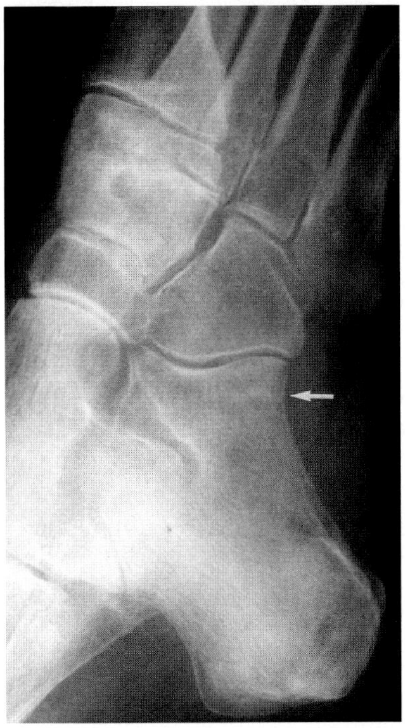

Fig. 9.16. Internal oblique projection of the mid-foot demonstrating a stress fracture of the calcaneum (*arrow*)

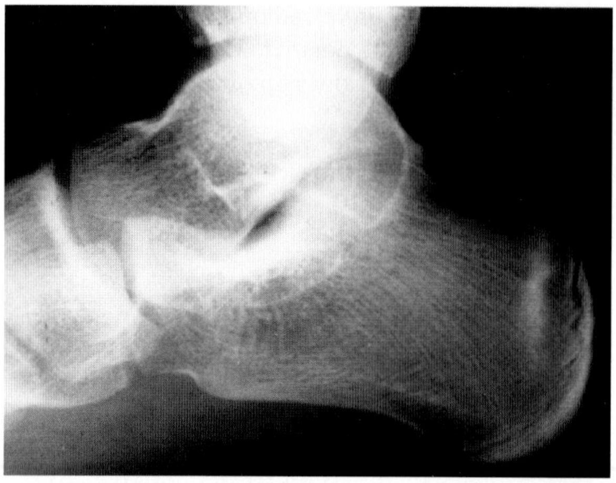

a

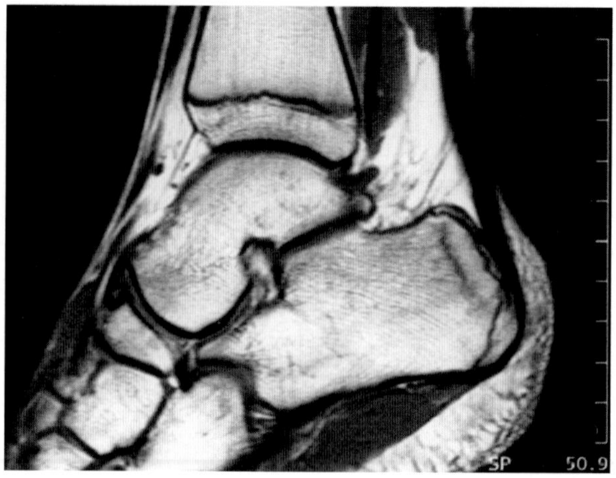

b

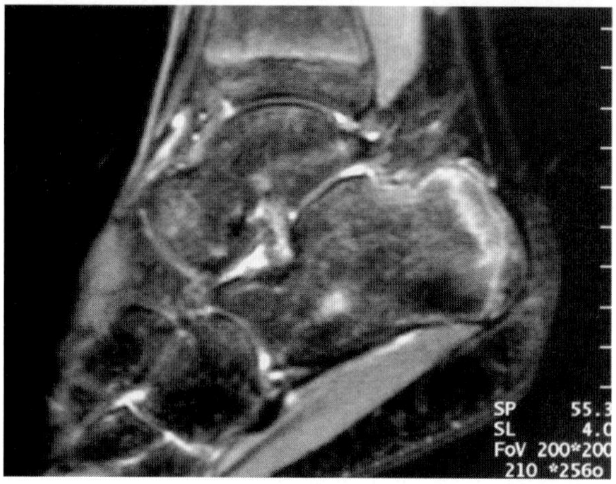

c

Fig. 9.17. a Lateral radiograph of the calcaneum demonstrating a stress fracture of the tuberosity. **b** Sagittal T1-weighted image demonstrates the fracture as linear low signal, while on a sagittal STIR image (**c**) this is seen as a linear high signal

graphs of the foot and ankle. The tibiotalar and calcaneocuboid joints remain aligned, but medial or lateral displacement of the calcaneum and navicular bones is evident. Such dislocations are often associated with talar or calcaneal osteochondral fracture. CT can be particularly helpful in evaluating these injuries (Fig. 9.18).

On occasion, a dislocation may essentially affect the subtalar joint alone, or alternatively the talonavicular joint alone. The latter is known as a 'swivel' dislocation and occurs more commonly medially than laterally. The principal injury is usually apparent, but there may be very slight widening of adjacent joint spaces with seemingly satisfactory alignment.

9.10.2 Tarsometatarsal (Lisfranc) Dislocation

Fracture-dislocation in the tarsometatarsal region is overlooked in 20% of cases. It can be a difficult region to evaluate on conventional radiographs, and careful scrutiny of this area is required (Myerson 1989). If a fracture in the region of the tarsometatarsal joints is seen, an associated dislocation should be strongly suspected (Fig. 9.13). If it is not obvious on radiographs, then further imaging with CT is warranted, the coronal plane being particularly valuable in the assessment of alignment.

9.11 Children

9.11.1 Fractures of the Distal Tibia and Fibula

The skeletal maturity of the patient determines the resulting bone, ligamentous or growth plate injury. The growth plate forms a plane of weakness which results in different patterns of injury to those in the adult. The ligaments of children are stronger than the growth plate, predisposing to physeal separa-

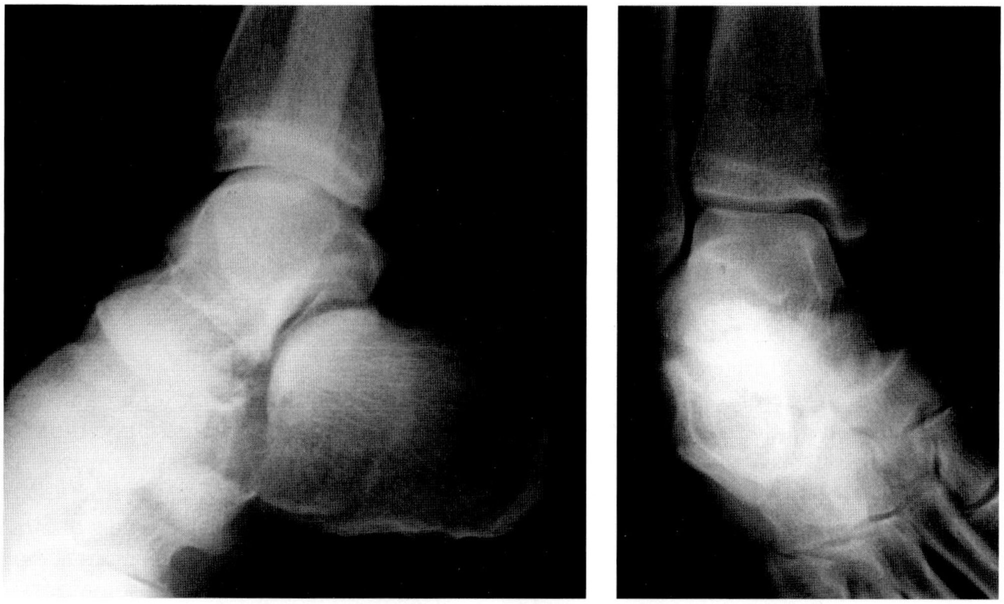

a b

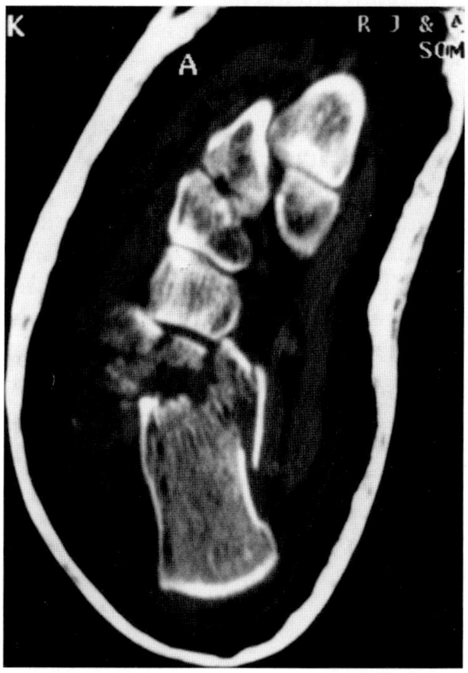

c

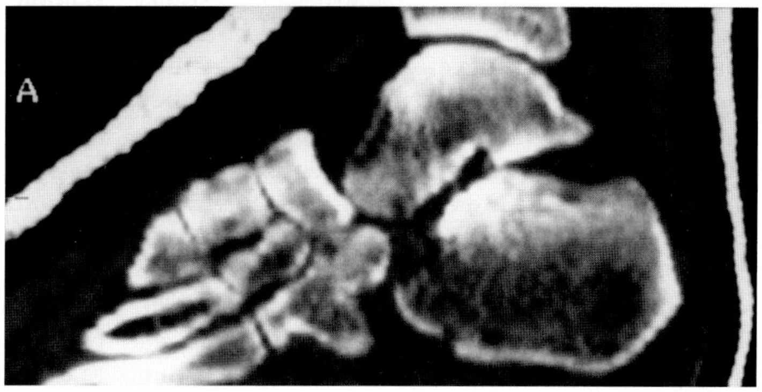

d

Fig. 9.18. **a** Lateral radiograph demonstrating a fracture of the calcaneum. The talonavicular and calcaneocuboid joints are not well seen. The posterior subtalar joint is abnormal. **b** AP radiograph demonstrates a fracture of the calcaneum and also subluxation of the talonavicular joint. **c** Axial CT image confirms the fracture through the anterior aspect of the calcaneum extending into the calcaneocuboid joint. **d** Sagittal CT reconstruction demonstrates marked posterior subluxation of the subtalar joint and subluxation of the talonavicular joint

tion in a child. Fractures in children rarely disturb the talotibial relationship (Rang 1983). The distal tibial epiphysis is the second most common site of epiphyseal injury in the entire skeleton after the distal radius. Tibial epiphyseal injuries often occur in the absence of injury to the fibula, indicative of the relative resilience of the fibula in children. As a result of an epiphyseal fracture, the growth plate frequently appears widened. Often there are thin, usually metaphyseal flakes of bone representing small avulsion fractures. When the epiphysis is minimally displaced, comparison with the opposite side may be necessary to confirm the diagnosis. The prognosis is dependent on the skeletal maturity of the patient, the severity of the injury, the fracture type, degree of comminution and displacement, and the adequacy of reduction.

9.11.2 Modified Lauge-Hansen Classification

A classification system of fractures can be anatomical or related to the mechanism of injury. An anatomical classification such as that used by SALTER and HARRIS (1963) (Fig. 9.19) is widely used. However, the classification on its own does not make reference to the mechanism of injury. The most widely accepted mechanism of injury classification of ankle fractures in children is that described by DIAS and TACHDJIAN (1978), who modified the adult-based Lauge-Hansen classification in their review of 71 fractures.

The classification of childhood ankle fractures is a complex area. VAHVANEN and AALTO (1980) compared their ability to classify 310 ankle fractures in children with the WEBER (1972), LAUGE-HANSEN (1954) and SALTER-HARRIS (1963) classifications. They found that they were 'largely unsuccessful' using the Weber and Lauge-Hansen classifications but could easily classify the fractures using the Salter-Harris system. They suggested that although ankle fractures in children can be extremely complex, they can be roughly divided into avulsional and epiphyseal fractures. Adequately reduced avulsional fractures can be expected to heal well, while epiphyseal fractures may give rise to late complications. SPIEGEL et al. (1978) followed 184 of a series of 237 fractures of the distal end of the tibia or fibula in children. Using the Salter-Harris classification they identified three groups according to the risk of developing subsequent complications including shortening of the leg, angular deformity of the bone or incongruity of the joint. According to SPIEGEL the low-risk group, which consisted of 89 patients, 6.7% of whom had complications, included all type I and II fibula fractures, all type I tibial fractures, type III and type IV tibial fractures with less than 2 mm of displacement, and epiphyseal avulsion injuries. The high-risk group consisted of 28 patients, 32% of whom had complications. This group included type III and type IV tibial fractures with 2 mm or more of displacement, juvenile Tillaux fractures, tri-plane fractures and comminuted tibial epiphyseal fractures (type V). The third and unpredictable group was made up 66 patients, 16.7% of them with complications. Only type II tibial fractures were included. Interestingly, in this review, the presence or absence of a fibula fracture in association with a tibial epiphyseal fracture had no prognostic significance as regards the incidence of complications. This is noteworthy since some classification systems centre around the presence and location of the fracture of the fibula (WEBER 1972). In the studies by both SPIEGEL and VAHVANEN and AALTO, different types of fractures tended to occur in different age groups, the data suggesting a relationship between skeletal maturity and the fracture pattern. VAHVANEN noted that malleolar and intra-articular tibial fractures occurred at a younger age than tibial epiphyseal fractures, two-plane or tri-plane fractures. Since the medial part of the distal tibial epiphyseal plate closes before the lateral part (KLEIGER and MANKIN 1964), this might explain the separation of the lateral part of the tibial epiphysis in tri-plane

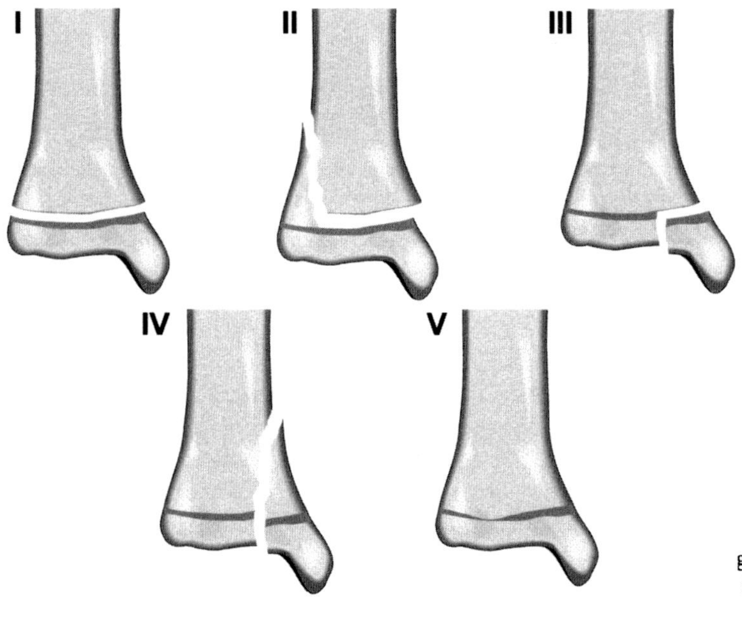

g. 9.19. The Salter-Harris classification as applied injuries of the distal tibial epiphysis fractures and in avulsion fractures of the tibiofibular syndesmosis.

Although there are a number of classification systems available for fractures of the ankle in children, the Salter-Harris classification with its consideration of the involvement of the epiphysis remains very important. Other systems may be helpful as regards management and approach to treatment.

9.11.3
Salter-Harris Fractures

Distal tibial epiphyseal injuries are usually Salter-Harris type I (Fig. 9.17). In the more common Salter-Harris type II injuries, the triangular corner fragment always arises from the side of the metaphysis towards which the epiphysis is displaced. Salter-Harris type III epiphyseal separations occur either medially or laterally (Fig. 9.20). Those of the medial portion of the epiphysis occur in adduction injuries or avulsion by the deltoid ligament when the ankle is injured with the foot in pronation. The medial fragment includes the medial malleolus. Type III fractures involving the lateral half of the epiphysis occur only after the growth plate has started to fuse since closure of the growth plate commences medially. This has been described as a juvenile Tillaux fracture (Kleiger and Mankin 1964). The fracture line extends from the articular surface, traverses the epiphysis and continues through the physis laterally. A variably sized piece of the anterolateral bony epiphysis is pulled off by the anterior talofibular ligament, which is either mildly or moderately displaced.

Salter-Harris type IV injuries of the distal tibial epiphysis occur as a result of adduction. This type of injury requires open reduction and accurate fixation to prevent growth arrest. Type V injuries are extremely rare, the radiographs are usually normal initially, and the diagnosis is usually made retrospectively when premature closure is seen on subsequent radiographs.

Most epiphyseal injuries can be adequately reduced by closed means, except the Salter-Harris type IV adduction injury of the medial portion of the distal tibial epiphysis. Type III injuries are occasionally displaced to such a degree that open reduction is required. Irreducible Salter-Harris type II separations of the distal tibial epiphysis due to interposition of the anterior tibial tendon and neurovascular bundle have been reported (Grace 1983).

9.11.4
Tri-plane Fracture

The tri-plane fracture described by Marmor in 1970 is an injury unique to the closure of the distal tibial physis. It is called this because there are fracture lines

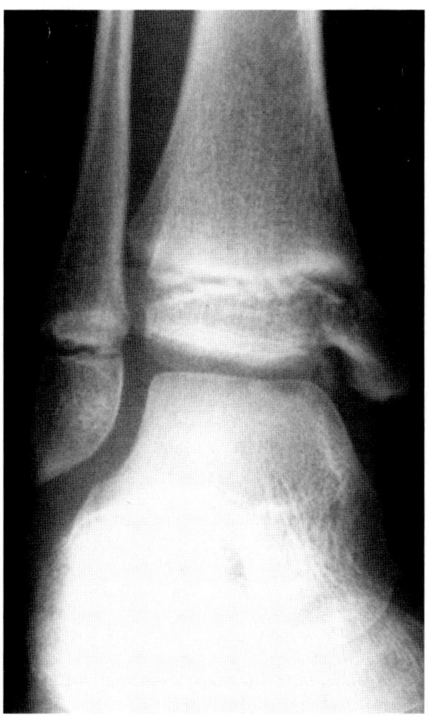

a

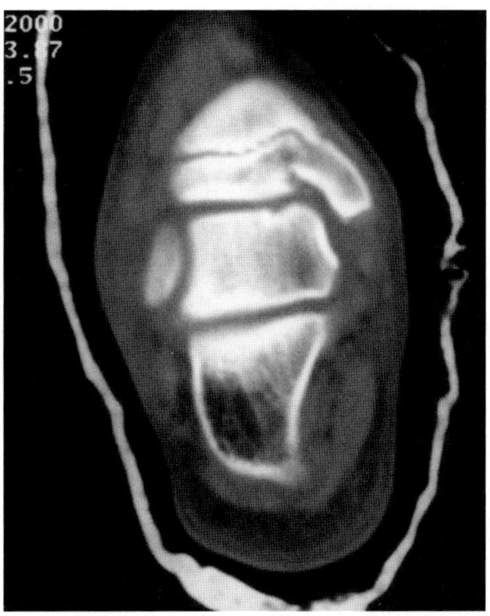

b

Fig. 9.20. a AP view demonstrating a Salter-Harris type III fracture of the distal tibia. Note also the osteochondral defect of the medial talar dome. **b** Coronal CT image demonstrates the Salter-Harris type III fracture, some tiny bone fragments and the osteochondral injury of the talar dome in three planes: a sagittal plane in the epiphysis, a horizontal plane within the physis, and an oblique vertical plane in the posterior distal metaphysis. This produces a multiplanar Salter-Harris type IV injury. There are two types of tri-plane fractures: ones with two fragments (Fig. 9.21) and ones with three fragments (Fig. 9.22). Both are due to plantar flexion and external rotation and may occur with or without an associated long oblique fracture of the distal fibula. The fracture appears as a Salter-Harris type III on the AP view and Salter-Harris type II on the lateral view (Fig. 9.23). The two-fragment tri-plane fracture usually occurs after the epiphysis has begun to unite, similar to the juvenile Tillaux fracture. Two sub-types of two-fragment tri-plane fractures have also been reported, a medial and a lateral. The lateral is the more common one, the medial malleolus remaining intact. The three-fragment tri-plane fractures are less common than the two-fragment fractures, and generally occur in younger children before the tibial epiphysis has begun to close (MacNealy et al. 1982; Dias and Giegerich 1983).

Three-part tri-plane fractures are more likely to require open reduction and internal fixation to restore and preserve the joint. In the three-part fracture, the entire epiphysis is usually displaced posteriorly as opposed to the two-part fracture in which only a portion of the epiphysis is displaced, the other portion remaining attached and properly aligned with the anterior tibial metaphysis. The entire distal tibial epiphysis is also displaced posteriorly in Salter-Harris type II plantar flexion and external rotational injuries. However, in these latter injuries, the distal tibial epiphysis remains intact without the vertical fracture at the epiphysis found in the tri-plane fracture.

9.12 Osteochondral Injuries

This type of injury most commonly affects the talar dome, both its medial and lateral aspect in equal proportions (Figs. 9.24, 9.25). It usually results from

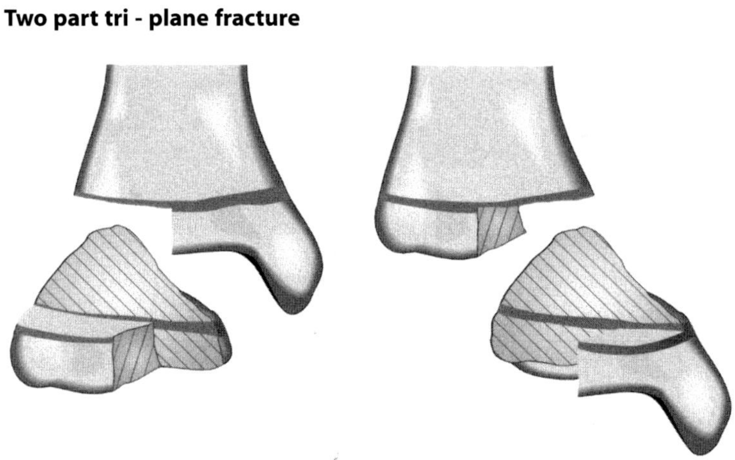

Fig. 9.21. Line diagram demonstrating the two-part tri-plane fracture

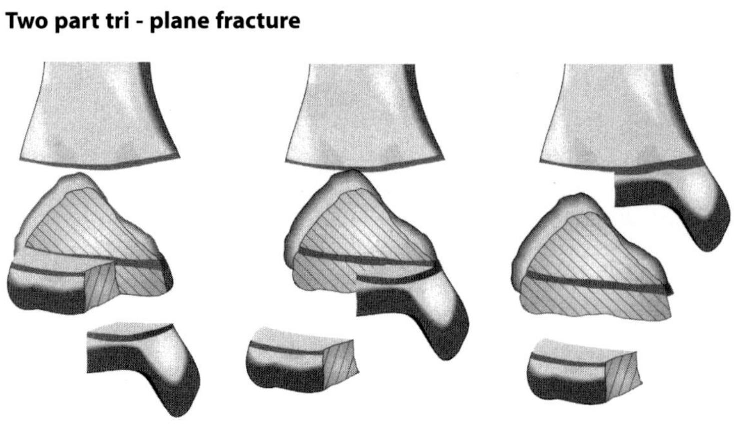

Fig. 9.22. Line diagram demonstrating the three-part tri-plane fracture

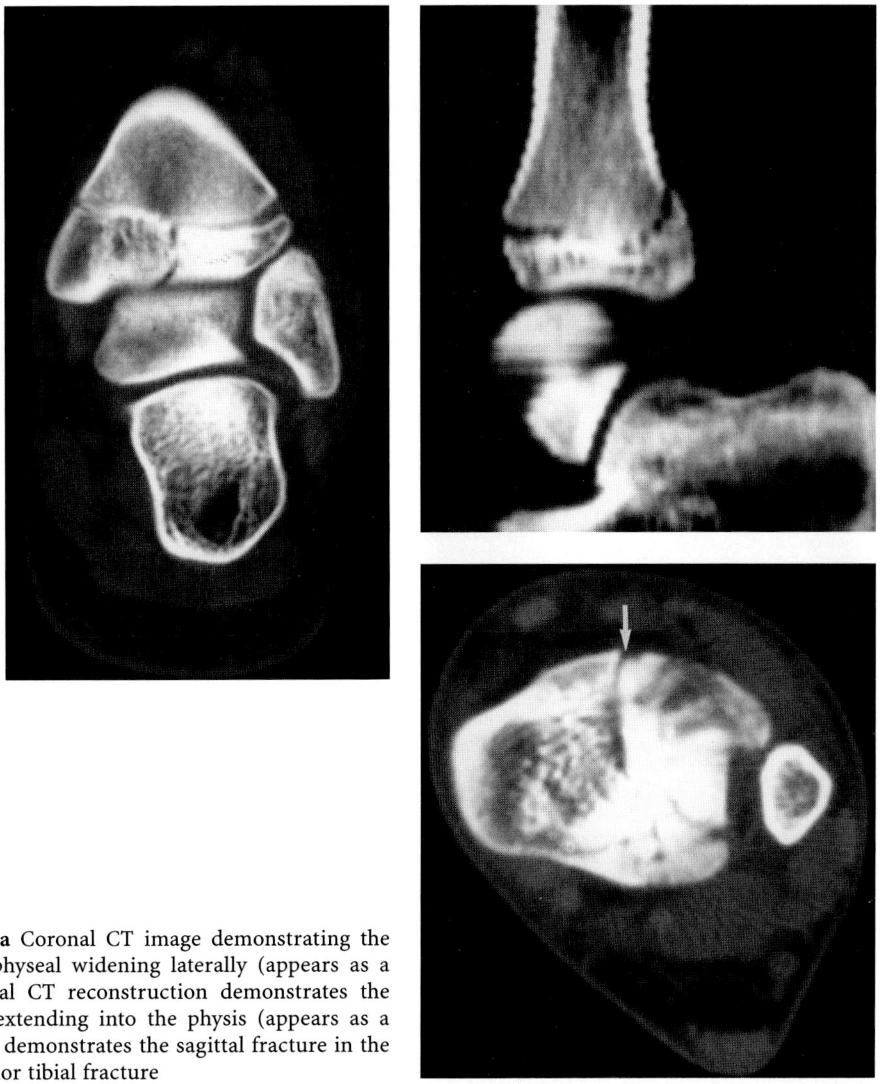

a b c

Fig. 9.23a–c. Tri-plane fracture. **a** Coronal CT image demonstrating the tibial epiphyseal fracture with physeal widening laterally (appears as a Salter-Harris type III). **b** Sagittal CT reconstruction demonstrates the posterior metaphyseal fracture extending into the physis (appears as a Salter-Harris type II). **c** Axial CT demonstrates the sagittal fracture in the epiphysis (*arrow*) and the posterior tibial fracture

an inversion injury. There is often associated rupture of the lateral ligamentous complex, usually involving the anterior talofibular ligament and sometimes also the calcaneofibular ligament. Talar dome injury is often missed (20%) or not visible on conventional radiographs which show evidence of soft-tissue lateral ligamentous injury, and CT or MRI is required for the diagnosis. Injury to the lateral portion of the dome is more common in men, whereas injury to the medial portion of the dome is more common in women. The lesion varies from indentation of the dome to partial detachment of the fragment, complete detachment without displacement, and complete detachment with displacement. The radiographic features are best demonstrated on AP and internal oblique projections. The osteochondral fragment is seen as a fine flake of bone at the lateral or medial edge of the talus. Where the fragment is not visible, further imaging with CT arthrography may be employed (Fig. 9.24). Very subtle osteochondral abnormalities can also be beautifully demonstrated by MRI (Bohndorf 1999).

9.13 Complications of Bone Injuries

Complications of bone injuries at the ankle are varied. The most common is post-traumatic osteoarthritis. Close attention to good reduction of fractures at the ankle can help to minimise this complication. It is a frequent problem following compressive fractures of the calcaneum, largely as a result of the complex nature

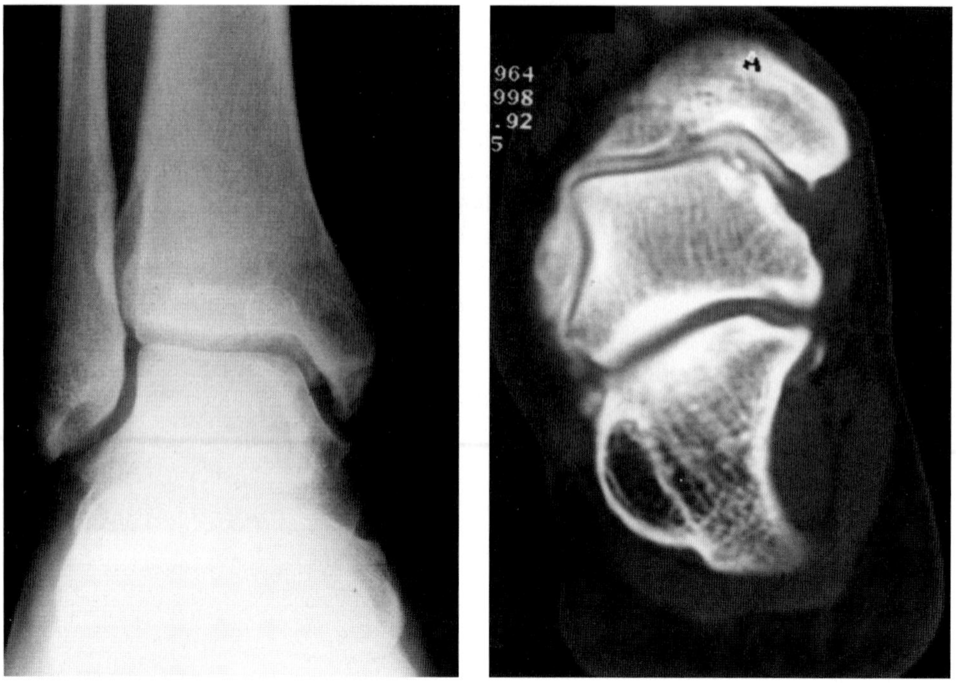

a b

Fig. 9.24. a AP radiograph of ankle demonstrating an osteochondral defect of the talar dome. **b** CT arthrogram of ankle demonstrates osteochondritis dissecans. Note contrast medium in the subtalar joint (there is a connection with the ankle joint in 10% of people)

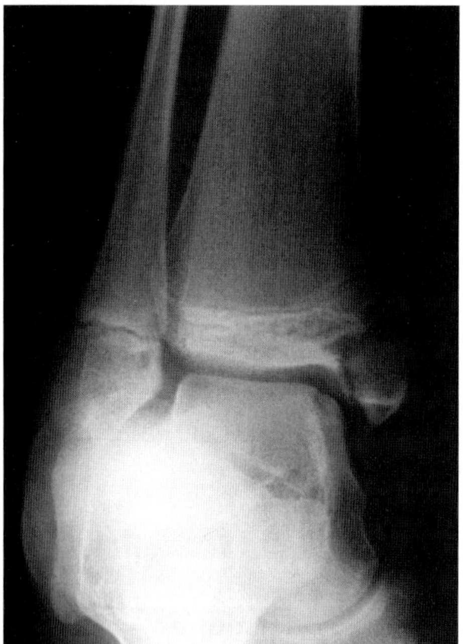

Fig. 9.25. Internal oblique radiograph of the ankle in an adolescent demonstrating a fracture of the medial malleolus and also of the medial aspect of the talar dome

of these injuries and the difficulties involved in achieving satisfactory realignment of all fragments.

Avascular necrosis is a particular complication associated with vertical fractures through the neck of the talus (Fig. 9.5). The majority of the arterial supply enters through the anterolateral portion of the neck of the talus, through the foramina in the sinus tarsi and tarsal canal, and through the foramina in the medial surface of the body (Haliburton et al. 1958; Kelly and Sullivan 1963). When the neck of the talus is fractured, the blood supply is easily disrupted, and the body is susceptible to avascular necrosis. This can also occur following dislocation associated with fracture of the neck. Radiologically, the appearances of avascular necrosis of the talus are similar to those elsewhere in the body. There is a geographical demarcation of increased density compared with adjacent bone (which is of normal or reduced density). This pattern can also be readily detected with CT or MRI. The body and talar dome can ultimately collapse with progression to arthritis.

Reflex sympathetic dystrophy (RSD) is a potential complication of any injury at the ankle. It is manifest clinically by pain, soft-tissue swelling and reduced movement. Radiographically, there may be soft-tissue swelling and osteoporosis. The radionuclide bone scan shows diffuse increased uptake on both the vascular (diffusion) and static (delayed) phases.

Ankle injury in the child and adolescent where the growth plate has been disturbed may be complicated by tethering (premature partial or complete fusion) across the growth plate with subsequent angular deformity secondary to asymmetric arrest. It can also rarely be found secondary to malunion. Growth problems can lead to leg length discrepancy, which accounts for about 20% of the indications for leg-lengthening procedures.

9.14 Summary

Bone injury affecting the ankle joint can be complex and difficult to classify. A classification system is usually used in order to facilitate comparison between different modes of management, but they can also sometimes help in directing the search for other associated or expected injuries. Not all injuries will fit neatly into a classification system. Furthermore, an injury classified on the basis of conventional radiographs is commonly re-classified when CT is employed.

In the mid-foot, where there are many bones tightly packed together and many overlapping shadows, a high index of suspicion of a possible Lisfranc fracture-dislocation is essential to reduce the risk of overlooking this injury.

This chapter has dealt principally with the radiograph in bone and joint injury, with emphasis on the value of CT particularly in hindfoot and mid-foot injuries. MRI will detect occult bone injury, marrow oedema and osteochondral injury but has its main role in the assessment of soft-tissue injury.

References

Ayeni JP (1988) Pilon fractures of the Tibia: a study based on 19 cases. Injury 19:109–114

Bohndorf K (1999) Imaging of acute injuries of the articular surfaces (chondral, osteochondral and subchondal fractures). Skeletal Radiol 28:545–560

Bonnin JG (1970) Injuries to the ankle. Hafner, New York

Canale ST, Kelly FB Jr (1978) Fractures of the neck of the talus: long-term evaluation of seventy one cases. JBJS 60 A:143–156

Cancelmo RP (1962) Isolated fracture of the anterior tibial tubercle. AJR 87:1064–1066

Dameron TB Jr (1975) Fractures and anatomical variations of the proximal portion of the fifth metatarsal. JBJS 57A: 788–792

Danis R (1949) Les fractures malleolaires. In: Danis R (ed) Theorie et pratique de l'osteosynthese. Masson, Paris, pp 133–165

Destot E (1911) Traumatismes du pied et rayons. X. Malleoles, astragale, calcaneum avantpied. Masson, Paris, pp 1–10

Dias LS, Giegerich CR (1983) Fractures of the distal tibial epiphysis in adolescence. JBJS 65A:438–443

Dias LS, Tachdjian MO (1978) Physeal injuries of the ankle in children classification. Clin Orthop 136:230–233

Eisele SA, Sammarco GJ (1993) Fatigue fractures of the foot and ankle in the athlete (review). J Bone Joint Surg 75A: 290–298

Essex-Lopresti P (1952) The mechanism, reduction technique, and results in fractures of the os calcis. Br J Surg 39:395–419

Grace DL (1983) Irreducible fracture-separations of the distal tibial epiphysis. JBJS 65B:160–162

Guyer BH, Levinsohn EM, Fredrickson BE, Bailey GL, Formikell M (1985) Computed tomography of calcaneal fractures: anatomy, pathology, dosimetry and clinical relevance. AJR 145:911–919

Haliburton RA, Sullivan CR, Kelly PJ, Peterson LFA (1958) The extra-osseous and intra-osseous blood supply of the talus. JBJS 40A:115–1120

Harper MC (1992) Ankle fracture classification systems; a case for integration of the Lauge-Hansen and AO-Danis-Weber Schemes. Foot Ankle 13:404–407

Harty M (1973) Anatomic considerations in injuries of the calcaneus. Orthop Clin North Am 4: 179–183

Hawkins LG (1970) Fractures of the neck of the talus. JBJS 52A:991–1002

Heger L, Wulff K, Seddiqi MSA (1985) Computed tomography of calcaneal fractures. AJR 145:131–137

Helal B, Gibb P (1987) Freiberg's disease: a suggested pattern of management. Foot Ankle 8:94–102

Henderson MS (1932) Trimalleolar fractures of the ankle. Surg Clin North Am 12:867–872

Hindman BW, Koss SDK, Sowerby MRR (1986) Fractures of the talus and calcaneus: evaluation by computed tomography CT. J Comput Tomogr 10:191–196

Isherwood I (1961) A radiological approach to the subtalar joint. JBJS 43B:566–574

Jones R (1902) Fracture of the base of the fifth metatarsal bone by indirect violence. Ann Surg 35:697–700

Kelly PJ, Sullivan CR (1963) Blood supply of the talus. Clin Orthop 30:37–44

Kleiger B, Mankin HJ (1964) Fracture of the lateral portion of the distal tibial epiphysis. JBJS 46A:25–32

Lauge-Hansen N (1949) "Ligamentous" ankle fractures, diagnosis and treatment. Acta Chir Scand 97:544–550

Lauge-Hansen N (1950) Fractures of the ankle II. Combined experimental-surgical and experimental-roentgenologic investigations. Arch Surg 60:957–985

Lauge-Hansen N (1954) Fractures of the ankle III. Genetic roentgenologic diagnosis of fractures of the ankle. AJR 71:456–471

Lorentzen JE, Christensen SB, Krogsoe O, Sneppen O (1977) Fractures of the neck of the talus. Acta Orthop Scand 48: 115–120

MacKinnon AP (1928) Fracture of the lower articular surface of the tibia in fracture dislocation of the ankle. JBJS 10: 352–362

MacNealy GA, Rogers LF, Hernandez R, Poznanski AK (1982) Injuries of the distal tibial epiphysis: systematic radiographic evaluation. AJR 138:683

Mainwaring BL, Daffner RH, Riemer BL (1988) Pylon fractures of the ankle: a distinct clinical and radiologic entity. Radiology 168:215–218

Maisonneuve JGT (1840) Recherches sur la fracture du perione. Arch Gen Med 7:165

Marmor L (1970) An unusual fracture of the tibial epiphysis. Clin Orthop 73:132–135

Meurman KOA (1981) Less common stress fractures in the foot. Br J Radiol 54:1–7

Myerson MS (1989) The diagnosis and treatment of injuries to the lisfranc joint complex. Orthop Clin North Am 20: 655–664

Pankovich AM, Shivaram MS (1979) Anatomical basis of variability in injuries of the medial malleolus and the deltoid ligament. Acta Orthop Scand 50:225–236

Protas JM, Kornblatt BA (1981) Fractures of the lateral margin of the distal tibia. The tillaux fracture. Radiology 138:55–57

Rang M (1983) Children's fractures, 2nd edn. Lippincott, Philadelphia

Rogers LF (1992) The Ankle. In: Rogers LF (ed) Radiology of skeletal trauma, chap 22. Churchill Livingstone, New York, pp 1376–1377

Rosenberg ZS, Feldman F, Singson RD (1987) Intra-articular calcaneal fractures: computed tomographic analysis. Skeletal Rad 16:105–113

Ruwe PA, Randall RL, Baumgaertner MR (1993) Pilon fractures of the distal tibia. Orthop Rev 22:987–996

Salter RB, Harris WR (1963) Injuries involving the Epiphyseal Plate. JBJS 45A:587–622

Spiegel PG, Cooperman DR, Laros GS (1978) Epiphyseal fractures of the distal ends of the tibia and fibula. A retrospective study of 237 cases in children. JBJS 60A:1046–1050

Stiell IG, Greenberg GH, McKnight RD, Nair RC, McDowell I, Worthington JR (1992) A study to develop clinical decision rules for the use of radiography in acute ankle injuries. Ann Emerg Med 21:384–390

Stiell IG, Greenberg GH, McKnight RD et al (1993) Decision rules for the use of radiography in acute ankle injuries: refinements and prospective validation. JAMA 269: 1127–1132

Stiell IG, McKnight RD, Greenberg GH, McDowell I, Nair RC, Wells GA, Johns C, Worthington JR (1994) Implementation of the Ottawa ankle rules. JAMA 271:827–832

Torg JS, Balduini FC, Zelko RR, Pavlov H, Peff TC, Das M (1984) Fractures of the base of the fifth metatarsal distal to the tuberosity. JBJS 66A:209–214

Vahvanen V, Aalto K (1980) Classification of ankle fractures in children. Arch Orthop Tr Surg 97:1–5

Van Hal ME, Keene JS, Lange TA, Clancy WG Jr (1982) Stress fractures of the great toe sesamoids. Am J Sports Med 10: 122–128

Verma S, Hamilton K, Hawkins HH, Kothari R, Singal B, Buncher R, Nguyen P, O'Neill M (1997) Clinical application of the Ottawa ankle rules for the use of radiography in acute ankle injuries. An independent site assessment. AJR 169:825–827

Weber BG (1972) Die Verletzungen des Oberen Sprunggelenkes. In: Aktuelle Probleme in der Chirugie, no 3, 2nd edn. Huber, Bern

10 Tendon Pathology

F. KAINBERGER, S. NEHRER, and H. IMHOF

CONTENTS

10.1 General Aspects of Injury of Tendons

The tendons of the ankle and the foot are part of the end of the functional chain of transmitting strength and weight on the ground, thus providing the stability to stand and the dynamics of gait. Therefore, they are specifically prone to overload, and overuse syndromes are a major cause of restricted movement and pain with the potential of rupture in some larger tendons (KANNUS and JOSZA 1991; PETERSON and RENSTRÖM 2001). Patients typically experience a tendon rupture as a sudden and striking blow (similar feelings to those described by the ancient hero Achilles hit by Apollo's arrow are today reported by contemporary high-ranking athletes). Nevertheless, in the majority of cases, tendon injuries are the result of prolonged abnormal training habits in sporting activities, use of improper footwear, overweight, or other lifestyle problems. The incidence and prevalence of tendon disease has been increasing dramatically over the past few decades, and a variety of distinct symptoms and signs are observed clinically, especially in patients involved in various sporting activities.

The different forms of degeneration, inflammation, necrosis, or rupture of tendon tissue can be regarded as stages of a process of progressive overuse and may be summarized under the term 'tendon overuse syndrome (TOS)' (KAINBERGER et al. 2001). In the first phase of TOS, painful functional impairment of movement occurs without any morphological changes. In the second stage, abnormalities of the gliding tissue in the form of bursitis, tendovaginitis, or peritendinitis are observed. Chronic inflammation of the tendon sheath may lead to stenosing tenosynovitis with fibrosis and tendon entrapment. In the third stage, such lesions are followed by degenerative changes of the tendon itself. Often, these changes present more clearly than during the early forms of TOS, and three types of tendon degeneration can be differentiated: tendinosis at distinct points along the course of the tendon, fibro-ostosis at the tendon insertion, and compression syndromes. Rupture of fibers following tendinosis may be considered as the last or fourth stage of TOS. Modulations in the course of tendon overuse depend on the location of certain areas of vulnerability of each tendon, so-called 'critical zones', and distinct periods of time during the course of the disease, the 'vulnerable phases'. Hence, typical forms of overuse can be described for many tendons (Table 10.1).

Other less common tendon disorders are due to rheumatic or metabolic diseases. Imaging findings generally show different patterns of distribution of the lesions, but because of the inherently high biomechanical load on tendon fibers, findings of degeneration predominate in the pathologic and clinical picture in these cases, too. Tumours of the tendons are rare except for ganglia that are commonly observed in the dorsal tendon sheaths of the foot. Giant cell

F. KAINBERGER, MD
Univ.-Klinik für Radiodiagnostik, AKH, Waehringer Guertel 18–20, 1090 Vienna, Austria
H. IMHOF, MD
Univ.-Klinik für Radiodiagnostik, AKH, Waehringer Guertel 18–20, 1090 Vienna, Austria
S. NEHRER, MD
Univ.-Klinik für Orthopaedie, AKH, Waehringer Guertel 18–20, 1090 Vienna, Austria

Table 10.1. Distinct forms of overuse for individual tendons of the ankle and the foot

Tendon	Overuse syndrome	Etiology
Achilles tendon	Peritendinitis, tendinosis	Ischemic and/or mechanical (hyperpronation)
	Haglund's heel (retrocalcaneal bursitis)	Compression due to prominent calcaneus and/or improper footwear
	Posterior calcaneal spur, fibro-ostosis	Increased traction at tendon attachment site
	Apophysitis (Sever's or Albert's disease, insertionitis)	Juvenile insertional tendinopathy
Plantar aponeurosis	Plantar fasciitis (subcalcaneal pain syndrome, calcaneal spur)	Microtrauma at insertion of plantar fascia
Tendon of tibialis posterior muscle	Tendovaginitis, tendinosis	Flatfoot deformity, hyperpronation
Tendon of flexor hallucis longus muscle	Tendovaginitis, checkrein deformity (stenosing tendovaginitis)	Friction between talar tubercles, specifically in ballet dancers
	Os trigonum syndrome (dancer's heel)	Posterior ankle impingement
	Hallux saltans	Friction at point where tendon of flexor digitorum longus crosses (Henry's knot)
Peroneal tendons	Tendovaginitis, tendinosis	Lateral ankle trauma, flatfoot deformity
	Peroneal split syndrome	Repetitive subluxations
	Os peroneum syndrome	Peroneal fracture, attrition, or rupture of peroneus longus tendon, hypertrophy of os peroneum
Tendon of tibialis anterior muscle	Tendovaginitis, tendinosis	Forceful dorsiflexion during running or jumping, flatfoot deformity
Tendon of extensor digitorum longus muscle	Extensor peritenonitis, tendinosis	Increased pressure from shoes, repetitive dorsiflexion

tumor of the tendon sheath also occurs in the ankle and the foot (Paez et al. 1999). As a generalization, all neoplasms that originate from the synovium may be observed in tendon sheaths.

10.2 Indications for Imaging of Tendons

Diagnostic imaging should be performed to characterize the type and stage of tendon overuse with the aims to initiate appropriate treatment and to prevent progression to a tendon rupture. The risk of a rupture is determined by intrinsic and extrinsic parameters (Table 10.2), and especially with ultrasound and MRI, it is possible to analyze many of the intrinsic factors in detail (Pecina and Bojanic 1993; Gibbon et al. 1999; Campbell and Grainger 2001; Nehrer et al. 1997). There are three main indications for imaging: Symptoms and signs of overuse or of inflammation with pain and impairment when walking or running, suspicion of a rupture, and posttherapeutic or postoperative check-up examinations to document the morphologic integrity of a tendon (Stoller and Ferkel 1997; Kainberger et al. 1997; Shalabi et al. 2001).

In general, ultrasound is the modality of first choice for tendon imaging. Often, however, radiographs are obtained because this has been routine practice for many years, and it is not limited by restrictions in access or by a small field-of-view. MR imaging is regarded to be the ideal modality to describe abnormalities of tendons, their gliding tissue, and their relationship to neighboring osseous and soft-tissue structures (Astrom et al. 1996; Movin et al. 1998; Peterson and Renström 2001). CT may be used to detect posttraumatic or postoperative bony abnormalities as is typically the case in peroneal tendon injury (Ho et al. 2001).

Invasive radiographic techniques like peroneal tenography or retrocalcaneal bursography have been superceded by MR imaging.

Kinematic MR imaging of the ankle may, despite the limited clinical experience with this technique, become a useful tool in evaluating certain pathologic conditions like subluxation of the peroneal tendons or complex functional impairment of the hindfoot (Shellock 1997).

Table 10.2. Extrinsic and intrinsic factors that influence the development of tendon overuse syndromes (modified after PETERSON and RENSTRÖM 2001)

Intrinsic factors
Malalignment of lower extremity:
leg length discrepancy
femoral anteversion
joint alignment abnormalities (varus, valgus, other)
foot abnormalities (flat or cavus foot)
Variants in the origin, course, or insertion of tendons:
shallow osseous canal
accessory muscle
accessory or atypically formed bone
Muscle tension imbalance with respect to flexibility or strength
Hypovascularization of tendon tissue
Underlying systemic metabolic or inflammatory disease
Psychological factors or psychiatric disease
Personal attributes:
gender, age, weight and height, growth
Extrinsic factors
Training errors:
excessive training
abrupt changes in intensity of training
unskilled athlete
doping[a]
Improper footwear or clothing
Environmental factors:
hard or uneven ground

[a] Effects of doping on tendon tissue are under discussion and not yet proven

10.3 Pathologic Findings

According to their anatomic arrangement in muscle compartments which form distinct functional units, four groups of the major tendons of the foot may be differentiated:

- the superficial plantar flexor tendons with the Achilles tendon and the much smaller tendon of the plantaris longus muscle. The plantar aponeurosis that originates at the medial process of the tuberosity of the calcaneus can be regarded as a structure that conveys strength from the calf muscles to the five metatarsal rays and the toes.
- the tendons of the deep plantar flexors of the calf that run behind the medial malleolus through fibro-osseous tunnels. They all act as supinators and are important stabilizers of the plantar arches.
- the peroneal tendons behind the lateral malleolus that support plantarflexion and pronation.
- the long extensor tendons that run ventrally to the ankle joint.

The tendons of the short flexor and extensor muscles may be afflicted in the form of tendovaginitis. Generally, this is a concomitant finding in association with disruption of the plantar plate, infection of the soft tissues, or other diseases of the forefoot.

It is not unusual that in certain foot deformities, tendon lesions may be observed in more than one compartment. Specifically important conditions include hyperpronation of the hindfoot and the flatfoot deformity. Hindfoot valgus or repetitive hyperpronation of the foot have been regarded as important intrinsic factors for the development of degeneration of the Achilles tendon with increased strain in the medial part of this tendon, lesions of the tibialis posterior tendon, plantar fasciitis, and associated abnormalities in the sinus tarsi (Fig. 10.1) (CLEMENT et al. 1984; BALEN and HELMS 2001).

10.3.1 Superficial Plantar Flexor Tendons

10.3.1.1 Achilles Tendon

The Achilles tendon is the largest tendon of the human body, measuring between 5 and 7 cm in length. At its proximal end, the tendon tapers into the superficial fascia of the muscles of the calf. As a normal variant, the soleus muscle junction may be located far distally, sometimes with the formation of an accessory soleus muscle, or m. soleus quartus. On axial images, the normal tendon has an asymmetric, kidney-shaped cross-section in its mid-third, with a major feeding vessel entering anteriorly. The longer axis of the tendon cross-section may form an angle between 0 and 30 deg to the coronal plane. Therefore, measurements of tendon thickness should be performed at the level of greatest thickness and by measuring the shorter axis of the tendon cross-section.

Achillodynia refers to pain at the posterior heel with or without impairment in walking or running. It is the typical clinical finding that indicates affliction of this tendon.

10.3.1.1.1 Peritendinitis and Bursitis

As the Achilles tendon is not covered by a tendon sheath, abnormal friction between the tendon and its surrounding structures is classified as peritendinitis or bursitis. In acute peritendinitis, swelling and edema

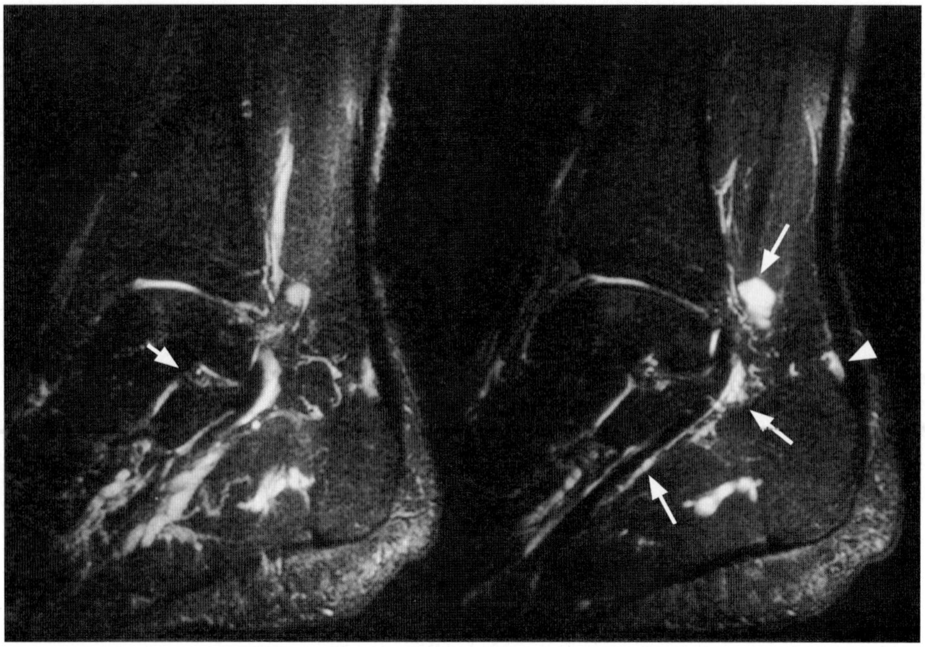

Fig. 10.1. A 29-year-old runner with Achilles bursitis (*arrowhead*), tendovaginitis at the medial malleolus (*long arrows*), and edema in sinus tarsi (*short arrow*), all indicating hyperpronation syndrome of his hindfoot

will result in thickening and T2-weighted hyperintense signal on MR images; in chronic forms, peritendineous fibrous adhesions may occur that could limit the Achilles tendon during its movements. With ultrasound, tiny irregularities of the tendon contours seem to be indicative of such chronic peritendinitis.

The subachilles bursa is located in the gap between the distal third of the tendon and the posterior aspect of the calcaneus. The normal bursa may form a small fluid collection up to 0.5 mm in size which is readily visible as a cystic structure on ultrasound images or as a bright hyperintense signal on T2-weighted MR images, respectively (Kainberger et al. 1990; Bottger et al. 1998). At the level of the calcaneus, there is a superficial Achilles tendon bursa.

10.3.1.1.2 Degenerative Tendon Disease

Tendinosis is a degeneration of the tendon fibers with accompanying repetitive inflammatory changes. It generally develops in the 'critical zone' of the mid-third of the tendon. With further overuse and especially in male patients up to a maximum age of 40 years, the 'vulnerable phase', tendinosis may progress to partial or complete rupture (Nehrer et al. 1997; Gibbon et al. 1999). There is no general agreement in the literature about whether tendinosis develops on the basis of biomechanical abnormalities in the tendon structure or of an impaired blood supply, or of both. Cummins hypothesized that in certain individuals, the tendon fibers that depend on the soleus muscle are under different tension than those that originate from the gastrocnemius muscle (Cummins et al. 1946). Other theories put forward the role of a hypovascular zone that lies between the distal and the mid-portion of the tendon, because its proximal part receives blood from the pretendineous fat pad whereas the distal part is supplied from the rete calcanei (Stein et al. 2000).

Signs of tendinosis include an anterior convexity that may be followed by a fusiform swelling in the mid-third with a shorter diameter of more than 6 mm (Table 10.3). With ultrasound, abnormalities of the tendon structure commonly manifest as irregular thickening of the internal peritendinea with a blurred hypoechoic nodular lesion (Fig. 10.2) (van Holsbeeck and Introcaso 2001). Such lesions are preferably located at the ventromedial aspect of the mid-third of the Achilles tendon (Kainberger et al. 1990; Gibbon et al. 1999). On axial and intermediate T2-weighted MR images, they manifest as irregular,

Table 10.3. Grading of Achilles tendon lesions (Fornage 1986; Kainberger et al. 1996; Astrom et al. 1996)

Grade	Measurements of shorter tendon diameter
Normal	4–6 mm
Low degree	6–8 mm and/or oval-shaped cross-section
Moderate	8–10 mm
High (=chronic rupture)	>10 mm

reticular, and hyperintense foci on all T2-weighted sequences (Fig. 10.3). High-resolution axial sequences are suitable to document the abnormal orientation of the internal peritendinea (MANTEL et al. 1996; SOILA et al. 1999; SCHWEITZER and KARASICK 2000).

Fibro-ostosis at the tendon insertion is caused by repeated strain with inflammation and is visible on radiographs as a bony spur. An inhomogeneity of the tendon structure in this region is detected with ultrasound much earlier than with conventional radiographs.

Apophysitis calcanei (Sever's or Albert's disease) is an overuse disease mainly observed in boys between 8 and 14 years old who are actively involved in soccer playing or similar sporting activities. On radiographs, fragmentation and sclerosis of the calcaneal apophysis with or without a soft-tissue swelling of the subachilles bursa is visible. Signs of bursitis may be readily detected with ultrasound or with MR imaging.

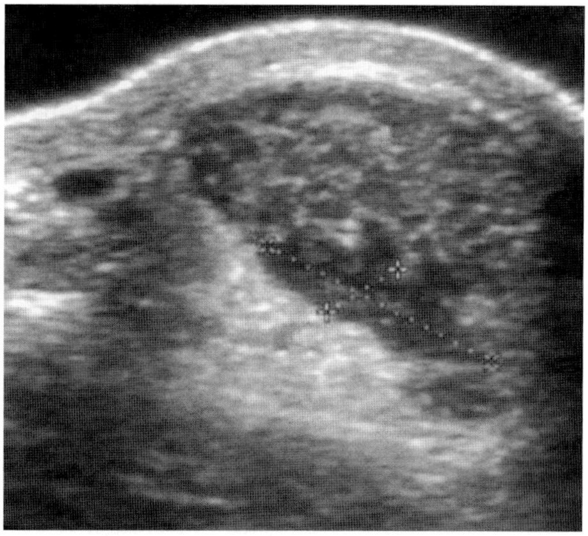

Fig. 10.2. A 33-year-old man with achillodynia. Irregular hypoechoic area in the ventromedial part of Achilles tendon indicates moderate tendinosis

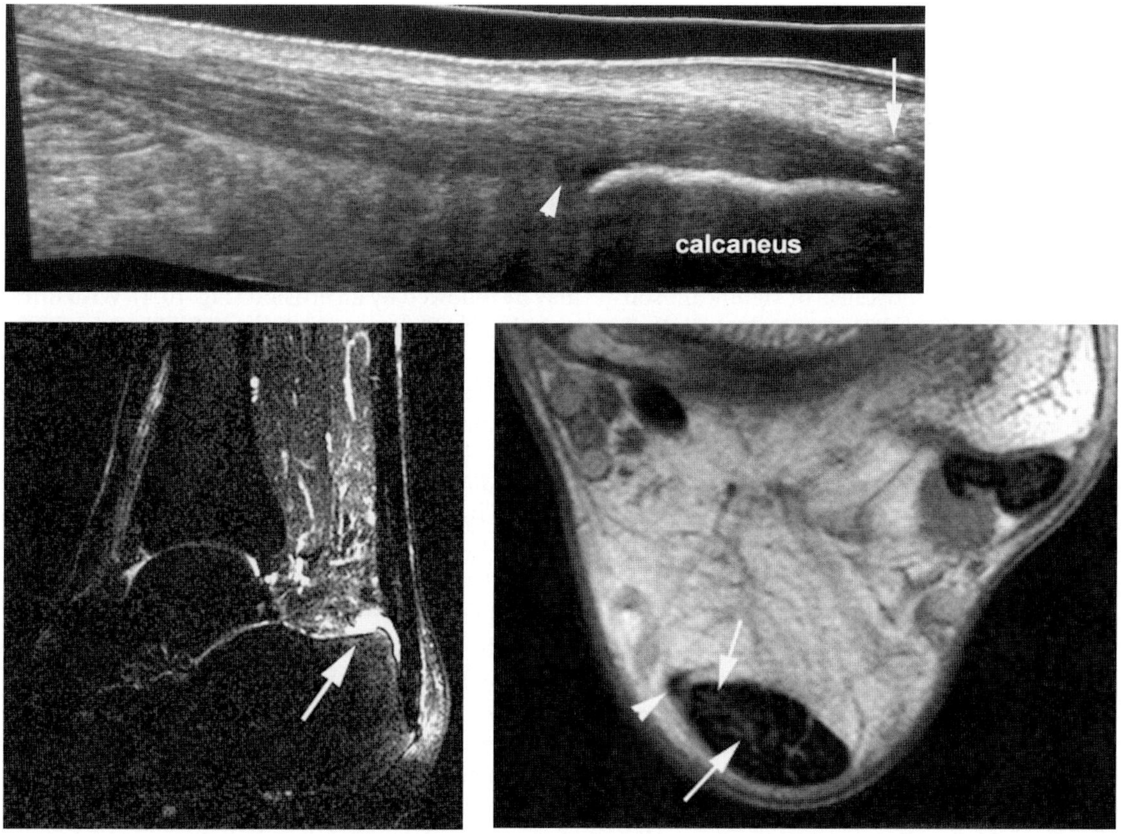

Fig. 10.3a–c. A 38-year-old patient with achillodynia in his left ankle. **a** Tendon shows fusiform hypoechoic thickening, a fluid-filled subachilles bursa, and a small calcified spur at insertion site (*arrow*). **b** On T2-weighted, fat-suppressed MRI, a subachilles bursitis is visible (*arrow*) along with tiny, linear hyperintensities within the tendon tissue. Hyperintense edema within the dorsal calcaneus and the soft tissues at the tendon insertion indicate chronic compression. **c** On axial, intermediate-weighted image, irregular thickening of the peritendinea (*arrows*) indicates severe degeneration of the tendon tissue. Small, hypointense structure medial of the Achilles tendon (*arrowhead*) is the normal tendon of the plantaris longus muscle

Haglund's disease is a compression syndrome due to improper footwear and/or a prominent tuber of the calcaneus. The latter, the calcaneus altus or latus, is a clinical diagnosis but may be detected with its voluminous posterior and proximal aspect on lateral radiographs of the hindfoot. Soft-tissue swelling with acute or chronic inflammation of the adjacent bursae may be followed by a localized tendinosis of the distal third which is not associated with an increased risk of rupture.

10.3.1.1.3 Rupture

Tendon rupture is in most cases associated with a minor trauma, suggesting that an underlying tendinopathy is the major causative factor. This observation is supported by microanatomic studies in which degeneration of collagen fibers could be documented in a large series of ruptured tendons (Kannus and Jozsa 1991). Ruptures are typically located in the 'critical zone' of the mid-third of the tendon but may also be observed more proximally at the myotendineous junction. The latter typically occurs after a heavy push-off with concomitant rotation of the lower leg ('tennis leg'). Other causes of tendon rupture are due to different forms of metabolic and rheumatic diseases. Clinical symptoms and signs are often suggestive of the diagnosis of a rupture. However, because the long deep flexor and the peroneal tendons may compensate dysfunction of the Achilles tendon and because of significant soft-tissue swelling, ruptures may be overlooked clinically (Saltzman and Tearse 1998).

Signs of rupture reflect the discontinuity of tendon fibers and are often associated with hemorrhage. With ultrasound, tendons can be investigated in real-time mode with dynamic stress tests in plantarflexion and extension, thus documenting dehiscence of torn fibers and pointing out the area of maximum intensity of pain. The diagnosis of a partial tear may be established if defects of the tendon contour and at least some intact tendon fibers are suggestive of an incomplete rupture. Relevant signs of complete tendon rupture are totally disrupted tendon fibers, posterior acoustic shadowing originating from a fibrillar-appearing tendon stump, and tendon retraction (Hartgerink et al. 2001). In many cases, a hypoechoic pseudomass due to hematoma is visible at the site of rupture. In old ruptures that were not treated surgically, repair mechanisms with granulation tissue mey lead to a concentrically layered 'onion skin' appearance of the Achilles tendon on axial ultrasound images (Kainberger et al. 1996).

On MR images, a tendinous gap can be detected and its extent described in detail on sagittal and axial T1-weighted images. Partial tendon tears can be defined as linear or focal regions of increased signal and thickening of fibers without a tendinous gap. In many cases, it may be difficult to distinguish areas of tendinosis from chronic intrasubstance tears without documenting either discontinuity in the tendon fibers or discrete hyperintense signal intensity on T2-weighted or STIR images with partial tears. Subacute hemorrhage generates high signal intensity on T1-weighted images.

10.3.1.1.4 Rheumatic and Metabolic Disorders

Rheumatoid arthritis is the most common form of rheumatic disorders occurring at this site, followed by various manifestations of seronegative arthritis like Reiter's or Bechterew's disease and by severe forms of systemic lupus erythematosus. Inflammation of the Achilles tendon due to tuberculosis or other infectious diseases is today an extremely rare finding.

A deep achillobursitis, which in many cases is associated with an erosive defect of the adjacent calcaneus, is a distinctive feature of rheumatic disease. On radiographs, an increased soft-tissue density in the corner between the tendon and the proximal and posterior aspect of the calcaneus is visible and may be followed by an erosion (Fig. 10.4). With ultrasound and MR imaging, signs of fluid accumulation with synovial thickening are visible. Additional bone marrow edema in the calcaneus is a typical finding of rheumatic disease on MR images. Concomitant signs of hypoechoic or hyperintense tendonitis may be visible. With increasing frequency, an achillobursitis is observed in high-ranking athletes which may be due to different immunologic reactions in such individuals with a higher capacity of anerobic metabolism.

Metabolic tendinopathy of the Achilles tendon occurs mainly after systemic treatment with corticosteroids or after local instillation of such preparations that leads to necrosis of the tendon tissue and the preachilles fat pad. Other metabolic changes of the tendon tissue occur with certain lipid storage diseases and with some drugs. In heterozygous familial hypercholesterolemia, bilateral Achilles' tendon xanthomas can be detected in many individuals before they are clinically apparent (Bude et al. 1998).

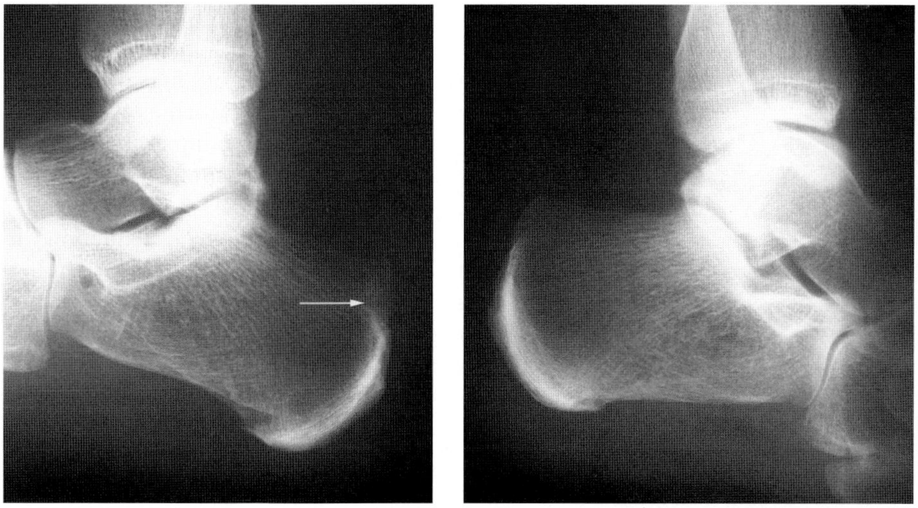

Fig. 10.4. Erosive 'Achilles bursitis defect' (*arrow*) on right posterior calcaneus in a patient with rheumatoid arthritis compared with normal left calcaneus

10.3.1.2
Tendon of the Plantaris Longus Muscle

The plantaris longus muscle originates at the posterior aspect of the proximal tibia and has a long, thin tendon that inserts on the medial aspect of the calcaneus (Fig. 10.3c). Rarely, partial or complete rupture that clinically simulates lesions of the Achilles tendon may occur during explosive sporting activities with hyperpronation and leads to intermuscular hematoma between the medial head of the gastrocnemius muscle and soleus muscle. On MR or ultrasound images, a fluid collection in the expected location of the plantaris tendon may be visible.

10.3.1.3
Plantar Aponeurosis

The plantar aponeurosis originates from the medial process of the calcaneal tuberosity and is the thick central portion of the fascia investing the plantar muscles.

The pain of plantar fasciitis is related to chronic inflammation at its attachment. It may be associated with a calcaneal spur, inflammatory changes, or thickening of the plantar aponeurosis. On MR studies, it frequently demonstrates hyperintense signal intensity changes within the fascia, the adjacent muscles, and the subcutaneous fat, especially on fat-suppressed T2-weighted images. In several studies, the value of ultrasound to describe hypoechoic thickening indicative of plantar fasciitis was shown (Gibbon and Long 1999; Tsai et al. 2000).

Fibro-ostosis at the base of the calcaneus is a typical finding in certain seronegative spondylarthropathies. On conventional radiographs, small erosions or sclerotic spurs may be observed. With MR imaging, these lesions are hyperintense on T2-weighted images.

Plantar fibromatosis is characterized by the development of fibrous nodules in the plantar aponeurosis similar to Dupuytren's contracture. On MR images, the nodules are hypointense on T1-weighted and T2-weighted images and may contain central areas of intermediate to increased signal intensity on T2*-weighted or STIR images (Morrison et al. 1994). The differential diagnosis includes a ganglion, neurofibroma, or fibrosarcoma, but they are hyperintense on T2-weighted images in most cases.

10.3.2
Deep Flexor Tendons of Medial Malleolus

The medial ankle tendons are formed from the deeper muscle group of the calf, i.e., tibialis posterior, flexor digitorum longus, and flexor hallucis longus muscles. The three tendons are important stabilizers of the plantar arches by crossing each other under the base of the first metatarsal and changing their sequence. The tendon sheaths of the three muscles communicate with the ankle joint in 10%–20% of normal individuals. Fluid collections in the tibiotalar joint may be distributed to the tendon sheaths, and the synovium of both the joint and the tendon sheaths may be inflamed in patients with rheumatic disease ('Baker's cyst of the ankle', Fig. 10.5). Minimal fluid collections within these tendon sheaths, however, are regarded as a normal finding (Premkumar et al. 2002).

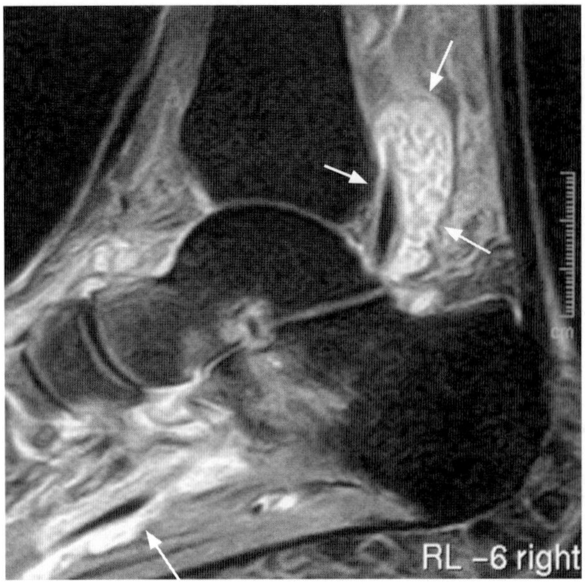

Fig. 10.5. Synovial sheath inflammation of tendons of medial malleolus (*arrows*) in a patient with seronegative arthritis. Typical inflammatory bone marrow edema in distal talus, navicular bone, and anterior part of calcaneus

10.3.2.1
Tibialis Posterior Tendon Injuries

The tibialis posterior tendon inserts at the medial tubercle of the navicular bone and may contain a sesamoid bone gliding on the medial side of the talar head. Prominence or hypertrophy of the tubercle or an accessory navicular bone are normal variants and may be associated with rupture of this tendon (Schweitzer et al. 1993). The tendon is exposed to stress due to compression within the malleolar groove, to hyperpronation of the foot, or to flatfoot deformity. Tendon overuse develops in its typical form, with functional impairment, tendovaginitis, tendinosis, and eventual partial and complete rupture. In the same fashion as with the Achilles tendon, theories exist about the development of tendinosis, referring to mechanical alteration, to insufficient blood supply, or to both possibilities (Frey et al. 1990; Holmes and Mann 1992).

In tenosynovitis, fluid in the tendon sheath may be observed that is hyperintense on T2-weighted MR images and hypoechoic with ultrasound. Intrinsic degeneration of the tendon typically develops in its distal part, with tendon hypertrophy that is best appreciated on axial images as an increased cross-sectional diameter. An increase in the central intrasubstance signal intensity may also be seen on T1-weighted and often on T2-weighted or STIR images (Fig. 10.6). Many of these abnormalities are readily visible with ultrasound (Miller et al. 1996; Premkumar et al. 2002). These findings of progressive degeneration have been regarded as type I rupture of this tendon, which can be differentiated from typeII (partial) and type III (complete) ruptures (Rosenberg et al. 1988).

In partial tears, a nonconcentric reduction in tendon width may give the tibialis posterior tendon an elongated appearance. Complete rupture of the tibialis posterior tendon may occur spontaneously and is reported to be often associated with prior synovitis or steroid injection. With MR imaging, a discontinuity and a fluid filled gap are visible on T2-weighted images. Traumatic dislocation of the tibialis posterior tendon is a rare injury attributed to forced dorsiflexion with inversion.

10.3.2.2
Flexor Hallucis Longus Abnormalities

The tendon of this muscle runs in a groove on the posterior surface of the lower end of the tibia, the posterior surface of the talus, and the undersurface of the sustentaculum tali of the calcaneus. In the sole of the foot, it crosses the tendon of the flexor digitorum longus muscle, to which it is connected by a fibrous slip.

Overuse and rupture of this tendon are rare and are typically associated with ballet dancing. Three

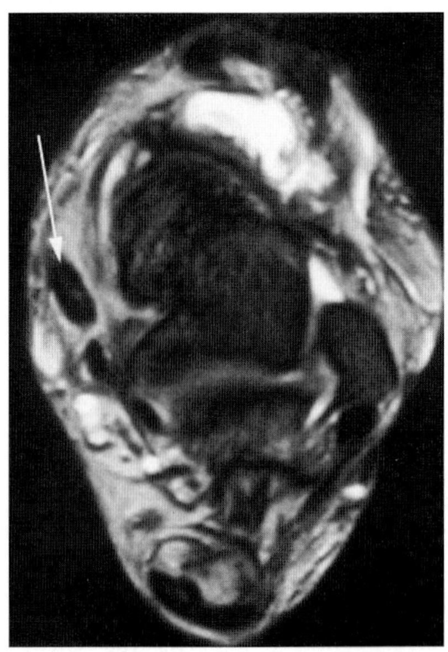

Fig. 10.6. A 52-year-old woman with flatfoot deformity. Degeneration of the tibialis posterior tendon with central hyperintensity (*arrow*) indicating intrasubstance tear

'critical zones' have been identified within this tendon. The first is where it passes behind the medial malleolus between the talar tubercles. T2-weighted axial images show areas of increased fluid signal intensity in the tendon sheath. In rare cases, a tethering of the flexor hallucis longus tendon proximal to the flexor retinaculum produces a 'checkrein deformity' with a flexion contracture of the interphalangeal joint of the greater toe and an extension contracture of the first metatarsophalangeal joint (JAHSS 1991).

Further, the flexor hallucis longus tendon can be involved in posterior ankle impingement due to an oversized os trigonum, which is an ossicle at the posterior process of the talus. The typical findings of tendovaginitis and hypertrophy of this ossicle are readily visible with MRI (TAMBURRINI et al. 1999).

Occasionally, tendinitis or rupture is found under the base of the first metatarsal where the flexor digitorum longus crosses over the flexor hallucis longus beneath the first metatarsal head between the sesamoids (MAMMONE 1997). Coronal images are necessary to detect such distal ruptures (STOLLER and FERKEL 1997).

10.3.3 Peroneal Tendons

The tendons of the peroneus longus and brevis muscles run within a tendon sheath behind the lateral malleolus in a groove of the fibula and beneath a retinaculum. The superficial peroneus brevis tendon inserts on the plantar side of the base of the fifth metatarsal bone. The tendon of the peroneus longus muscle is located deeper in close vicinity to the calcaneofibular ligament and inserts at the first metatarsal bone by crossing the entire plantar dome through a fibro-osseous tunnel. With MR imaging, the peroneal tendons as well as the fibular and retinacular anatomy can be analyzed in detail. The os peroneale is a sesamoid bone within this tendon that may glide over the surface of the cuboid's tuberosity at the point where the tendon changes its direction. Because of the tight fixation of the tendons to the adjacent bones, the typical forms of overuse are relatively rare compared with deterioration of tendon tissue in association with osseous fractures (Fig. 10.7) (EBRAHEIM et al. 1991). Peroneal tendon entrapment or impingement is associated with a depressed fracture of the calcaneus with narrowing of the calcaneofibular space (BOLES et al. 1997).

Tendovaginitis and tendinosis at the level of the lateral malleolus is often associated with dislocation of the peroneal tendons and an insufficient retinaculum. Fluid within the sheath of the peroneal tendons and, possibly, altered tendon size and intratendinous increased signal intensity may be observed (MINK 1992). A shallow fibular tendon groove, a congenital absence of the retinaculum, or its laxity due to chronic hyperpronation of the hindfoot may predispose to

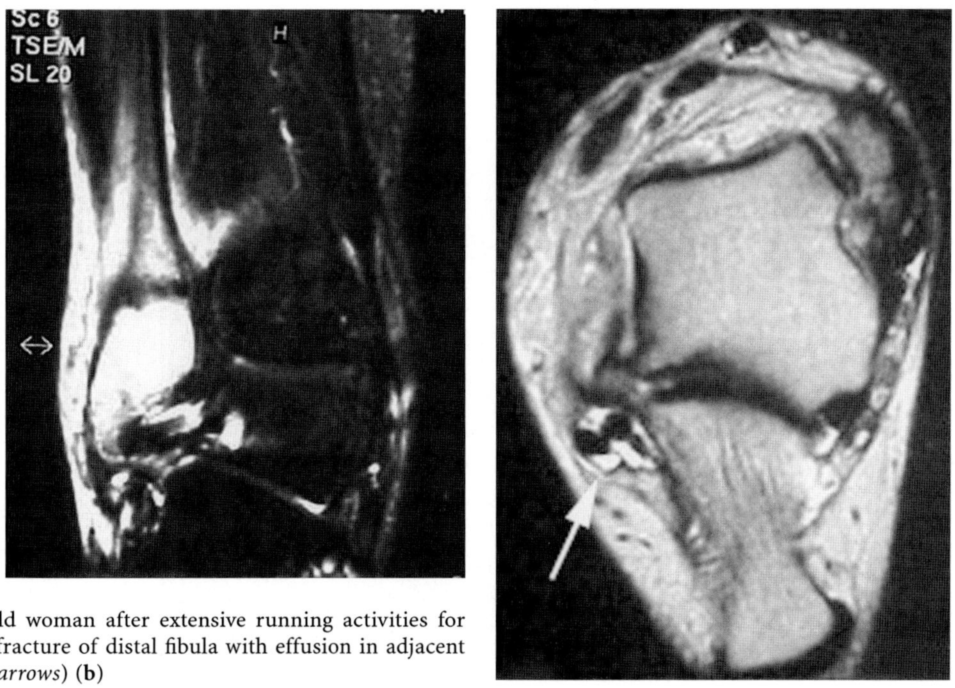

a b

Fig. 10.7a,b. A 32-year-old woman after extensive running activities for several months. **a** Stress fracture of distal fibula with effusion in adjacent peroneal tendon sheath (*arrows*) (**b**) subluxation or luxation (Clarke et al. 1998). Causes of abnormal fluid within the tendon sheath include traumatic dislocation of the tendons, systemic rheumatic disorders, tarsal coalition, congenital or acquired hypertrophy of the peroneal tubercle, altered foot mechanics, and improper footwear.

Furthermore, tears of the calcaneofibular ligament allow communication of the ankle and the peroneal tendon sheath, accounting for fluid in the sheath in some patients who have had ankle trauma.

Ruptures may occur spontaneously or may be associated with an acute injury with laceration of the lateral aspect of the ankle. The peroneus brevis tendon was shown to be degenerated in 11% of specimens in an autopsy study (Sobel et al. 1990). With MR imaging, longitudinal splits, hypertrophy, and fluid within partial tears of this tendon were demonstrated at the level of the lateral malleolus. Lateral ligament tears with associated laxity of the superior peroneal retinaculum may lead to peroneus brevis tendon splits and anterolateral subluxation of both peroneal tendons. Reactive lateral calcaneal marrow edema is sometimes associated with acute rupture of the peroneus brevis tendon (Fig. 10.8). Ruptures of the peroneus longus tendon are in most cases associated with lacerations of the peroneus brevis tendon.

10.3.4 Tendons of the Long Extensor Muscle Group

The group of the long extensor tendons acts as dorsal flexors of the foot and include those from the tibialis anterior muscle and from the extensor hallucis longus muscle.

Clinical signs of overuse with anterior ankle swelling and local pain occur in athletes secondary to forced plantar flexion and ankle eversion (Mink 1992). Spontaneous ruptures are rare and are generally observed in individuals over 50 years old.

The tibialis anterior tendon passes through the anterior crural retinaculum and inserts on the medial cuneiform and the adjacent base of the first metatarsal. Abnormal fluid within the synovial sheath of this tendon may be associated with tendon rupture or rheumatoid disease, or it may occur idiopathically (Fig. 10.9). Rupture of the tibialis anterior tendon can occur in its distal part between the extensor retinaculum and the insertion. Traumatic lacerations may also occur, related to the superficial and anterior location of this tendon. A distal rupture of this tendon has been explained to be related to a dorsal osteophyte (Jahss 1991).

The extensor hallucis longus is a thin muscle, situated between the tibialis anterior and the extensor digitorum longus muscles. Effusion in the tendon sheath may be observed due to abnormal compression from shoes or following repetitive dorsiflexion of the foot.

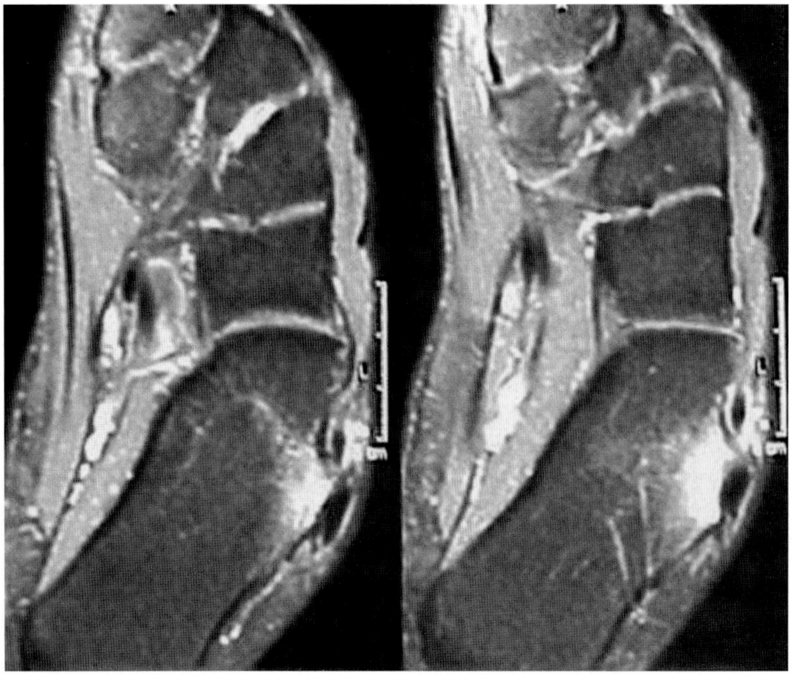

Fig. 10.8. Abnormal fluid within peroneal tendon sheath and adjacent bone marrow edema indicating severe form of tendon overuse

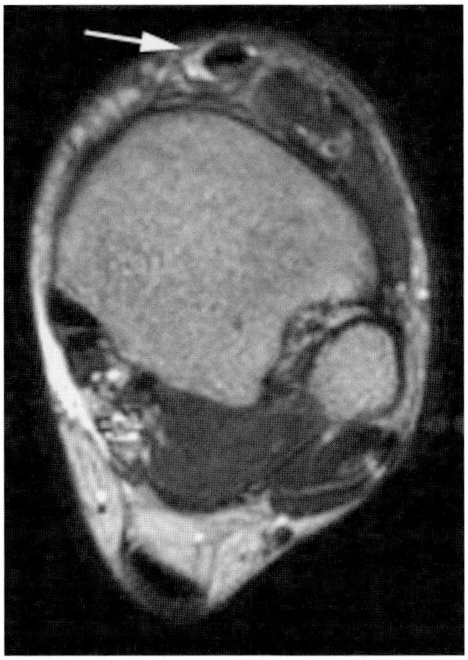

Fig. 10.9. A 27-year-old runner with painful swelling anterior to his ankle joint. T2-weighted MRI with effusion in tendon sheath of tibialis anterior tendon (*arrow*)

10.4 Conclusion

Diagnostic imaging of tendons should be performed with the aim to clarify the reasons for a painful overuse syndrome. Compared with muscles and bones, the bradytrophic tendons have a relatively long time of adaptation and regeneration with consequences in training and living habits. Especially in the field of sports medicine, the imaging findings have to be correlated with individual patterns of overuse in order to stop the progressive course of tendon disease from functional impairments, which carry a good prognosis of healing, to manifest rupture.

References

Archambault JM, Wiley JP, Bray RC, Verhoef M, Wiseman DA, Elliott PD (1998) Can sonography predict the outcome in patients with achillodynia? J Clin Ultrasound 26:335–339

Astrom M, Gentz CF, Nilsson P, Rausing A, Sjoberg S, Westlin N (1996) Imaging in chronic achilles tendinopathy: a comparison of ultrasonography, magnetic resonance imaging and surgical findings in 27 histologically verified cases. Skeletal Radiol 25:615–620

Balen PF, Helms CA (2001) Association of posterior tibial tendon injury with spring ligament injury, sinus tarsi abnormality, and plantar fasciitis on MR imaging. AJR Am J Roentgenol 176:1137–1143

Boles MA, Lomasney LM, Demos TC, Sage RA (1997) Enlarged peroneal process with peroneus longus tendon entrapment. Skeletal Radiol 26:313–315

Bottger BA, Schweitzer ME, El-Noueam KI, Desai M (1998) MR imaging of the normal and abnormal retrocalcaneal bursae. AJR Am J Roentgenol 170:1239–1241

Bude RO, Nesbitt SD, Adler RS, Rubenfire M (1998) Sonographic detection of xanthomas in normal-sized Achilles' tendons of individuals with heterozygous familial hypercholesterolemia. AJR Am J Roentgenol 170:621–625

Campbell RS, Grainger AJ (2001) Current concepts in imaging of tendinopathy. Clin Radiol 56:253–267

Clarke HD, Kitaoka HB, Ehman RL (1998) Peroneal tendon injuries. Foot Ankle Int 19:280–288

Clement DB, Taunton JE, Smart GW (1984) Achilles tendinitis and peritendinitis: etiology and treatment. Am J Sports Med 12:179–184

Cummins EJ, Anson BJ, Carr BW, Wright RR (1946) The structure of the calcaneal tendon (of Achilles) in relation to orthopedic surgery. Surg Gynecol Obstet 93:107–116

Ebraheim NA, Zeiss J, Skie MC, Jackson WT (1991) Radiological evaluation of peroneal tendon pathology associated with calcaneal fractures. J Orthop Trauma 5:365–369

Fornage B (1986) Achilles tendon: US examination. Radiology 159:759–764

Frey C, Shereff M, Greenidge N (1990) Vascularity of the posterior tibial tendon. J Bone Joint Surg Am 72:884–888

Gibbon WW, Long G (1999)Ultrasound of the plantar aponeurosis (fascia). Skeletal Radiol 28:21–26

Gibbon WW, Cooper JR, Radcliffe GS (1999) Sonographic incidence of tendon microtears in athletes with chronic Achilles tendinosis. Br J Sports Med 33:129–130

Hartgerink P, Fessell DP, Jacobson JA, van Holsbeeck MT (2001) Full- versus partial-thickness achilles tendon tears: sonographic accuracy and characterization in 26 cases with surgical correlation. Radiology 220:406–412

Ho RT, Smith D, Escobedo E (2001) Peroneal tendon dislocation: CT diagnosis and clinical importance. AJR Am J Roentgenol 177:1193

Holmes GB Jr, Mann RA (1992) Possible epidemiological factors associated with rupture of the posterior tibial tendon. Foot Ankle13:70–79

Jahss MH (1991) Tendon disorders of the foot and ankle. In: Jahss MH (ed) Disorders of the foot and ankle. Saunders, Philadelphia, pp 1461–1492

Kainberger FM, Engel A, Barton P, Hübsch P, Neuhold A, Salomonowitz E (1990) Injury of the Achilles tendon: diagnosis with sonography. AJR Am J Roentgenol 155: 1031–1036

Kainberger F, Nehrer S, Breitenseher M, Seidl G, Baldt M, Rand T, Imhof H (1996) Ultrasound morphology of the Achilles tendon and differential diagnosis. Ultraschall Med 17: 212–217

Kainberger F, Mittermaier F, Seidl G, Parth E, Weinstabl R (1997) Imaging of tendons – adaptation, degeneration, rupture. Eur J Radiol 25:209–222

Kainberger F, Ulreich N, Bernhard C, Müllner T, Nehrer S, Imhof H (2001) Tendon overuse syndrome (TOS): imaging diagnosis. Wien Med Wochenschr 151:509–512

Kannus P, Jozsa L (1991) Histopathological changes preceeding spontaneous rupture of a tendon. J Bone Joint Surg (Am) 73:1507–1525

Mammone JF (1997) MR imaging of tendon injuries about the foot and ankle. Clin Podiatr Med Surg 14: 313–335

Mantel D, Flautre B, Bastian D, Delforge PM, Delvalle A, Leclet H (1996) Étude structurale du tendon d'Achille en IRM. Corrélation avec la microanatomie et l'histologie. Structural MRI study of the Achilles tendon. Correlation with microanatomy and histology. J Radiol 77:261–265

Miller SD, Van Holsbeeck M, Boruta PM, Wu KK, Katcherian DA (1996) Ultrasound in the diagnosis of posterior tibial tendon pathology. Foot Ankle Int 17:555–558

Mink JH (1992) Tendons. In: Deutsch AL, Mink JH, Kerr R (eds) MRI of the foot and ankle. Raven, New York, pp 135–152

Morrison WB, Schweitzer ME, Wapner KL, Lackman RD (1994) Plantar fibromatosis: a benign aggressive neoplasm with a characteristic appearance on MR images. Radiology 193:841–845

Movin T, Kristoffersen-Wiberg M, Shalabi A, Gad A, Aspelin P, Rolf C (1998) Intratendinous alterations as imaged by ultrasound and contrast medium-enhanced magnetic resonance in chronic achillodynia. Foot Ankle Int 19: 311–317

Nehrer S, Breitenseher M, Brodner W, Kainberger F, Fellinger EJ, Engel A, Imhof H (1997) Clinical and sonographic evaluation of the risk of rupture in the Achilles tendon. Arch Orthop Trauma Surg 116:14–18

Paez H, Vuletin JC, Soave RL, Sellitto RV (1999) Pedal giant cell tumor of tendon sheath. J Am Podiatr Med Assoc 89: 368–372

Pecina MM, Bojanic I (1993) Overuse injuries of the skeletal system. CRC Press, Boca Raton, p 31

Peterson L, Renström P (2001) Sports Injuries. Their prevention and treatment. Dunitz, London, pp 331–392

Premkumar A, Perry MB, Dwyer AJ, Gerber LH, Johnson D, Venzon D, Shawker TH (2002) Sonography and MR imaging of posterior tibial tendinopathy. AJR Am J Roentgenol 178:223–232

Rosenberg ZS, Cheung Y, Jahss MH, Noto AM, Norman A, Leeds NE (1988) Rupture of posterior tibial tendon: CT and MR imaging with surgical correlation. Radiology 169: 229–235

Saltzman CL, Tearse DS (1998) Achilles tendon injuries. J Am Acad Orthop Surg 6:316–325

Schweitzer ME, Karasick D (2000) MR imaging of disorders of the Achilles tendon. AJR Am J Roentgenol 175:613–625

Schweitzer ME, Caccese R, Karasick D, Wapner KL (1993) Posterior tibial tendon tears: utility of secondary signs for MR imaging diagnosis. Radiology 188:655–659

Shalabi A, Kristoffersen-Wiberg M, Aspelin P, Movin T (2001) MR evaluation of chronic Achilles tendinosis. A longitudinal study of 15 patients preoperatively and two years postoperatively. Acta Radiol 42:269–276

Shellock FG (1997) Kinematic magnetic resonance imaging. In: Stoller DW (ed) MRI in orthopaedics and sports medicine. Lippincott / Williams and Wilkins, Philadelphia, pp 1023–1058

Sobel M, Bohne WH, Levy ME (1990) Longitudinal attrition of the peroneus brevis tendon in the fibular groove: an anatomic study. Foot Ankle 11:124–128

Soila K, Karjalainen PT, Aronen HJ, Pihlajamaki HK, Tirman PJ (1999) High-resolution MR imaging of the asymptomatic Achilles tendon: new observations. AJR Am J Roentgenol 173:323–328

Stein V, Laprell H, Tinnemeyer S, Petersen W (2000) Quantitative assessment of intravascular volume of the human Achilles tendon. Acta Orthop Scand 71:60–63

Stoller DW, Ferkel RD (1997) The ankle and foot. In: Stoller DW (ed) MRI in orthopaedics and sports medicine. Lippincott / Williams and Wilkins, Philadelphia, pp 443–596

Tamburrini O, Porpiglia H, Barresi D, Bertucci B, Console D (1999) The role of magnetic resonance in the diagnosis of the os trigonum syndrome. Radiol Med (Torino) 98: 462–467

Tsai WC, Chiu MF, Wang CL, Tang FT, Wong MK (2000) Ultrasound evaluation of plantar fasciitis. Scand J Rheumatol 29:255–259

Van Holsbeeck MT, Introcaso JH (2001) Musculoskeletal ultrasound. Elsevier Science Health Science, St Louis, pp 77–129

11 Ligament Pathology

A. KATZ and S. J. ERICKSON

CONTENTS

It is not surprising that the ankle joint receives so much clinical attention. It bears more weight than any other joint in the body and is subject to equilibrating proprioceptive and mechanical forces with every step. Ankle sprain is the most common sports-related injury, responsible for up to 10% of all emergency room visits. There is an estimated daily incidence of 1 per 10,000 individuals. With a cost ranging from $300 to $900 per patient per incident and an estimated annual cost of 2 billion dollars, its monetary burden to the health care system is equal to that of coronary artery bypass surgery (FALLAT et al. 1998; KANNUS and RENSTROM 1991).

A. KATZ, MD; S. J. ERICKSON, MD
Department of Radiology, Froedtert East Clinics - 2nd Floor, 9200 West Wisconsin Avenue, Milwaukee, WI 53226-3596, USA

In this chapter, we shall first briefly discuss the various imaging modalities, focusing on the utility of each in the evaluation of the ankle ligaments. Second, the normal gross and MR imaging anatomy and functional significance of the ankle ligaments will be presented. Third, specific ligamentous injuries and the MR imaging findings will be discussed. Treatment options are presented where relevant.

11.1 Diagnostic Techniques

11.1.1 Physical Examination

In the evaluation of the injured ankle, physical examination may be helpful in localizing the point of maximal tenderness and in identifying soft-tissue swelling. Although this evaluation is subjective in nature, criteria have been reported to establish the probability of the existence of ligament injury. Circumferential swelling of greater than 4 cm compared with the normal ankle is 70% sensitive for the presence of a ligamentous injury. Point tenderness over the calcaneofibular ligament is 72% sensitive for tear. Physical examination of the anterior talofibular ligament, however, is less accurate, with point tenderness over this structure 52% sensitive for ligament rupture. If all of the above physical findings are present, there is a 91% likelihood of ligamentous rupture (BORUTA et al. 1990).

11.1.2 Radiography

Ankle radiography shows sites of soft-tissue swelling and provides high specificity as to the absence of fracture. Specific avulsion fractures provide indirect evidence for ligamentous injury. For example, an avulsion fracture of the inferiormost aspect of the lateral malleolus implies a calcaneofibular ligament injury, whereas a posterior malleolar fracture implies a posterior tibiofibular ligament avulsive injury.

11.1.3 Stress Radiography

Stress radiography has been used in the evaluation of ligamentous injury. This modality operates under the premise that the absence of static joint support enables predictable variance from the normal relationship between the talus, tibia, and fibula. The anterior drawer test has been used to assess the status of the anterior talofibular ligament. There has been much disagreement about the normal value of the distance between the tibial plafond and the talar dome (Boruta et al. 1990; Breitenscher et al. 1997; Chandnani et al. 1994). The talar tilt test employs an inversion stress at the calcaneal cuboid joint to evaluate the relationship between the tibial plafond and the talar dome. Comparison to radiographs of the unstressed, ipsilateral ankle and to the stressed and unstressed contralateral side is made. A wide range of normal values is cited in the literature. Sauser et al. (1983) reported a specificity of 99%, but a sensitivity of only 38% using this technique. The inaccuracy of stress radiography was further demonstrated by Cardone et al. (1993), who reported that 12 of 23 patients with normal stress radiographs were subsequently shown to have ligament tears by MR imaging.

11.1.4 Arthrography

In the past, conventional ankle arthrography had been used to assess ligamentous integrity. Typically, ligamentous tears result in compromise of the ankle joint capsule, resulting in extravasation of the contrast material. Since the anterior talofibular ligament represents an anterolateral thickening of the ankle joint capsule, it can be expected that a tear of this ligament would disrupt the capsule and a provide a pathway for anterolateral extravasation above the level of the lateral malleolus (Sauser et al. 1983). Similarly, a tear of the calcaneofibular ligament, which is in close proximity to the peroneal tendons, can result in contrast extravasation around and into the peroneal tendon sheaths. It has been recommended that ankle arthrography be performed between 24 h and 5 days after the injury (Boruta et al. 1990). After this time, fibrosis may seal the site of disruption, decreasing the negative predictive value of the study. This examination fell out of favor because the false-negative rates were high, particularly if the examination was not performed within the narrow time window.

11.1.5 Peroneal Tenography

The presumed pathologic communication between the peroneal tendon sheaths and the ankle joint resulting from a calcaneofibular ligament tear prompted investigators to utilize peroneal tenography in the evaluation of ligamentous injury. Initial reports described 95% accuracy in the diagnosis of calcaneofibular ligament tears, with a positive predictive value of nearly 100% (Black et al. 1978). It was later discovered that a communication between the peroneal tendon sheaths and ankle joint can be a normal finding.

11.1.6 Ultrasound and CT

Ultrasound has been used by some investigators to evaluate the ankle ligaments (Milz et al. 1996). A discussion of this modality is beyond the scope of this chapter. Computed tomography can show avulsion fractures but is not widely used in the direct evaluation of ligaments.

11.1.7 MR Imaging

MR imaging provides the benefits of global assessment, excellent tissue contrast, and superior spatial resolution. It is now accepted as the single best modality for the evaluation of joints.

A 1.5-Tesla magnet is preferable for an optimum signal-to-noise ratio, but diagnostic information can be obtained using lower field strength units with careful attention to technique. The patient is positioned supine on the MR table using a local extremity coil selected to provide an optimum balance between anatomic coverage and spatial resolution. Schneck et al. (1992) have described the ideal ankle position and imaging plane for optimal visualization of each of the ankle ligaments (Table 11.1). In actual practice, however, repositioning is seldom employed more than once during the examination. Furthermore, many imagers perform the entire examination with

Table 11.1. Optimum position for evaluation of ligamentous structures (adapted from Schneck et al. 1992)

Ankle position	Plane of imaging	Ligaments evaluated
Full dorsiflexion	Axial	Tibiofibular, talofibular, deltoid, and spring ligaments
Full dorsiflexion	Coronal	Tibiospring, tibiocalcaneal, posterior tibiofibular
Full plantarflexion	Axial	Calcaneofibular ligament
Full plantarflexion	Coronal	Tibionavicular and anterior tibiotalar
Full dorsiflexion	Sagittal	Lower spring

the ankle in one fixed orientation – neutral, plantarflexion, or slight dorsiflexion (Muhle et al. 1999).

At our institution, the generic ankle protocol consists of axial proton density, axial T2-weighted fat-suppressed, sagittal T2-weighted fat-suppressed, and oblique coronal proton-density fat-suppressed sequences with the foot in neutral position; an oblique axial T1-weighted sequence prescribed at an angle of approximately 45 deg in relation to the inferior surface of the plantarflexed foot is performed last. This protocol evaluates the ankle tendons, the bones, and the ankle (talocrural), subtalar, talonavicular, and calcaneocuboid joints in addition to the ligaments. A global evaluation of the ankle is needed because unexpected associated findings are common (see Table 11.2). At our institution, we utilize 10–12 cm fields-of-view with 3–4 mm slice thicknesses.

Some authors have advocated the use of a 3D technique, with a slice thickness of 1 mm or less (Verhaven et al. 1991). Acquisition of isotropic voxels permits subsequent multiplanar reformation with little, if any, degradation in spatial resolution. Because of the amount of data involved, viewing at a workstation is necessary.

MR arthrography has been advocated for the assessment of the ligaments of the ankle. This procedure developed in response to the relatively large percentage of nonvisualized ligaments initially reported with MR imaging (Mink 1992).

Table 11.2. Posttraumatic causes of ankle pain (adapted from Helgason and Chandnani 1998)

Ankle sprain/ligament injury/impingement
Peroneus tendon subluxation/tear
Osteochondral injury
Fracture
Sinus tarsi syndrome
Subtalar instability

11.2 Ligaments: Normal Histology, Anatomy, and Function

Histologically, ligaments are composed of collagen bundles aligned parallel to the long axis of the structure. There are proprioceptor and pressure receptors in proximity to the ligaments, which provide positional information. Intervening fat is often present in variable quantities. The relative amount of intraligamentous fat will render the ligament either homogeneously hypointense or striated. It is particularly important that normal striations are not confused with ligamentous pathology.

The ligaments of the ankle joint proper can be divided into three major complexes. These include the lateral collateral ligamentous complex, the medial collateral (deltoid) ligament, and the syndesmotic ligamentous complex. Other ligaments of interest include those of the sinus tarsi, the spring ligament, and Lisfranc's ligament.

11.2.1 Lateral Collateral Ligament

The lateral collateral ligament is composed of three individual ligaments: the anterior talofibular ligament, the calcaneofibular ligament, and the posterior talofibular ligament (Fig. 11.1). The anterior talofibular ligament courses in a horizontal orientation and is, therefore, best visualized on axial projections with the foot in neutral position (Fig. 11.1a,b). In this projection, it possesses a predominantly flat shape extending from the anterior aspect of the fibula to the lateral talar body. The anterior talofibular ligament is composed of two discrete bands, the superior band being the larger of the two. The superior band reaches the fibular origin of the anterior tibiofibular ligament and the inferior band, the fibular origin of the calcaneofibular ligament (Sarrafian 1993). The anterior talofibular ligament can be considered contiguous with the joint capsule, representing an area of relative thickening. This structure courses upward with the ankle in dorsiflexion, and inferiorly with the foot in plantarflexion. The ligament is homogeneously low in signal intensity and is seen in virtually 100% of ankle MR examinations utilizing modern imaging techniques (Fig. 11.2) (Muhle et al. 1999).

The calcaneofibular ligament, in contrast to the anterior talofibular ligament, has a relatively cord-like appearance (Fig. 11.1). It can be identified imme-

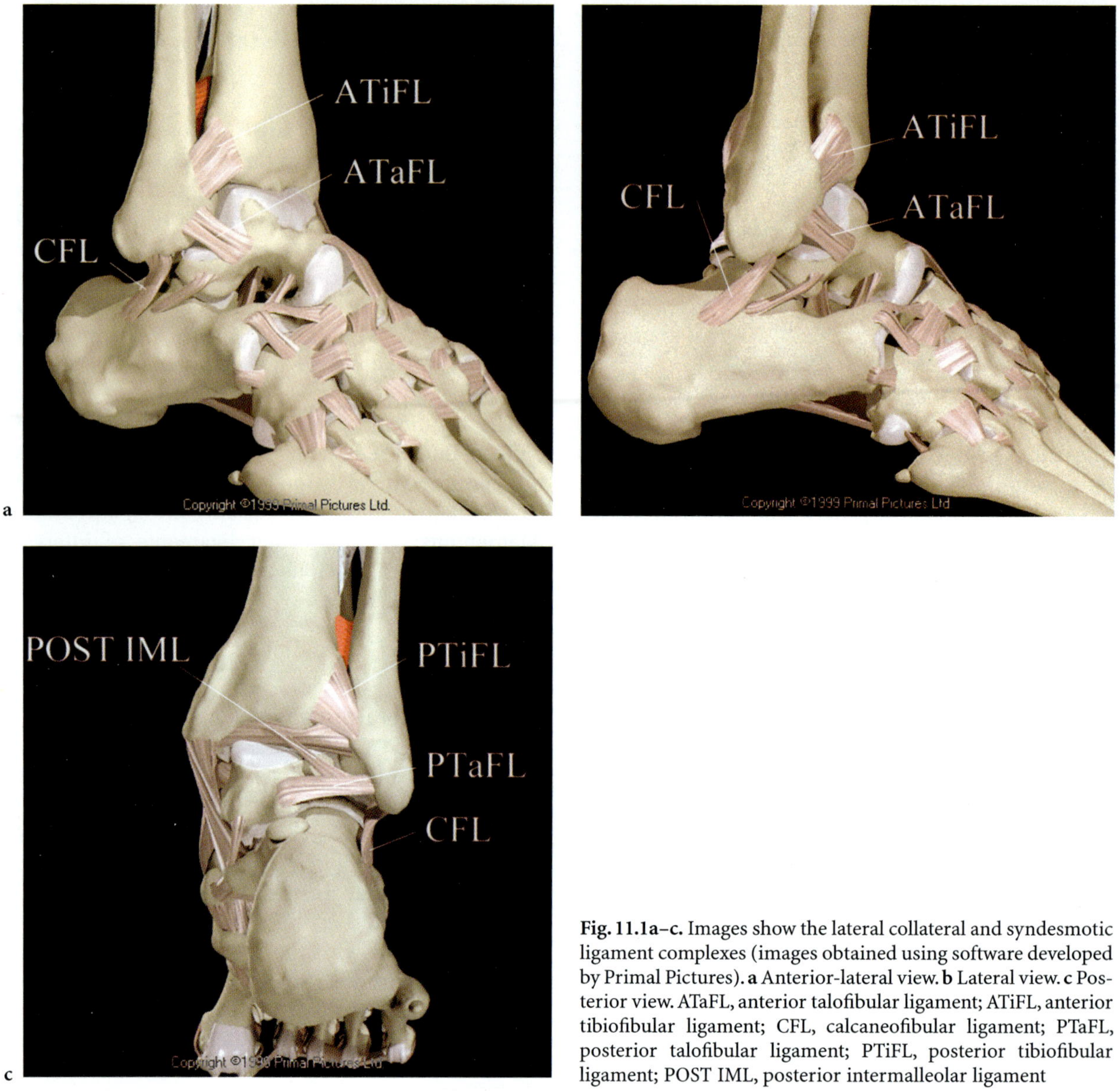

Fig. 11.1a–c. Images show the lateral collateral and syndesmotic ligament complexes (images obtained using software developed by Primal Pictures). **a** Anterior-lateral view. **b** Lateral view. **c** Posterior view. ATaFL, anterior talofibular ligament; ATiFL, anterior tibiofibular ligament; CFL, calcaneofibular ligament; PTaFL, posterior talofibular ligament; PTiFL, posterior tibiofibular ligament; POST IML, posterior intermalleolar ligament

diately deep to the peroneal tendons and is indented by them (Fig. 11.3). The calcaneofibular ligament courses from its origin on a small tubercle situated on the lateral aspect of the calcaneus anteromedially to insert onto the lower aspect (but not the tip) of the anterior border of the lateral malleolus. Ruth (1961) noted a wide variation in the precise course of this structure in a study of 30 dissected ankles and 55 ankles during surgery. It can be imaged using an oblique axial plane with the ankle in neutral position or in the axial, or slightly off axial, plane with the foot in full plantar flexion. The normal calcaneofibular ligament is homogeneous in signal intensity (Fig. 11.4) (Muhle et al. 1999).

The posterior talofibular ligament is a very strong ligament which extends from the distal fibular malleolar fossa to its broad attachment onto the lateral tubercle of the posterior talar process (Figs. 11.1c, 11.5). It can be visualized at the same axial level as the anterior talofibular ligament (Fig. 11.2). This structure serves as a border between the ankle joint and the posterior subtalar joint. Morphologically, the posterior talofibular ligament is fan-shaped with a medial base and lateral apex. Because it is fasciculated, on MR imaging it has a striated appearance (Muhle et al. 1999).

The lateral collateral ligament provides lateral support to the ankle joint with the anterior talofibular ligament and calcaneofibular ligament providing the

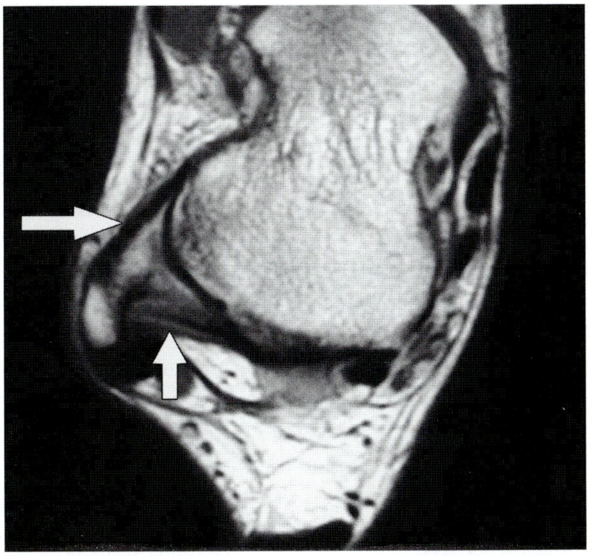

Fig. 11.2. Axial MR image shows the anterior talofibular ligament (*long arrow*) and posterior talofibular ligament (*short arrow*)

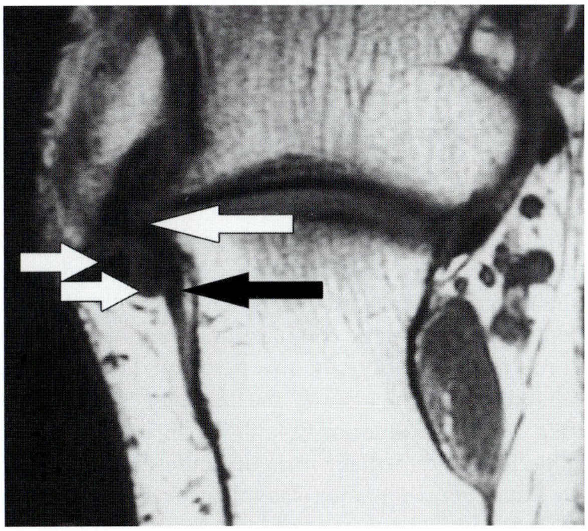

Fig. 11.4. Oblique axial image shows the calcaneofibular ligament (*long arrows*) and the overlying peroneal tendons (*short arrows*) (reprinted with permission from Erickson et al. 1991)

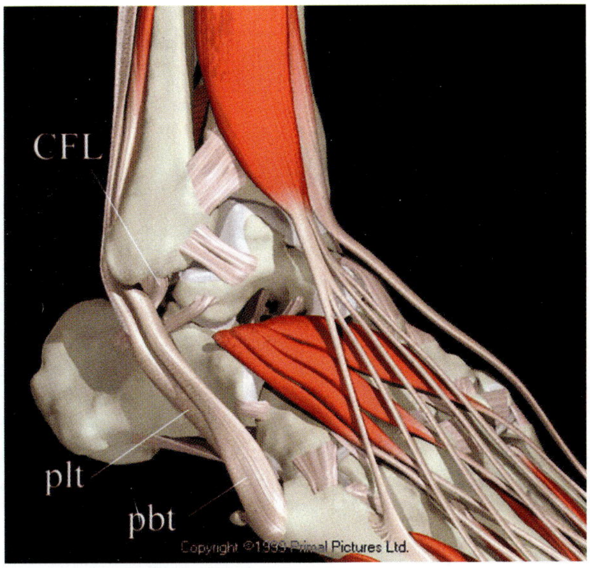

Fig. 11.3. Anterolateral image of the ankle shows the calcaneofibular ligament (*CFL*) and the overlying peroneus brevis (*pbt*) and peroneus longus (*plt*) tendons (image obtained using software developed by Primal Pictures)

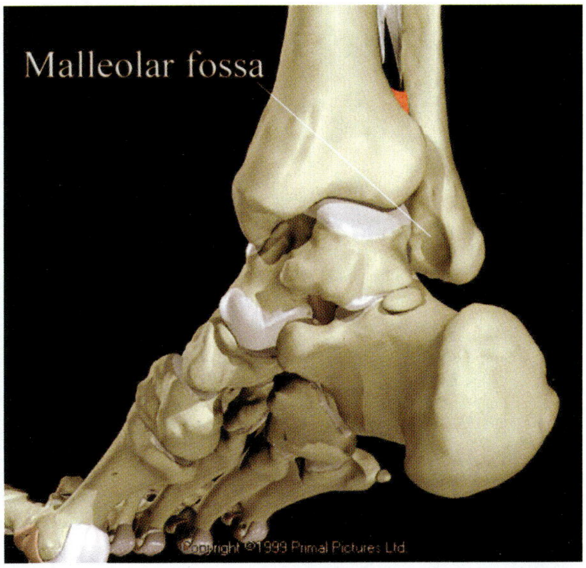

Fig. 11.5. Posteromedial image of the ankle shows the indentation within the distal, medial aspect of the fibula known as the malleolar fossa (image obtained using software developed by Primal Pictures)

critical support in different ankle positions. The calcaneofibular ligament lies perpendicular to the talar long axis. Its anterior fibers accept greater tension with increasing ankle dorsiflexion. The calcaneofibular ligament is the primary restraint in unloaded external rotation. In the neutral position, the anterior talofibular ligament is in a relaxed state with fibers paralleling the long axis of the talus. With plantarflexion, the anterior talofibular ligament receives the primary tensile forces upon the ankle and is therefore the primary stabilizer to ankle inversion injuries with the ankle in the unloaded position. Along with the deltoid ligament, the anterior talofibular ligament provides restraint in unloaded internal rotation injuries (Boruta et al. 1990). With the ankle in weight-bearing, the articular surface of the ankle mortise provides stability. From an imaging standpoint, the lateral collateral ligament is the most relevant ligamentous structure.

11.2.2 Tibiofibular Syndesmotic Complex

The tibiofibular syndesmotic complex is defined by the group of ligaments joining the distal fibula and the concave lateral distal tibia. Anatomically, the tibiofibular syndesmotic complex can be subdivided into three main constituents: the posterior and anterior tibiofibular ligaments and the interosseous ligament (Fig. 11.1). The anterior tibiofibular ligament extends superiorly and medially from the anterior distal fibula to insert upon the anterolateral tubercle of the tibia (Fig. 11.1a,b). The anterior tibiofibular ligament is multifascicular and is best seen on axial sections within 1 cm of the tibial plafond (Fig. 11.6). The most inferior fascicle contacts the anterolateral aspect of the talar dome and is sometimes referred to as Bassett's ligament (Bassett et al. 1990). The extensor digitorum longus tendon passes anterior to the anterior tibiofibular ligament and can be used as a reliable landmark in its identification.

The posterior tibiofibular ligament is significantly stronger than the anterior tibiofibular ligament and consists of superficial and deep components (Fig. 11.6) (Sarrafian 1993). The superficial component extends from the posterior aspect of the lateral malleolus superiorly and medially to the posterolateral portion of the tibial tubercle. The deep component arises near the superficial component and initially courses superiorly, medially, and posteriorly; then it assumes a more transverse course along the posterior aspect of the tibial articular surface, some fibers reaching the medial malleolus. This structure forms a 'posterior labrum'. The posterior tibiofibular ligament is closely related to the flexor hallucis longus and the peroneal tendons.

The interosseous ligament constitutes the lower portion of the interosseous membrane between the

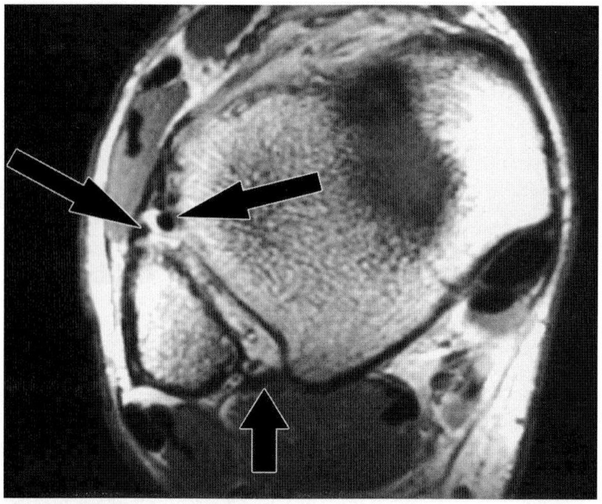
a

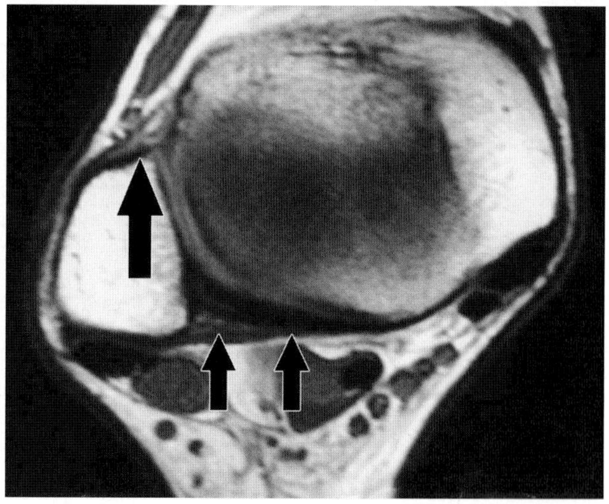
b

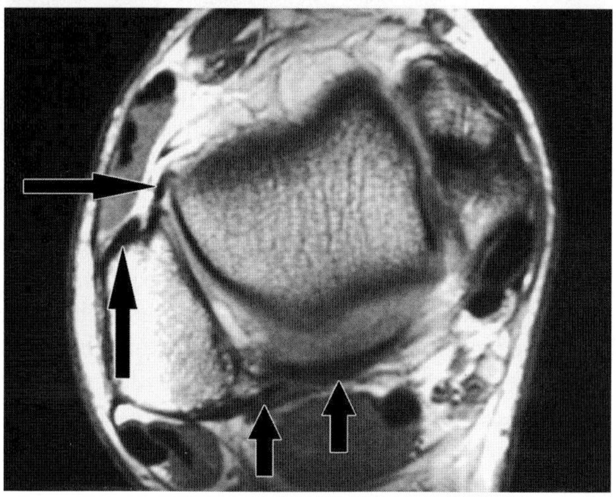
c

Fig. 11.6a–c. Anterior (*long arrows*) and posterior tibiofibular ligaments (*short arrows*). **a** Axial image above the ankle joint. **b** Axial image at the level of the tibial plafond showing the deep portion of the posterior tibiofibular ligament. **c** Axial image obtained at the level of the talus tibia and fibula (Fig. 11.7). The fibers of this structure form the superior border of the tibiofibular synovial recess, an extension of the ankle joint.

Two imaging features assist in the differentiation of the tibiofibular from the talofibular ligaments. First, the syndesmotic ligaments insert upon the rounded anterior and posterior portions of the fibula at levels in which the medial aspect of the fibula appears flat. In contrast, the talofibular ligaments reside at the level of the mesially concave portion of the distal fibula known as the malleolar fossa (Figs. 11.2, 11.6, 11.8, 11.9) (Erickson et al. 1991). Second, on axial images the anterior aspect of the talus appears 'squared' at the level of the tibiofibular ligaments, whereas it assumes a more rounded contour at the level of the talofibular ligaments (Rosenberg et al. 2000).

A variable fourth component of the tibiofibular syndesmotic complex, the posterior intermalleolar ligament or marsupial meniscus, has been reported in 56% of cadaveric specimens and in 19% of MR

a b

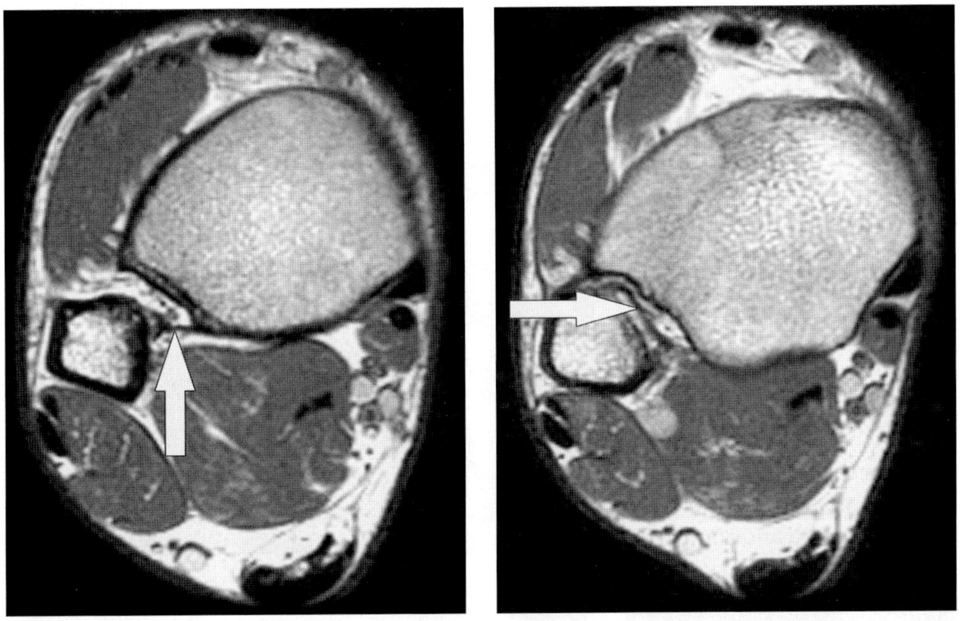

Fig. 11.7a,b. Interosseous ligament (*arrows*). **a** Axial image shows the syndesmotic region. **b** Axial image obtained at a more caudal level

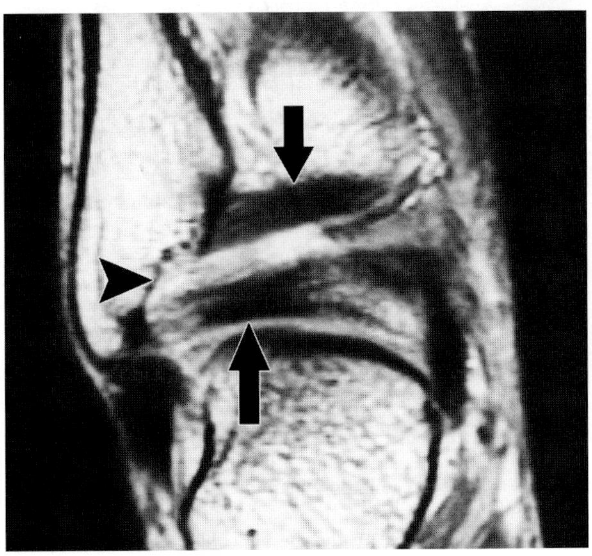

Fig. 11.8. Posterior tibiofibular (*short arrow*) and posterior talofibular ligaments (*long arrow*) on oblique coronal image. Note the malleolar fossa (*arrowhead*)

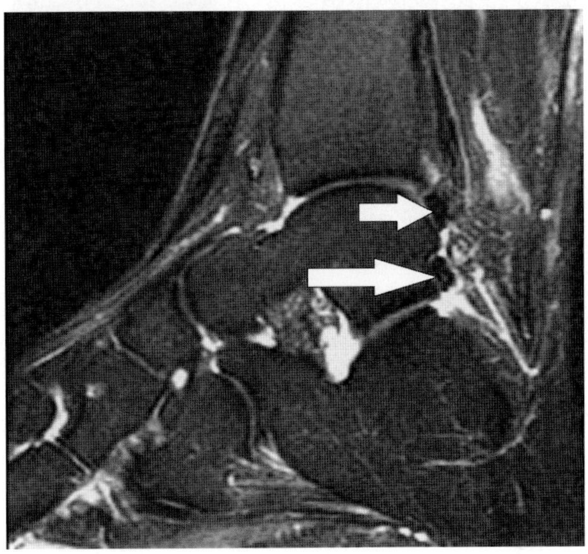

Fig. 11.9. Posterior talofibular (*long arrow*) and posterior tibiofibular (*short arrow*) ligaments on sagittal image

examinations (Rosenberg et al. 1995). It lies inferior to the posterior tibiofibular ligament, separating it from the posterior talofibular ligament (Fig. 11.1c).

11.2.3 Medial Collateral (Deltoid) Ligament

The medial collateral ligamentous complex provides ligamentous support to the medial ankle. This structure is divided into superficial and deep components, each of which can be further subdivided into individual constituents. The alternative name, the deltoid ligament, is based on the triangular shape of the superficial component. The apex of the triangle lies at the medial malleolus, with the insertions fanning out inferiorly (Sarrafian 1993).

The superficial component is usually subdivided into three contributions, though Sarrafian (1993) states that this component is actually a solid lamina and that any such division is artificial (Fig. 11.10). The tibionavicular ligament courses anteriorly and inferiorly, crossing both the ankle joint and the talonavicular joint to insert onto the navicular tuberosity. This structure contributes to both of these joint capsules.

The tibiocalcaneal contribution is the strongest superficial component. This ligament inserts onto the medial border of the sustentaculum tali and comprises a portion of both the ankle and subtalar joint capsules. The tibio-spring ligament (Schneck et al. 1992), also called the superomedial calcaneonavicular ligament (Sarrafian 1993), extends from the medial malleolus to the upturned lateral edge of the calcaneonavicular (spring) ligament. Similar to its tibiocalcaneal counterpart, the tibio-spring ligament crosses both the ankle and the anterior subtalar joints.

The posterior tibiotalar contribution originates from the posterior aspect of the medial malleolus and courses posteriorly, inferiorly, and laterally to insert onto the posteromedial talar tubercle. All three constituents of the superficial component appear relatively hypointense and homogeneous on MR images (Figs. 11.11, 11.12).

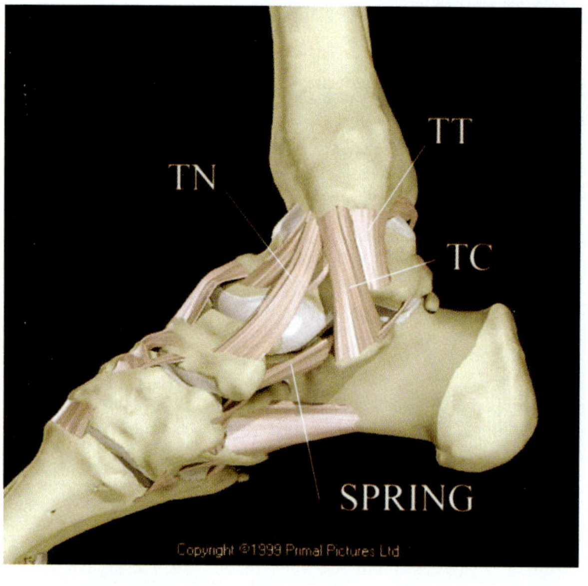

Fig. 11.10. Image of the medial aspect of the ankle shows the three superficial components of the medial collateral ligament and the spring ligament. TC, tibiocalcaneal ligament; TN, tibionavicular ligament; TT, posterior tibiotalar ligament. (Image was obtained using software developed by Primal Pictures)

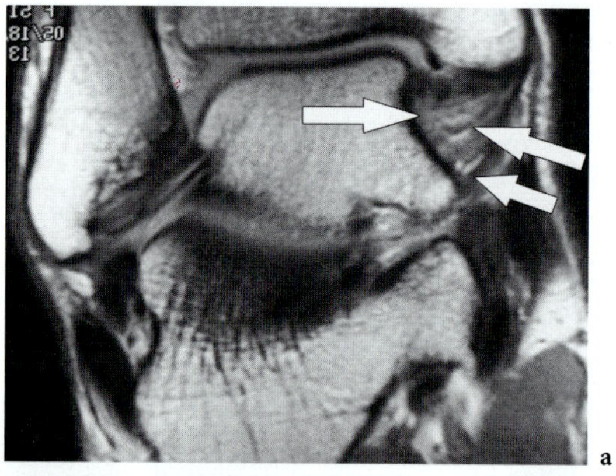
a

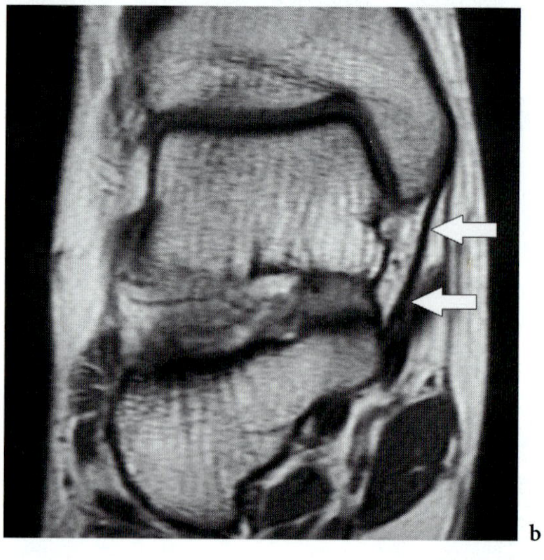
b

Fig. 11.11a,b. Medial collateral ligament. **a** Coronal image shows the striated appearance of the posterior tibiotalar constituent of the deep component of the medial collateral ligament (*long arrows*) and overlying tibiotalar constituent of the superficial component (*short arrow*). **b** Oblique coronal image obtained at a more anterior level shows portions of the superficial component of the medial collateral ligament (*arrows*)

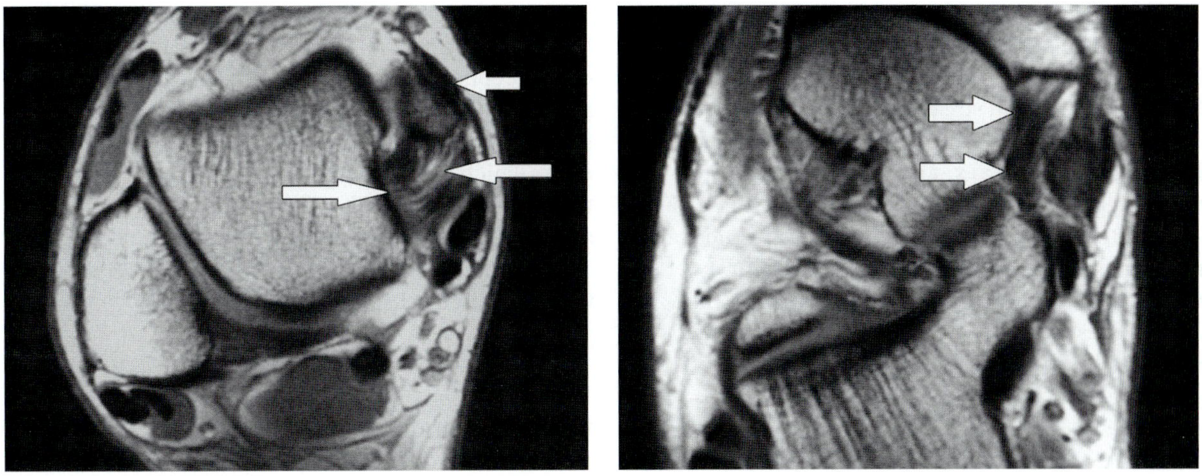

Fig. 11.12a,b. Medial collateral ligament. **a** Axial image shows the striated posterior tibiotalar constituent of the deep component (*long arrows*) as well as the proximal aspect of the superficial component (*short arrow*). **b** Axial image obtained at a more caudal level shows the superficial component of the medial collateral ligament (*arrows*)

The deep component of the deltoid ligament is composed of the anterior tibiotalar ligament and the posterior tibiotalar ligament (Fig. 11.13). The anterior tibiotalar ligament is variably present. When seen, it is a structure of heterogeneous signal intensity, which inserts at the anterior body and neck of the talus.

The posterior tibiotalar ligament is intraarticular and relatively thick in morphology. It is the strongest single constituent of the medial collateral ligament. It courses from its broad attachment onto the medial malleolus posteriorly to its insertion onto the medial talar body. It is partially overlain by the posterior tibiotalar contribution of the superficial component. This ligament appears heavily striated and is well seen on both coronal and axial images (Figs. 11.11, 11.12).

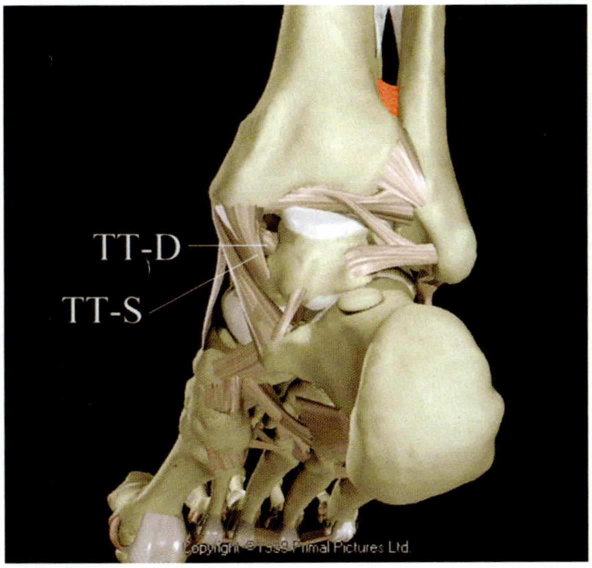

Fig. 11.13. Medial collateral ligament. Posterior medial image of the ankle shows the relationship of the posterior tibiotalar constituent of the deep component (*TT-D*) in relation to the posterior tibiotalar constituent of the superficial component (*TT-S*). (Image was obtained using software developed by Primal Pictures)

11.2.4 Sinus Tarsi

This anatomic region constitutes a cone-shaped space bounded by the neck of the talus and the anterior superior aspect of the calcaneus (Fig. 11.14).

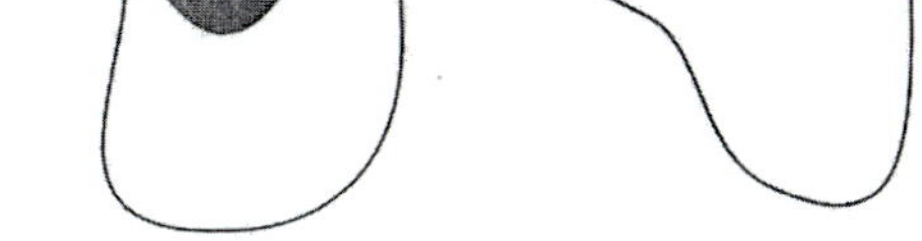

Fig. 11.14. Two schematic images of the sinus tarsi. 1, cervical ligament; 3, interosseous talocalcaneal ligament; 2/4/5, the medial, intermediate, and lateral roots of the inferior extensor retinaculum, respectively. (Image is reprinted with permission from Lektrakul et al. 2001)

The tarsal sinus is represented by the larger, lateral opening, the tarsal canal by the medial, narrower portion. Normally, the sinus tarsi is predominately filled with fat. Blood vessels, nerves, and joint recesses also reside within this region, but are relatively inconspicuous (Klein and Spreitzer 1993). The major ligamentous structures within the tarsal sinus include the cervical ligament, interosseous talocalcaneal ligament, and the roots of the inferior extensor retinaculum (Figs. 11.15, 11.16) (Lektrakul et al. 2001). These extracapsular ligaments serve as further stabilizers of the lateral ankle and hindfoot and provide support for the subtalar joint.

11.2.5 Spring (Plantar Calcaneonavicular) Ligament

The spring ligament, or plantar calcaneonavicular ligament, is vital in the support of the arch of the foot. It creates an acetabulum for the talar head. It arises from the undersurface of the talar sustentaculum, attaching to the inferior and medial surfaces of the navicular (Figs. 11.10, 11.16c). Its medial border curves cephalad to become contiguous with the tibiospring ligament. Laterally, the spring ligament is contiguous with the medial band of the bifurcate ligament, which joins the superior and anterior calcaneus to the adjacent cuboid and navicular bones (Davis et al. 1996; Rule et al. 1993). The medial aspect of this ligament is more reliably assessed with MR imaging than the plantar aspect (Yao et al. 1999).

11.2.6 Lisfranc's Ligament

The Lisfranc (tarsometatarsal) joint separates the row of tarsal bones from the bases of the five metatarsals. The triangular-shaped base of the second metatarsal articulates with the recessed middle cuneiform to form a mortise joint. Lisfranc's ligament extends anteriorly and laterally from the lateral face of the medial cuneiform to the medial face of the second metatarsal.

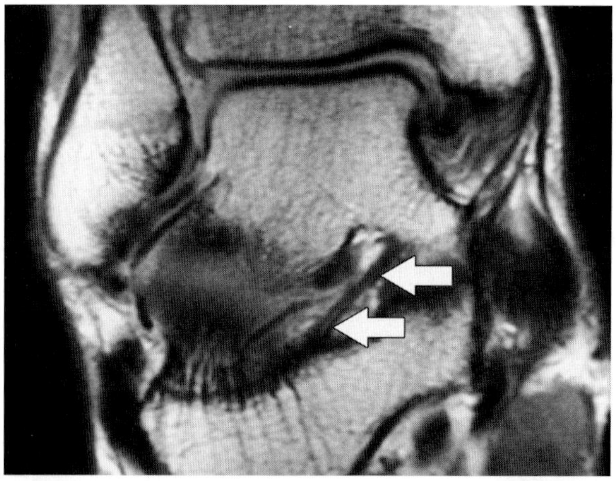

a

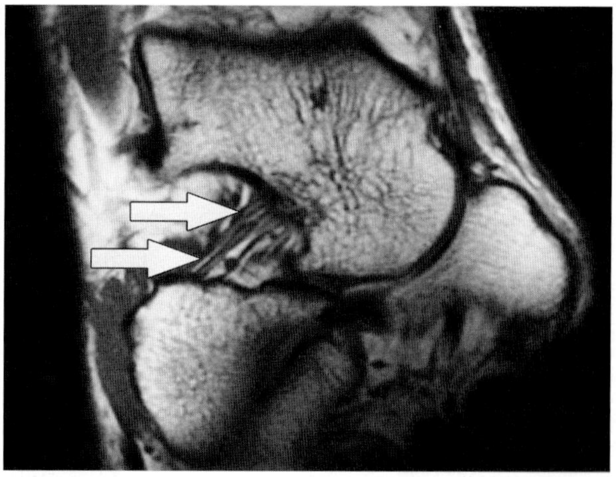

b

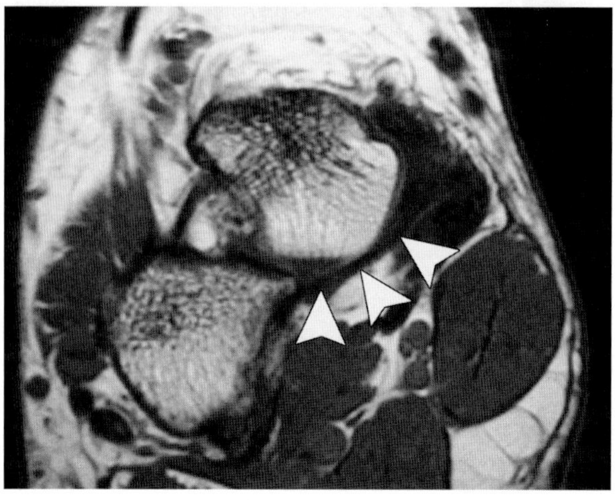

c

Fig. 11.15a–c. Coronal images showing the sinus tarsi proceeding from posterior to anterior (**a–c**, respectively). Short arrows, the interosseous talocalcaneal ligament; long arrows, the cervical ligament; arrowheads, the spring ligament and tibiospring portion of the medial collateral ligament

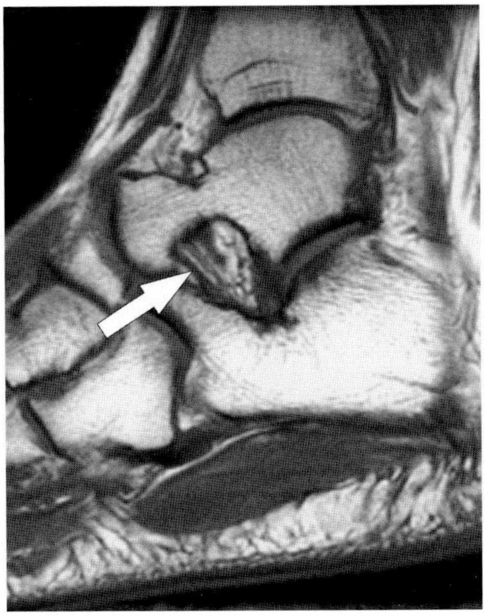

a

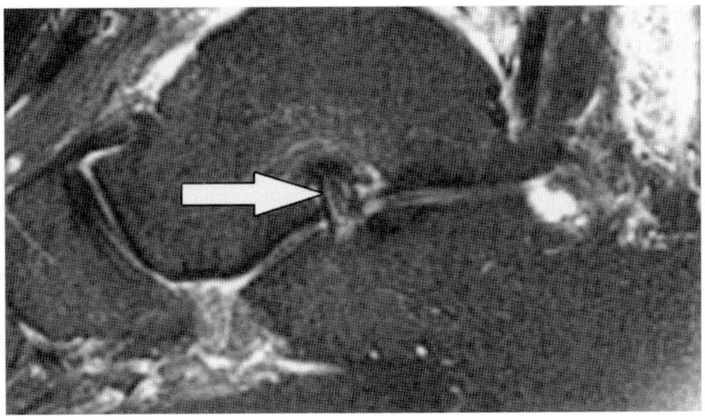

b

Fig. 11.16a,b. Sinus tarsi. **a** Sagittal image shows the cervical ligament (*arrow*). **b** Sagittal image obtained more medially shows the interosseous talocalcaneal ligament (*arrow*)

This ligament is best visualized using a special double oblique plane – an initial oblique coronal plane perpendicular to the metatarsal shafts is prescribed from a representative sagittal image; next, an oblique plane parallel to the metatarsal shafts is prescribed from a representative oblique coronal image. This structure displays a prominent striated appearance (Fig. 11.17). Other tarsal-metatarsal and intermetatarsal ligaments complete the support of the Lisfranc joint.

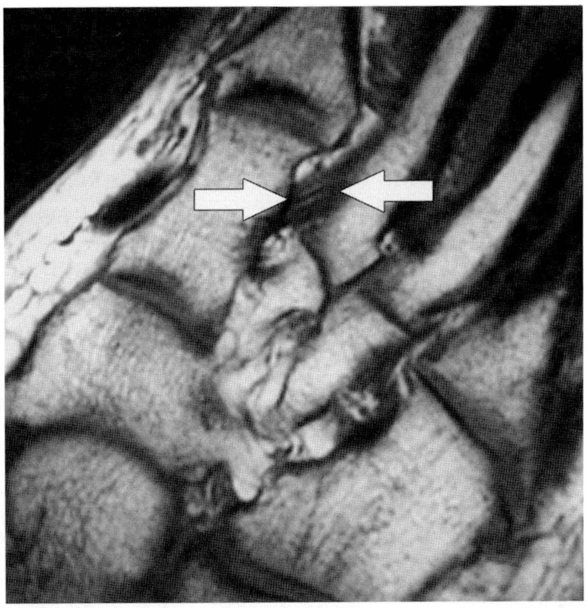

Fig. 11.17. Oblique axial image shows the striated Lisfranc's ligament coursing from the lateral aspect of the medial cuneiform to the base of the second metatarsal (*arrows*)

11.3 Ligament Pathology

11.3.1 General Considerations

Ankle sprains can be classified into clinical grades (Cass and Morray 1984; Boruta et al. 1990). Grade 1 sprain is characterized by a lack of instability on clinical stress testing. This correlates histologically with a microscopic ligamentous tear. The patient presents with pain, focal tenderness, and mild swelling. Grade 2 tear is characterized by mild instability, indicating a partial ligament tear. More pronounced swelling and tenderness are observed on physical examination. In a grade 3 tear, there is complete disruption of the ligament and gross instability. Physical examination shows either no endpoint or a soft endpoint to stress testing.

The MR imaging findings of torn ankle ligaments reflect the grade and age of injury. Acute injuries are manifested by ligament discontinuity, thickening, thinning, or contour irregularity. A normally homogeneous, hypointense ligament may appear heterogeneous, with foci of increased signal intensity observed on T1-weighted and T2-weighted images. A normally striated ligament may, on the other hand, appear atypically homogeneous. A joint effusion may be present, and fluid may extravasate into the adjacent soft tissues. Periligamentous edema, subcutaneous edema, and bone contusions are routinely observed.

Chronic injuries are manifested by thickening, attenuation, or absence of the ligament. Frequently, the ligament exhibits a wavy contour (Cardone et al. 1993). Intermediate signal intensity within a chronically torn ligament may reflect residual edema, fat, or synovitis. The acute findings of edema and hemarthrosis will have resolved, but small joint effusions may be present. In addition, there can be signs of synovial proliferation or scarring, evident as areas of decreased signal intensity on T1-weighted and T2-weighted images.

Accepted indications for MR imaging of the ankle following injury include chronic ankle pain, instability, or both in those patients in whom conservative therapeutic measures fail. In a high performance athlete, ankle MR imaging can be used in the acute setting to evaluate the prognosis as well to aid in determining if surgery is warranted.

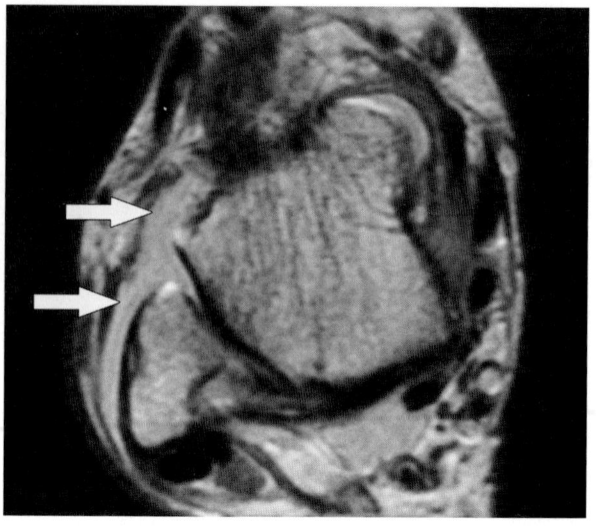

Fig. 11.19. Anterior talofibular ligament injury. Axial proton-density-weighted image shows disruption of the anterior talofibular ligament with joint fluid extending into the adjacent soft tissues (*arrows*)

11.3.2 Lateral Collateral Ligament

The lateral collateral ligament is the most commonly injured ligamentous complex following an inversion injury (Erickson and Johnson 1997). Its constituents are typically affected in a progressive, predictable manner with increasing inversion forces. The anterior talofibular ligament, being biomechanically the weakest constituent, is the first ligament to be injured in the sequence (Figs. 11.18–11.21). Because the anterior talofibular ligament is pulled along the ridge of the talar neck with tearing of the related joint capsule, ruptures occur in the mid-substance of the ligament 45% of the time (Mink 1992). Some 50% of the time there is an associated talar avulsion fracture. The calcaneofibular ligament, which is involved in 20%–25% of ligament injuries to the ankle, is affected next in turn with increasing inver-

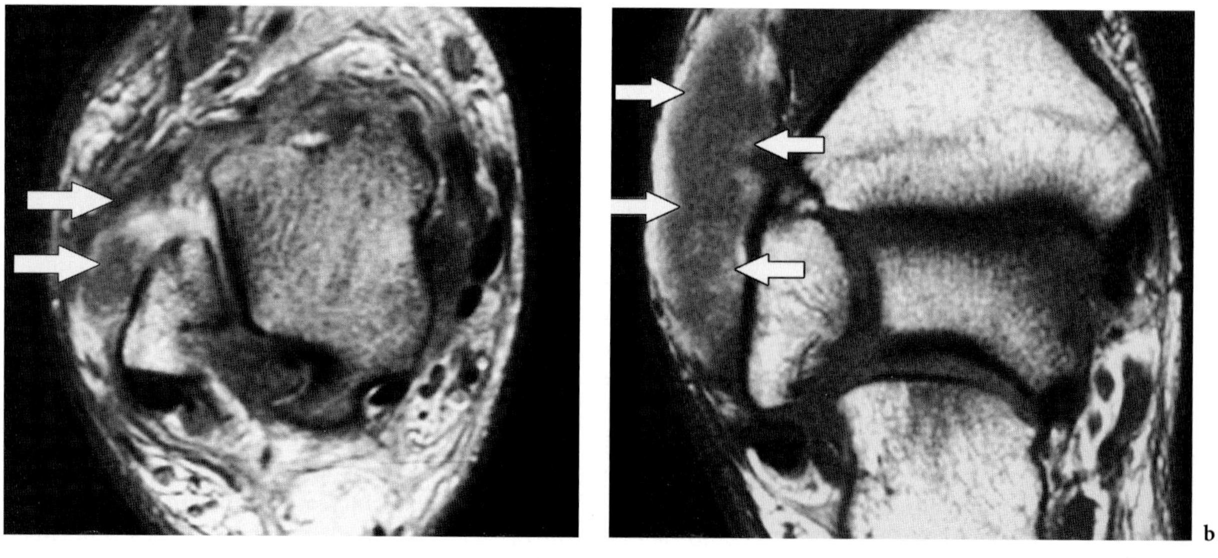

Fig. 11.18a,b. Anterior talofibular ligament injury. **a** Axial proton-density-weighted image shows gross disruption of the anterior talofibular ligament (*arrows*) with subacute soft-tissue changes. **b** Oblique axial T1-weighted image shows a large, lateral, soft-tissue focus consistent with a hematoma (*arrows*)

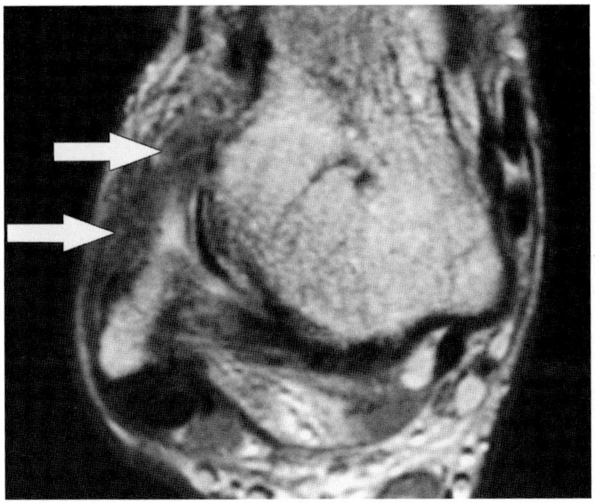

Fig. 11.20. Chronic anterior talofibular ligament injury. Axial proton-density-weighted image shows a markedly indistinct and irregular anterior talofibular ligament, consistent with chronic injury (*arrows*)

sion stress (Fig. 11.22–11.24). Complete rupture of this structure is believed to place the patient at high risk for future ankle instability (Oloff et al. 1992). The third lateral ligament, the posterior talofibular ligament, is rarely injured following inversion injury.

Initially, there were reports of a limited role for MR imaging in the evaluation of the ankle ligaments. As recently as 1998, Helgason and Chandnani reported only a 50% sensitivity of MR imaging for anterior talofibular ligament and calcaneofibular ligament injuries. In a retrospective analysis performed by Kreitner et al. (1999), however, MR imaging was found to be 100% accurate in the diagnosis of anterior talofibular ligament tears. In Kreitner's investigation, MRI correctly identified an intact calcaneofibular ligament in all 10 cases in which the ligament was shown to be normal at surgery. Two partial calcaneofibular ligament tears were also accurately diagnosed; of 6 complete tears proven surgically, 2 were misdiagnosed as partial tears. A second series consisting of 15 cases with surgical correlation reported 100% sensitivity and 50% specificity for complete anterior talofibular ligament tears and 92% sensitivity and 100% specificity for calcaneofibular ligament tears (Breitenseher et al. 1997). Verhaven et al. (1991), in their study using 3D gradient-echo technique, reported 100% sensitivity, 50% specificity, and 94.4% accuracy for anterior talofibular ligament tears. For calcaneofibular ligament injuries, 91.7% sensitivity, 100% specificity, and 94.4% accuracy were reported.

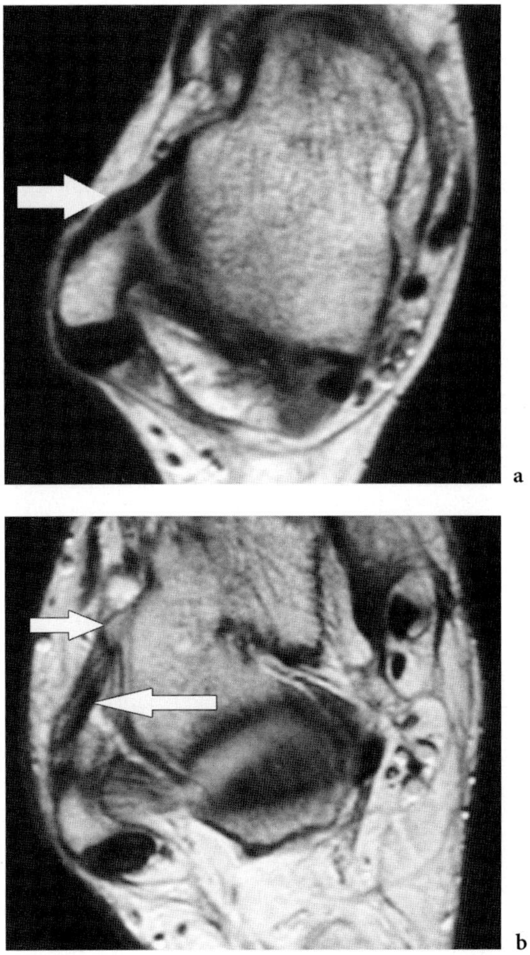

Fig. 11.21a,b. Chronic anterior talofibular ligament injuries with more subtle MR findings. **a** Axial proton-density-weighted image shows thickening of the anterior talofibular ligament (*arrow*). **b** Axial proton-density-weighted image in a different patient shows thickening and increased signal intensity in the anterior talofibular ligament (*large arrow*) in combination with an excrescence arising from the talar attachment site (*small arrow*)

Chandnani et al. (1994) published a prospective study of 17 patients in which stress radiography, MR imaging, and MR arthrography were compared with surgical or arthroscopic findings. Fourteen anterior talofibular and 10 calcaneofibular ligament tears were found at surgery. MR arthrography diagnosed 100% of the anterior talofibular ligament and 83% of the calcaneofibular ligament tears. In addition to the primary MR imaging findings, secondary arthrographic signs of ligamentous tear may improve the diagnostic accuracy. A tear of the anterior talofibular ligament can be associated with transcapsular contrast extravasation from the joint adjacent to the anterior talofibular ligament. Findings indicative of

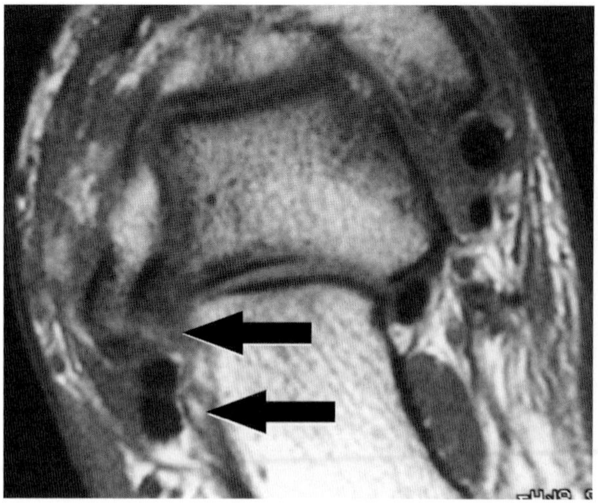

Fig. 11.22. Calcaneofibular ligament injury. Oblique axial T1-weighted image shows a wavy, attenuated, and relatively hyperintense calcaneofibular ligament (*arrows*)

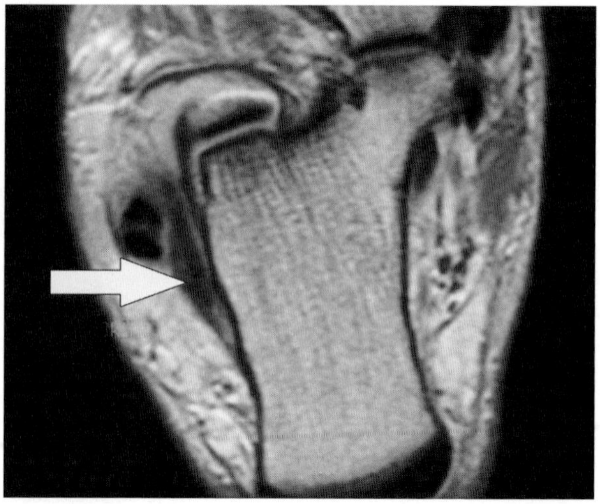

Fig. 11.24. Calcaneofibular ligament injury. Axial proton-density-weighted image shows thickening of the calcaneofibular ligament, particularly adjacent to its calcaneal attachment site (*arrow*)

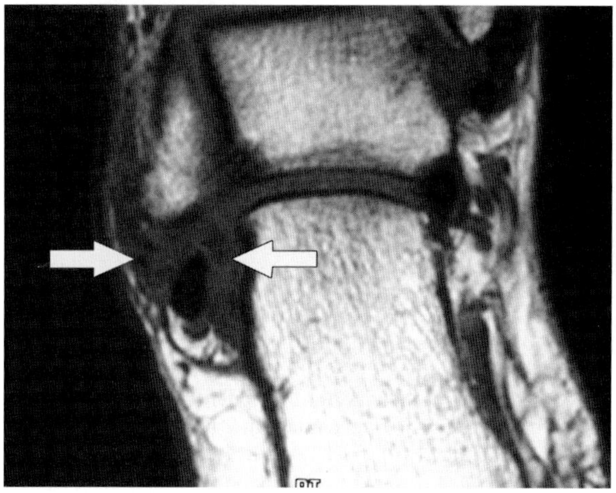

Fig. 11.23. Calcaneofibular ligament injury. Oblique axial T1-weighted image demonstrates hypointense soft tissue adjacent to an enlarged calcaneofibular ligament (*arrows*)

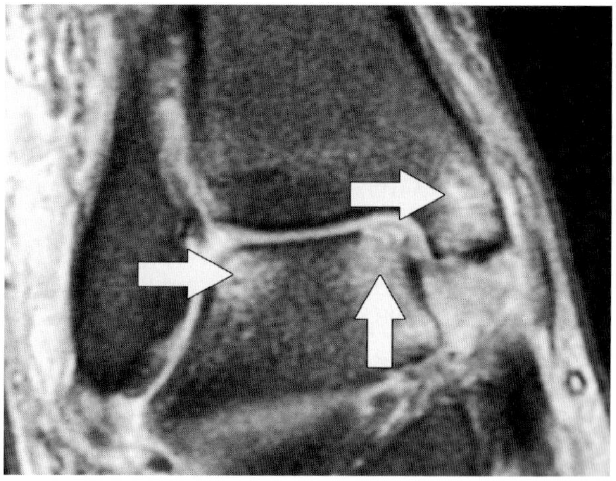

Fig. 11.25. Bone contusions associated with ankle sprain. Oblique coronal proton-density-weighted fat-suppressed image shows contusions involving the medial malleolus and both the medial and lateral aspects of the talar dome (*arrows*). There is associated soft-tissue edema

calcaneofibular ligament tear with MR arthrography include extravasation lateral to the calcaneofibular ligament or into the peroneal tendon sheaths. For the rare posterior talofibular ligament tear, extravasation posterior to this structure would be expected.

Recently, the presence, pattern, and significance of bone contusions acquired during ankle sprains have been addressed. Nishimura et al. (1996) evaluated patterns of bone bruising following lateral collateral ligament injuries (Fig. 11.25). Four basic patterns were observed. First, posterolateral talar dome contusions were associated with inversion/dorsiflexion injuries. Second, bone contusions involving the posterior talus and/or medial malleolus were associated with inversion/ plantarflexion mechanisms of injury. Anterior shift of the talus was believed to cause impingement of the posterior aspect of the talus upon the medial malleolus. Third, contusions of the anteromedial talus were seen with inversion/dorsiflexion injuries, in which the talus was hypothesized to translate posteriorly, causing impingement of the anterior aspect of the talus upon the medial malleolus. Fourth, a combination of the second and third bone contusion patterns was seen with more complex mechanisms of injury.

Sijbrandij et al. (2000) reported an 18% incidence of talar and tibial bone contusions following trauma. 'Kissing' lesions were commonly identified.

11.3.3 Treatment

Conservative management is generally indicated for the initial treatment of all types of injuries. The time honored regimen of rest, immobilization, compression, and elevation/early mobilization (RICE) is initially recommended (Boruta et al. 1990; Fallat et al. 1998; Karlsson and Lansinger 1990). For grade 2 sprains, immobilization followed by early rehabilitation may be indicated. It is felt that proprioceptive exercises and peroneal strengthening aid in preventing future instability. Even most grade 3 injuries will heal with conservative therapy.

Chronic sequelae following ankle sprain injury are common. Approximately 30%–40% of patients develop chronic ankle pain (Fallat et al. 1998; Karlsson and Lansinger 1990) and 10%–20%, chronic instability (Chandnani et al. 1994). There are several hypothesized mechanisms for chronic instability (Hertel 2000; Karlsson and Lansinger 1990). First, persistently torn ligaments can result in loss of static support of the ankle. Second, injury to proprioceptors and mechanoreceptors might interfere with the reflex loop; delayed contraction of the peroneal muscles would hinder dynamic stabilization of the ankle, and ultimately create a sensation of instability. Third, there can be alteration in the length or strength of the supporting ligaments. The differential diagnosis for chronic instability/pain is described in Table 11.3.

If initial conservative therapy is unsuccessful, ligament reconstruction or repair can be performed. Ligament reconstruction initially involves recruitment of half of the peroneus brevis tendon. This segment is then re-routed through a drill hole in the lateral malleolus, its exact course and site of attachment being dependent upon the specific procedure or procedural modification employed (Fig. 11.26). Some of the more common reconstructive procedures include the Evans, modified Evans, Watson-Jones, and Chrisman-Snook operations (Shereff 1993). The aim of these surgeries is to recreate the vector forces of the injured anterior talofibular and calcaneofibular ligaments.

An alternative approach used for the treatment of chronic instability is that of delayed primary repair (Shereff 1993). The modified Brostrum procedure addresses the injured anterior talofibular and calcaneofibular ligaments directly. The remnants of these structures are divided in half, the two ends are overlapped, and then these ends are sutured together. The extensor retinaculum is mobilized and then sutured to the periosteum of the fibula for reinforcement.

11.3.4 Anterolateral Impingement Syndrome

The anterolateral gutter is a space bounded by the anterolateral aspect of the talus, anteromedial aspect of the distal fibula, and the anterolateral aspect of the distal tibia (Fig. 11.27). Anterolateral impingement syndrome (ALIS) can be defined as abnormal soft tissue within the anterolateral gutter in the presence of symptoms of entrapment. Etiologies include prior anterior talofibular ligament tear, nonspecific synovial hyperplasia, or scarring (Rubin et al. 1996). An accessory fascicle of the anterior tibiofibular ligament may also produce similar symptoms (Bassett's ligament).

ALIS presents clinically as point tenderness over the region of the anterior talofibular ligament with pain elicited on forced or passive ankle dorsiflexion. Occasionally, a click may be elicited with dorsiflexion and eversion (Rubin et al. 1996; Farooki et al. 1998). A 'meniscoid lesion' situated within the anterolateral gutter may be seen at surgery. The clinical differential diagnosis is listed in Table 11.4.

Table 11.3. Differential diagnosis for chronic pain/instability (adapted from Helgason and Chandnani 1998)

Peroneus tendon subluxation or tear
Anterior talofibular ligament injury
Osteochondritis dissecans
Avulsion fracture
Sinus tarsi syndrome
Subtalar instability
Transverse talar instability

Table 11.4. Differential diagnosis for anterolateral impingement syndrome (ALIS) (adapted from Rubin et al. 1997)

Ankle instability
Peroneal tendon tear or subluxation
Loose body
Stress fracture
Degenerative joint disease
Sinus tarsi syndrome

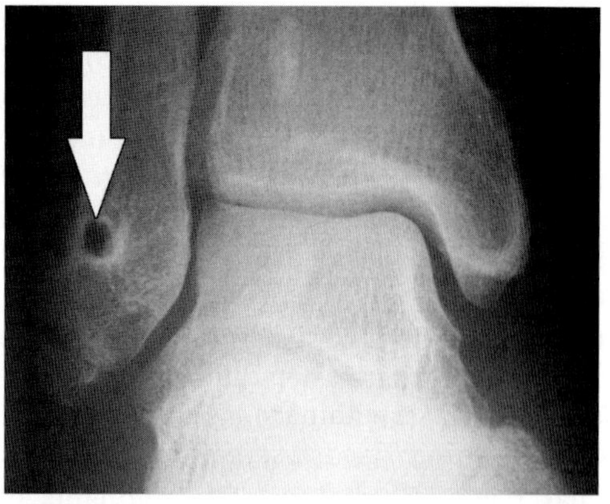

a

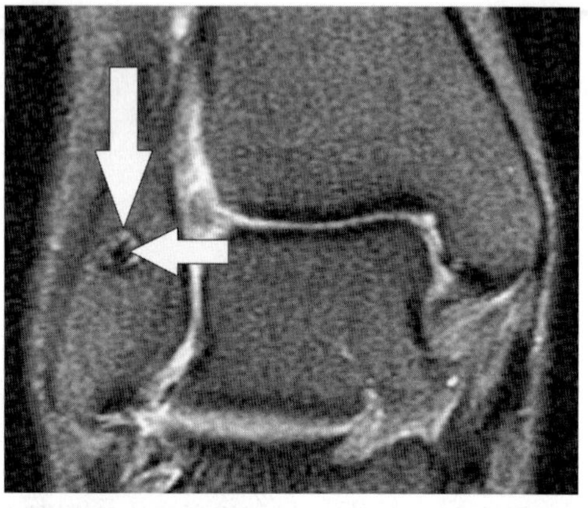

b

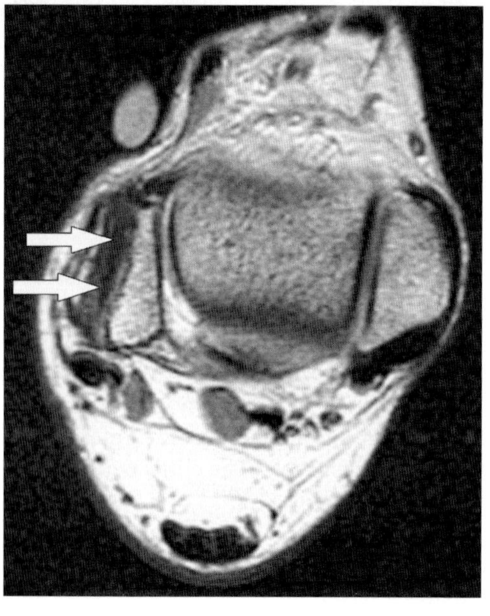

c

Fig. 11.26a–c. Ankle reconstruction. **a** Mortise view of the ankle shows a drill hole within the distal fibula (*arrow*). **b** Oblique coronal proton-density-weighted MR image of the ankle shows the drill hole within the distal fibula (*large arrow*) and the recruited segment of the peroneus brevis tendon coursing through it (*small arrow*). **c** Axial proton-density-weighted image shows the recruited portion of the peroneus brevis tendon (*arrows*) coursing through the drill hole

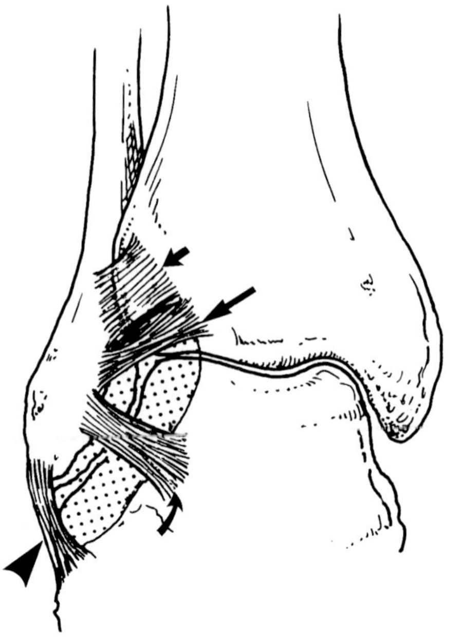

Fig. 11.27. Anterolateral gutter is represented by the *stippled pattern* in this image. Straight arrows, anterior tibiofibular ligament; curved arrow, anterior talofibular ligament; arrowhead, calcaneofibular ligament. (Reprinted with permission from MINK 1992)

FAROOKI et al. (1998) reported sensitivity, specificity, and accuracy of 42%, 85%, and 69%, respectively, for MRI in the the diagnosis of ALIS. RUBIN et al. (1996) described MR and arthroscopic findings in patients with ALIS. Arthroscopic findings included an accessory anterior inferior tibiofibular ligament (n=5), an abnormal meniscoid scar or soft-tissue collection (n=9), and synovial hyperplasia (n = 4). Radiographic imaging of the ankle occasionally demonstrated mild anterior tibial spurring. MR imaging findings included joint fluid and abnormal, relatively hypointense soft tissue in the anterolateral gutter (Fig. 11.28). Without a joint effusion, no cases of abnormal soft tissue were seen. The torn end of the anterior talofibular ligament may result in a false-positive diagnosis of ALIS. Therefore, in the presence of an intact anterior talofibular ligament, abnormal soft tissue in the anterolateral gutter suggests the diagnosis of ALIS. MR imaging can be used to confirm the diagnosis of ALIS as well as to evaluate other abnormal structures preoperatively. Patients deemed appropriate for intervention may undergo arthroscopic debridement and partial synovectomy. This procedure is 84% effective in returning patients to their baseline activity level (FERKEL et al. 1991).

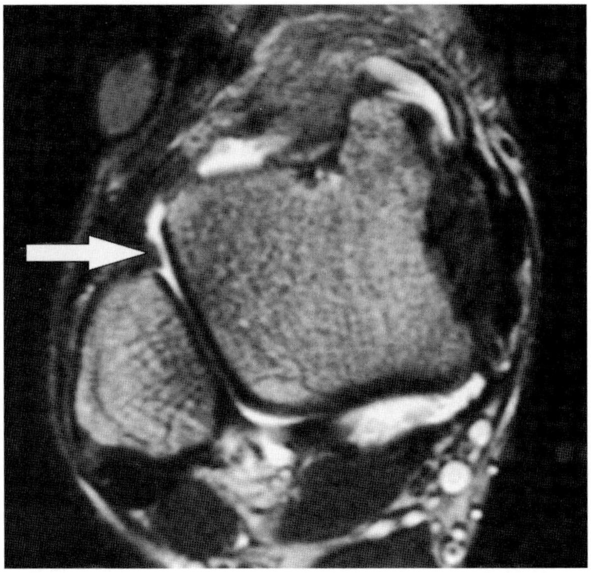

Fig. 11.28. Anterior lateral impingement. Axial T2-weighted image shows a triangular focus protruding into the anterior lateral gutter (*arrow*)

11.3.5 Syndesmotic Ligament Injury

Syndesmotic injuries occur in up to 10% of all ankle injuries and may contribute to ankle instability (Vogl et al. 1997). Two mechanisms of injury are proposed (Mink 1992; Timins 2000). First, lateral rotation of the talus with the axis of rotation around the posterior tibiofibular ligament can produce a proximal fibular fracture above the level of the ankle mortise. Tension upon the anterior tibiofibular ligament and interosseous ligament may result in tears of these structures or in a posterior malleolar fracture. Alternatively, medial malleolar fractures or deltoid ligament ruptures may occur. Second, an eversion stress will cause the talus to abduct against the fibula, which can result in a fibular fracture above the level of the tibial plafond, either with a Dupuytren fracture or a Maisonneuve fracture (Vogl et al. 1997). Syndesmotic ligament complex rupture and medial ligamentous/osseous injury are commonly present.

High fibular fractures as well as posterior tibial fractures can be identified radiographically. Routine or stress radiography may be required to evaluate the distal tibiofibular relationship. Routine MR imaging or MR arthrography can be used to diagnose syndesmotic complex injury; the latter uses the finding of contrast extravasation cephalad to the level of the syndesmotic recess as a diagnostic sign (Resnick 1988).

Findings of MR imaging related to syndesmotic complex injury have been reported by Vogl et al. (1997) (Fig. 11.29). In that study, ankle injuries were classified as sprains, incomplete tears, or ruptures (Table 11.5). Treatment was primarily conservative. Surgical repair was indicated with findings of tibiofibular diastasis and mortise widening, fibular shortening, or a displaced medial malleolar fracture. Treatment consisted of internal fixation of the distal tibia to the fibula. With high ankle sprains, abnormal soft tissue may be visualized within the interosseous space. Ossification can be identified in severe, chronic cases.

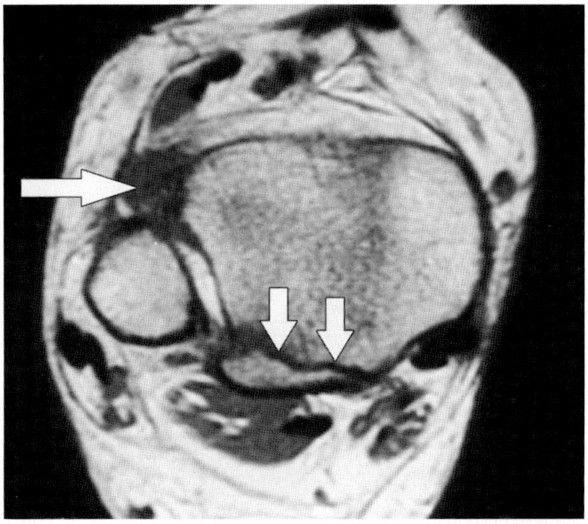

Fig. 11.29. Syndesmotic ligament injury. Axial proton-density-weighted image shows a tear of the anterior tibiofibular ligament (*large arrow*) as well as a posterior tibial avulsive fracture, related to the insertion of the posterior tibiofibular ligament (*small arrows*)

Table 11.5. Classification of syndesmotic ligament injuries

Sprain	Incomplete tear	Rupture
Normal shape and contour	Tibiofibular joint diastasis	Prolapse of fat (20%) or joint fluid (20%)
	Ligament nonvisualization (20%)	
Increased internal signal (enhancement)[a]	Wavy, irregular contour	
	Increased signal on T2-weighted (47%) and T1-weighted (60%) images (enhancement 100%)[a]	

Adapted from Vogl et al. 1997. [a]Enhancement indicates finding seen only on enhanced T1-weighted fat-saturated images. Percentages in parentheses indicate frequency of findings

11.3.6 Medial Collateral Ligament Injuries

Normally, the medial collateral ligament (MCL) functions as a primary restraint against internal rotation and eversion stress in the unloaded ankle (Boruta et al. 1990). Due to its inherent strength, avulsion fractures of the medial malleolus are significantly more common than injury to the ligament. Although isolated MCL injuries can occur with pure eversion stress, they are more commonly associated with lateral collateral ligament or syndesmotic injuries (Timins 2000).

Clinical findings suggesting MCL injury include swelling, ecchymosis, and point tenderness just below the medial malleolus. Radiography aids in the diagnosis of medial malleolar fracture. MR findings include loss of striations with homogenous intermediate signal intensity within the deep portion, discontinuity of either the deep or superficial component, or reactive fluid within the posterior tibial tendon sheath (Figs. 11.30, 11.31) (Rosenberg et al. 2000).

11.3.7 Spring Ligament Injury

The spring ligament is one of the key static stabilizers of the longitudinal arch. Injury to this structure may result in pes planovalgus. Yao et al. (1999) reported 54%–77% sensitivity and 100% specificity for MR imaging in the diagnosis of spring ligament injury.

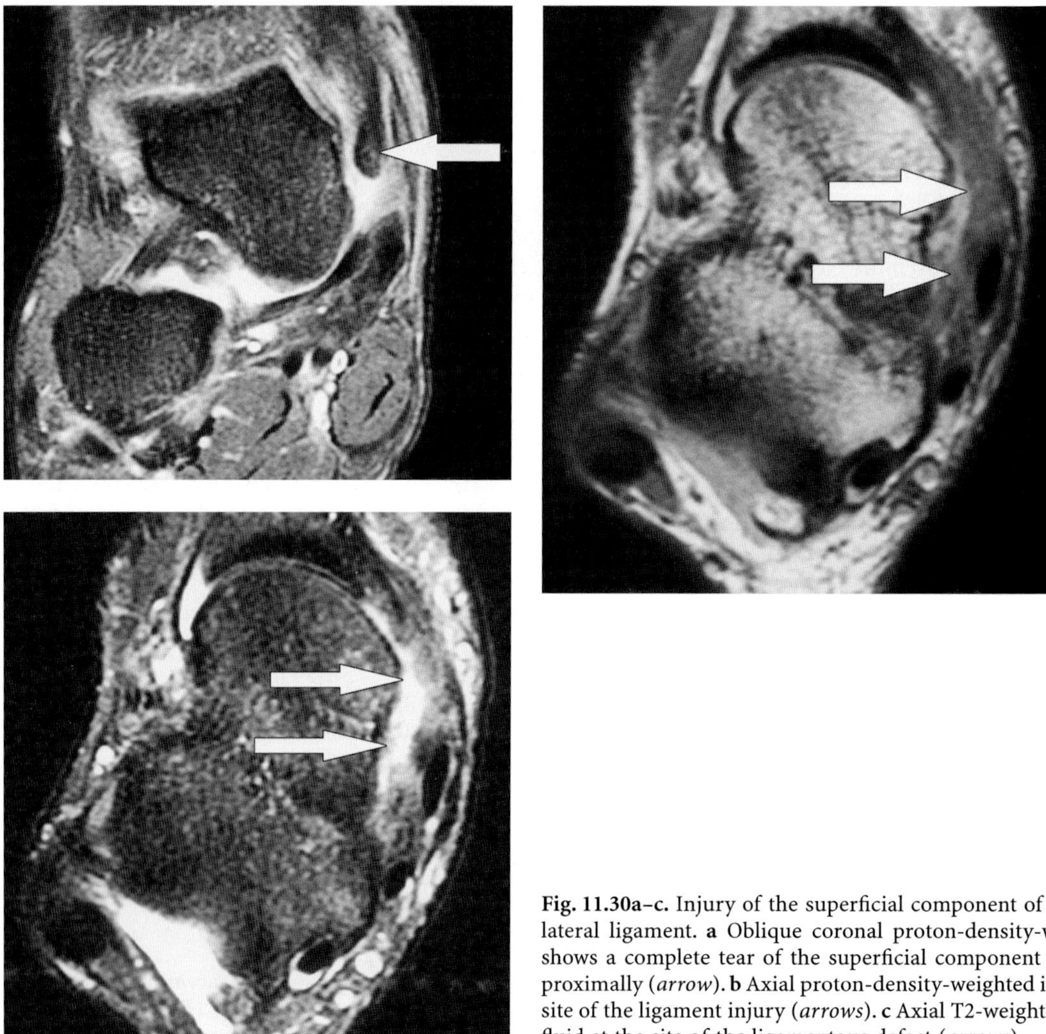

a b c

Fig. 11.30a–c. Injury of the superficial component of the medial collateral ligament. **a** Oblique coronal proton-density-weighted image shows a complete tear of the superficial component with retraction proximally (*arrow*). **b** Axial proton-density-weighted image shows the site of the ligament injury (*arrows*). **c** Axial T2-weighted image shows fluid at the site of the ligamentous defect (*arrows*)

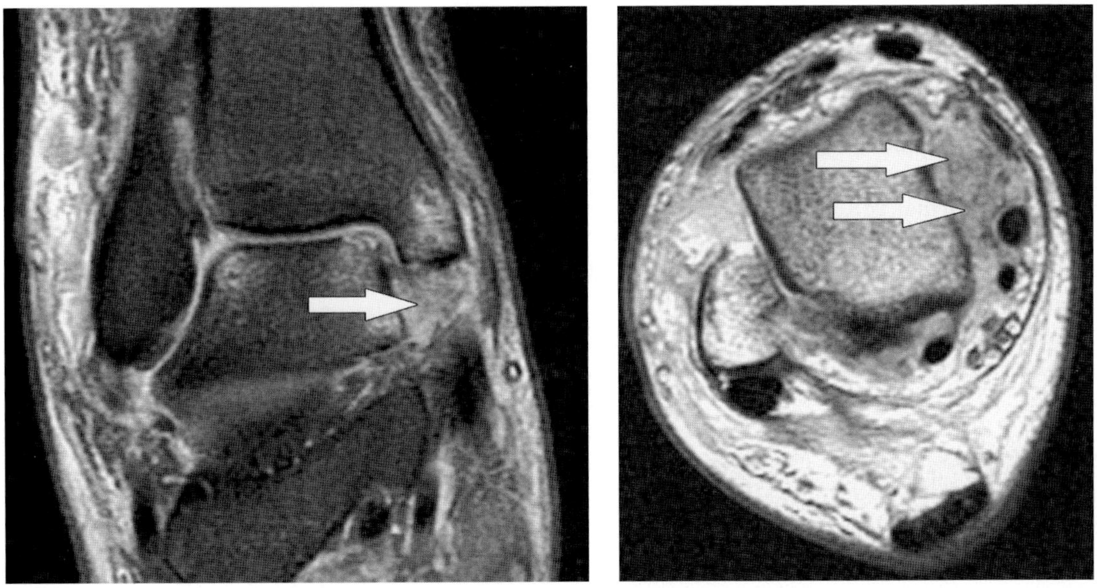

a b

Fig. 11.31a,b. Injury of the deep component of the medial collateral ligament. **a** Oblique coronal proton-density-weighted image with fat suppression shows a tear of the deep component (*arrow*). Note multiple bone contusions. **b** Axial proton-density-weighted image shows markedly distorted architecture in the expected location of the posterior constituent of the deep component of the medial collateral ligament (*arrows*)

11.3.8 Subtalar Ligament Injury

The ligaments of the sinus tarsi are injured in a significant proportion of ankle sprains. A study by TOCHIGI et al. (1998) described the relative importance of ligament injury in the spectrum of ankle sprains. These investigators provided a prospective analysis of 24 patients with acute ankle sprains, all of whom underwent MR imaging. Attention was paid to the lateral collateral ligament and subtalar complex. Tears were correlated with outcome on clinical follow-up. Thirteen of 24 patients demonstrated injuries of the interosseous talocalcaneal ligament. The presence of interosseous talocalcaneal ligament injury correlated with a poor clinical outcome. Injury to the cervical ligament was seen in 10 of 24 patients and was also associated with a poor clinical outcome. In contrast, lateral collateral ligament injury did not have a significant association with a poor clinical outcome.

11.4 Sinus Tarsi Syndrome

The term sinus tarsi syndrome was originally coined by O'CONNOR in 1958 to describe the association between ankle sprain and lateral tarsal sinus tenderness. Patients present with lateral foot pain and focal tenderness over the tarsal sinus. Some 70% of patients give a history of prior inversion trauma. The remainder of cases are attributed to inflammatory conditions, cysts, and foot deformities. The diagnosis is confirmed when pain relief is noted following anesthetic injection of the tarsal sinus. Pathologic analysis of surgical specimens obtained from patients with sinus tarsi syndrome demonstrates any or all of the following: fibrosis, nonspecific inflammatory changes, chronic synovitis, synovial cysts. KLEIN and SPREITZER (1993) studied 33 patients with symptoms of sinus tarsi syndrome with MR imaging (Table 11.6).

Twenty-six of the 33 patients were noted to have lateral collateral ligament injury. In 11 of 33 patients, low signal intensity on T1-weighted images and increased signal intensity on T2-weighted images

Table 11.6. Findings defining an abnormal tarsal sinus (adapted from KLEIN and SPREITZER 1993)

Decreased signal intensity on T1-weighted images
Increased or decreased signal intensity on T2-weighted images
Thickened or wavy ligaments
Abnormal fluid collection

were observed in the tarsal sinus (Figs. 11.32, 11.33). This was believed to indicate nonspecific inflammation or synovitis. In 17 of 33 patients, decreased signal intensity, most likely attributable to fibrosis, was observed on both T1- and T2-weighted images. Abnormal fluid collections were seen in 5 of 33 cases. No patients with a normal MR appearance of the tarsal sinus had sinus tarsi syndrome, suggesting that a normal tarsal sinus on MR imaging effectively excludes the diagnosis. There is evidence that a limited number of patients with sinus tarsi syndrome respond to conservative measures (Kuwada 1994).

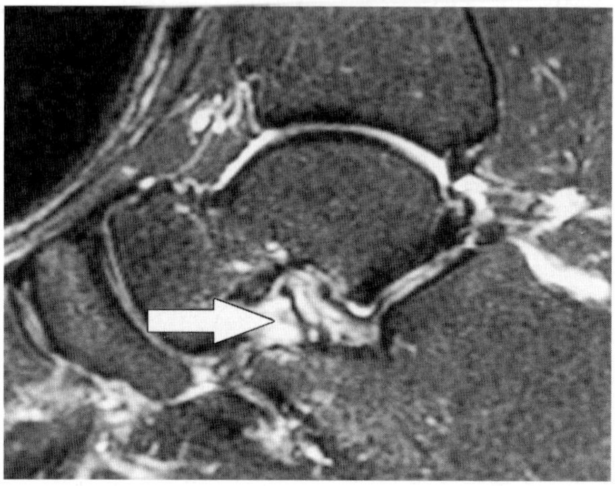

Fig. 11.32. Sinus tarsi pathology. Sagittal T2-weighted image with fat suppression shows increased signal intensity within the sinus tarsi, adjacent to the sinus tarsi (subtalar) ligaments (*arrow*)

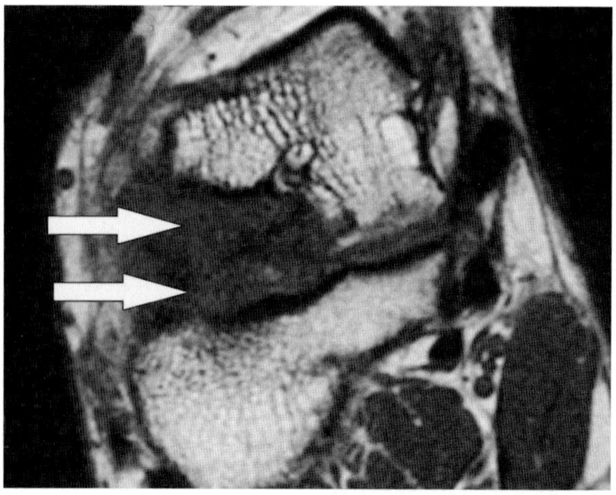

Fig. 11.33. Sinus tarsi injury. Oblique coronal T1-weighted image shows amorphous, hypointense soft tissue within the sinus tarsi (*arrows*). Normally, this region contains predominantly fat, as well as vascular and ligamentous structures

This investigator used injection of the tarsal sinus, rehabilitation, and placement of foot orthotics in his conservative treatment regimen. Surgical debridement, he found, was successful in 66 of 88 patients. There were no associated significant complications.

11.4.1 Lisfranc Injuries

Most Lisfranc fracture-dislocations occur as a result of plantarflexion with focal pronation or supination (Vuori and Aro 1993) (Table 11.7). Traumatic forces tend to be distributed around the second metatarsal, which acts as the fulcrum for rotational injury.

Lisfranc injuries can be characterized as homolateral, partial, and divergent. Homolateral trauma involves lateral fracture-dislocations at all tarsal-metatarsal joints. Partial injury implies that not all rays are involved. With divergent Lisfranc injuries, the more lateral rays are dislocated or displaced laterally, and the more medial rays are displaced medially. Some 30% of Lisfranc injuries are associated with additional midfoot injuries, commonly other metatarsal fractures or cuboid fractures. Most of these additional injuries occur in the setting of high-energy trauma.

Radiographs are the first-line diagnostic imaging study and are often sufficient for the diagnosis. CT is ideal for demonstrating small chip fractures that could be missed radiographically. Using the benefits of multiplanar reformations, subtle dorsal and plantar subluxations may become more obvious. CT has been recommended as a routine work-up for patients with significant hyperflexion injury to the foot (Preidler et al. 1999). A prospective study of 49 patients sustaining hyperflexion foot injuries was performed comparing radiographs, CT, and MR imaging. Radiographs of the foot were obtained in three planes with weight bearing. CT was performed with 2–3-mm-thick slices parallel to the dorsum of the foot. MR imaging sequences utilized triplanar spin-echo T1-weighted, fast spin-echo T2-weighted, and inversion recovery sequences with 2–3 mm slices (Table 11.8).

Table 11.7. Mechanism of injury for Lisfranc fracture-dislocations (adapted from Vuori and Aro 1993)

Low energy trauma (32%)
Fall from a height (14%)
Crush (21%)
Motor vehicle collision (33%)

Table 11.8. Comparison of imaging modalities in the detection of Lisfranc fracture-dislocations

Imaging modality	Metatarsal fractures detected	Tarsal fractures detected	Tarsometatarsal dislocations	Other
Radiography	33	20	8	
CT	53	41	16	
MRI	41 & 18 MT bone bruises	39 with 9 tarsal bone bruises	16	11 Lisfranc's ligament disruptions

(adapted from Preidler et al. 1999)

With the addition of an additional imaging modality – CT or MR imaging – significantly more treatable injuries were detected. Comparing CT to MRI, CT detected a greater number of fractures, while MRI was able to detect bone contusions and other soft-tissue injuries. Cross-sectional imaging modalities were equivalent in identifying tarsal-metatarsal malalignment.

The added benefit of MR was statistically evaluated in a paper by Preidler et al. (1996). These investigators concluded that while MR imaging reliably demonstrated ligaments of the Lisfranc joint, there was no detectable added benefit to the patient in terms of clinical management and long-term outcome.

References

Bassett FH III, Gates HS III, Billys JB, Morris HB, Nikolaou PK (1990) Talar impingement by the anteroinferior tibiofibular ligament. J Bone Joint Surg 72A:55–59

Black H, Brand R, Eichelberger M (1978) An improved technique for evaluation of ligamentous injury in severe ankle sprains. Am J Sports Med 6:276–282

Boruta PM, Bishop JO, Braly G, Tullos HS (1990) Acute lateral ankle ligament injuries: a literature review. Foot Ankle 11: 107–113

Breitenseher MJ, Trattnig S, Kukla C, Gaebler C, Kaider A, Baldt MM, Haller J, Imhof H (1997) MRI versus lateral stress radiography in acute lateral ankle ligament injuries. J Comput Assist Tomogr 21:280–285

Cardone BW, Erickson SJ, Hartog BDD, Carrera GF (1993) MRI of injury to the lateral collateral ligamentous complex of the ankle. J Comput Assist Tomogr 17:102–107

Cass JR, Morray BF (1984) Ankle instability: current concepts, diagnosis and treatment. Mayo Clin Proc 59:165–170

Chandnani VP, Harper MT, Ficke JR, Gagliardi JA, Rolling L, Christensen KP, Hansen MF (1994) Chronic ankle instability: evaluation with MR arthrography, MR imaging and stress radiography. Radiology 192:189–194

Davis WH, Sobel M, DiCarlo EF, Torzilli PA, Deng X, Geppert MJ, Patel MB, Deland J (1996) Gross, histological, and microvascular anatomy and biomechanical testing of the spring ligament complex. Foot Ankle Int 17:95–102

Erickson SJ, Johnson JE (1997) MR imaging of the ankle and foot. Radiol Clin North Am 35:163–192

Erickson SJ, Smith JW, Ruiz ME, Fitzgerald SW, Kneeland JB, Johnson JE, Shereff MJ, Carrera GF (1991) MR imaging of the lateral collateral ligament of the ankle. AJR 156: 131–136

Fallat L, Grimm DJ, Saracco JA (1998) Sprained ankle syndrome: prevalence and analysis of 639 acute injuries. J Foot Ankle Surg 37:280–285

Farooki S, Yao L, Seeger LL (1998) Anterolateral impingement of the ankle: effectiveness of MR imaging. Radiology 207: 357–360

Ferkel RD, Karzel RP, Del Pizzo W, Friedman MJ, Fischer SP (1991) Arthroscopic treatment of anterolateral impingement of the ankle. Am J Sports Med 19:440–446

Helgason JW, Chandnani VP (1998) MR arthrography of the ankle. Radiol Clin North Am 36:729–738

Hertel G (2000) Functional instability following lateral ankle sprain. Sports Med 29:361–371

Kannus P, Renstrom P (1991) Treatment for acute tears of the lateral ligaments of the ankle. J Bone Joint Surg [Am] 73: 305–312

Kammus P, Renstrom P (1991) Tratment for acute tears of the lateral ligaments of the ankle. J Bone Joint Surg [Am] 73: 305–312

Karlsson J, Lansinger O (1990) Lateral instability of the ankle joint. Clin Orthop Relat Res 276:253–261

Klein MA, Spreitzer AM (1993) MR imaging of the tarsal sinus and canal: normal anatomy, pathologic findings, and features of the sinus tarsi syndrome. Radiology 186:233–240

Kreitner K-F, Ferber A, Grebe P, Runkel M, Berger S, Thelen M (1999) Injuries of the lateral collateral ligaments of the ankle: assessment with MR imaging. Eur Radiol 9:519–524

Kuwada GT (1994) Long-term retrospective analysis of the treatment of sinus tarsi syndrome. J Foot Ank Surg 33: 28–29

Lektrakul N, Chung CB, Yeon-man L et al (2001) Tarsal sinus: arthrographic, MR imaging, MR arthrographic, and pathologicalfindings in cadavers and retrospective study data in patients with sinus tarsi syndrome. Radiology 219: 802–810

Milz P, Milz S, Putz R et al (1996) 13 mHz high-frequency sonography of the lateral ankle joint ligaments and the tibiofibular syndesmosis in anatomic specimens. J Ultrasound Med 15:227–284

Mink JH (1992) Ligaments of the ankle. In: Deutsch AL, Mink JH, Kerr R (eds) MRI of the foot and ankle. Raven, New York, pp 173–197

Muhle C, Frank LR, Rand T, Yeh L-R, Wong EC, Skaf A, Dantas

RWM, Haghighi P, Trudell D, Resnick D (1999) Collateral ligaments of the ankle: high-resolution MR imaging with a local gradient coil and anatomic correlation in cadavers. Radiographics 19:673–683

Nishimura G, Yamato M, Togawa M (1996) Trabecular trauma of the talus and medial malleolus concurrent with lateral collateral ligamentous injuries of the ankle: evaluation with MR imaging. Skeletal Radiol 25:49–54

O'Conner D (1958) Sinus tarsi syndrome: a clinical entity. J Bone Joint Surg 40:720–726

Oloff LM, Sullivan BT, Heard GS, Thornton MC (1992) Magnetic resonance imaging of traumatized ligaments of the ankle. J Am Pod Med Assoc 82:25–32

Preidler KW, Wang Y-C, Brossmann J, Trudell D, Daenen B, Resnick D (1996) Tarsometatarsal Joint: anatomic details on MR images. Radiology 199:733–736

Preidler KW, Peicha G, Lajtai G, Seibert FJ, Fock C, Szolar DM, Raith H (1999) Conventional radiography, CT and MR imaging in patients with hyperflexion injuries of the foot: diagnostic accuracy in the detection of bony and ligamentous changes. AJR 173:1673–1677

Resnick D (1988) Arthrography, tenography and bursography. In: Resnick D, Niwayama G (eds) Diagnosis of bone an joint disorders. Saunders, Philadelphia

Rosenberg ZS, Cheung YY, Beltran J et al (1995) Posterior intermalleolar ligament of the ankle: normal anatomy and MR imaging features. AJR 165:387–390

Rosenberg ZS, Beltran J, Bencardino JT (2000) MR imaging of the ankle and foot. Radiographics 20:S153–S179

Rubin DA, Tishkoff NW, Britton CA, Conti SF, Towers JD (1997) Anterolateral soft-tissue impingement in the ankle: diagnosis using MR imaging. AJR 169:829–835

Rule J, Yao L, Seeger LL (1993) Spring ligament of the ankle: normal MR anatomy. AJR 161:1241–1244

Ruth CJ (1961) The surgical treatment of injuries of the fibular collateral ligaments of the ankle. J Bone Joint Surg [Am] 43:229

Sarrafian S (1993) Anatomy of the foot and ankle, 2nd edn. Lippincott, Philadelphia

Sauser DD, Nelson RC, Lavine MH, Wu CW (1983) Acute injuries of the lateral ligaments of the ankle: comparison of stress radiography and arthrography. Radiology 148:653–657

Schneck CD, Mesgarzadeh M, Bonakdarpour A, Ross GJ (1992) MR imaging of the most commonly injured ankle ligaments, part I. Normal anatomy. Radiology 184:499–506

Shereff MJ (1993) Atlas of foot and ankle surgery. Saunders, Philadelphia

Sijbrandij ES, van Gils APG, Louwerens JWK, de Lange EE (2000) Post-traumatic subchondral bone contusions and fractures of talotibial joint: occurrence of "kissing" lesions. AJR 175:1701–1710

Timins ME (2000) MR imaging of the foot and ankle. Foot Ankle Clin 5:83–101

Tochigi Y, Yoshinaga K, Wada Y, Moriya H (1998) Acute inversion injury of the ankle: magnetic resonance imaging and clinical outcomes. Foot Ankle Int 19:730–734

Verhaven EFC, Shahabpour M, Handelberg FWJ, Vaes PHEG, Opdecam PJE (1991) The accuracy of three-dimensional magnetic resonance imaging in the diagnosis of ruptures of the lateral ligaments of the ankle. Am J Sport Med 19: 583–587

Vogl TJ, Hochmuth K, Diebold T, Lubrich J, Hofmann R, Stockle U, Sollner O, Bisson S, Sudkamp N, Maeurer J, Haas N, Felix R (1997) Magnetic resonance imaging in the diagnosis of acute injured distal tibiofibular syndesmosis. Invest Radiol 32:401–409

Vuori J-P, Aro HT (1993) Lisfranc joint injuries: trauma mechanisms and associated injuries. J Trauma 35:40–45

Yao L, Gentili A, Cracchiolo A (1999) MR imaging findings in spring ligament insufficiency. Skel Radiol 28:245–250

12 Compressive Neuropathies and Plantar Fascial Lesions

J. S. Yu

CONTENTS

Heel pain is a common complaint, and there are a number of pathologic processes that can produce this symptom. The multitude of disorders that can present with heel pain is compounded by the difficulty in differentiating these conditions clinically. As such, MR imaging has become virtually indispensable for the making of a diagnosis. Disorders that cause compression of the nerves are often difficult to diagnose noninvasively, and two important conditions in this respect that will be discussed in detail in this chapter are tarsal tunnel syndrome and sinus tarsi syndrome. One of the most recognizable causes of heel pain is plantar fasciitis. Yet there are a number of other disorders that affect the plantar fascia that may elicit similar symptoms. These entities include acute plantar fasciitis, chronic plantar fasciitis, traumatic rupture, fibromatosis, normal postsurgical changes, and pathologic postfasciotomy conditions.

J. S. Yu, MD
Associate Professor of Radiology, Chief, Musculoskeletal Division, Department of Radiology, S-255 Rhodes Hall, 450W. 10th Ave., Columbus, Ohio 43210, USA

12.1 Compressive Neuropathies

12.1.1 Sinus Tarsi Syndrome

The sinus tarsi describes a funnel-shaped space between the talus and calcaneus, its narrow opening located just posterior to the middle subtalar joint and its wider lateral opening seen just superior to the anterior calcaneal process. The artery of the tarsal canal, end nerves, ligaments (interosseous and cervical), and the medial fibers of the inferior extensor retinaculum are found within this space. The ligaments of the sinus tarsi contribute to hindfoot stabilization. In a recent investigation, it was suggested that the sinus tarsi may function also as a source of nociceptive and proprioceptive information on the movement of the foot and ankle (Akiyama et al. 1999).

The sinus tarsi syndrome describes a painful condition characterized by pain over the lateral aspect of the hindfoot, often accompanied by a sensation of instability and weakness (Beltran 1994; Brown 1960; O'Conner 1958; Steinbach 1998; Taillard et al. 1981). Pain relief with injection of a local anesthetic agent into the sinus tarsi is diagnostic of the syndrome. In nearly 75% of cases, this syndrome is caused by disruption of the interosseous and/or cervical ligament(s) acquired during an inversion injury. Nearly one-half of cases are associated with tears of the lateral ligaments of the ankle (Breitenseher et al. 1997). The injury can lead to the development of hyperplastic synovial and fibrous tissue, which then becomes a space-occupying process in the tarsal sinus (Frey et al. 1999). On MR images, the condition has a characteristic appearance. The interosseous and cervical ligaments are best depicted on coronal and sagittal images. When the interosseous ligament tears, the formation of scar tissue and gross hyalinization of the torn ligament ends occur, with subsequent impingement of the anterior aspect of the posterior subtalar joint by the hyperplastic tissue (Frey et al. 1999) (Fig. 12.1). Poor definition of the ligaments, edema in the

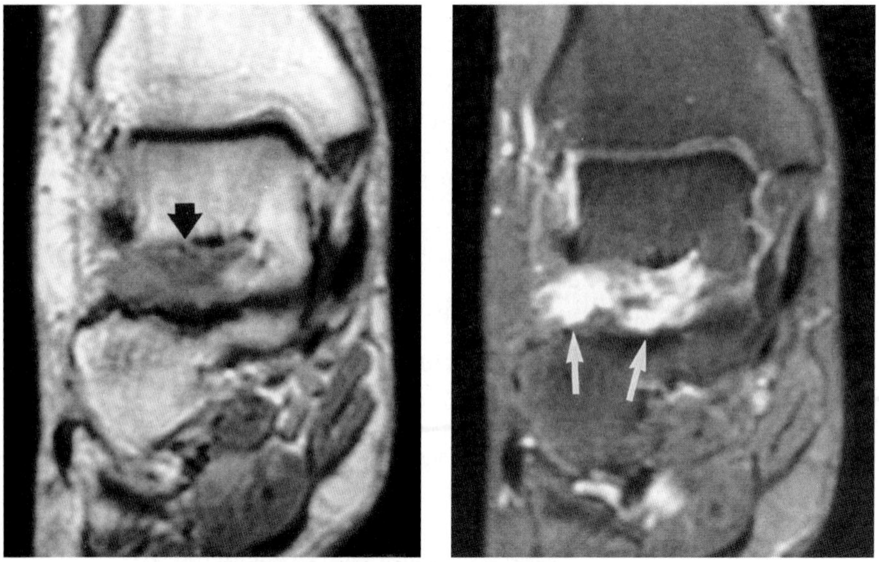

a b

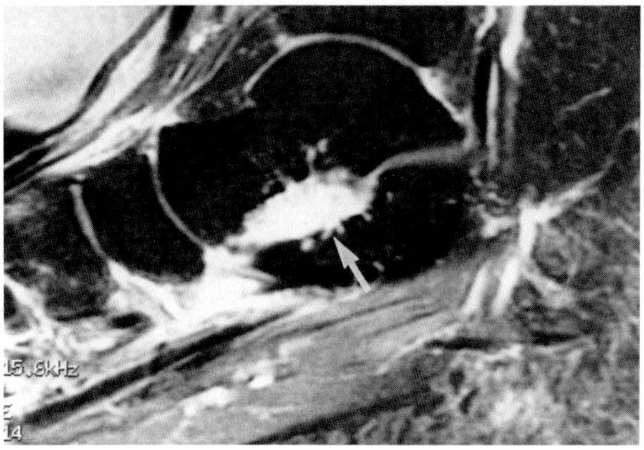

c

Fig. 12.1a–c. Post-traumatic sinus tarsi syndrome. Coronal proton-density-weighted image (**a**) shows disrupted interosseous and cervical ligaments in the sinus tarsi (*arrow*). Coronal (**b**) and sagittal (**c**) fat-saturated T1-weighted images show marked enhancement of hyperplastic synovial tissue (*arrows*) that now resides in this space

soft tissues in the sinus tarsi, and marked enhancement of hypertrophic tissue after administration of intravenous gadolinium are typical findings. Replacement of the fat tissue in the sinus tarsi is a useful observation (Breitenseher et al. 1997). If the posterior subtalar joint is injected with contrast material, one would expect to see extravasation of contrast into the sinus tarsi if the interosseous ligament is disrupted.

Other conditions can cause sinus tarsi syndrome, however, and these include synovial inflammatory diseases such as rheumatoid arthritis and gout, peroneal nerve entrapment, ganglion cysts (Fig. 12.2), tumors, and osteoarthritis (Frey et al. 1999).

12.1.2 Tarsal Tunnel Syndrome

The tarsal tunnel refers to a space in the foot that contains the medial tendons of the ankle, posterior tibial nerve, and medial vascular structures. The tarsal tunnel is a continuation of the deep posterior compartment of the leg and extends from the level of the medial malleolus to the tarsal navicular. The floor of this fibro-osseous space is comprised of the tibia, medial talar surface, sustentaculum tali, and medial calcaneal wall (Lau and Daniels 1999). Its roof is formed by the laciniate ligament of the flexor retinaculum, which is a continuation of the superficial and deep fascia of the lower extremity (Havel et al. 1988; Lau and Daniels 1999). The origin of the laciniate ligament is on the medial malleolus, and its insertion occurs posteriorly and inferiorly to the calcaneal tuberosity (Dellon and Mackinnon 1984). The base of the flexor retinaculum corresponds to the superior border of the abductor hallucis muscle (Sarrafian 1993). The tendons of the posterior tibial, flexor digitorum longus, and flexor hallucis longus muscles reside within the tarsal tunnel and are separated from the neurovascular bundle by

a b

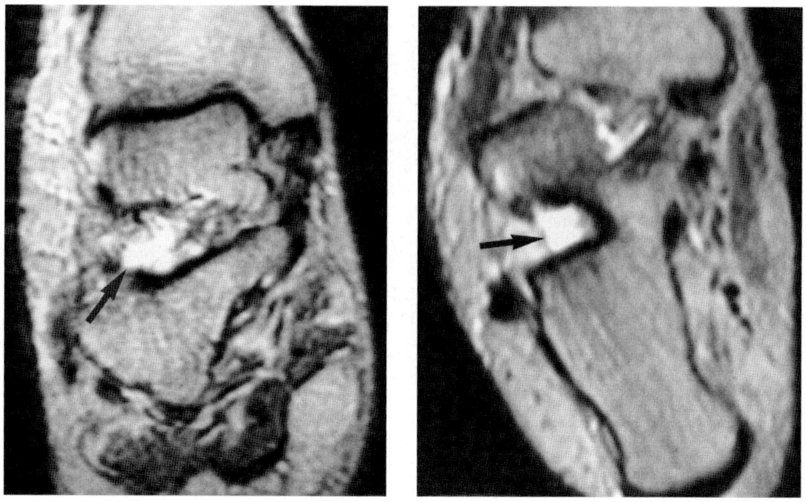

Fig. 12.2a,b. Sinus tarsi syndrome caused by a ganglion. Coronal (**a**) and transaxial T2-weighted (**b**) images show a fluid-filled structure in the sinus tarsi (*arrow*). Surgery revealed a ganglion

fibrous septations. The septae are attached to the neurovascular bundle by a layer of dense areolar tissue, causing it to be relatively immobile.

The posterior tibial nerve, accompanied by an artery and vein, trifurcates into the medial calcaneal, medial plantar,and lateral plantar nerves. The location at which the nerve divides is variable (DELLON and MACKINNON 1984; HAVEL et al. 1988; SARRAFIAN 1993). In the majority of feet, the tibial nerve bifurcates into the medial and lateral plantar nerves within the tarsal tunnel, and these nerves are separated by the transverse interfascicular septum (HEIMKES et al. 1987). These terminal branches innervate the intrinsic muscles and skin of the sole of the foot. The medial plantar nerve supplies the muscles of the great toe and is sensory to the medial three and one-half digits, resembling the distribution of the median nerve of the hand. The lateral plantar nerve supplies the remaining muscles of the sole of the foot and is sensory to the lateral one and one-half digits, resembling the distribution of the ulnar nerve of the hand (SARRAFIAN 1993).

Tarsal tunnel syndrome refers to an entrapment neuropathy of the posterior tibial nerve or one of its branches. Pain, paresthesia, sensory deficits, and weakness are characteristic symptoms of this syndrome (O'MALLEY et al. 1985). Patients often complain of a burning sensation along the plantar surface of the foot that is exacerbated by long periods of weight-bearing. The pain may radiate proximally in 33% of patients, along the medial aspect of the leg, a finding that is referred to as the Valleix phenomenon (KECK 1962). Percussion of the tibial nerve behind the medial malleolus may elicit similar symptoms (BABA et al. 1997; BAILIE and KELIKIAN 1998). MR imaging is the single best method for diagnosing this condition since this technique allows unimpeded visualization of the tarsal tunnel and its contents (ZEISS et al. 1990). It is extremely sensitive to changes related to the contents of the tarsal tunnel, the flexor retinaculum, and the tibial nerve (KERR and FREY 1991). The cause of tarsal tunnel syndrome can be identified in 60%–80% of patients. Common causes include trauma, space-occupying lesions (Fig. 12.3), and congenital abnormalities.

Displaced fractures of the distal tibia, talus, or calcaneus may elicit the syndrome (CIMINO 1990; STEFKO et al. 1994), as well as ankle sprains involving the deltoid ligament (LAU and DANIELS 1999). Posttraumatic synovitis of the posterior tibialis, flexor digitorum longus, or flexor hallucis longus may also compress the contents of the tarsal tunnel (JACKSON and HAGLUND 1992; SCHON 1994). Many different space-occupying lesions have been reported as an etiology of tarsal tunnel syndrome, including ganglia, lipoma, neurilemmoma, hypertrophic flexor retinaculum, hypertrophic abductor hallucis muscle, accessory flexor digitorum longus muscle (Fig. 12.4), and varicosities (Fig. 12.5) (BIENEMAN and SUNDARAM 2000; CHEUNG et al. 1999; CIMINO 1990; JANECKI and DOVBERG 1977; KENZORA et al. 1982; O'MALLEY et al. 1985; NAGAOKA and SATOU 1999; SAMMARCO and STEPHENS 1990). Certain congenital conditions may predispose a person to tarsal tunnel syndrome. When there is a varus deformity of the heel, compensatory forefoot pronation effectively shortens the abductor hallucis muscle, decreasing the cross-sectional area of the tarsal tunnel and stretching the plantar nerve (LAU and DANIELS 1999; RADIN 1983). When there is a valgus heel, abduction of the forefoot in a pes planus deformity can increase tension on the tibial nerve (DANIELS et al. 1998).

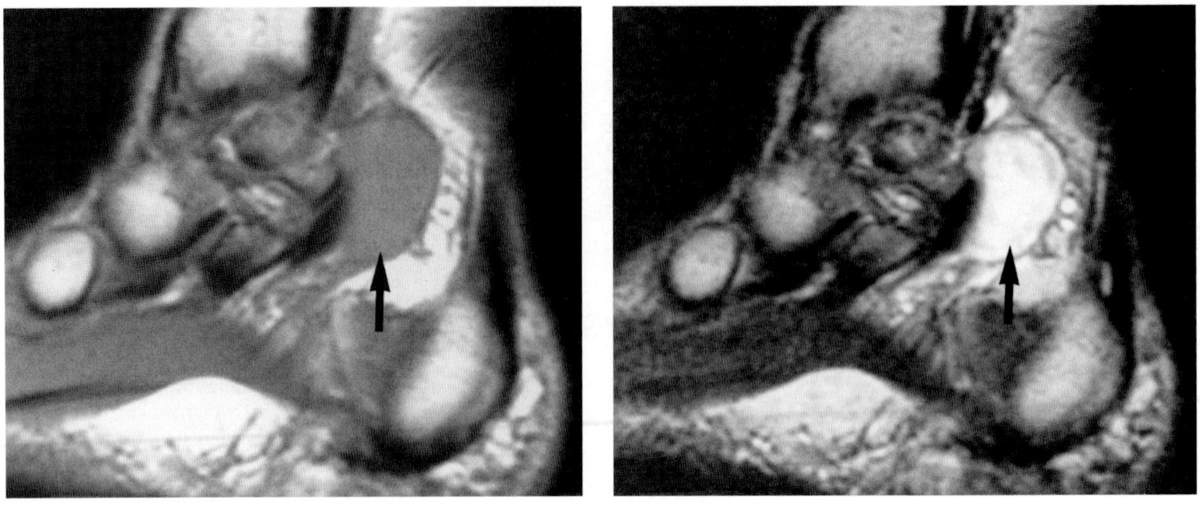

Fig. 12.3a,b. Tarsal tunnel syndrome caused by a tumor. Sagittal proton-density (**a**) and T2-weighted (**b**) images show a large fusiform mass within the tarsal tunnel just posterior to the flexor hallucis longus tendon (*arrow*) that proved to be a neurofibroma at surgery

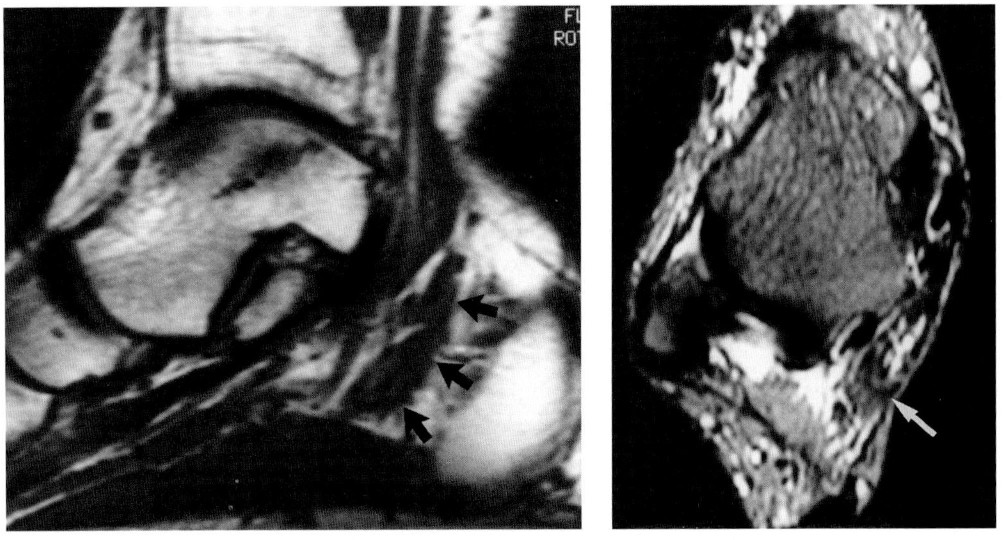

Fig. 12.4a,b. Tarsal tunnel syndrome caused by an anomalous muscle. **a** Sagittal T1-weighted image shows a tubular soft-tissue mass (*arrows*) posterior to the flexor hallucis longus muscle, which is typical of the accessory flexor digitorum longus muscle. **b** Transaxial T2-weighted image shows how much space this anomalous muscle (*arrow*) occupied in this patient

Decompression of the flexor retinaculum or resection of the causative lesion is the most optimal treatment. Common causes of failed tarsal tunnel decompression include epineural fibrosis of the tibial nerve, inadequate tarsal tunnel release, chronic disease, and a double crush syndrome (Cimino 1990; Dos Remedios and Jolly 2000; Skalley et al. 1994; Upton and McComas 1973; Zeiss et al. 1991). A double crush syndrome refers to a situation in which an entrapped nerve is associated with a second nerve lesion located more proximally owing to mechanical compression, mechanical tension, or a diffuse axonal abnormality (Upton and McComas 1973).

12.2 Plantar Fascia Disorders

The plantar fascia, composed of both collagen and elastic fibers, contributes to the support of the longitudinal arch of the foot along with the midfoot

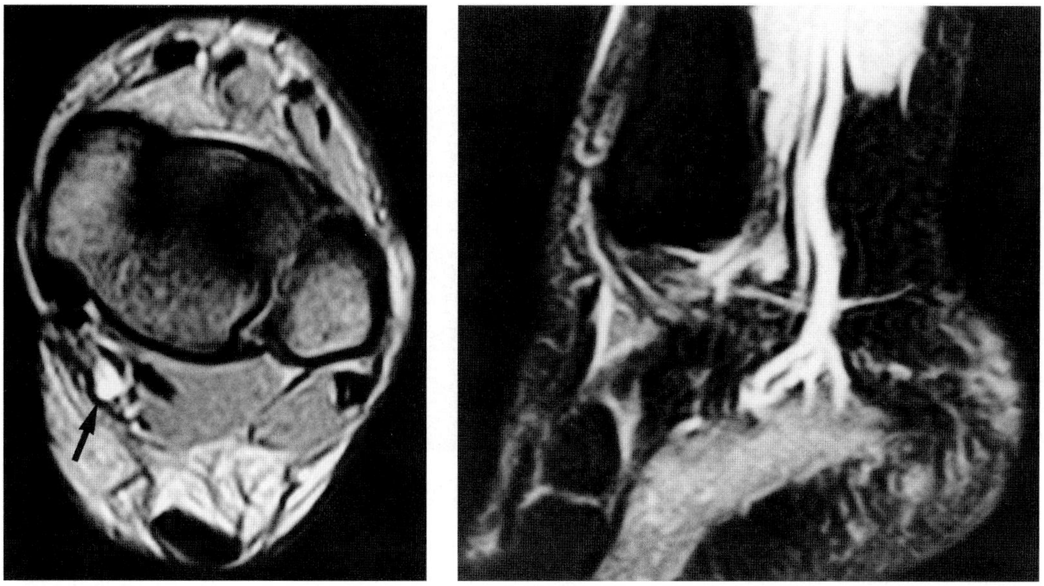

a b

Fig. 12.5a,b. Tarsal tunnel syndrome caused by varicosities. Transaxial (**a**) and sagittal (**b**) T2-weighted images show prominent varicosities (*arrow* in **a**) in the tarsal tunnel. Varicosities are a relatively common cause of tarsal tunnel syndrome

ligaments and the intrinsic and extrinsic muscles of the foot (Bojsen-Mller and Fagstad 1976; Hedrick 1996; Hicks 1954; Huang et al. 1993; Kim and Voloshin 1995; Kitaoka et al. 1997b). This dense connective tissue band resides in the inferior aspect of the foot and is comprised of three variably developed components: the central, lateral, and medial cords. The central cord is the most important biomechanical component, arising from the medial aspect of the medial calcaneal tubercle and extending distally in a fan-like configuration while enveloping the aponeurosis of the flexor digitorum brevis muscle. Five distinct bands interconnect with the plantar plates, plantar interdigital ligaments, and the sagittal septae underneath the metatarsophalangeal joints (Bojsen-Moller and Flagstad 1976; Hedrick 1996; Hicks 1954). The lateral cord arises from the lateral margin of the medial calcaneal tubercle and extends to the cuboid and base of the fifth metatarsal bone, enveloping the aponeurosis of the abductor digiti minimi muscle. The medial cord is very thin and invests the abductor hallucis muscle.

MR imaging is ideal for the detection of ankle pathology (Yu and Vitellas 1996; Long et al. 1998). The MR appearance of a normal plantar fascia on sagittal images is a thin, linear band of low signal intensity in the plantar aspect of the foot measuring an average of 3.2–3.4 mm thick (Berkowitz et al. 1991). The sharp fascial margins are well depicted, interfacing with the deep plantar muscles and superficial subcutaneous fat. On cross-section, the plantar fascia has a semilunar configuration that is concave in its deep surface and convex superficially. Proximally, it has a cuff-like appearance and is primarily comprised of the central and lateral cords, whereas distally the three cords may be seen accompanying the intrinsic foot muscles.

12.2.1
Acute and Chronic Plantar Fasciitis

Plantar fasciitis, a condition caused by chronic microtrauma at the enthesis of the plantar fascia, is a common source of heel pain. Several etiologic factors have been described, including a pes cavus deformity, enthesopathy from systemic diseases, overuse including excessive loading from obesity, trauma, and altered gait (DeMaio et al. 1993; Furey 1975; Leach et al. 1986). The central cord is the component most commonly affected, and fascial and perifascial inflammation become evident as microtears of the fascia develop. During the acute phase of the disorder, marked thickening of the plantar fascia associated with areas of high signal intensity from inflammatory changes in the fascia are conspicuous findings on T2-weighted and inversion-recovery MR images (Berkowitz et al. 1991) (Fig. 12.6). Edema at the fascia-muscle (deep) and fascia-fat (superficial) interfaces and inflammation of the adjacent subcutaneous fat are also notable findings.

The majority of patients with acute plantar fasciitis respond to conservative therapy consisting of

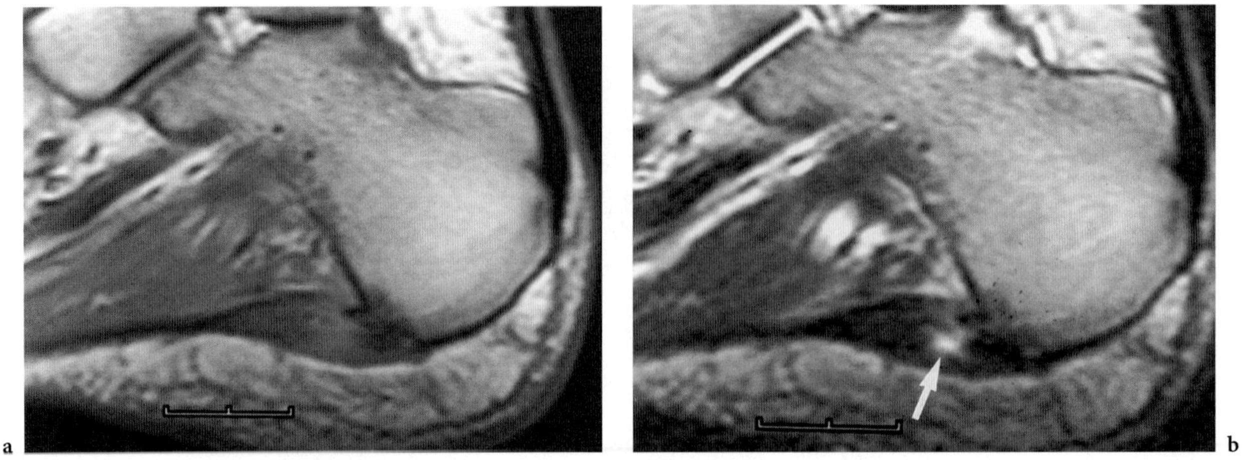

Fig. 12.6a,b. Acute plantar fasciitis. Sagittal proton-density (a) and T2-weighted (b) images show a markedly thickened plantar fascia. Perifascial edema is noted on the T2-weighted image as well as a focus of high signal intensity (*arrow* in b)

rest, ice packs, orthosis, antiinflammatory medication, and occasionally steroid injection (Snider et al. 1983; Kwong et al. 1988). In most instances, the duration of treatment seldom exceeds a few weeks before noticeable improvement is observed.

Persons who experience recurrent episodes of fasciitis suffer from chronic plantar fasciitis (Yu 2000) (Fig. 12.7). These patients complain of chronic heel pain characterized by periods of exacerbation and periods of relief for a duration that exceeds 6 months, and obesity may be a significant contributing factor in the development of the disease process (Furey 1975; Powell et al. 1998; Hill and Cutting 1989; Lapidus and Guidotti 1965). The MR imaging findings in patients with chronic fasciitis are more subtle than in patients with the acute form of the disease. The fascia generally appears thickened; however, the signal alteration within the aponeurosis may not be evident unless an inversion-recovery sequence or fat-suppressed T2-weighted sequence is performed (Yu 2000). Perifascial edema tends to be subdued as well. In a large percentage of patients, a heel spur may be detected on the inferior aspect of the calcaneus. Most experts agree that these spurs are a reactive phenomenon to increased tensile forces at the enthesis of the fascia, and not the inciting cause of the inflammatory process (McCarthy and Gorecki 1979). This opinion is based on the observation that patients with heel pain frequently do not have a spur on the initial radiographs but subsequently develop them on follow-up.

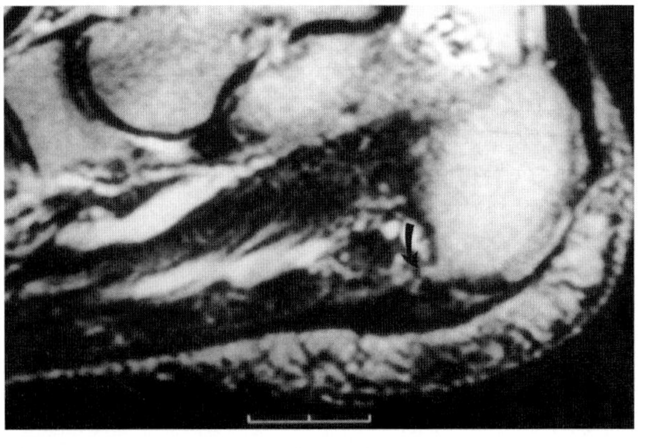

Fig. 12.7. Chronic plantar fasciitis. Sagittal T2-weighted image shows an enthesophyte (*arrow*) at the insertion of the central cord of a thickened plantar fascia. Edema tends to be less conspicuous in chronic cases than in patients with acute fasciitis. (Used with permission from Yu 2000)

12.2.2 Rupture of the Plantar Fascia

A spontaneous rupture of the plantar fascia is an unusual injury. This particular injury has its highest prevalence in athletes who have had repeated injections of corticosteroids into the fascia, although it has also been reported as an isolated finding in people who have had no prior history of plantar fascia pathology (Ahstrom 1988; Herrick and Herrick 1983; Leach et al. 1978; McElgun and Cavaliere 1994; Pai 1996; Rolf et al. 1997; Sellman 1994). The most common mechanism of injury leading to a ruptured fascia is forced plantar flexion of the foot during the act of rapid acceleration, occurring when the foot is planted and actively pushing against the ground (McElgun and Cavaliere 1994). When there is an underlying abnormality of the plantar fascia, a sustained and prolonged activity such as walking may be sufficient to rupture the plantar fascia (PAI 1996). A recent study has indicated that rupture of the plantar fascia may also occur as a complication of a plantar fasciotomy (YU et al. 1999b). Clinically, patients experience a sensation of a 'snap' followed by intense focal pain in the heel. On physical examination, a lump associated with swelling and tenderness along the plantar fascia and ecchymosis are notable findings.

The MR appearance of an acutely ruptured plantar fascia is a gap with frayed free ends associated with interstitial edema (Fig. 12.8). Edema at the muscle and subcutaneous fat interfaces is also a common finding. When there is an incomplete tear of the fascia, its appearance on MR imaging may mimic the findings of acute plantar fasciitis, and therefore, the clinical presentation is an important distinguishing feature. An acute tear is heralded by an antecedent traumatic event, whereas the clinical presentation of acute plantar fasciitis is more indolent.

Another condition that mimics plantar fasciitis is a chronic rupture, and these cases require a high index of suspicion. The most common presentation is a mass in the bottom of the foot. Characteristic MR findings include nodular thickening on both sides of the plantar fascia at the site of rupture (Fig. 12.9). Arriving at the correct diagnosis begins with obtaining a careful history and performing a thorough examination (SELLMAN 1994).

12.2.3 Plantar Fascia Fibromatosis

Fibromatoses comprise a group of soft-tissue lesions that may occur either as a superficial nodular mass (plantar fibromatosis) or as a deep infiltrative mass (aggressive fibromatosis) that may mimic a malignant process in the soft tissues of the foot. Clinically, pain and swelling are also notable findings. Histologically, this pathologic process is characterized by benign proliferation of well differentiated fibroblasts and myofibroblasts within the plantar fascia (DE PALMA et al. 1999). When superficial, a small nodule is often palpable, but deeper lesions tend to be more insidious and may not be detected until they elicit a mass effect on the adjacent musculature or neurovascular structure (LEE et al. 1993). When conservative therapy fails to relieve the symptoms in patients who have fibromatosis, surgical excision is recommended using a wide margin because the recurrence rate for simple excision is high, ranging from 60% to 100% (WAPNER et al. 1995).

a

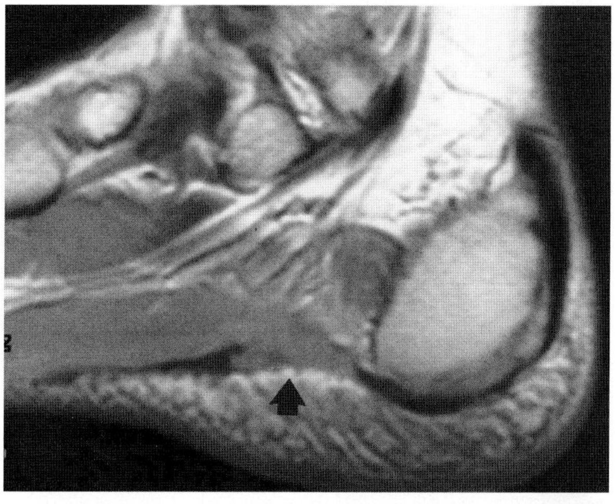

b

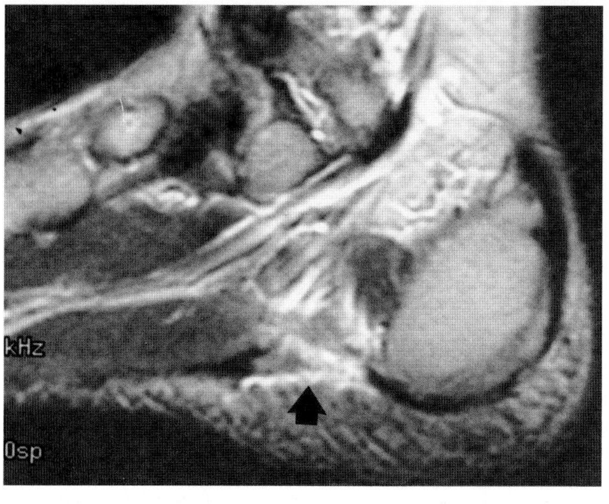

Fig. 12.8a,b. Acute rupture of plantar fascia. Sagittal proton-density (**a**) and T2-weighted (**b**) images show frayed free ends of an acutely ruptured fascia. Note the large gap (*arrow*) in the fascia and the extensive edema in and around the site of rupture

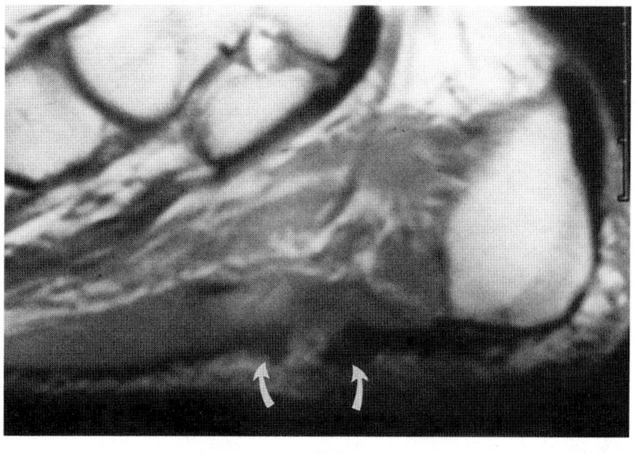

Fig. 12.9. Chronic rupture of plantar fascia. Sagittal T1-weighted image shows nodular thickening of the plantar fascia at the site of chronic rupture (*arrows*). This patient presented with an enlarging 'mass'. (Used with permission from YU 2000)

A plantar fibroma, also known as Ledderhose disease, is a superficial form of fibromatosis and occurs in middle-aged people with a genetic predisposition for other fibromatous conditions including Dupuytren's contracture (palmar fibromatosis) and Peyronie disease (penile fibromatosis) (Quinn et al. 1991). There is also an association with diabetes, alcoholism, epilepsy, and frozen shoulder (De Palma et al. 1999). This lesion characteristically presents in the medial aspect of the plantar fascia near the first metatarsal midshaft and neck region and has a tendency to be multinodular or an aggregate of multiple nodules (Fig. 12.10). Bilateral lesions occur in 10%–25% of cases (Lee et al. 1993; Wetzel and Levine 1990). Deep or aggressive fibromatosis is less common than its superficial counterpart and may occur anywhere along the plantar fascia. It is highly aggressive and tends to infiltrate the adjacent musculature (Fig. 12.11). This lesion is similar to an abdominal desmoid.

MR imaging is important because it is able to delineate the full extent of the disease process. On MR imaging, fibromatosis may have a variety of appearances, reflecting the tissue composition and cellularity of a lesion (Quinn et al. 1991). On T1-weighted images, lesions are either isointense or slightly hyperintense in comparison to the signal intensity of muscle (Durr et al. 1999; Morrison et al. 1995). Areas of low signal intensity represent dense clusters

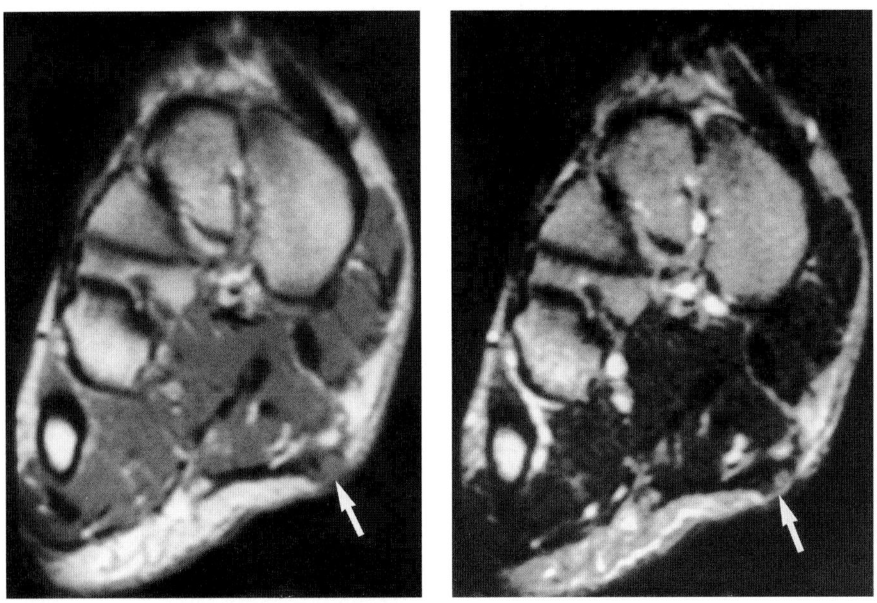

a b

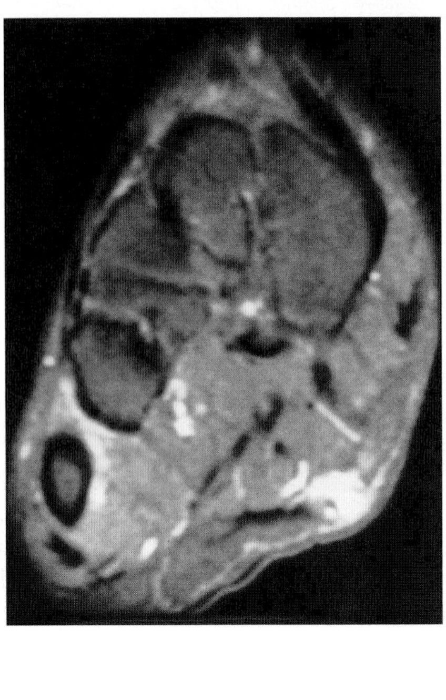

c

Fig. 12.10a–c. Superficial plantar fascia fibroma. Coronal proton-density (**a**) and T2-weighted (**b**) images show a round soft-tissue mass (*arrow*) involving the medial fibers of the central cord of the plantar fascia below the level of the first tarsometatarsal joint. **c** Coronal fat-saturated T1-weighted image shows intense enhancement of the fibroma after intravenous administration of gadolinium. (Used with permission from Yu 2000)

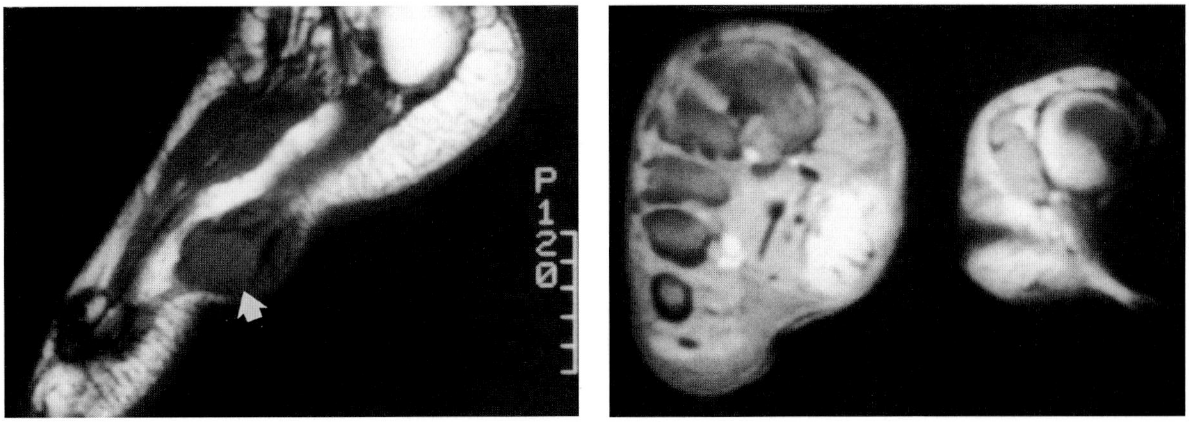

a b

Fig. 12.11a,b. Plantar fascia fibromatosis. **a** Sagittal T1-weighted image shows a large soft-tissue mass in the distal aspect of the plantar fascia (*arrow*). **b** Coronal fat-saturated T1-weighted image after intravenous administration of gadonium shows intense homogeneous enhancement of the lesion. (Used with permission from Yu 2000)

of collagen. Occasionally, lesions may appear quite bright on T1-weighted images. In many fibromas, the shortening of T1 relaxation occurs from the presence of fat, but in other lesions, fat is conspicuously absent. An as yet unidentified protein has been hypothesized as the cause of the shortened T1 relaxation (Quinn et al. 1991). On T2-weighted images, a wide spectrum of signal intensity has been observed (Morrison et al. 1994; Quinn et al. 1991; Wetzel and Levine 1990). In comparison to the signal intensity of muscle, lesions may appear homogeneously low in signal intensity, isointense to slightly hyperintense, or heterogeneously bright. Higher signal intensity on T2-weighted images may be a sign of more aggressive growth (Feld et al. 1990). Aggressive fibromatosis, therefore, demonstrates high signal intensity on T2-weighted images more often than superficial fibromatosis. Enhancement patterns after the administration of intravenous contrast have been equally variable, ranging from no enhancement of the lesion to marked heterogeneous enhancement (Morrison et al. 1994).

The initial treatment is aimed at relieving symptoms to tolerable levels (De Palma et al. 1999; Sammarco and Mangone 2000). There is, however, a high incidence of recurrence after both local and wide excision (Aluisio et al. 1996).

12.2.4 Normal Postfasciotomy Appearance

Patients who suffer from intractable pain caused by plantar fasciitis have been purported to benefit from a partial plantar fasciotomy when conservative therapy fails. The success rate of this procedure varies; however, most surgeons report improvement in symptoms in 90%–95% of patients who have been followed for a short period after surgery (Daly et al. 1992; Gormley and Kuwada 1992; Leach et al. 1978; Lester and Buchanan 1984; Schepsis et al. 1991; Snider et al. 1983). The plantar fascia may be released either through an open incision or endoscopically. With the latter technique, a puncture incision is used to create a portal through which an endoscope is introduced. The aim of both procedures is to transect 80% of the cuff portion of the plantar fascia medially (Baxter and Thigpen 1984; Hofmeister et al. 1995; Lewis et al. 1991; Reeve et al. 1997). There are several reasons for performing a partial fasciotomy instead of a complete transection, including the risk of injury to the nerve of the abductor digiti minimi muscle and potentially deleterious effects on the longitudinal arch of the foot with a complete fasciotomy (Murphy et al. 1998; Thordarson et al. 1997).

A recent study investigated the expected MR appearance of the plantar fascia after a fasciotomy has been performed (Yu et al. 1999a). The plantar fascia does not resume its normal native appearance after a fasciotomy. The enthesis of the fascia remains thickened, on average two to three times the normal thickness. The most notable observations are complete absence of edema in the fascia or the surrounding soft tissues and indistinctness of the surface morphology owing to perifascial fibrosis (Yu et al. 1999a) (Fig. 12.12). Residual areas of intermediate signal intensity are also a common finding on proton-density-weighted images and most likely indicate the presence of degenerative changes in the fascia. The appearance of the fascia is similar in patients who have had an open or endoscopic fasciotomy. About

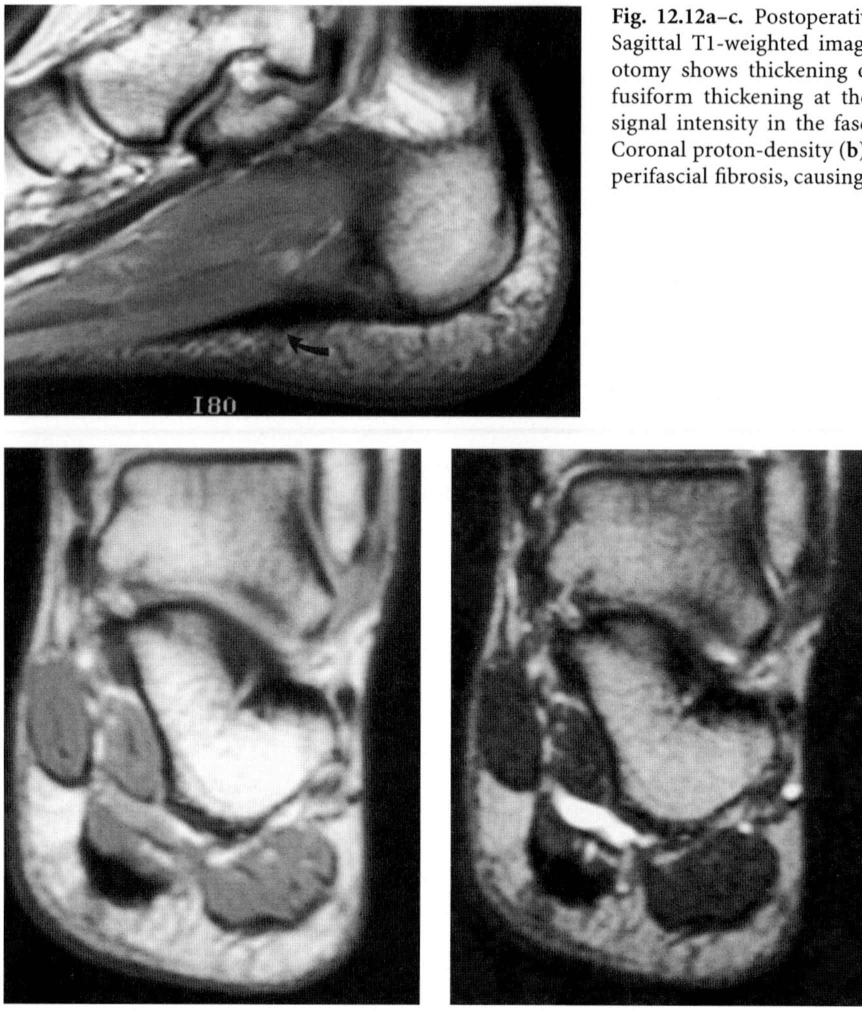

a b c

Fig. 12.12a–c. Postoperative appearance of a fasciotomy. **a** Sagittal T1-weighted image 30 months after an open fasciotomy shows thickening of the plantar fascia enthesis and fusiform thickening at the site of surgery (*arrow*). Altered signal intensity in the fascia corresponded to degeneration. Coronal proton-density (**b**) and T2-weighted (**c**) images show perifascial fibrosis, causing the margins to appear indistinct

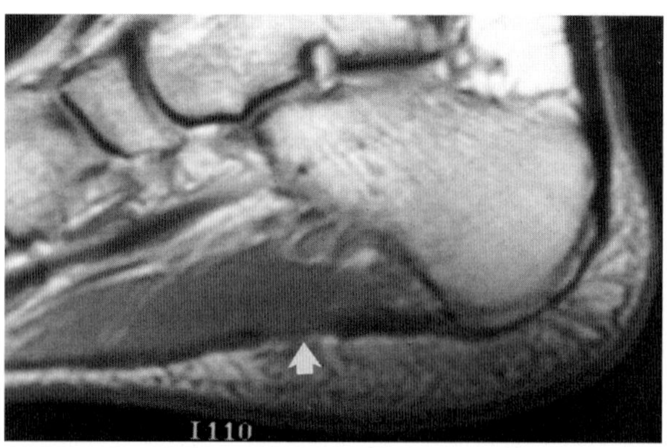

Fig. 12.13. Postoperative gap. Sagittal T1-weighted image taken 23 months after a endoscopic fasciotomy shows a persistent gap in the fascia (*arrow*)

one-fifth of people demonstrates a persistent gap at the fasciotomy (Fig. 12.13).

12.2.5 Failed Plantar Fasciotomy

A plantar fasciotomy yields excellent pain relief and rapid return to activities in a majority of patients, but recent long-term evaluations have been more critical of this procedure. Although a majority of patients who undergo this procedure do not require any further intervention, a small but growing percentage of patients has required subsequent follow-up either owing to a persistence or recurrence of foot pain.

A recent investigation correlating foot pain with MR findings in patients with foot pain who have undergone fasciotomies suggested that symptoms could be classified into one of three pathologic processes (Yu et al. 1999b). The most common condition was either persistent or recurrent plantar fasciitis. In some feet, classic MR findings of acute plantar fasciitis were noted, including thickening of the fascia, intrafascial edema, and perifascial soft-tissue edema (Fig. 12.14). In others, the MR findings were more difficult to detect, and the predominant finding in these feet was the presence of perifascial edema only evident on inversion recovery images. A second common cause of pain was related to midfoot instability (Yu et al. 1999b). The plantar fascia has been experimentally shown to carry as much as 14% of the total static load on the foot (Kim and Voloshin 1995). With a plantar fasciotomy, a 10% reduction of the dynamic loading capacity on the foot may occur. When the height of the longitudinal arch decreases, it accentuates loading on the posterior tibial tendon as well as the peroneus brevis and longus tendons (Kitaoka et al. 1997a,b; Sellman 1994; Karasick and Schweitzer 1993) (Fig. 12.15). Two important effects on the foot when the arch height decreases are an increased incidence of acute tears of these tendons that support the arch and an increased incidence of midtarsal joint degeneration (Kitaoka et al. 1997; Murphy et al. 1998; Thordarson et al. 1997; Yu et al. 1999b). Alterations in the midfoot mechanics most likely contributed to a third common cause of pain, which was related to pathologically increased forces that ultimately caused the breakdown of soft-tissue and osseous structures. The most common failure was an acute rupture of the plantar fascia at or near the fasciotomy (Yu et al. 1999b). It is likely, however, that other factors such as alterations in gait, shift in the distribution of stresses, and the cumulative effect of abnormal stresses in different areas of the foot also contribute to tissue breakdown, but these factors are virtually impossible to quantify.

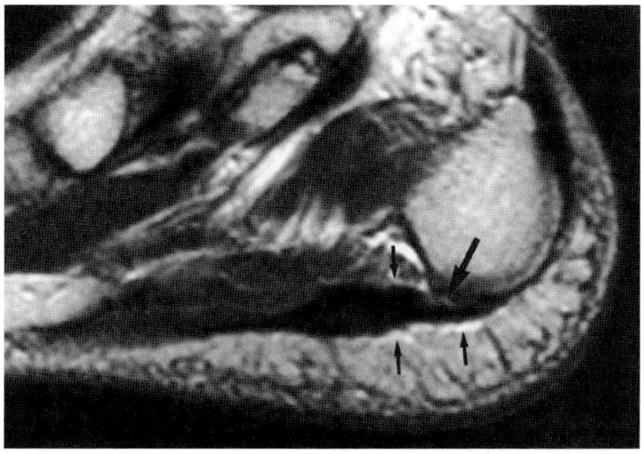

Fig. 12.14. Perifascial edema. Sagittal T2-weighted image taken 26 months after an open fasciotomy show a thin layer of edema at both the fascia-muscle and fascia-subcutaneous fat interfaces (*small arrows*). There is also a focus of high signal intensity at the enthesis (*larger arrow*). This patient had recurrence of her original symptoms of plantar fasciitis. (Used with permission from Yu et al. 1999b)

12.3 Conclusion

The power of MR imaging in the evaluation of patients with heel pain lies in its ability to resolve the complicated anatomy of the hindfoot clearly and

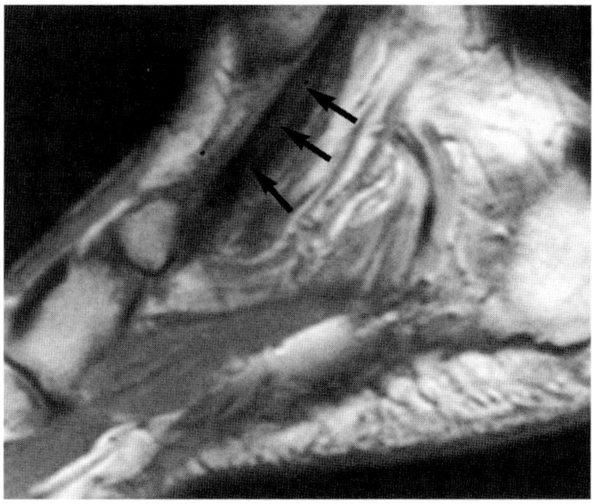

a

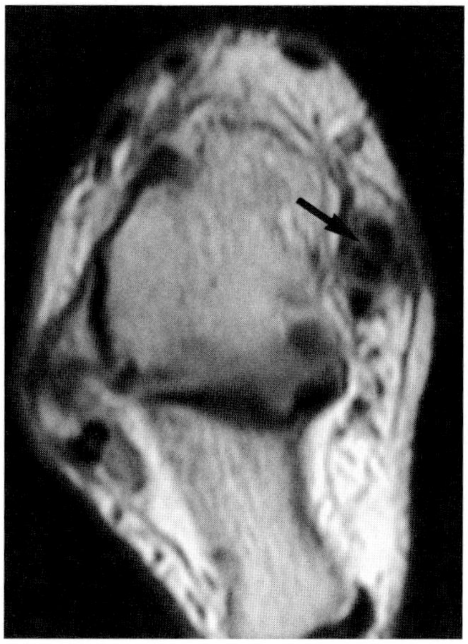

b

Fig. 12.15a,b. Longitudinal tear of the posterior tibialis tendon. Sagittal (**a**) and transaxial (**b**) proton-density-weighted images show a longitudinal cleft (*arrows*) of the posterior tibialis tendon that developed 31 months after this patient underwent an open fasciotomy. This patient presented with new onset pain in the midfoot unequivocally. Whether it depicts normal anatomy or a pathologic finding, MR imaging virtually eliminates the guessing that frequently accompanies a clinical evaluation. Utilization of MR imaging in patients with heel pain in whom conservative therapy fails will often help direct the further course of management.

Reference

Ahstrom JP (1988) Spontaneous rupture of the plantar fascia. Am J Sports Med 16:306–307

Akiyama K, Takakura Y, Tomita Y, Sugimoto K, Tanaka Y, Tamai S (1999) Neurohistology of the sinus tarsi and sinus tarsi syndrome. J Orthop Sci 4:299–303

Aluisio FV, Mair SD, Hall RL (1996) Plantar fibromatosis: treatment of primary and recurrent lesions and factors associated with recurrence. Foot Ankle 17:672–678

Baba H, Wada M, Annen S, Azuchi M, Imura S, Tomita K (1997) The tarsal tunnel syndrome: evaluation of surgical results using multivariate analysis. Int Orthop 21:67–71

Bailie DS, Kelikian AS (1998) Tarsal tunnel syndrome: diagnosis, surgical technique, and functional outcome. Foot Ankle 19:65–72

Baxter DE, Thigpen CM (1984) Heel pain: operative results. Foot Ankle 5:16–25

Beltran J (1994) Sinus tarsi syndrome. Magn Reson Imaging Clin North Am 2:59–65

Berkowitz JF, Kier R, Rudicel S (1991) Plantar fasciitis: MR imaging. Radiology 179:665–667

Bieneman BK, Sundaram M (2000) Fibrous mass compressing the posterior tibial neurovascular bundle. Orthopedics 23: 165–168

Bojsen-Moller F, Flagstad KE (1976) Plantar aponeurosis and internal architecture of the ball of the foot. J Anat 121: 599–611

Breitenseher MJ, Haller J, Kukla C et al (1997) MRI of the sinus tarsi in acute ankle sprain injuries. J Comput Assist Tomogr 21:274–279

Brown JE (1960) The sinus tarsi syndrome. Clin Orthop 18: 231–233

Cheung YY, Rosenberg ZS, Colon E, Jahss M (1999) MR imaging of flexor digitorum accessorius longus. Skeletal Radiol 28:130–137

Cimino WR (1990) Tarsal tunnel syndrome: review of the literature. Foot Ankle 11:47–52

Daly PJ, Kitaoka HB, Chao EY (1992) Plantar fasciotomy for intractable plantar fasciitis: clinical results and biomechanical evaluation. Foot Ankle 13:188–195

Daniels T, Lau J, Hearn T (1998) The effects of foot position and load on tibial nerve tension. Foot Ankle 19:73–78

De Palma L, Santucci A, Gigante A, Di Giulio A, Carloni S (1999) Plantar fibromatosis: an immunohistochemical and ultrastructural study. Foot Ankle 20:253–257

Dellon AL, Mackinnon SE (1984) Tibial nerve branching in the tarsal tunnel. Arch Neurol 41:645–646

DeMaio M, Paine R, Mangine RE, Drez D Jr (1993) Plantar fasciitis. Orthopedics 16:1153–1163

Dos Remedios ET, Jolly GP (2000) The accessory soleus and recurrent tarsal tunnel syndrome: case report of a new surgical approach. J Foot Ankle Surg 39:194–197

Durr HR, Krodel A, Lienemann A, Refior HJ (1999) Fibromatosis of the plantar fascia: diagnosis and indications for surgical treatment. Foot Ankle 20:13–17

Feld R, Burk DL, McCue P, Mitchell DG, Lackmann R, Rifkin MD (1990) MRI of aggressive fibromatosis: frequent appearance of high signal intensity on T2-weighted images. Magn Reson Imaging 8:583–588

Frey C, Feder KS, DiGiovanni C (1999) Arthroscopic evaluation of the subtalar joint: does sinus tarsi syndrome exist? Foot Ankle Int 20:185–191

Furey JG (1975) Plantar fasciitis: the painful heel syndrome. J Bone Joint Surg 57-A:672–673

Gormley J, Kuwada GT (1992) Retrospective analysis of calcaneal spur removal and complete fascial release for the treatment of chronic heel pain. J Foot Surg 31:166–169

Havel PE, Ebraheun NA, Clark SE, Jackson WT, DiDio L (1988) Tibial nerve branching in the tarsal tunnel. Foot Ankle 9: 117–119

Hedrick MR (1996) The plantar aponeurosis. Foot Ankle 17: 646–649

Heimkes B, Posel P, Stotz S, Wolf K (1987) The proximal and distal tarsal tunnel syndromes: an antomical study. Int Orthop 11:193–196

Herrick RT, Herrick S (1983) Rupture of the plantar fascia in a middle-aged tennis player, a case report. Am J Sports Med 11:95–96

Hicks JH (1954) The mechanics of the foot. II. The plantar aponeurosis and the arch. J Anat 88:25–31

Hill JJ, Cutting PJ (1989) Heel pain and body weight. Foot Ankle 9:254–255

Hofmeister EP, Elliott MJ, Juliano PJ (1995) Endoscopic plantar fascia release: an anatomical study. Foot Ankle 11:719–723

Huang CK, Kitaoka HB, An KN, Chao KN (1993) Biomechanical evaluation of longitudinal arch stability. Foot Ankle 14: 353–357

Jackson DL, Haglund BL (1992) Tarsal tunnel syndrome in runners. Sports Med 13:146–149

Janecki CJ, Dovberg JL (1977) Tarsal tunnel syndrome caused by neurilemoma of the medial plantar nerve. J Bone Joint Surg 59-A:127–128

Karasick D, Schweitzer ME (1993) Tear of the posterior tibial tendon causing asymmetric flatfoot: radiologic findings. AJR 161:1237–1240

Keck C (1962) The tarsal tunnel syndrome. J Bone Joint Surg 44-A:180–182

Kenzora JE, Lenet MD, Sherman M (1982) Synovial cyst of the ankle joint as a cause of tarsal tunnel syndrome. Foot Ankle 3:181–183

Kerr R, Frey C (1991) MR imaging in tarsal tunnel syndrome. J Comput Assist Tomogr 15:280–286

Kim W, Voloshin AS (1995) Role of plantar fascia in the load bearing capacity of the human foot. J Biomech 28: 1025–1033

Kitaoka HB, Luo ZP, An KN (1997a) Effect of the posterior tibial tendon on the arch of the foot during simulated weithbearing: biomechanical analysis. Foot Ankle 18: 43–46

Kitaoka HB, Luo ZP, An KN (1997b) Mechanical behavior of the foot and ankle after plantar fascia release in the unstable foot. Foot Ankle 18:8–15

Kwong PK, Kay D, Voner RT, White MW (1988) Plantar fasciitis: mechanics and pathomechanics of treatment. Clin Sports Med 7:119–126

Lapidus PW, Guidotti FP (1965) Painful heel: report of 323 patients with 364 painful heels. Clin Orthop 39:178–186
Lau JTC, Daniels TR (1999) Tarsal tunnel syndrome: a review of the literature. Foot Ankle 20:201–209
Leach R, Jones R, Silva T (1978) Rupture of the plantar fascia in athletes. J Bone Joint Surg 60-A:537–539
Leach RE, Seavey MS, Salter DK (1986) Results of surgery in athletes with plantar fasciitis. Foot Ankle 7:156–161
Lee TH, Wapner KL, Hecht PJ (1993) Current concepts review: plantar fibromatosis. J Bone Joint Surg 75-A:1080–1084
Lester DK, Buchanan JR (1984) Surgical treatment of plantar fasciitis. Clin Orthop 186:202–204
Lewis G, Gatti A, Barry LD, Greenberg PM, Levenson M (1991) The plantar approach to heel surgery: a retrospective study. J Foot Surg 30:542–546
Long D, Yu JS, Vitellas KM (1998) Imaging of ankle trauma. Crit Rev Diagn Imaging 39:393–445
McCarthy DJ, Gorecki GE (1979) The anatomical basis of inferior calcaneal lesions: a cryomicrotomy study. J Am Podiatr Assoc 69:527–536
McElgun T, Cavaliere R (1994) Sequential bilateral rupture of plantar fascia in a tennis player. Sports Med 84:137–141
Morrison WB, Schweitzer ME, Wapner KL, Hecht PJ, Gannon FH, Behm WR (1995) Osteomyelitis in feet of diabetics: clinical accuracy, surgical utility and cost-effectiveness of MR imaging. Radiology 196:557–564
Murphy GA, Pneumaticos SG, Kamaric E, Noble PC, Trevino SG, Baxter DE (1998) Biomechanical consequences of sequential plantar fascia release. Foot Ankle 19:149–152
Nagaoka M, Satou K (1999) Tarsal tunnel syndrome caused by ganglia. J Bone Joint Surg 81-B:607–610
O'Conner D (1958) Sinus tarsi syndrome: a clinical entity. J Bone Joint Surg 40-A:720–729
O'Malley GM, Lambdin CS, McCleary GS (1985) Tarsal tunnel syndrome. Orthopedics 8:758–760
Pai VS (1996) Rupture of the plantar fascia. J Foot Ankle Surg 35:39–40
Powell M, Post WR, Keener J, Wearden S (1998) Effective treatment of chronic plantar fasciitis with dorsiflexion night splints: a crossover prospective randomized outcome study. Foot Ankle 19:10–18
Quinn SF, Erickson SJ, Dee PM et al (1991) MR imaging of fibromatosis: results in 26 patients with pathologic correlation. AJR 156:539–542
Radin EL (1983) Tarsal tunnel syndrome. Clin Orthop 181: 167–170
Reeve F, Laughlin RT, Wright DG (1997) Endoscopic plantar fascia release: a cross-sectional anatomic study. Foot Ankle 18:398–401
Rolf C, Guntner P, Ericsater J, Turan I (1997) Plantar fascia rupture: diagnosis and treatment. J Foot Ankle Surg 36: 112–114
Sammarco GJ, Mangone PG (2000) Classification and treatment of plantar fibromatosis. Foot Ankle 21:563–569
Sammarco GJ, Stephens MM (1990) Tarsal tunnel syndrome caused by the flexor digitorum accessorius longus. J Bone Joint Surg 72-A:453–454
Sarrafian SK (1993) Nerves. In: Sarrafian SK (ed) Anatomy of the foot and ankle: descriptive, topographic, functional, 2nd edn. Lippincott, Philadelphia, pp 365–383
Schepsis AA, Leach RE, Gorzyca J (1991) Plantar fasciitis. Etiology, treatment, surgical results, and review of the literature. Clin Orthop 266:185–196
Schon LC (1994) Nerve entrapment, neuropathy, and nerve dysfunction in athletes. Orthop Clin. North Am 25: 47–59
Sellman JR (1994) Plantar fascia rupture associated with corticosteroid injection. Foot Ankle 15:376–381
Skalley TC, Schon LC, Hinton RY, Myerson MS (1994) Clinical results following revision tibial nerve release. Foot Ankle 15:360–367
Snider MP, Clancy WG, McBeath AA (1983) Plantar fascia release for chronic plantar fasciitis in runners. Am J Sports Med 11:215–219
Stefko RM, Lauerman WC, Heckman JD (1994) Tarsal tunnel syndrome caused by an unrecognized fracture of the posterior process of the talus. J Bone Joint Surg 76-A: 116–118
Steinbach LS (1998) Painful syndromes around the ankle and foot: magnetic resonance imaging evaluation. Top Magn Reson Imaging 9:311–326
Taillard W, Meyer J, Garcia J, Blanc Y (1981) The sinus tarsi syndrome. Int Orthop 5:117–130
Thordarson DB, Kumar PJ, Hedman TP, Ebramzadeh E (1997) Effect of partial versus complete plantar fasciotomy on the windlass mechanism. Foot Ankle 18:16–20
Upton AR, McComas AJ (1973) The double crush syndrome in nerve-entrapment syndromes. Lancet 2:359–361
Wapner KL, Ververeli PA, Moore JH, Hecht PJ, Becker CE, Lackman RD (1995) Plantar fibromatosis: a review of primary and recurrent surgical treatment. Foot Ankle 16: 548–551
Wetzel LH, Levine E (1990) Soft-tissue tumors of the foot: value of MR imaging for specific diagnosis. AJR 155: 1025–1030
Yu JS (2000) Pathologic and post-operative conditions of the plantar fascia: review of MR imaging appearances. Skeletal Radiol 29:491–501
Yu JS, Vitellas KM (1996) The calcaneus: applications of magnetic resonance imaging. Foot Ankle 17:771–780
Yu JS, Smith G, Ashman C, Kaeding CC (1999a) The plantar fasciotomy: MR imaging findings in asymptomatic volunteers. Skeletal Radiol 28:447–452
Yu JS, Spigos D, Tomczak R (1999b) Foot pain after a plantar fasciotomy: an MR analysis to determine potential causes. J Comput Assist Tomogr 23:707–712
Zeiss J, Ebraheim N, Rusin J (1990) Magnetic resonance imaging in the diagnosis of tarsal tunnel syndrome. Case report. Clin Imaging 14:123–126
Zeiss J, Fenton P, Ebraheim N, Coombs RJ (1991) Magnetic resonance imaging for ineffectual tarsal tunnel surgical treatment. Clin Orthop 264:264–266

13 Infection

H. P. Ledermann, W. B. Morrison, and M. E. Schweitzer

CONTENTS

13.1 Introduction

Infection can involve the foot and ankle via contiguous spread, direct implantation, or hematogenous spread. Hematogenous osteomyelitis is most frequently encountered in children and adolescents. In adults, the vast majority of foot and ankle infections result from an ulcer with contiguous spread of infection or from direct implantation such as a puncture wound or surgery (Ledermann et al. 2002a). Most foot infections occur in adults with predisposing conditions such as vascular disease, altered biomechanics, or neuropathy. Diabetic patients are especially prone to foot ulceration and infection. The diabetic foot will be discussed in detail in Chapter 14.

Manifestations of infection commonly seen in the foot and ankle include: skin ulceration, sinus tracts, soft-tissue infection and necrosis, abscess formation, septic tenosynovitis, osteomyelitis, and septic arthritis. The following discussion considers each of these entities separately.

13.2 Skin Ulceration

Skin ulceration is seen on MR images as an interruption of the cutaneous signal line and can be very subtle when only superficial skin erosion is present. Whereas ulcers of the plantar aspect of the toes and the metatarsophalangeal joints are generally easily diagnosed by MR imaging, ulcerations at the medial and lateral aspect of the toes and the dorsum may be more difficult to recognize (Fig. 13.1) (Ledermann et al. 2002a). Most ulcers display a marginal rim enhancement after contrast administration (Morrison et al. 1998), and the interruption of the skin line is often best seen on postcontrast images.

Callus represents focal thickening of skin at areas of increased pressure or friction. Breakdown of callus can lead to ulceration, and this is discussed and illustrated in more detail in the chapter on diabetic foot infections. Deep ulceration is frequently associated with underlying osteomyelitis (Fig. 13.2) or septic arthritis (Ledermann et al. 2002a). This is analogous to the clinical concept that the ability to pass a probe to the bone through a skin ulcer is virtually diagnostic of osteomyelitis (Grayson et al. 1995; Newman et al. 1991). This does not appear to be entirely accurate, since in our experience air occasionally extends to bone through an ulceration while the bone marrow signal is normal (Fig. 13.3). However, if this finding is seen on MR images with a questionable marrow signal abnormality in the adjacent bone, it should be considered highly suspicious of osteomyelitis.

H. P. Ledermann, MD; W. B. Morrison, MD;
M. E. Schweitzer, MD
Thomas Jefferson University Hospital, Department of Radiology, 111 S. 11th St., #3390 Gibbon, Philadelphia, PA 19107, USA

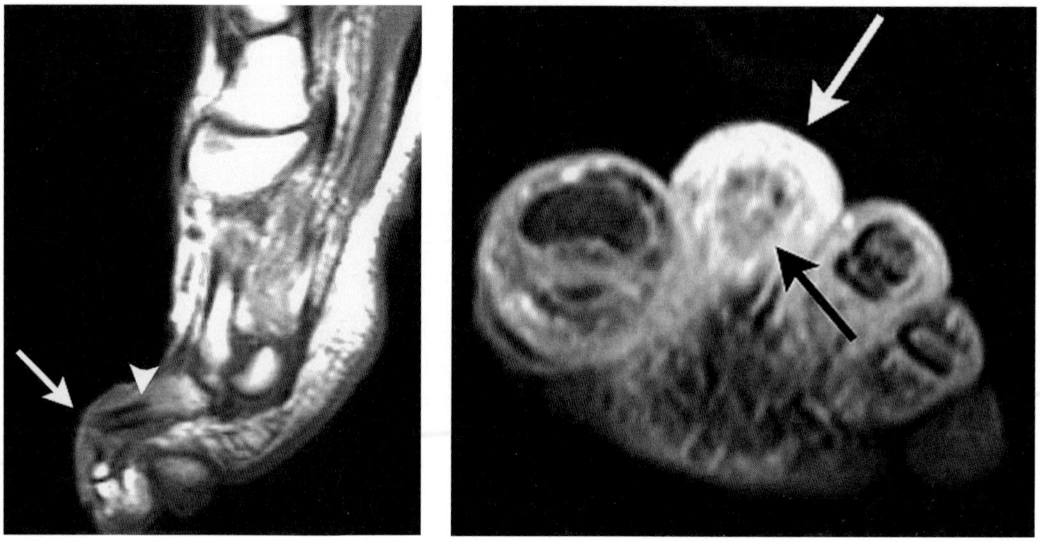

Fig. 13.1a,b. Hammertoe deformity with shallow ulcer over the proximal interphalangeal joint. **a** Sagittal T1-weighted image shows destruction of the proximal interphalangeal joint (*arrow*) and low signal intensity in the bone marrow (*arrowhead*) of the proximal phalanx indicative of osteomyelitis. The ulcer is not clearly visible on MR imaging due to underlying soft-tissue swelling. **b** Axial T1-weighted, contrast-enhanced, fat-suppressed image with extensive cellulitis (*white arrow*) on the dorsum of the toe and enhancement of the bone marrow of the proximal phalanx (*black arrow*), confirming osteomyelitis

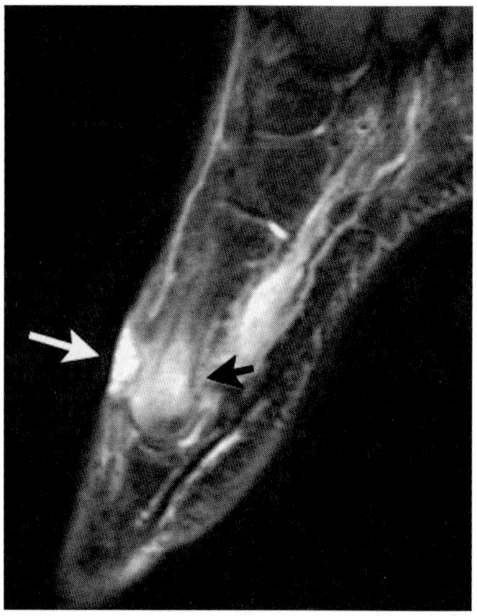

Fig. 13.2. Deep ulceration (*white arrow*) with underlying osteomyelitis (*black arrow*) on a T2-weighted fat-suppressed image

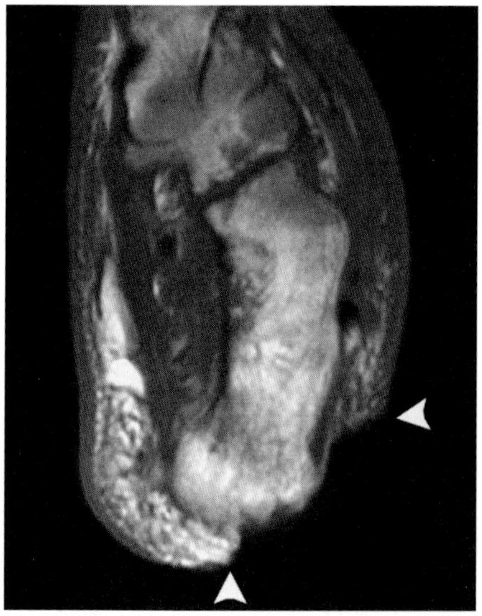

Fig. 13.3. Exposed calcaneal bone with large heel ulcer (*between arrowheads*). Note normal bone marrow of the calcaneus on this T1-weighted image

13.3 Sinus Tracts

Sinus tracts are a common finding in cases with osteomyelitis and adjacent skin ulceration (Morrison et al. 1998). On MR imaging, a thin line of signal approximating fluid is generally seen (Fig. 13.4) (Boutin et al. 1998; Morrison et al. 1993); however, if the tract is not actively draining, the fluid signal may not be apparent. The most sensitive method for detecting sinus tracts is with postcontrast fat-suppressed T1-weighted images, on which the tract will be visualized as parallel lines of enhancement in a tram-track pattern (Fig. 13.4) (Morrison et al. 1993).

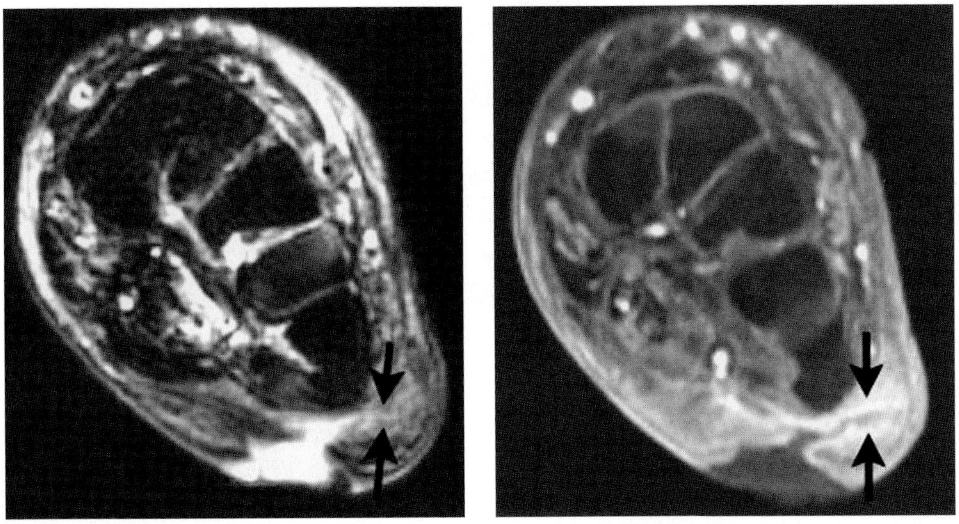

a b

Fig. 13.4a,b. MR signal characteristics of a sinus tract. **a** Axial T2-weighted fat-suppressed image with a large ulcer and fine sinus tract seen as a subtle hyperintense line (*between arrows*). **b** On a contrast-enhanced image, the sinus tract is now much more obvious, displaying a typical tram-track pattern (*between arrows*)

13.4 Cellulitis and Foreign Bodies

Cellulitis is most commonly seen adjacent to areas of skin ulceration, cuts, and puncture wounds with contiguous spread of organisms into the subcutaneous fat. Radiographs and CT display soft-tissue swelling and are often performed to detect opaque foreign bodies such as certain types of glass or metal (Fig. 13.5). Nonopaque foreign bodies are more difficult to localize with radiographs and may require CT or ultrasound examination (Jacobson et al. 1998). MR signal characteristics of cellulitis are swelling of the involved soft tissues, loss of the fat signal in subcutaneous tissues, and high signal, though less marked than fluid, on T2-weighted images (Ledermann et al. 2002b). There is diffuse enhancement following contrast administration (Fig. 13.6) (Tang et al. 1988; Unger et al. 1988). The margins are poorly defined. Foreign-body granulomas display focal plantar cellulitis, and contrast-enhanced images may reveal a nonenhancing center which represents exudate around the foreign body (Fig. 13.7).

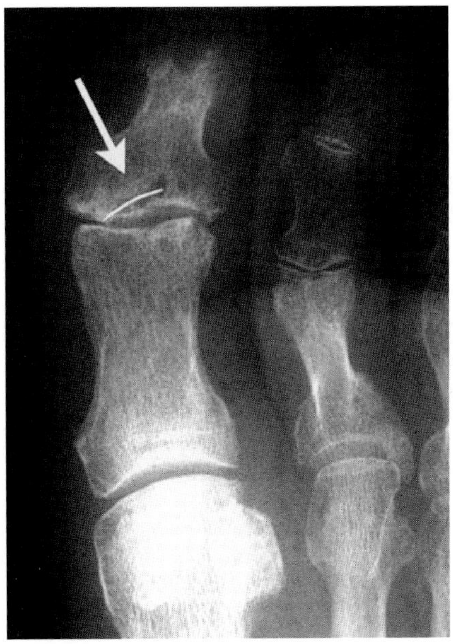

Fig. 13.5. Radiographic localization of a metallic needle tip (*arrow*) in the base of the first distal phalanx. Note sharply defined bony defects around the foreign body with subtle surrounding sclerosis compatible with localized chronic infection

Cellulitis must be differentiated with MR imaging from diffuse diabetic pedal edema and from necrotic tissue: In diabetics with vascular disease, diffuse edema is common (Moore et al. 1991; Yuh et al. 1989), but this type of edema enhances minimally or not at all and usually does not replace the normal soft-tissue fat signal. Diabetic edema is discussed and illustrated in detail in Chapter 14.

Three-phase bone scintigraphy will display increased activity in the area of cellulitis during the angiographic and blood pool phases, but there will be relatively normal bone activity on the delayed images.

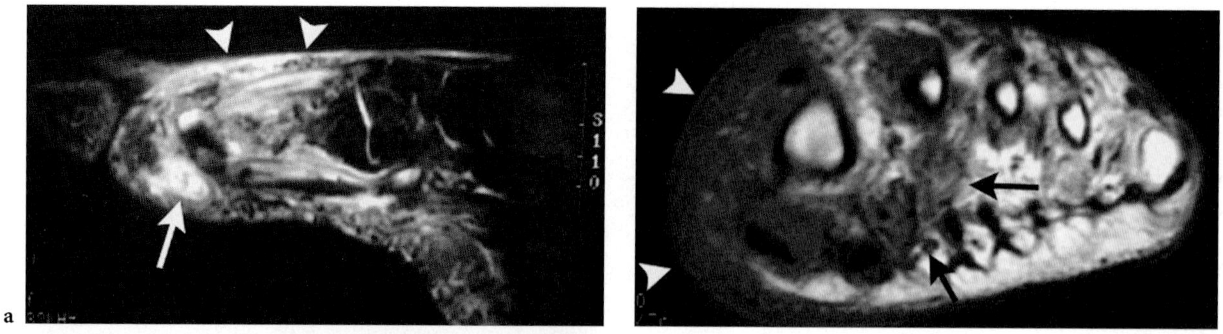

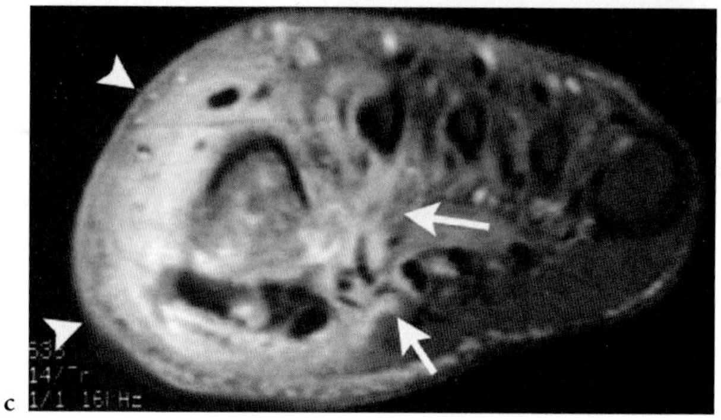

Fig. 13.6a–c. MR signal characteristics of soft-tissue infection. **a** T2-weighted image reveals a small collection (*arrow*) and diffuse hyperintense signal in the soft tissues of the first ray (*arrowheads*). **b** T1-weighted image with replacement of fat signal in the area of cellulitis (*arrowheads*). Note extension of the soft-tissue infection into the central compartment (*arrows*). **c** T1-weighted, contrast-enhanced, fat-suppressed image with diffuse contrast enhancement (*arrowheads*) confirming infection. Note extension of enhancement into the central compartment (*arrows*)

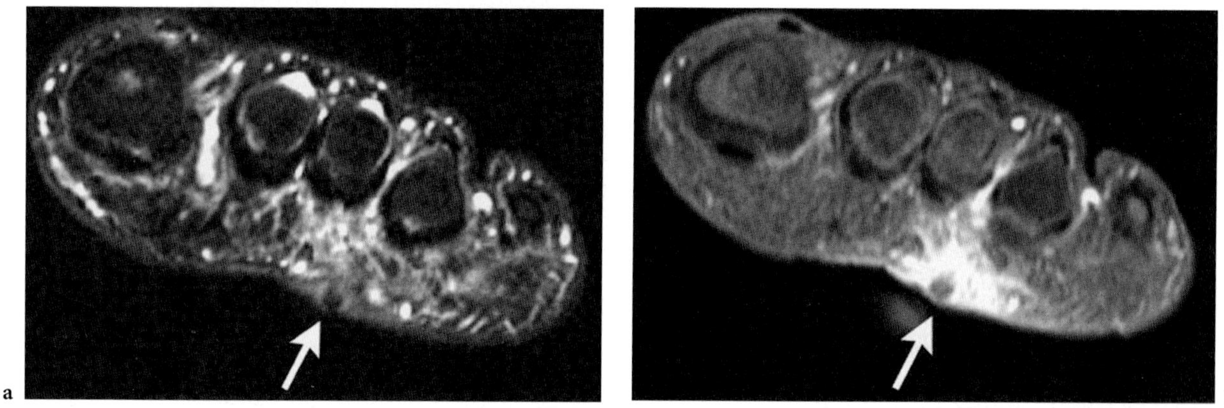

Fig. 13.7a,b. Foreign-body granuloma. **a** T2-weighted fat-suppressed image reveals a small, round, hypointense lesion (*arrow*) in the cutis of the sole with discrete blooming. **b** Contrast-enhanced fat-suppressed image with localized cellulitis and nonenhancing center (*arrow*) corresponding to the foreign body

13.5 Soft-Tissue Infection and Devitalization

It is very important to evaluate the extent of soft-tissue and osseous infection on MR images, since this can significantly alter plans for medical or surgical management (Nigro et al. 1992). Surgeons have recognized that extensive amputation of the foot leads to more rapid progression of disease in the contralateral foot due to shifting of the weight-bearing stresses (Waters et al. 1976). Therefore, in recent years, there has been increased emphasis on foot-preserving amputations, in which optimally only the infected tissue is removed (Tan et al. 1996; Wieman et al. 1998). This has in part been facilitated by the development of MRI, which can provide a surgical 'map' of the infected and viable tissue (Craig et al. 1997; Durham et al. 1991; Horowitz et al. 1993; Moore et al. 1991; Morrison et al. 1995; Nigro et al. 1992).

Pedal infection readily spreads into and across joints, through tendons, and across fascial planes (Fig. 13.6)

(LEDERMANN et al. 2002b). Soft-tissue involvement often progresses more rapidly than osseous disease, so the radiologist should carefully examine the soft tissues extending proximally from the source of the infection; if this tissue is not debrided, the patient may fail their foot-sparing procedure and require more extensive amputation.

Injured tissues in the critically ischemic extremity are more likely to proceed to gangrene because the metabolic requirements to heal an injury are far greater than those required to maintain normal tissue viability (FRY et al. 1998). Soft-tissue necrosis is commonly seen in infections of diabetic feet due to underlying microvascular disease. A more detailed discussion of MR imaging of devitalized tissue is provided in the chapter on diabetic foot infection. Necrotic tissue is seen on MR imaging with signal isointense to muscle on T1-weighted images, with a range of signal characteristics on T2-weighted images from mildly hyperintense to near fluid signal. On contrast-enhanced images, there is no enhancement of the devitalized tissue, with a relatively sharp cut-off at the border of normal surrounding soft-tissue enhancement (LEDERMANN etal. 2002c). At the border of the necrotic tissue, a brightly enhancing cellulitic tissue (Fig. 13.8) is often seen which may represent granulation tissue. Gas can also be seen in the soft tissues, particularly in devitalized areas; this process does not follow the same rapid progression associated with fasciitis due to gas-forming organisms, but rather is often related to communication of air through deep ulcers and sinus tracts into the soft tissues or to nonclostridial gas gangrene (BESSMAN and WAGNER 1975). Soft-tissue gas can also be seen after debridement. The presence and extension of soft-tissue gas are easily evaluated on plain radiographs (Fig. 13.9). On MR images, gas is seen as tiny foci of signal void, often with a slight marginal susceptibility artifact (Fig. 13.10). Small gas collections may be less obvious on MR images compared with CT (BOUTIN et al. 1998; WYSOKI et al. 1997).

13.6 Necrotizing Fasciitis

Necrotizing fasciitis is a rare soft-tissue infection characterized by necrosis of subcutaneous tissue and fascia and usually accompanied by severe systemic toxicity (FISHER et al. 1979; SCHMID et al. 1998). Predisposing conditions for necrotizing fasciitis in the lower leg or ankle include diabetes mellitus or soft-tissue ischemia (FISHER et al. 1979; FRY et al. 1998; WYSOKI et al. 1997). Clinically, progressive necrosis of the skin and subcutaneous tissues is seen. Blisters and bullae are common with group A streptococcal infections. However, subcutaneous necrosis and severe infection extend well beyond the edges of

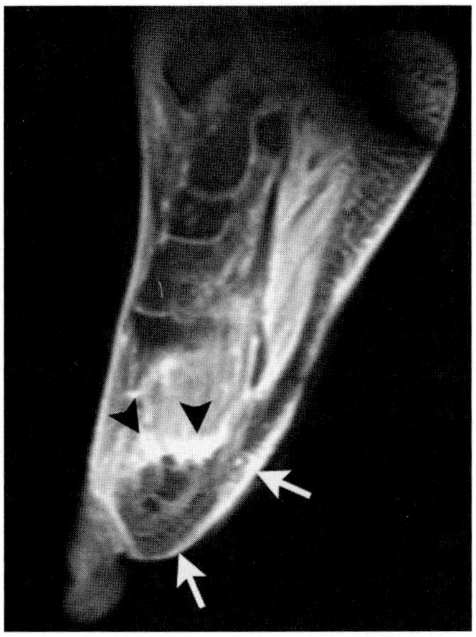

Fig. 13.8. Diagnosis of necrotic tissue by MR imaging. Contrast-enhanced fat-suppressed image reveals nonenhancing tissue at the plantar aspect of the forefoot (*arrows*). Note sharp demarcation of nonenhancing area and rim of enhancement (*arrowheads*) at the periphery of nonenhancing tissue

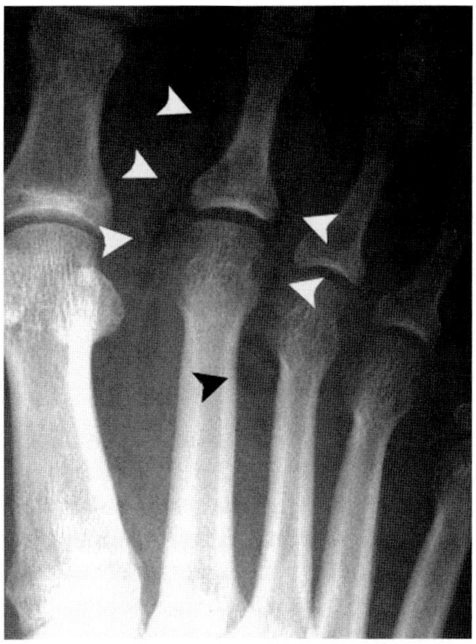

Fig. 13.9. Nonclostridial gas-forming infection of the second toe with extension of gas bubbles (*arrowheads*) proximally into the forefoot

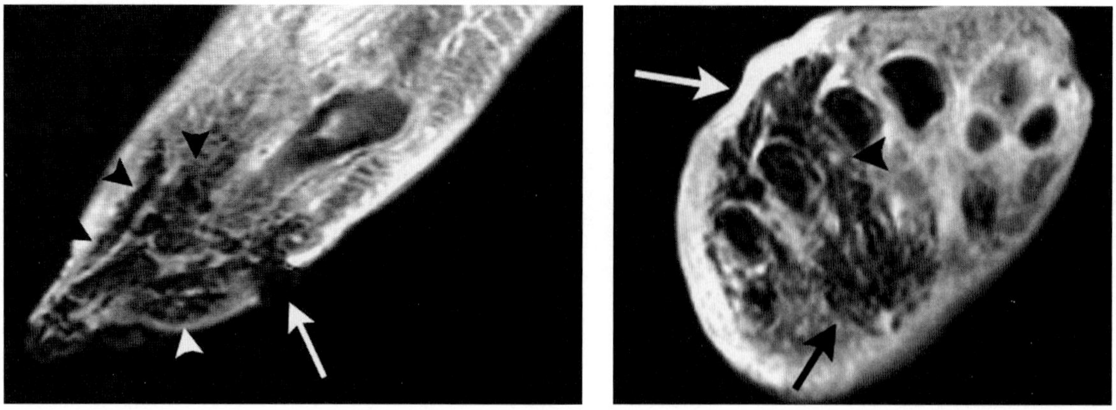

a b

Fig. 13.10a,b. MR signal characteristics of a gas-producing infection. **a** T1-weighted, contrast-enhanced, fat-suppressed image with an ulcer (*arrow*) below the fifth metatarsophalangeal joint. Note extensive gas inclusions on the plantar (*white arrowhead*) and dorsal (*black arrowheads*) aspect of the forefoot. **b** T1-weighted, contrast-enhanced, fat-suppressed image shows gas inclusions in the central plantar compartment (*black arrow*), the interosseous compartment (*arrowhead*), and the dorsal compartment (*white arrow*)

the superficially apparent wound necrosis. Plain radiographs may reveal soft-tissue thickening and gas inclusion (Fisher et al. 1979). CT studies exhibit asymmetric fascial thickening and fat stranding in 80% of patients and may additionally disclose abscesses in approximately one-third of patients (Walshaw and Deans 1996; Wysoki et al. 1997). MR imaging criteria for the diagnosis of necrotizing fasciitis include thickening of fascia with fluid collections and enhancement after contrast administration (Fig. 13.11) (Schmid et al. 1998). These signs are, however, not specific and may also be seen in other conditions such as cellulitis, abscess, dermatomyositis, and posttraumatic states (Arslan et al. 2000; Loh et al. 1997; Schmid et al. 1998).

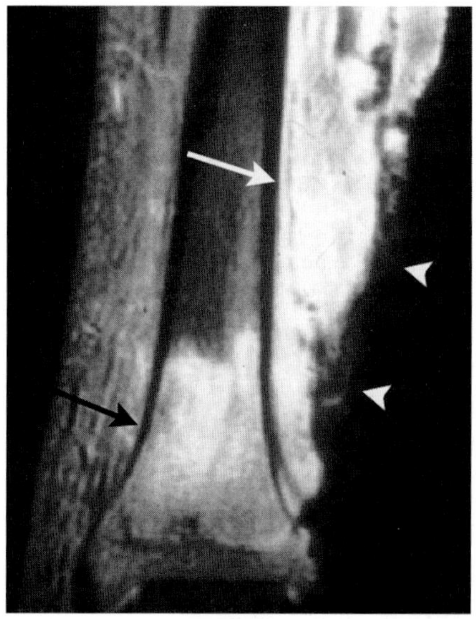

Fig. 13.11. Extensive infection of the lower leg in a patient with necrotizing fasciitis. There is a large soft-tissue defect with necrotic nonenhancing tissue (*arrowheads*) on the wound surface and diffuse enhancement of the muscle compartment (*white arrow*). Note also osteomyelitis of the distal tibia (*black arrow*)

13.7 Abscess Formation

13.7.1 Soft-Tissue Abscess

Abscess formation is generally seen in more indolent or long-standing infections but can also be seen in aggressive disease. The incidence in patients with foot infections referred for MR imaging ranges from 10% (Croll et al. 1996) to 50% (Beltran et al. 1990; Cook et al. 1996; Ledermann et al. 2002d) depending on the patient selection. Soft-tissue abscesses generally form in proximity to the entry site of infection or adjacent to fascial planes (Ledermann et al. 2002d); however, as infection spreads along the compartments, abscesses can develop far from the skin ulcer. On MR images, abscess is seen as a focal collection of signal which approximates fluid, with thick rim enhancement on postcontrast images (Fig. 13.12) (Dangman et al. 1992; Paajanen et al. 1987). However, as discussed earlier, this rim enhancement will not be seen in areas of tissue devitalization or severe ischemia (Ledermann et al. 2002c); in this setting, focal fluid signal will be seen on T2-weighted images in a broader region with

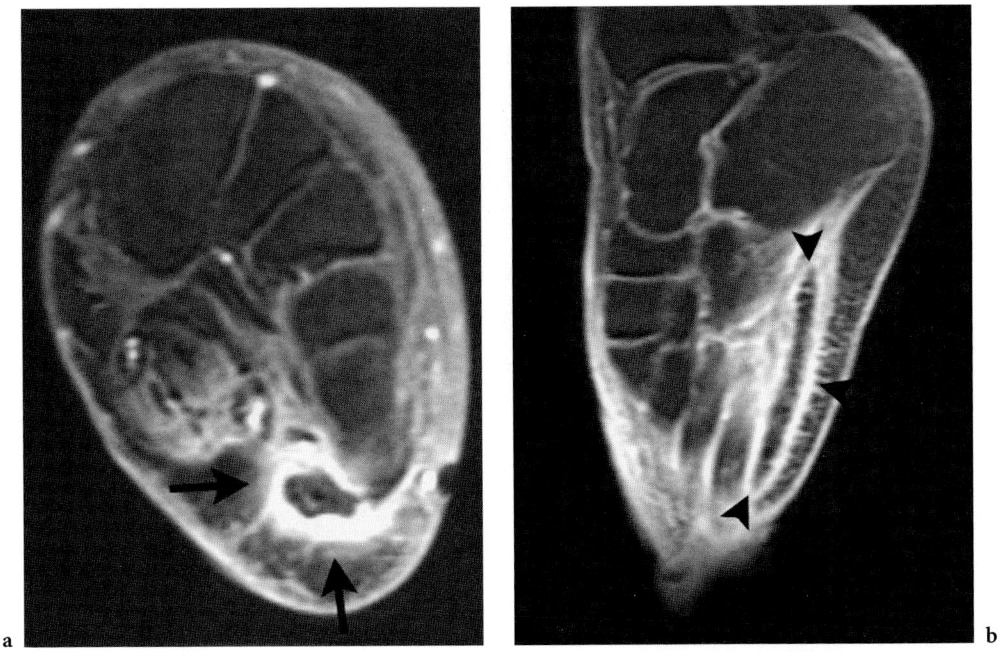

Fig. 13.12a,b. Lateral plantar space abscess. **a** Axial T1-weighted, contrast-enhanced, fat-suppressed image reveals thick rim enhancement (*arrows*) around the abscess which is confined to the lateral plantar compartment. **b** Sagittal T1-weighted, contrast-enhanced, fat-suppressed image reveals that the abscess (*arrowheads*) occupies the entire length of the lateral plantar compartment

absence of enhancement compared with the surrounding tissue. This represents liquified necrotic tissue. Abscesses often communicate with sinus tracts which extend to bones, joints, tendon sheaths, or the skin surface.

13.7.2 Intraosseous Abscess

Intraosseous abscesses can originate from hematogenous infection or more commonly from spread of infection from an adjacent skin ulcer. Hematogenous intraosseous abscesses, also known as Brodie's abscesses, typically occur in children and young adults, with *Staphylococcus aureus* as the organism most commonly isolated (Waldvogel et al. 1970). The metaphyseal regions of growing ends of long bones of the lower extremities are typically affected, such as the femur, tibia, and fibula (Winters 1960). Since most patients present with equivocal clinical symptoms, a radiologic work-up is critical in assessing the diagnosis (Alter and Sprinkle 1995). Classic radiographic findings of a Brodie's abscess include a well-defined lytic lesion with a geographic pattern of destruction and absence of bone enlargement, matrix, or cortical break (Lopes et al. 1997). However, atypical presentations have been reported including diaphyseal location (33%), associated cortical thickening (50%), periosteal reaction (40%), and sequestra (20%) (Miller et al. 1979). Therefore, atypical presentations of Brodie's abscesses can be mistaken for osteoid osteoma due to the extensive sclerotic reaction (Miller et al. 1979; Sim et al. 1975) or aggressive lesions due to periosteal reaction or mottled bone destruction in more aggressive infection (Miller et al. 1979). On MR imaging, typical findings of Brodie's abscess include a 'target' appearance with a center of low signal intensity on T1-weighted images and high signal on T2-weighted images (Fig. 13.13) (Marti-Bonmati et al. 1993). More peripherally, two concentric rings may be seen: An inner ring corresponding to granulation tissue with isointense signal to muscle on T1-weighted images and high signal on T2-weighted images and contrast enhancement (Fig. 13.13). The outer ring, which is hypointense on T1-weighted and T2-weighted images, probably represents eburnated bone or fibrotic reaction (Marti-Bonmati et al. 1993). However, the appearance of intraosseous abscesses in part depends on the aggressiveness of the infection. A more indolent infection will display the typical findings of a Brodie's abscess (Azouz et al. 1993; Dangman et al. 1992; Tang et al. 1988). In a rapidly progressive infection, however, the signal may not be equivalent to fluid on T2-weighted images, and rather than rim enhancement, an ill-defined region of

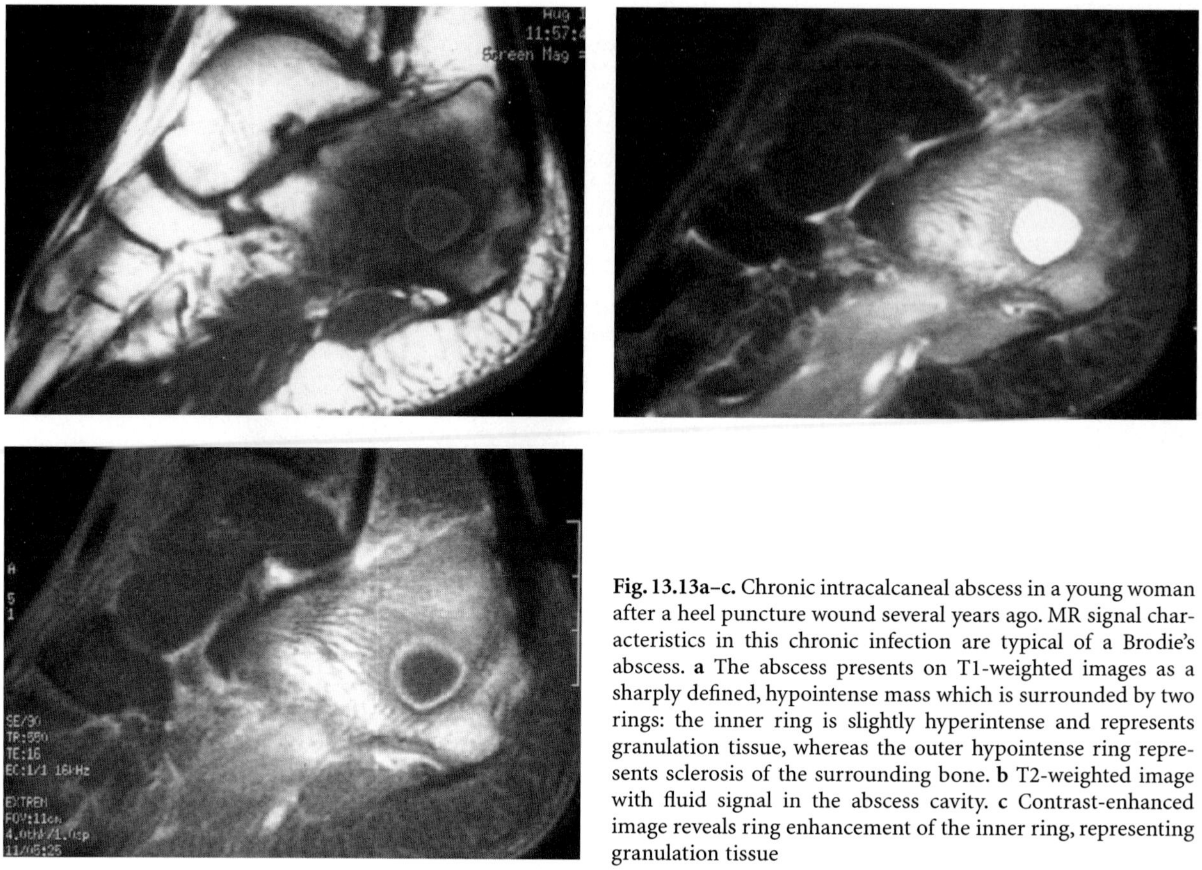

Fig. 13.13a–c. Chronic intracalcaneal abscess in a young woman after a heel puncture wound several years ago. MR signal characteristics in this chronic infection are typical of a Brodie's abscess. **a** The abscess presents on T1-weighted images as a sharply defined, hypointense mass which is surrounded by two rings: the inner ring is slightly hyperintense and represents granulation tissue, whereas the outer hypointense ring represents sclerosis of the surrounding bone. **b** T2-weighted image with fluid signal in the abscess cavity. **c** Contrast-enhanced image reveals ring enhancement of the inner ring, representing granulation tissue

nonenhancement is seen, representing a more acute area of devitalization.

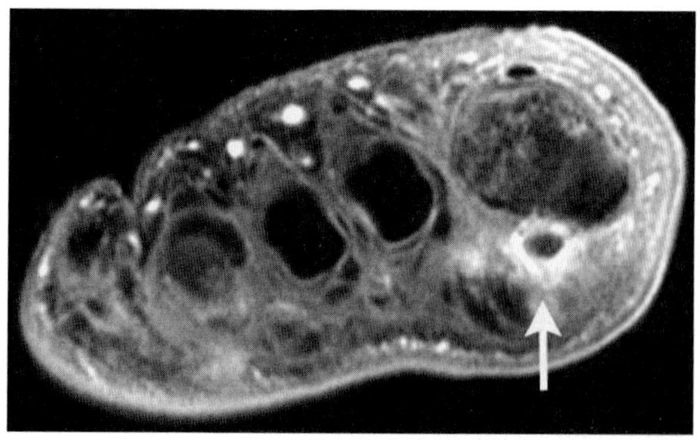

Fig. 13.14. Axial T1-weighted, contrast-enhanced, fat-suppressed image with thick contrast enhancement of the tendon sheath of the first flexor tendon (*arrow*) compatible with septic tenosynovitis

13.8 Septic Tenosynovitis

Similar to septic arthritis, septic tenosynovitis of the foot and ankle is typically a result of contiguous spread (Boutin et al. 1998; Ledermann et al. 2002e). The tendons of the toes course directly below frequently ulcerated areas such as the metatarsophalangeal and interphalangeal joints and are often involved in deep infection. However, infection of the flexor hallicus longus sheath can also result from septic arthritis of the ankle or subtalar joint with which it communicates. MR imaging reveals disproportionate fluid within the sheath which is often complex. Post-contrast images show a thick rim of enhancement representing the proliferative, inflamed synovium (Fig. 13.14) (Jaovisidha et al. 1996). Radiographic signs consist of soft-tissue swelling and, occasionally, subjacent osteomyelitis (Boutin et al. 1998). An often cited complication of septic tenosynovitis of the flexor tendons of the toes is proximal spread of infection into the central plantar compartment with abscess formation (Fig. 13.15) (Bernhard et al. 1984; Bose 1979). In the hindfoot, proximal spread of infection along the flexor tendons from the central plantar compartment into the lower leg has also been reported

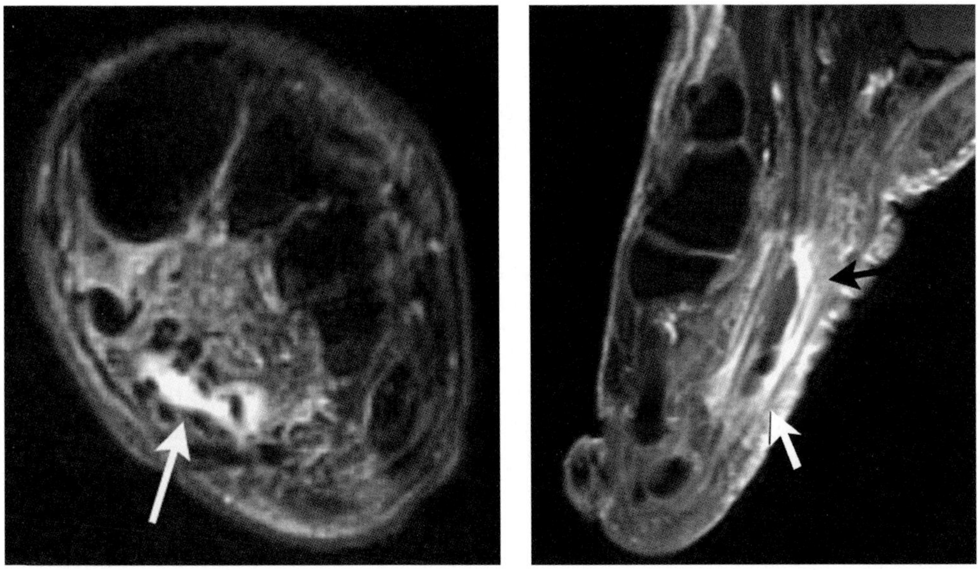

a b

Fig. 13.15a,b. Central plantar space abscess originating from a second toe infection. **a** Axial T2-weighted fat-suppressed image demonstrates a fluid collection (*arrow*) in the central plantar space. **b** Sagittal T1-weighted, contrast-enhanced, fat-suppressed image confirms the presence of an abscess with rim enhancement (*arrows*)

(Loeffler and Ballard 1980; Manoli and Weber 1990). This potential route of spread of infection along the flexor tendons of the hindfoot has been confirmed by direct injections into the plantar compartment of cadaveric feet with ascension of the injected material into the lower leg (Feingold et al. 1977; Kamel and Sakla 1961). In our experience, most cases of pedal septic tenosynovitis remain confined to the area of infection (Ledermann et al. 2002e). Development of a plantar space abscess along the flexor tendons of the toes or proximal spread of infection into the lower leg is rarely seen in our practice on MR imaging (Ledermann et al. 2002e).

13.9 Osteomyelitis

Osteomyelitis can involve the foot and ankle via contiguous spread, direct implantation, or hematogenous spread. Although hematogenous spread is the most common route in other areas of the body such as the spine, contiguous spread and direct implantation are much more common in the foot and ankle because they are susceptible to vascular disease, neuropathy, and trauma. Direct implantation is the second most common route of spread and can occur from puncture wounds, deep lacerations, open fractures, surgery, and injection procedures. However, the vast majority of cases of osteomyelitis involving the foot and ankle occur through contiguous spread from adjacent soft-tissue infection (Ledermann et al. 2002a; Lipsky et al. 1990).

13.9.1 Radiography

For patients with the clinical suspicion of foot or ankle infection, radiographs are typically the initial radiologic study obtained (Boutin et al. 1998; Gold et al. 1995; Schauwecker et al. 1990). Plain radiographs provide information regarding postoperative changes, calcifications, foreign bodies, soft-tissue gas, arthritis, neuropathic disease, and deformities, and are very useful for comparison with MR images. However, radiographic findings of osteomyelitis do not appear for 10–14 days and until 35%–50% of the bone has been destroyed (Curtiss 1973; Dalinka et al. 1975). Radiographic changes are not only delayed (Capitanio and Kirkpatrick 1970; David et al. 1987; Schauwecker et al. 1990), but sensitivity is poor (Newman et al. 1991; Wang et al. 1990; Weinstein et al. 1993; Yuh et al. 1989). The first signs of contiguous spread of infection to adjacent bone on plain radiographs include soft-tissue swelling and periosteal reaction. These signs are nonspecific, however, and can also be seen in the presence of soft-tissue infection or after traumatic irritation of periosteal bone (Boutin et al. 1998). With progression of the infectious process, cortical disruption and medullary involvement ensue (Fig. 13.16).

13.9.2 Computed Tomography

MR imaging has largely replaced CT in the evaluation of pedal infections. CT may, however, be useful to evaluate the presence of sequestra and involucra in chronic osteomyelitis (Ledermann et al. 2000). A sequestrum is a piece of necrotic bone which is separated from living bone by granulation tissue. An involucrum is a layer of living bone which has formed about the sequestrum. Since CT offers exceptional detail of the bony architecture in a cross-sectional display, it can also be used to evaluate cortical destruction, periosteal new bone formation, and the presence of intraosseous gas (Azouz 1981; Gold et al. 1991, 1995; Magid and Fishman 1992; Maurer et al. 1992; Seltzer 1984; Wing et al. 1985), all of which are less conspicuous on MR images.

13.9.3 Magnetic Resonance Imaging

Utilization of MRI for the evaluation of infection of the foot and ankle has increased dramatically over the past decade. Numerous studies have investigated the utility of MR imaging for the evaluation of osteomyelitis of the foot and ankle (Beltran et al. 1990; Cook et al. 1996; Craig et al. 1997; Croll et al. 1996; Durham et al. 1991; Horowitz et al. 1993; Ledermann et al. 2002a; Levine et al. 1994; Lipman et al. 1998; Morrison et al. 1995; Newman et al. 1992; Nigro et al. 1992; Seabold et al. 1990; Wang et al. 1990; Weinstein et al. 1993; Wrobel and Connolly 1998; Yuh et al. 1989). In studies which included more than 25 patients, sensitivity ranged from 77% (Levine et al. 1994) to 100% (Weinstein et al. 1993; Yuh et al. 1989), and specificity ranged from 79% (Ledermann et al. 2002a) to 100% (Croll et al. 1996; Levine et al. 1994). A summary of all studies which included at least 25 patients and provided data concerning sensitivity, specificity, and accuracy is provided in Table 13.1.

The diagnosis of osteomyelitis on MR images is based on identification of an altered bone marrow signal. Infection of the marrow compartment results in loss of the normal fatty marrow signal on T1-weighted images, with edema on T2-weighted or STIR images and enhancement on post-gadolinium T1-weighted images (Fig. 13.17) (Morrison et al. 1993). Identification of this finding away from the subchondral bone results in high sensitivity for osteomyelitis; however, other entities can alter the bone marrow signal in a similar fashion, including fracture, tumor, severe inflammatory arthritis or neuropathic disease, or recent postoperative change (Beltran et al. 1990; Daffner et al. 1986; Gold

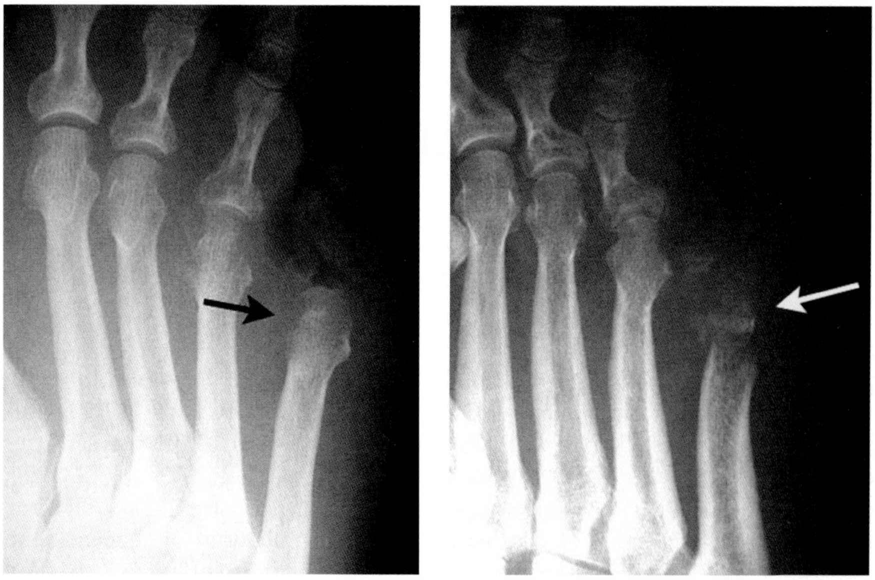

Fig. 13.16a,b. Osteomyelitis of the fifth metatarsal head after amputation of the fifth toe. **a** Cortical destruction (*arrow*) of the medial aspect of the fifth metatarsal head proves the presence of bone infection. **b** Follow-up radiograph after 2 months of conservative treatment reveals progression of osteomyelitis with total destruction of the fifth metatarsal head (*arrow*)

Table 13.1. Utility of MR imaging for the evaluation of osteomyelitis of the foot and ankle. Only reports that included at least 25 patients and provided data concerning sensitivity, specificity, and accuracy in the diagnosis of osteomyelitis were included

Author	Year	Patients/path. or culture proven	Sensitivity	Specificity	Accuracy	Comments
CROLL et al.	1996	27/21	88%	100%	95%	1.5 Tesla, no gadolinium
MORRISON et al.	1995	59/41	82% diabetic	80% diabetic	89%	53 patients with gadolinium and fat-supression
			89% not diabetic	94% not diabetic		
LEVINE et al.	1994	27/18	77%	100%	90%	1.5 Tesla, no gadolinium
WEINSTEIN et al.	1993	47/32	100%	81%	95%	0.5 Tesla (n=20) and 1.5 Tesla (n=27), no gadolinium, prospective
NIGRO et al.	1992	44/34	100%	95%	98%	1.5 Tesla, no gadolinium
LEDERMANN et al.	2002	158/158	90%	79%	87%	158 patients with gadolinium, 1.5 Tesla
WANG et al.	1990	50/32	99%	81%	94%	0.5 Tesla (n=23), 1.5 Tesla (n=27), no gadolinium

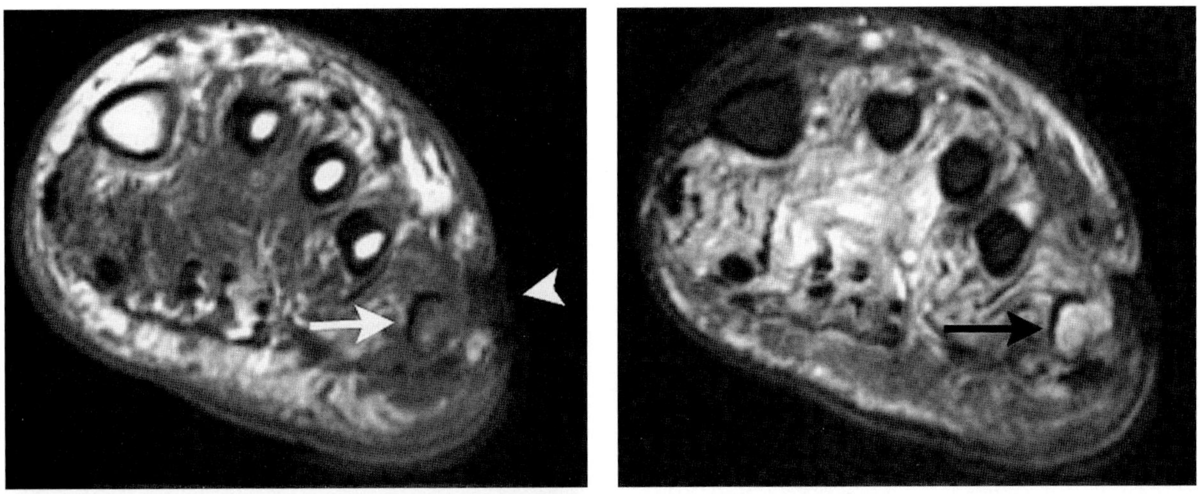

a b

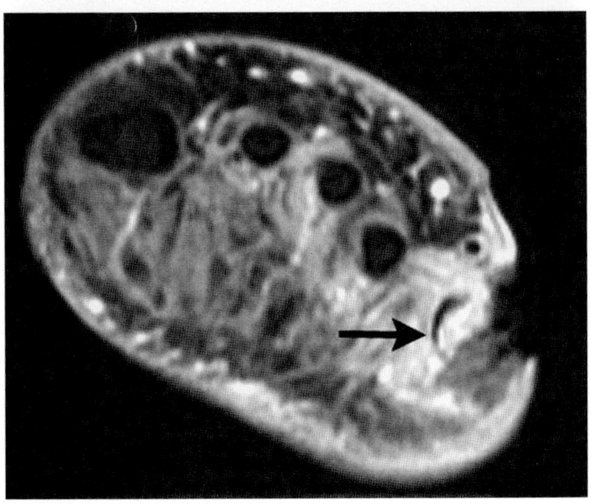

c

Fig. 13.17a–c. Osteomyelitis of the fifth metatarsal shaft. **a** T1-weighted image reveals an ulcer (*arrowhead*) at the lateral forefoot and hypointense signal in the bone marrow of the fifth metatarsal bone (*arrow*) indicative of osteomyelitis. **b** T2-weighted fat-suppressed image with hyperintense signal in the bone marrow of the fifth metatarsal bone (*arrow*) compatible with osteomyelitis. **c** T1-weighted, contrast-enhanced, fat-suppressed image with contrast enhancement of the fifth metatarsal confirming osteomyelitis et al. 1995; Jelinek et al. 1996; Moore et al. 1991; Morrison et al. 1993; Seabold et al. 1990). Evaluation of the pattern of signal abnormality helps distinguish infection from these other entities, and identification of a fracture line, a discrete lesion, adjacent arthritis or neuropathic disease, or postoperative metal artifact improves the specificity; in this regard, correlation with radiographs and the clinical history is important. Over 90% of cases of osteomyelitis of the foot and ankle are a result of contiguous spread through the skin (Bamberger et al. 1987; Lipsky et al. 1990); therefore, the majority of cases of osteomyelitis also have some combination of adjacent skin ulceration, cellulitis, soft-tissue abscess, and sinus tract (Craig et al. 1997; Ledermann et al. 2002a). These signs can be thought of as 'secondary signs' of osteomyelitis and can also improve the specificity (Morrison et al. 1998). Secondary signs are also important in situations where findings on different MR imaging sequences are discordant; for example, a minority of cases of osteomyelitis demonstrate normal or near-normal marrow signal on T1-weighted images but show edema and enhancement (Morrison et al. 1998). This would not be unexpected in the pathogenesis of osteomyelitis, since the fatty marrow is not immediately destroyed, but rather is probably metabolized at a rate dependent on the extent of inflammation. Similarly, infected marrow may show fat replacement and edema, but little or no enhancement if the vascular supply is compromised (Park et al. 1982). In these situations, identification of associated soft-tissue infection improves the reader's confidence about the diagnosis of osteomyelitis.

Some manifestations of osteomyelitis may have atypical signal characteristics; these include chronic osteomyelitis and sclerosing osteomyelitis as well as gangrene (Gold et al. 1995). Gangrene will be discussed in Chapter 14. Chronic osteomyelitis and sclerosing osteomyelitis are indolent processes with areas of bone necrosis and sclerosis; as a result, MR imaging may show areas of low signal on T1-weighted and T2-weighted images (Erdman et al. 1991; Tang et al. 1988). Foci of granulation tissue are often seen, with intermediate to high T2 signal and enhancement. The activity of the infection can be difficult to determine unless there are ill-defined areas of marrow edema and enhancement and bone erosion or destruction (Dangman et al. 1992). In this regard, comparison with previous studies is very important to document stability. Biopsy should be directed to the areas of enhancement or bone destruction but is often culture-negative despite active infection.

13.9.4 Radionuclide Studies

Technetium-99 m methylene diphosphonate (MDP) three-phase bone scans have a high sensitivity for osteomyelitis (Fig. 13.18) (Crim and Seeger 1994; Israel et al. 1987; Keenan et al. 1989; Larcos et al. 1991; Maurer et al. 1986; Newman et al. 1991; Seldin et al. 1985; Weinstein et al. 1993; Yuh et al. 1989) and are excellent for excluding bone infection in the presence of a normal radiograph, but their specificity is low (Graham et al. 1983; Knight et al. 1988; Larcos et al. 1991; Morrison et al. 1993; Seabold et al. 1989; Yuh et al. 1989). Increased accumulation

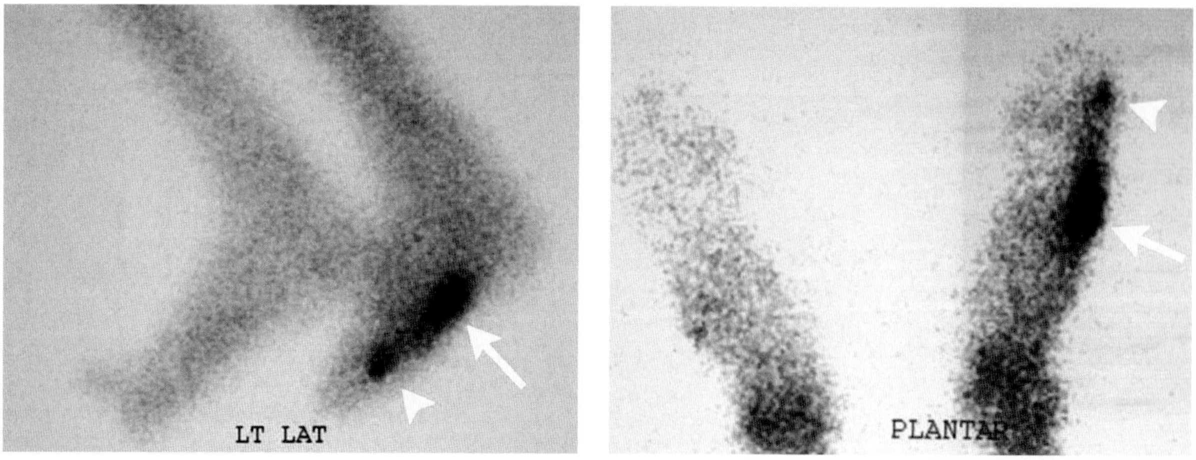

a b

Fig. 13.18a,b. Bone scan (Tc-99 m MDP) of a patient with an ulcer at the tip of the fifth toe and at the lateral forefoot. **a** Blood-pool phase with increased tracer activity in the region of the lateral forefoot (*arrow*) and at the tip of the fifth toe (*arrowhead*) indicating hyperemia. **b** A 24-h delayed phase with increased tracer activity in the distal fifth phalanx and the fifth metatarsal, confirming osteomyelitis in both locations of tracer can be seen in other conditions such as bone tumors, neuropathic osteoarthropathy, fractures, and following trauma and surgery. One advantage of Tc-99 m MDP studies over radiography is that they can detect osteomyelitis within 24–48 h of onset (Gold et al. 1991). Gallium-67 scans are also used to diagnose pedal osteomyelitis. However, abnormal uptake is also seen in neoplasms, hematomas, and areas of increased bone turnover such as healing fractures, surgical sites, and neuropathic arthropathy (Alazraki et al. 1985; Boutin et al. 1998; Deysine et al. 1975; Donohoe 1998; Rosenthall et al. 1979).

Further disadvantages of gallium-67 scans are the physical characteristics of the radiopharmaceutical, with high energies and long physical half-life and the necessity to image patients up to 72–96 h after injection.

Labeled white blood cell scans have a higher specificity (Maurer et al. 1986) to detect osteomyelitis and may be helpful in excluding infection in a Charcot joint (Schauwecker 1995). The drawbacks of this method are: time consuming preparation and handling of blood products, poor spatial resolution (Jacobson et al. 1991; McAfee and Samin 1985), and reduced sensitivity in detecting chronic osteomyelitis (Schauwecker et al. 1984; Schauwecker 1989). Since both gallium-67 citrate and indium-111-labeled leukocyte studies are usually combined with technetium-99 m scans, studies require up to 3 days to complete (Boutin et al. 1998). Therefore, the costs can be greater than that of MR imaging (Donohoe 1998).

13.10 Septic Arthritis

Septic arthritis in the foot and ankle may arise via hematogenous spread but is more commonly seen as a complication of adjacent soft-tissue infection (Brower 1996; Ledermann et al. 2002a). In the phalanges, this is often due to breakdown of callus at the dorsal aspect of the toes (Armstrong and Lavery 1998). At the MTP joints, septic arthritis is usually due to communication with plantar ulcers (or medial ulceration at the first MTP joint) (Ledermann et al. 2002a). Septic arthritis at the midfoot is not as common but may be seen in patients with foot deformity related to neuropathic disease; with loss of the arch, ulcers can form directly under the Lisfranc or Chopart joint. Ankle or subtalar joint involvement is often related to infection arising over the malleoli or over the posterior calcaneal tubercle. Since the ankle and subtalar joints communicate in approximately 20% of feet, infection can spread to both joints simultaneously.

13.10.1 Radiography

Radiographs will first demonstrate symmetric periarticular soft-tissue swelling, which represents cellulitis and joint effusion (Butt 1973). This finding is often seen in infections of the ankle joint (Fig. 13.19) (Brower 1996) but may not be as obvious in infections of smaller joints such as the interphalangeal joints. Marginal juxtaarticular bone erosion and joint space loss due to cartilage destruction are seen with further progression (Fig. 13.20) (Brower 1996). Involvement of adjacent osseous structures results in moth-eaten bony destruction and periostitis.

13.10.2 Magnetic Resonance Imaging

On MR images of a septic joint, an effusion is typically seen, although it may be decompressed by drainage through the skin and may not be large (Ledermann et al. 2002a). Synovial thickening and enhancement are present but may be subtle, especially in the small joints of the digits. Unfortunately, MR imaging cannot definitively discern between septic arthritis and other causes of joint inflammation. However, the

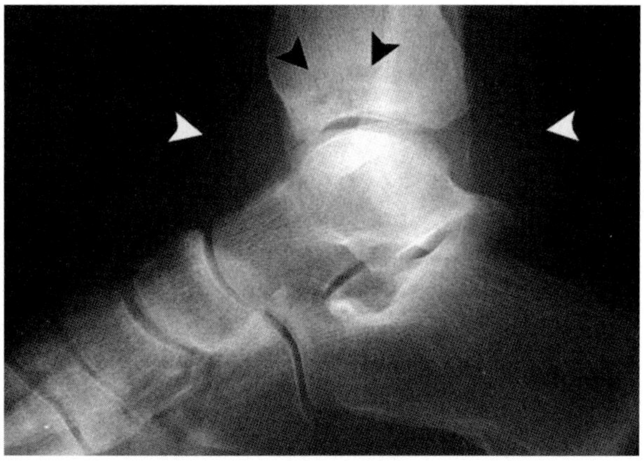

Fig. 13.19. Septic arthritis of the ankle joint with soft-tissue swelling (*white arrowheads*) due to joint effusion and surrounding cellulitis. Note also ill-defined bone destruction (*black arrowheads*) in the anterior distal tibial epiphysis due to an intraosseous abscess

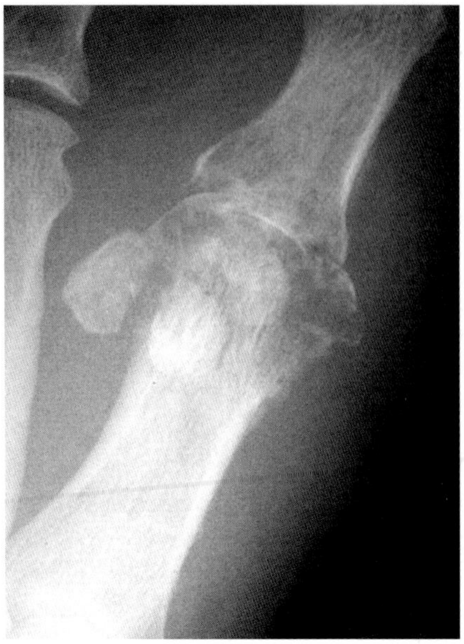

Fig. 13.20. Septic arthritis of the first metatarsophalangeal joint. Note joint space narrowing, periarticular bone resorption, marginal bone erosion, and surrounding soft-tissue swelling

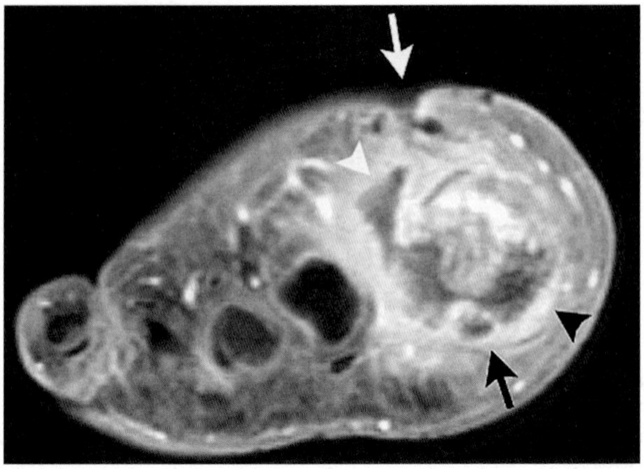

Fig. 13.21. Septic arthritis of the first metatarsophalangeal joint due to dorsal ulceration (*white arrow*). T1-weighted, contrast-enhanced, fat-suppressed image reveals an interdigital sinus tract (*white arrowhead*) with communication to the infected joint. Note thick synovial enhancement (*black arrowhead*) and ring enhancement of the flexor hallucis tendon compatible with septic tenosynovitis (*black arrow*)

combination of bone erosions with marrow edema is highly suggestive of a septic articulation on MR imaging (Fig. 13.21) (Graif et al. 1999). The coexistence of synovial thickening, synovial edema, soft-tissue edema, or bone marrow enhancement increases the level of confidence (Graif et al. 1999). MR diagnosis of a septic joint in pedal infection may be more specific than in other parts of the body since there will be adjacent skin ulceration in the vast majority of cases (Ledermann et al. 2002a). Additionally, sinus tracks can sometimes be seen extending to the infected joint (Fig. 13.21). If bone marrow edema is confined to a thin rim beneath the cortex, it is not indicative of secondary osteomyelitis. However, if the edema or enhancement extends into the medullary bone, osteomyelitis should be considered.

13.10.3 Radionuclide Studies

Bone scintigraphy using technetium-99 m MDPwill display pathologic uptake around the involved joint during the vascular and blood pool phases. During the third 'bone' phase, uptake in the adjacent articular bone can be seen (Brower 1996; Donohoe 1998). Although bone scintigraphy is very sensitive, it is not specific because any inflammatory arthropathy or a neuropathic joint results in similar changes. Extensive purulent joint effusion may lead to decreased perfusion of the synovium with a cold scan (Mitchell et al. 1988). Gallium-67 citrate is not accumulated by the epiphyseal plate, unlike diphosphonates, and is therefore helpful in pediatric arthritis but is also a nonspecific test. Other disadvantages of gallium-67 scintigraphy were mentioned earlier in this chapter in Section 13.9.4. Additional 111-oxine labeled leukocyte scan improves the specificity (Boutin et al. 1998), but chronic infections with predominant lymphocytic infiltration may lead to decreased uptake.

13.11 MR Imaging Protocols in Pedal Infection

MR imaging protocols vary widely, but attention to some general principles can help optimize the examination. If the primary site of infection is known, coil selection and imaging planes should be tailored; for example, an extremity coil is excellent for imaging the ankle but often results in suboptimal examination of the toes. For toe imaging, 3-inch or 5-inch surface coils are preferred. However, if the main concern is extent of proximal spread, the small surface coils may not provide adequate coverage. A minimum of two planes should be acquired; plane selection should also be tailored to the situation. For the toes, images coronal to the body should be included since the tiny bones easily volume average in the sagittal and axial planes.

Fat suppression is important to use when performing T2-weighted sequences; otherwise edema will not be apparent. If fat suppression is suboptimal or unavailable, a STIR sequence should be acquired. Some studies recommend intravenous contrast (Dangman et al. 1992; Morrison et al. 1993), whereas others question its benefit (Craig et al. 1997; Marcus et al. 1996; Miller et al. 1997). It remains controversial whether contrast improves the accuracy for the diagnosis of osteomyelitis. However, it is clear that contrast improves the detection of soft-tissue pathology (Dangman et al. 1992; Hopkins et al. 1995). It differentiates cellulitis from diabetic soft-tissue edema and improves evaluation of the soft-tissue extent (Craig et al. 1997; Morrison et al. 1995). It helps detect sinus tracts and abscesses (Ledermann et al. 2002d) as well as areas of devitalization or necrosis (Ledermann et al. 2002c). Therefore, despite the increased cost, its use is essential if the patient is being considered for surgical management. Fat suppression is also important when acquiring post-contrast T1-weighted images (Morrison et al. 1993).

References

Alazraki N, Fierer J, Resnick D (1985) Chronic osteomyelitis: monitoring by 99mTc phosphate and 67 Ga citrate imaging. AJR. 145:767–771

Alter SA, Sprinkle RW (1995) Brodie's abscess: a case report. J Foot Ankle Surg 34:208–214

Armstrong DG, Lavery LA (1998) Diabetic foot ulcers: prevention, diagnosis and classification. Am Fam Physician 57: 1325–1328

Arslan A, Pierre-Jerome C, Borthne A (2000) Necrotizing fasciitis: unreliable MRI findings in the preoperative diagnosis. Eur J Radiol 36:139–143

Azouz EM (1981) Computed tomography in bone and joint infections. J Can Assoc Radiol 32:102–106

Azouz EM, Greenspan A, Marton D (1993) CT evaluation of primary epiphyseal bone abscesses. Skeletal Radiol 22:17–23

Bamberger DM, Daus GP, Gerding DN (1987) Osteomyelitis in the feet of diabetic patients. Long-term results, prognostic factors, and the role of antimicrobial and surgical therapy. Am J Med 83:653–660

Beltran J, Campanini DS, Knight C et al (1990) The diabetic foot: magnetic resonance imaging evaluation. Skeletal Radiol 19:37–41

Bernhard LM, Bakst M, Coleman W et al (1984) Plantar space abscesses in the diabetic foot: diagnosis and treatment. J Foot Surg 23:283–290

Bessman AN, Wagner W (1975) Nonclostridial gas gangrene. Report of 48 cases and review of the literature. JAMA 233: 958–963

Bose K (1979) A surgical approach for the infected diabetic foot. Int Orthop 3:177–181

Boutin RD, Brossmann J, Sartoris DJ et al (1998) Update on imaging of orthopedic infections. Orthop Clin North Am 29:41–66

Brower AC (1996) Septic arthritis. Radiol Clin North Am 34: 293–309

Butt WP (1973) Radiology of the infected joint. Clin Orthop 96:136–149

Capitanio MA, Kirkpatrick JA (1970) Early roentgen observations in acute osteomyelitis. Am J Roentgenol Radium Ther Nucl Med 108:488–496

Cook TA, Rahim N, Simpson HC et al (1996) Magnetic resonance imaging in the management of diabetic foot infection. Br J Surg 83:245–248

Craig JG, Amin MB, Wu K et al (1997) Osteomyelitis of the diabetic foot: MR imaging-pathologic correlation. Radiology 203:849–855

Crim JR, Seeger LL (1994) Imaging evaluation of osteomyelitis. Crit Rev Diagn Imaging 35:201–256

Croll SD, Nicholas GG, Osborne MA et al (1996) Role of magnetic resonance imaging in the diagnosis of osteomyelitis in diabetic foot infections. J Vasc Surg 24:266–270

Curtiss PH Jr (1973) Some uncommon forms of osteomyelitis. Clin Orthop 96:84–87

Daffner RH, Lupetin AR, Dash N et al (1986) MRI in the detection of malignant infiltration of bone marrow. AJR 146:353–358

Dalinka MK, Lally JF, Koniver G et al (1975) The radiology of osseous and articular infection. CRC Crit Rev Clin Radiol Nucl Med 7:1–64

Dangman BC, Hoffer FA, Rand FF et al (1992) Osteomyelitis in children: gadolinium-enhanced MR imaging. Radiology 182:743–747

David R, Barron BJ, Madewell JE (1987) Osteomyelitis, acute and chronic. Radiol Clin North Am 25:1171–1201

Deysine M, Rafkin H, Teicher I et al (1975) Diagnosis of chronic and postoperative osteomyelitis with gallium 67 citrate scans. Am J Surg 129:632–635

Donohoe KJ (1998) Selected topics in orthopedic nuclear medicine. Orthop Clin North Am 29:85–101

Durham JR, Lukens ML, Campanini DS et al (1991) Impact of magnetic resonance imaging on the management of diabetic foot infections. Am J Surg 162:150–153

Erdman WA, Tamburro F, Jayson HT et al (1991) Osteomyelitis: characteristics and pitfalls of diagnosis with MR imaging. Radiology 180:533–539

Feingold ML, Resnick D, Niwayama G et al (1977) The plantar compartments of the foot: a roentgen approach I. Experimental observations. Invest Radiol 12:281–288

Fisher JR, Conway MJ, Takeshita RT et al (1979) Necrotizing fasciitis. Importance of roentgenographic studies for soft-tissue gas. JAMA 241:803–806

Fry DE, Marek JM, Langsfeld M (1998) Infection in the ischemic lower extremity. Surg Clin North Am 78:465–479

Gold RH, Hawkins RA, Katz RD (1991) Bacterial osteomyelitis: findings on plain radiography, CT, MR, and scintigraphy. AJR 157:365–370

Gold RH, Tong DJ, Crim JR et al (1995) Imaging the diabetic foot. Skeletal Radiol 24:563–571

Graham GD, Lundy MM, Moreno AJ et al (1983) The role of Tc-99 m MDP and Ga-67 citrate in predicting the cure of osteomyelitis. Clin Nucl Med 8:344–346

Graif M, Schweitzer ME, Deely D et al (1999) The septic versus nonseptic inflamed joint: MRI characteristics. Skeletal Radiol 28:616–620

Grayson ML, Gibbons GW, Balogh K et al (1995) Probing to

bone in infected pedal ulcers. A clinical sign of underlying osteomyelitis in diabetic patients. JAMA 273:721–723
Hopkins KL, Li KC, Bergman G (1995) Gadolinium-DTPA-enhanced magnetic resonance imaging of musculoskeletal infectious processes. Skeletal Radiol 24:325–330
Horowitz JD, Durham JR, Nease DB et al (1993) Prospective evaluation of magnetic resonance imaging in the management of acute diabetic foot infections. Ann Vasc Surg 7: 44–50
Israel O, Gips S, Jerushalmi J et al (1987) Osteomyelitis and soft-tissue infection: differential diagnosis with 24 hour/4 hour ratio of Tc-99 m MDP uptake. Radiology 163:725–726
Jacobson AF, Harley JD, Lipsky BA et al (1991) Diagnosis of osteomyelitis in the presence of soft-tissue infection and radiologic evidence of osseous abnormalities: value of leukocyte scintigraphy. AJR 157:807–812
Jacobson JA, Powell A, Craig JG et al (1998) Wooden foreign bodies in soft tissue: detection at US. Radiology 206: 45–48
Jaovisidha S, Chen C, Ryu KN et al (1996) Tuberculous tenosynovitis and bursitis: imaging findings in 21 cases. Radiology 201:507–513
Jelinek J, Pearl AB, Kominsky SJ et al (1996) Magnetic resonance imaging of the foot. Rheumatologic disorders mimicking osteomyelitis. J Am Podiatr Med Assoc 86:228–231
Kamel R, Sakla F (1961) Anatomical compartments of the sole of the human foot. Anat Rec 140:57–60
Keenan AM, Tindel NL, Alavi A (1989) Diagnosis of pedal osteomyelitis in diabetic patients using current scintigraphic techniques. Arch Intern Med 149:2262–2266
Knight D, Gray HW, McKillop JH et al (1988) Imaging for infection: caution required with the Charcot joint. Eur J Nucl Med 13:523–526
Larcos G, Brown ML, Sutton RT (1991) Diagnosis of osteomyelitis of the foot in diabetic patients: value of 111In-leukocyte scintigraphy. AJR 157:527–531
Ledermann HP, Kaim A, Bongartz G, Steinbrich W (2000) Pitfalls and limitations of magnetic resonance imaging in chronic posttraumatic osteomyelitis. Eur Radiol 10:1815–1823
Ledermann HP, Morrison WB, Schweitzer ME (2002a) MR image analysis of pedal osteomyelitis: distribution, patterns of spread, and frequency of associated ulceration and septic arthritis. Radiology 223:747–755
Ledermann HP, Morrison WB, Schweitzer ME (2002b) Is soft-tissue inflammation in pedal infection contained by fascial planes? MR analysis of compartmental involvement in 115 feet. AJR Am J Roentgenol 178:605–612
Ledermann HP, Schweitzer ME, Morrison WB (2002c) Non-enhancing tissue on MR imaging of pedal infection: characterization of necrotic tissue and associated limitations for diagnosis of osteomyelitis and abscess. AJR Am J Roentgenol 178:215–222
Ledermann HP, Morrison WB, Schweitzer ME (2002d) MR analysis of abscesses in patients with suspected pedal osteomyelitis. Radiology 224 (n press)
Ledermann HP, Morrison WB, Schweitzer ME (2002e) Tendon involvement in pedal infection: MR analysis of frequency, distribution and spread of infection along tendons. AJR Am J Roentgenol 179 (in press)
Levine SE, Neagle CE, Esterhai JL et al (1994) Magnetic resonance imaging for the diagnosis of osteomyelitis in the diabetic patient with a foot ulcer. Foot Ankle Int 15: 151–156
Lipman BT, Collier BD, Carrera GF et al (1998) Detection of osteomyelitis in the neuropathic foot: nuclear medicine, MRI and conventional radiography. Clin Nucl Med 23: 77–82
Lipsky BA, Pecoraro RE, Wheat LJ (1990) The diabetic foot. Soft tissue and bone infection. Infect Dis Clin North Am 4:409–432
Loeffler RD Jr, Ballard A (1980) Plantar fascial spaces of the foot and a proposed surgical approach. Foot Ankle 1: 11–14
Loh NN, Ch'en IY, Cheung LP et al (1997) Deep fascial hyperintensity in soft-tissue abnormalities as revealed by T2-weighted MR imaging. AJR 168:1301–1304
Lopes TD, Reinus WR, Wilson AJ (1997) Quantitative analysis of the plain radiographic appearance of Brodie's abscess. Invest Radiol 32:51–58
Magid D, Fishman EK (1992) Musculoskeletal infections in patients with AIDS: CT findings. AJR 158:603–607
Manoli A, Weber TG (1990) Fasciotomy of the foot: an anatomical study with special reference to release of the calcaneal compartment. Foot Ankle 10:267–275
Marcus CD, Ladam-Marcus VJ, Leone J et al (1996) MR imaging of osteomyelitis and neuropathic osteoarthropathy in the feet of diabetics. Radiographics 16:1337–1348
Marti-Bonmati L, Aparisi F, Poyatos C et al (1993) Brodie abscess: MR imaging appearance in 10 patients. J Magn Reson Imaging 3:543–546
Maurer AH, Millmond SH, Knight LC et al (1986) Infection in diabetic osteoarthropathy: use of indium-labeled leukocytes for diagnosis. Radiology 161:221–225
Maurer J, Lehmann BD, Vosshenrich R et al (1992) The place of computed tomography and magnetic resonance tomography in the diagnosis of bone sequestra. Aktuel Radiol 2: 345–349
McAfee JG, Samin A (1985) In-111 labeled leukocytes: a review of problems in image interpretation. Radiology 155:221–229
Miller TT, Randolph-DA J, Staron RB et al (1997) Fat-suppressed MRI of musculoskeletal infection: fast T2-weighted techniques versus gadolinium-enhanced T1-weighted images. Skeletal Radiol 26:654–658
Miller WB Jr, Murphy WA, Gilula LA (1979) Brodie abscess: reappraisal. Radiology 132:15–23
Mitchell M, Howard B, Haller J et al (1988) Septic arthritis. Radiol Clin North Am 26:1295–1313
Moore TE, Yuh WT, Kathol MH et al (1991) Abnormalities of the foot in patients with diabetes mellitus: findings on MR imaging. AJR 157:813–816
Morrison WB, Schweitzer ME, Bock GW et al (1993) Diagnosis of osteomyelitis: utility of fat-suppressed contrast-enhanced MR imaging. Radiology 189:251–257
Morrison WB, Schweitzer ME, Wapner KL et al (1995) Osteomyelitis in feet of diabetics: clinical accuracy, surgical utility, and cost-effectiveness of MR imaging. Radiology 196:557–564
Morrison WB, Schweitzer ME, Batte WG et al (1998) Osteomyelitis of the foot: relative importance of primary and secondary MR imaging signs. Radiology 207:625–632
Newman LG, Waller J, Palestro CJ et al (1991) Unsuspected osteomyelitis in diabetic foot ulcers. Diagnosis and monitoring by leukocyte scanning with indium in 111 oxyquinoline. JAMA 266:1246–1251
Newman LG, Waller J, Palestro CJ et al (1992) Leukocyte scan-

ning with 111In is superior to magnetic resonance imaging in diagnosis of clinically unsuspected osteomyelitis in diabetic foot ulcers. Diabetes Care 15:1527–1530

Nigro ND, Bartynski WS, Grossman SJ et al (1992) Clinical impact of magnetic resonance imaging in foot osteomyelitis. J Am Podiatr Med Assoc 82:603–615

Paajanen H, Grodd W, Revel D et al (1987) Gadolinium-DTPA enhanced MR imaging of intramuscular abscesses. Magn Reson Imaging 5:109–115

Park HM, Wheat LJ, Siddiqui AR et al (1982) Scintigraphic evaluation of diabetic osteomyelitis: concise communication. J Nucl Med 23:569–573

Rosenthall L, Lisbona R, Hernandez M et al (1979) 99mTc-PP and 67 Ga imaging following insertion of orthopedic devices. Radiology 133:717–721

Schauwecker DS (1989) Osteomyelitis: diagnosis with In-111-labeled leukocytes. Radiology 171:141–146

Schauwecker DS (1995) Differentiation of infected from noninfected rapidly progressive neuropathic osteoarthropathy. J Nucl Med 36:1427–1428

Schauwecker DS, Park HM, Mock BH et al (1984) Evaluation of complicating osteomyelitis with Tc-99 m MDP, In-111 granulocytes, and Ga-67 citrate. J Nucl Med 25:849–853

Schauwecker DS, Braunstein EM, Wheat LJ (1990) Diagnostic imaging of osteomyelitis. Infect Dis Clin North Am 4: 441–463

Schmid MR, Kossmann T, Duewell S (1998) Differentiation of necrotizing fasciitis and cellulitis using MR imaging. AJR 170:615–620

Seabold JE, Nepola JV, Conrad GR et al (1989) Detection of osteomyelitis at fracture nonunion sites: comparison of two scintigraphic methods. AJR 152:1021–1027

Seabold JE, Flickinger FW, Kao SC et al (1990) Indium-111-leukocyte/technetium-99m-MDP bone and magnetic resonance imaging: difficulty of diagnosing osteomyelitis in patients with neuropathic osteoarthropathy. J Nucl Med 31:549–556

Seldin DW, Heiken JP, Feldman F et al (1985) Effect of soft-tissue pathology on detection of pedal osteomyelitis in diabetics. J Nucl Med 26:988–993

Seltzer SE (1984) Value of computed tomography in planning medical and surgical treatment of chronic osteomyelitis. J Comput Assist Tomogr 8:482–487

Sim FH, Dahlin CD, Beabout JW (1975) Osteoid-osteoma: diagnostic problems. J Bone Joint Surg [Am] 57:154–159

Tan JS, Friedman NM, Hazelton-Miller C et al (1996) Can aggressive treatment of diabetic foot infections reduce the need for above-ankle amputation? Clin Infect Dis 23:286–291

Tang JS, Gold RH, Bassett LW et al (1988) Musculoskeletal infection of the extremities: evaluation with MR imaging. Radiology 166:205–209

Unger E, Moldofsky P, Gatenby R et al (1988) Diagnosis of osteomyelitis by MR imaging. AJR 150:605–610

Waldvogel FA, Medoff G, Swartz MN (1970) Osteomyelitis: a review of clinical features, therapeutic considerations and unusual aspects. N Engl J Med 282:198–206

Walshaw CF, Deans H (1996) CT findings in necrotising fasciitis–a report of four cases. Clin Radiol 51:429–432

Wang A, Weinstein D, Greenfield L et al (1990) MRI and diabetic foot infections. Magn Reson Imaging 8:805–809

Waters RL, Perry J, Antonelli D et al (1976) Energy cost of walking of amputees: the influence of level of amputation. J Bone Joint Surg [Am] 58:42–46

Weinstein D, Wang A, Chambers R et al (1993) Evaluation of magnetic resonance imaging in the diagnosis of osteomyelitis in diabetic foot infections. Foot Ankle 14:18–22

Wieman TJ, Mercke YK, Cerrito PB et al (1998) Resection of the metatarsal head for diabetic foot ulcers. Am J Surg 176: 436–441

Wing VW, Jeffrey-RB J, Federle MP et al (1985) Chronic osteomyelitis examined by CT. Radiology 154:171–174

Winters JLCI (1960) Acute hematogenous osteomyelitis: a review of 66 cases. J Bone Joint Surg [Am] 42:691–704

Wrobel JS, Connolly JE (1998) Making the diagnosis of osteomyelitis. The role of prevalence. J Am Podiatr Med Assoc 88:337–343

Wysoki MG, Santora TA, Shah RM et al (1997) Necrotizing fasciitis: CT characteristics. Radiology 203:859–863

Yuh WT, Corson JD, Baraniewski HM et al (1989) Osteomyelitis of the foot in diabetic patients: evaluation with plain film, 99mTc-MDP bone scintigraphy, and MR imaging. AJR 152:795–800

14 The Diabetic Foot

H. P. Ledermann, W. B. Morrison, and M. E. Schweitzer

CONTENTS

14.1 Background and Epidemiology

The worldwide population suffering from diabetes mellitus is increasing steadily: In 1995, it was estimated that there were 135 million individuals with this disease and for 2025 it is projected that there will be 300 million patients (King et al. 1998). An estimated 15 million people in the USA are diabetic (Boulton and Vileikyte 2000).

Diabetic foot ulceration is associated with significant morbidity and mortality (Mayfield et al. 1998; Reiber et al. 1998). In a recent report (Ramsey et al. 1999), 15% of patients with ulcers developed osteomyelitis, and 15.6% required amputation. Up to one-fifth of diabetic patients will be hospitalized at some point in their lives for a foot-related complication (Smith et al. 1987), primarily consisting of ulceration, infection, and ischemia. It has in fact been shown that more days are spent in hospital for the treatment of diabetic foot infections than any other complication of diabetes (Bild et al. 1989; Boutin et al. 1998; Caputo et al. 1994).

Diabetic foot complications lead to considerable health care expenses: In a recent retrospective cohort study lasting 2 years, the costs for a 40–65-year-old man with a new foot ulcer were nearly US$ 28,000 for the first 2 years after diagnosis (Ramsey et al. 1999). More than 50,000 lower extremity amputations are required annually for patients with diabetic foot ulcers in the USA, corresponding to direct annual costs that exceed one billion US dollars (Apelqvist et al. 1994). Diabetes is, in fact, the major cause of nontraumatic amputation, with the rate being 15–40 times higher than in the nondiabetic population (Humphrey et al. 1994; Most and Sinnock 1983). Estimated total costs, including rehabilitation for amputation, were estimated nearly 10 years ago to amount to between US$ 20,000 to 65,000 per person (Apelqvist et al. 1994; Reiber 1992).

In recent years, the complications and disadvantages of amputation have been increasingly recognized; there is a 50% incidence of serious complications in the contralateral foot within 2 years, and a 50% (Hoar and Torres 1962) to 66% (Goldner 1960) incidence of contralateral lower extremity amputation (LEA) within 5 years, at least in part due to shifting of weight-bearing to the other extremity. Furthermore, the quality of life decreases after an amputation (Pell et al. 1993). These issues have resulted in a shift in the treatment paradigm for diabetic foot complications. The emphasis is now placed on preventative foot care (Lavery and Gazewood 2000; Sumpio 2000). Early complications are treated with revascularization procedures, and partial, foot-sparing amputations instead of more extensive amputations, designed to preserve foot functional-

H. P. Ledermann, MD; W. B. Morrison, MD; M. E. Schweitzer, MD
Department of Radiology, Thomas Jefferson University Hospital, 111 S. 11th St., # 3390 Gibbon, Philadelphia, PA 19107, USA

ity (Holstein and Sorensen 1999; Karchmer and Gibbons 1994; Pinzur 1999; Tan et al. 1996). Radiologic techniques, especially MR imaging, play an important role in guiding this aggressive management of diabetic foot complications (Durham et al. 1991; Horowitz et al. 1993; Morrison et al. 1995; Nigro et al. 1992).

14.2 Pathophysiology of the Diabetic Foot

Diabetic foot ulceration is a multifactorial disease in which several diabetic complications (peripheral neuropathy, neuropathic osteoarthropathy, foot deformity, peripheral vascular disease, and immunopathy) act in concert.

14.2.1 Peripheral Neuropathy

Peripheral neuropathy is one of the most important causes of diabetic foot ulceration; the annual incidence of ulceration rises from less than 1% in patients who do not have neuropathy to more than 7% in patients with established neuropathy (Abbott et al. 1998; Young et al. 1994). In a recent 2-center study analyzing causes for diabetic ulceration, neuropathy was the most common component cause (Reiber et al. 1999). The most common casual pathway leading to ulceration involved the combination of neuropathy (resulting in insensitivity), deformity (claw toes, neuropathic osteoarthropathy), and trauma (toenail cutting, unrecognized injury, inappropriate footwear) (Reiber et al. 1999). Peripheral motor neuropathy results in muscle imbalance and atrophy which can alter weight-bearing and plantar pressures and (in addition to deformities) lead to callus formation and ulceration (Cavanagh et al. 1996; Lavery and Gazewood 2000; Lavery et al. 1998). Sensory neuropathy leads to a predisposition to and decreased perception of minor trauma to the foot, including friction, cuts, skin breakdown and ulceration (Deanfield et al. 1980; Levin 1995; Mueller et al. 1990; Reiber et al. 1999), tendon/ligament injury, joint injury, and fractures. Autonomic dysfunction, vascular fragility, ischemia, and reduced muscular activity result in deposition of fluid in the soft tissues and diffuse swelling and edema on MRI, which is diffuse and characteristic of advanced diabetes (Goodwin et al. 1995; Moore et al. 1996).

14.2.2 Neuropathic Osteoarthropathy (Charcot Arthropathy)

Neuropathic osteoarthropathy is common in advanced diabetic disease. A cascade of repetitive micro- and macro-trauma to joints and supporting ligaments (Johnson 1967; Sella and Barrette 1999), neuropathy with diminished perception of injury (Jeffcoate et al. 2000), and ischemia with poor healing results in joint instability, with subluxation (Newman 1979), deformity, and surrounding bone production (sclerosis and osteophytes) (Clouse et al. 1974). Charcot arthropathy can produce significant deformities that predispose the foot to ulceration. Midfoot or hindfoot involvement may result in plantar and medial prominences with subsequent ulceration. The Lisfranc joint (common tarsometatarsal joint) is the most common site of neuropathic osteoarthopathy in diabetics. Typically, the metatarsal bases are displaced superiorly, and the tarsal bones, especially the cuboid, may become weight-bearing, resulting in abnormal plantar pressures; this collapse of the longitudinal arch results in a 'rocker bottom' deformity. In this situation, the metatarsal bases may also form a source of excess friction, either at the dorsum of the foot related to superior displacement of the bones or medially and laterally due to 'splaying' of the metatarsal bases in the transverse plane. The Chopart joint (transverse intertarsal joint) is also commonly involved, and deformity of this articulation can result in abnormal plantar pressures and medial-lateral widening. Subtalar joint and ankle joint involvement is less common but may result in derangement of the joints and collapse of the weight-bearing structures such that unusual pressure is imposed on the calcaneus, talus, or malleoli. Neuropathic osteoarthropathy is uncommon in the forefoot but may occur in the metatarsophalangeal joints.

Neuropathic osteoarthropathy is typically seen in diabetic patients who have dense, distal, symmetrical neuropathy and have had diabetes for more than 10 years (Armstrong et al. 1997; Cofield et al. 1983). Considerable variation exists in the literature on the overall prevalence of neuropathic arthropathy due to different inclusion criteria; prevalences from 0.8% to 13% have been reported (Armstrong et al. 1997; Cavanagh et al. 1994; Cofield et al. 1983). Among diabetic patients with peripheral neuropathy, 29% were found to have neuropathic arthropathy (Cofield et al. 1983). It is assumed that diabetic neuropathic osteoarthropathy is related to a neural-initiated vascular reflex that leads to increased blood flow (Edelman et al. 1987). Several studies of the arterial circulation in the foot have documented a significant increase in vascularity (Archer et al. 1984; Edmonds 1986) and increased blood flow to bone (Edmonds et al. 1985; Eymontt et al. 1981; Zlatkin et al. 1987) which may be the result of sympathetic denervation. Such hypervascularity accompanied by arteriovenous shunting (Ward 1982) may lead to bone resorption, osteopenia, and bone fragility (Cundy et al. 1985; Edelman et al. 1987; Young et al. 1995). Cartilage damage leads to progression of the arthropathy, with the formation of erosions, subchondral cysts, and intraarticular bodies (Brower and Allman 1981). The current consensus supports the prominent role of misuse or abuse of insensitive joints in the pathogenesis of neuropathic osteoarthropathy (Myerson 2000; Resnick 1995). Cumulative minor trauma, when superimposed on bony and ligamentous changes, leads to diastasis, subluxation, dislocation, and fragmentation of the unprotected, insensate joints. Joint destruction due to diabetic neuroarthropathy is therefore primarily seen in patients who are ambulatory. An episode of trauma may not be necessary to initiate the destructive changes in this disease (Armstrong et al. 1997; Sella and Barrette 1999).

14.2.3 Foot Deformity

Foot deformity is an essential component of diabetic ulceration. Deformities can occur related to muscle atrophy/imbalance, neuropathic osteoarthropathy, tendon/ligament tear, or dysfunction. Motor neuropathy leads to atrophy of the intrinsic muscles, with subluxation and dislocation of the metatarsophalangeal joints and claw deformities (Lavery and Gazewood 2000). As the metatarsophalangeal joint subluxes, the fat pad that is normally directly under the ball of the foot is pulled distally, so the metatarsal head prominences are unprotected (Green and Brekke 1996; Grumbine and King 1996). Hallux valgus may occur, particularly after amputation of the second toe. Ulceration may form over the eminence because of pressure from footwear or on the medial aspect of the interphalangeal joint as this becomes weight-bearing because of pronation of the hallux.

Limited joint mobility is also associated with a higher risk of foot ulceration in diabetic patients (Armstrong et al. 1998; Armstrong and Lavery 1998; Birke et al. 1995; Frykberg et al. 1998; Lavery et al. 1995; Mueller et al. 1989). Limitation of the range of motion of the ankle joint, subtalar joint, and metatarsophalangeal joints increases the risk of developing foot ulcers in persons with diabetes who have peripheral sensory neuropathy (Armstrong et al. 1999; Lavery et al. 1998; Mueller et al. 1989). Limited joint motion decreases shock absorption of the lower extremity during walking and causes higher pressures on the sole of the foot (Lavery and Gazewood 2000).

14.2.4 Peripheral Vascular Disease

Peripheral vascular disease is more prevalent in patients with diabetes mellitus (Rosenbloom et al. 1988). Diabetic patients with peripheral vascular disease are at increased risk of foot ulceration (Criqui et al. 1992; Newman et al. 1993). Vascular disease causes calcification of the vessel walls (Edmonds 2000; Mozes et al. 1998) and stenoses, which result in chronic lower extremity ischemia. Thickening of the basement membrane of the capillaries furthermore inhibits perfusion of adjacent tissues (Siperstein et al. 1968; Tooke 1995). Ischemia causes poor wound healing (Stadelmann et al. 1998) and results in gangrene of the digits and forefoot in more advanced disease (Hill et al. 1999). Feet with an adequate vascular supply will develop a draining sinus in the face of infection, whereas those with a poor vascular supply will develop gangrene if challenged with an infectious process (Fry et al. 1998; Hill et al. 1999). Infarcts can occur in the bone marrow more proximally. Ischemia also affects other structures and may be an etiology for the progression of tendon degeneration/tear (Holmes and Mann 1992) as well as arthritis, including neuropathic disease (Younger and Bronfin 1996). Edema within confined compartments of the foot increases intracompartmental pressures (Lower and Kenzora 1994) and can accentuate the ischemic cascade.

14.2.5 Immunopathy

Immunopathy is also a feature of diabetic disease (Joshi et al. 1999; Stadelmann et al. 1998). However, the association between diabetes mellitus and increased susceptibility to infection in general is not supported by strong evidence (Joshi et al. 1999;

Thornton 1971; Wheat 1980). Nevertheless, several aspects of immunity are altered in patients with diabetes mellitus: leukocyte function is depressed, and leukocyte adherence, chemotaxis, and phagocytosis may be affected (Gallacher et al. 1995; Muchova et al. 1999; Rassias et al. 1999). These findings have not been fully confirmed in clinical studies, and the actual impact of immunopathy on diabetic foot infection still has to be evaluated.

14.3 Radiologic Findings

14.3.1 Ulceration and Callus

More than 90% of cases of diabetic pedal osteomyelitis result from contiguous spread of infection from foot ulcers (Bamberger et al. 1987; Cicchinelli and Corey 1993; Gold et al. 1995; Ledermann et al. 2002a). Skin callus and subsequent ulceration are predominantly seen in areas of excess friction or abnormal pressures: below the metatarsal heads, at the tips of the toes, over digital foot deformities (hammer toe, claw toe), on the heel, and over the malleoli (Gold et al. 1995). Ulceration can occur from cuts or friction-related skin erosion as well as from breakdown of callus (Boulton 1996; Pitei et al. 1999). Skin ulceration is seen on MR images as an interruption of the cutaneous signal with rim enhancement after contrast administration (Table 14.1) (Morrison et al. 1998). Deep ulceration leads to obvious skin and soft-tissue defects on MR images and is often associated with underlying osteomyelitis (Ledermann etal. 2002a). As a result, the MR imaging protocol should be planned with the ulcer location in mind, and interpretation of images should begin with a search for the ulcer and progress to the surrounding soft tissues and underlying bone.

Callus is seen as a focal cutaneous and subcutaneous soft-tissue prominence on MR images; the skin and subcutaneous signals blend imperceptibly in most calluses, although some calluses are centered in a subdermal location (especially inferior to the calcaneus) and may not affect the skin to a great degree. Calluses present low signal intensity on T1-weighted images, but show variable T2 signal based on the degree of granulation tissue and vascularity (Fig. 14.1) (Table 14.1). More vascular calluses (which may have a reddish appearance on visual inspection) demonstrate a high T2 signal and enhance diffusely after gadolinium administration (Fig. 14.1). In the absence of infection, the margins of the callus are fairly well defined. Common sites of involvement

Table 14.1. MR signal characteristics of conditions affecting the diabetic foot

	T1	T2	T1 postcontrast	Comments
Marrow signal:				
Osteomyelitis	Low	High	High	Adjacent soft-tissue infection
Infarction	Low, sharp margins	High, rim well defined	Marginal enhancement	
Neuropathic:				
Acute	Low	Low	High	To differentiate from osteomyelitis, see Table 14.2
Chronic	Normal to low	Normal to high	Subchondral enhancement	
Soft-tissue signal:				
Devitalization	Normal to low	Mixed to high	Regional absence of enhancement	Osteomyelitis, abscesses, cellulitis may not enhance
Diabetic edema	Normal to slightly low	High diffusely	No or little enhancement	Associated with muscle atrophy
Cellulitis	Low regionally	High diffusely	Enhancement regionally	
Callus	Focally low SQ	Low to intermediate	+/-enhancement	Blends with skin
Ulcer	Low	High	Marginal enhancement of crater	Focal discontinuity of skin signal
Sinus tract	Low	Linear high	'Tram-track' linear enhancement	Connects to skin or abscess
Abscess	Low	Focal fluid	Rim enhancement	

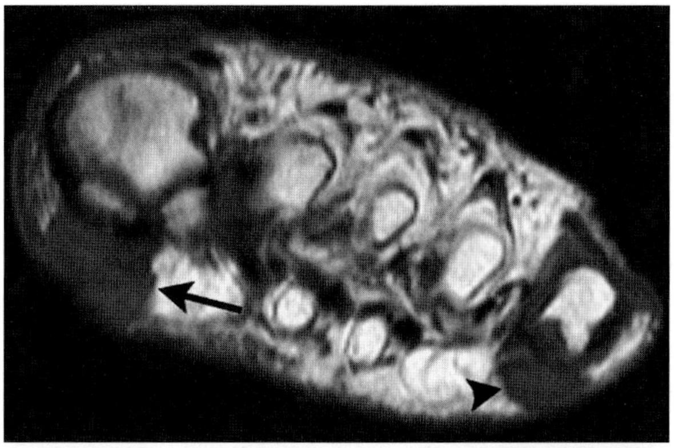
a
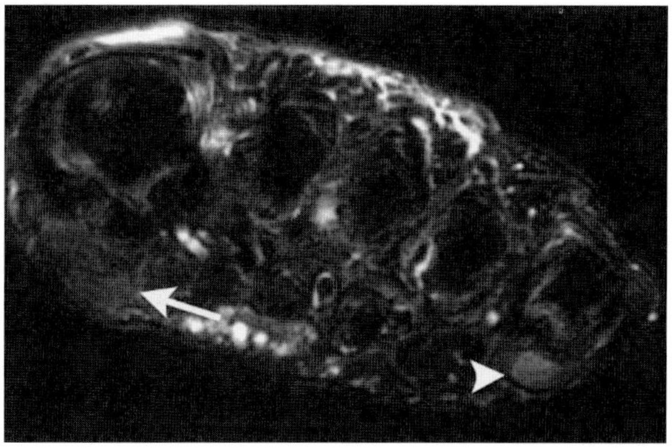
b
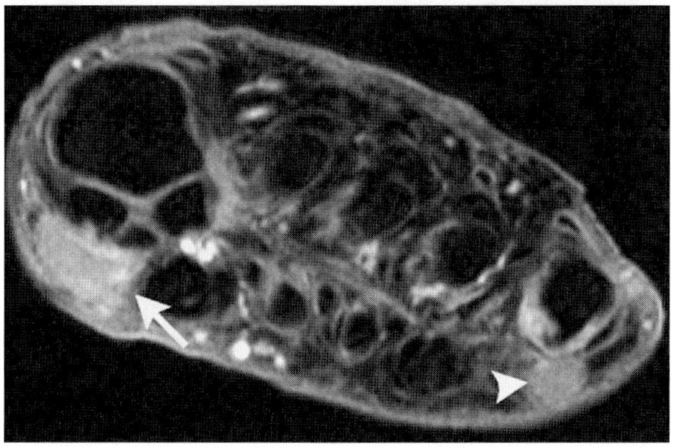
c

Fig. 14.1a–c. MR signal characteristics of callus in a patient with two subcutaneous calluses under the first (*arrow*) and fifth (*arrowhead*) metatarsal head. **a** On T1-weighted images, both calluses display isointense signal compared to muscle. **b** On T2-weighted fat-suppressed image, the medial callus is hypointense (*arrow*), whereas the lateral callus (*arrowhead*) is slightly hyperintense. **c** Contrast-enhanced images reveal homogenous contrast enhancement of both calluses with greater signal increase of the medial callus (*arrow*)

are areas of increased friction or abnormal pressure as described above. The most common site of callus formation is adjacent to the first or fifth metatarsal heads and may be related to ill-fitting shoes, hallux valgus deformity, bunionette deformity, or shifting of the plantar fat pad. With clawtoe or hammertoe deformity, callus often forms dorsally adjacent to the PIP or DIP joint (Lavery et al. 1998; Sumpio 2000). In the setting of deformity from neuropathic osteoarthropathy or posterior tibialis tendon dysfunction, calluses can arise in atypical locations, most commonly beneath the cuboid and adjacent to the calcaneus (Armstrong et al. 1997). The chronic friction that leads to callus formation can also result in adventitial bursitis, seen on MR images as a focus of fluid, usually thin and elongated or ovoid, in the subcutaneous tissues adjacent to a callus.

Detection of ulcerated callus is straightforward on MR images. Generally, a large skin defect is seen with rounded or 'heaped up' margins (Fig. 14.2); in this situation, the ulceration may even be visible radiographically as a focal area of air-type lucency overlying the soft tissues. Minor skin disruption or superficial skin erosion is more difficult to detect; a focal discontinuity of the skin signal may be subtle on MR images.

14.3.2 Diabetic Edema

In diabetic feet, diffuse soft-tissue swelling is common and may be easily detectable on radiographs. On MR images of diabetic feet, this is a common finding and is seen as soft-tissue edema (Goodwin et al. 1995; Moore et al. 1996). The distribution of edema is diffuse, seen within muscles, subcutaneous fat, or both,

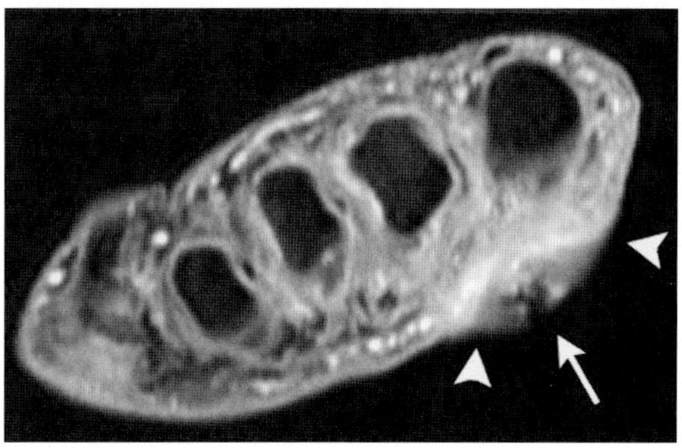

Fig. 14.2. Callus (*between arrowheads*) under the first metatarsal head with central ulceration (*arrow*) (contrast-enhanced fat-suppressed image)

and is characterized by high signal on T2-weighted or STIR images (Fig. 14.3). Subcutaneous fat signal is generally preserved, or at most there is patchy low signal on T1-weighted images. On gadolinium-enhanced images, the edematous tissue shows minimal enhancement, unlike cellulitis (Table 14.1) (Fig. 14.3). In advanced diabetes, the muscles of the foot are frequently atrophied, with decreased size and fatty infiltration seen best on T1-weighted images (Fig. 14.4) (Lower and Kenzora 1994).

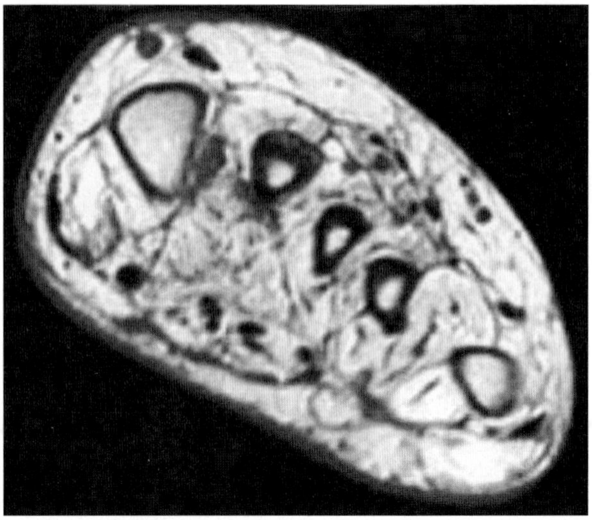

Fig. 14.4. Fatty atrophy of the intrinsic foot muscles in a patient with long-standing diabetes mellitus

14.3.3 Vascular Disease

Conventional angiography (Fig. 14.5) (Alson et al. 1997; Oser et al. 1995) and MR angiography (Fig. 14.6) (Baum et al. 1995; Kreitner et al. 2000; Lee et al. 1998; Owen et al. 1992) have been used for the diagnosis of diabetic vascular disease. Both techniques are highly effective for the diagnosis of diabetic macrovascular disease and to help plan revascularization procedures (Carpenter et al. 1996; Pomposelli et al. 1995), consisting of surgical bypass, angioplasty, or stenting. The use of angiography is limited in the evaluation of distal, small-vessel microvascular disease, which predominates in diabetics. Soft-tissue ischemia and devitalization related to this microvascular disease can be evaluated on MR images if both pre- and post-contrast sequences are performed (Ledermann et al. 2002b). Scanning is begun 1–2 min after a conventional intravenous dose of gadolinium contrast (0.1 mmol/kg) is administered. Fat-suppressed T1-weighted sequences are obtained, either using the spin-echo or gradient-echo technique. It is not generally necessary to perform postcontrast imaging in dynamic or rapid fashion; in fact, doing so may result in imaging prior to bolus

a

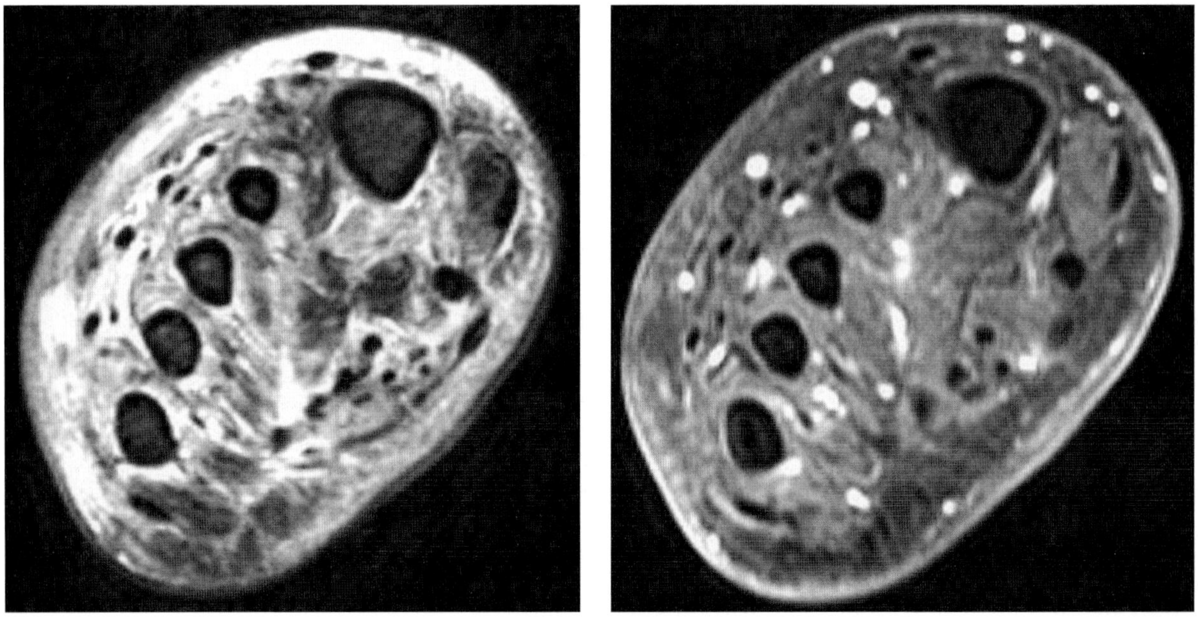

b

Fig. 14.3a,b. Diabetic pedal edema. **a** T2-weighted fat-suppressed image of the forefoot of a diabetic patient reveals diffuse subcutaneous and muscular edema. **b** After contrast administration, no abnormal enhancement of the edematous areas is seen, consistent with absence of infection

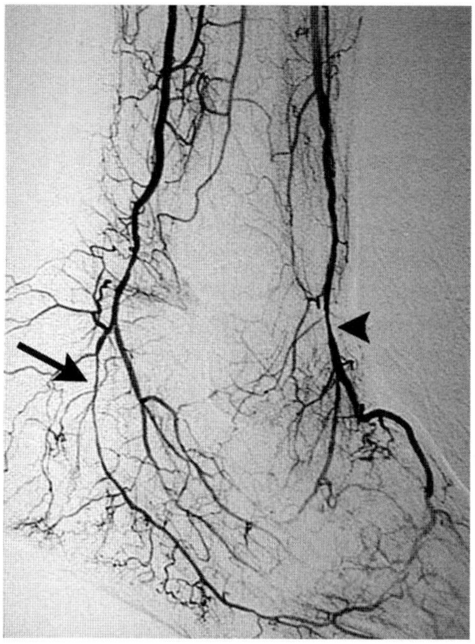

Fig. 14.5. Digital subtraction angiography with moderate concentric stenosis of the anterior tibial artery (*arrowhead*) and diffusely attenuated lumen of the plantar branch (*arrow*) of the posterior tibial artery

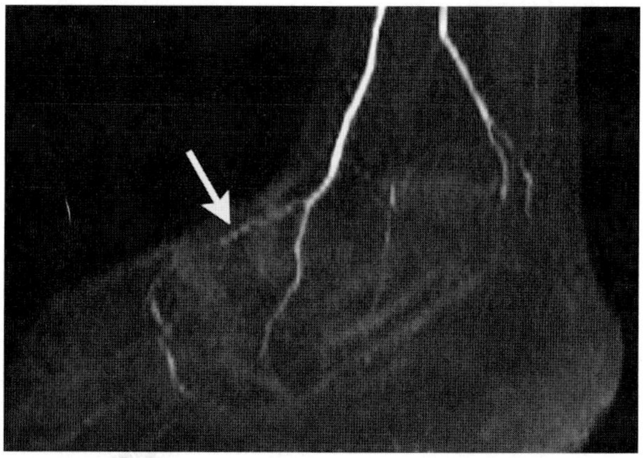

Fig. 14.6. MR angiography of the foot in a patient with gangrene of the great toe. The posterior tibial artery and the anterior branch of the peroneal artery have no flow signal and are occluded. Note also diffusely diminished signal of the dorsalis pedis artery compatible with diffuse attenuation of its lumen

arrival due to macrovascular disease more proximally. The injection quality can be assessed by comparing the vascular signal on pre- and post-contrast images. However, the imaging parameters and display window/level should be nearly identical on the pre- and post-contrast images in order to validate comparison.

Small-vessel disease of the foot will be observed as regional differences in soft-tissue contrast enhancement. Devitalization (foot 'infarction') often shows dramatic regional differences in contrast enhancement and may have sharp margins delineated by an ill-defined rim of increased enhancement (Fig. 14.7) (Ledermann et al. 2002b), representing reparative tissue or tissue-at-risk. This is analogous to the pattern of infarction of other organ systems. Within these zones, intravenous contrast does not penetrate or diffuses in with marked delay; therefore, it should be recognized that within these zones, osteomyelitis will not enhance, and abscesses will not rim-enhance (Ledermann et al. 2002b). In this setting, T1-weighted and T2-weighted images should be relied upon. Recognition of this phenomenon improves the sensitivity for the detection of osteomyelitis in the ischemic foot.

Ischemic tissue can result in more subtle MR imaging findings. These regions may merely enhance slightly less than surrounding tissue; region-of-interest (ROI) values of various areas of muscle and subcutaneous tissue can be obtained on a workstation to detect subtle areas of ischemia. Documentation of the presence and extent of ischemic and devitalized areas can facilitate surgical planning for debridement and limited, foot-sparing amputations. T2-weighted sequences and noncontrast T1-weighted sequences show variable signal within these areas of soft-tissue necrosis and may be misleading (Table 14.1). Chronic devitalization of the toes can result in a dramatic loss of tissue, which if uninfected is generally low signal on T2-weighted images and normal to low signal on T1-weighted images; this represents gangrene. If superinfected, a high T2 signal may be observed, but without contrast enhancement due to the regional devitalization.

Infarction of bone can also be seen within regions of ischemia. The MR imaging pattern is similar to infarction of other bones of the body (Table 14.1). Well-defined regions of signal abnormality are observed in the central medullary cavity, with a sharp, serpiginous pattern (Fig. 14.8) (Munk et al. 1989; Umans et al. 2000). The internal signal is variable, with areas of fat, fibrous tissue, or edema, often seen concurrently. The classic 'double line sign' of alternating marginal high and low T2 signal (Mitchell et al. 1987) may not be evident in the small bones of the foot. Often, infarction is present within multiple bones in a region of chronic ischemia.

14.3.4 Tendon Degeneration and Dysfunction

Tenosynovitis and tendon degeneration, dysfunction, and tear are also common in the diabetic foot. Teno-

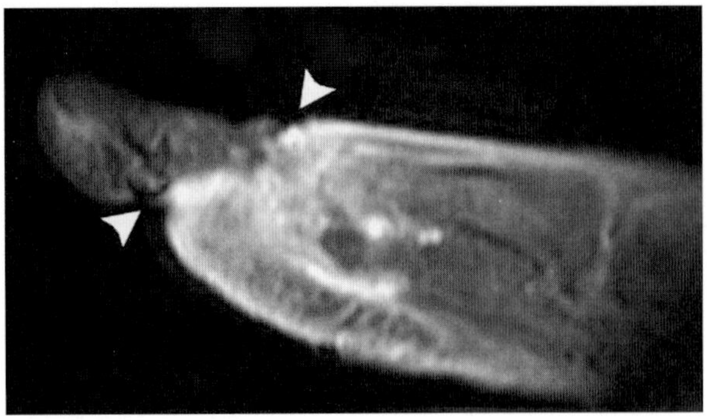

a

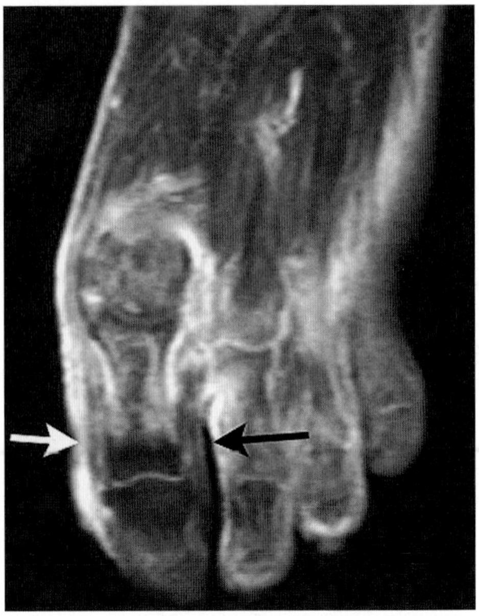

b

Fig. 14.7a,b. Gangrene of the great toe. **a** Contrast-enhanced fat-suppressed sagittal image with sharp demarcation (*arrowheads*) of contrast enhancement. Note discrete rim enhancement at the border of the necrotic tissue. **b** Axial image reveals a clearly defined cut-off of contrast enhancement (*arrows*) in the bone marrow of the proximal phalanx

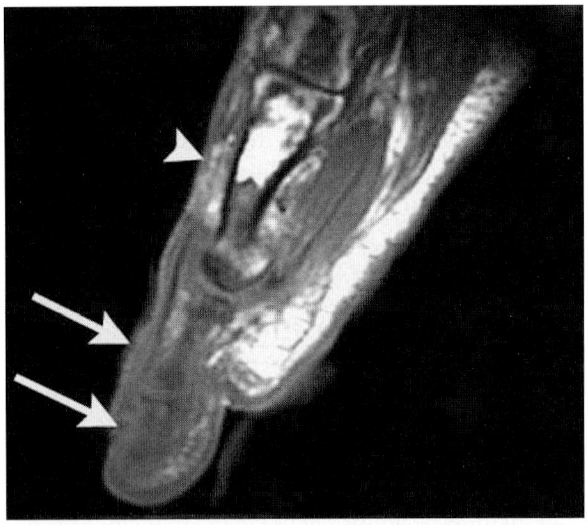

a

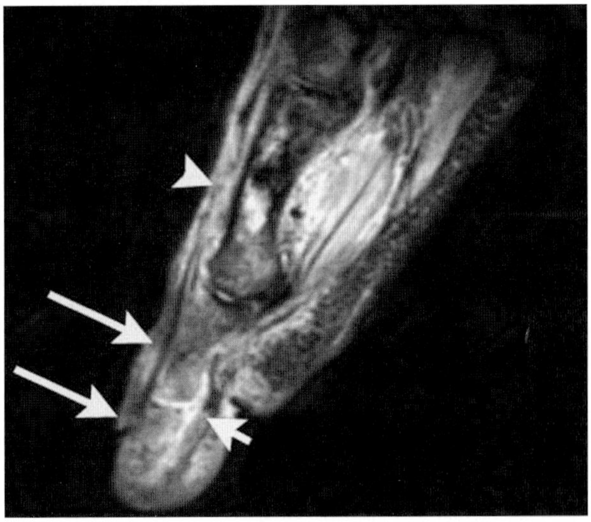

b

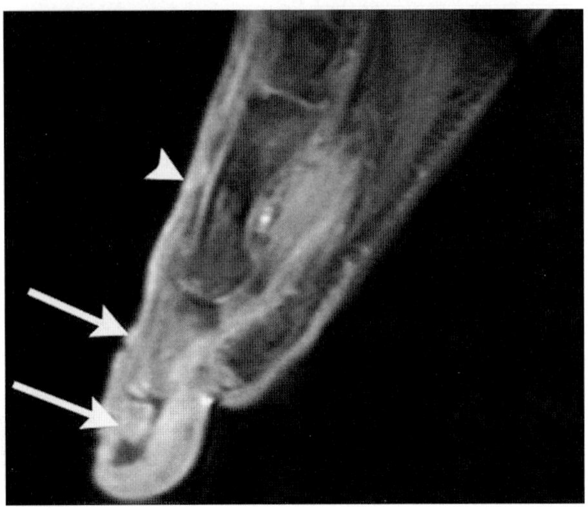

c

Fig. 14.8a–c. Infarction of the first metatarsal bone and osteomyelitis of the phalanges. **a** On the T1-weighted image, the infarction of the metatarsal bone presents as a patchy marrow signal alteration with hypointense areas and regions with fatty marrow (*arrowhead*). Complete fat signal loss in the proximal and distal phalanges is indicative of osteomyelitis (*arrows*). **b** On the T2-weighted image, the infarction is seen with geographic, sharply defined areas of hyperintentense signal (*arrowhead*). Diffuse bone marrow edema in the phalanges (*long arrows*) is indicative of osteomyelitis. Note joint effusion in the interphalangeal joint (*short arrow*) compatible with septic arthritis. **c** Contrast-enhanced fat-suppressed image without enhancement of the infarcted bone marrow (*arrowhead*) and diffuse enhancement of the infected phalanges (*arrows*) synovitis is discussed in Chapter 13. The etiology of tendon dysfunction and degeneration is multifactorial: Decreased sensation results in recurrent tendon injury, poor vascularity causes tendon ischemia and slow healing, while foot deformity and altered gait place additional stress on the tendons. The posterior tibialis tendon is particularly susceptible; it functions to invert the ankle as well as plantarflex the foot, but also supports the medial arch and restricts pronation and forefoot abduction (Schweitzer and Karasick 2000). Dysfunction of this tendon results in a characteristic deformity pattern that includes pes planus, overpronation and forefoot abduction, hindfoot valgus, and collapse of the medial arch (Schweitzer et al. 1993).

14.3.5 Neuropathic Osteoarthropathy

Neuropathic osteoarthropathy is most common at the Lisfranc joint (Armstrong et al. 1997; Clouse et al. 1974; Cofield et al. 1983; Schon et al. 1998) but can occur at any joint (Armstrong et al. 1997; Cofield et al. 1983; Schon et al. 1998); multiple joints in a region may be involved. Traditionally, neuropathic osteoarthropathy has been divided into an atrophic and hypertrophic form (Allman et al. 1988; Resnick 1995). However, diabetic Charcot arthropathy has been shown to progress from an acute inflammatory process, which may resemble the atrophic form, to a chronic stage which often shows productive changes (Armstrong et al. 1997). Since atrophic and hypertrophic stages resulting in a 'mixed' pattern can occur in the same joint during the development of a Charcot joint, we prefer to divide the following discussion into acute and chronic presentations of neuropathic osteoarthropathy.

14.3.5.1 Acute Neuropathic Osteoarthropathy

The acute form presents clinically as a warm, swollen, erythematous foot that may simulate infection (Sella and Barrette 1999). Radiographs may only reveal soft-tissue swelling and joint effusion in this stage (Katz et al. 1961; Sella and Barrette 1999; Thomasson and Sundaram 1985). However, slight offset of the joints may be observed: For example, at the Lisfranc joint, the medial margin of the second metatarsal shaft should align precisely with the medial margin of the second cuneiform. Offset of this junction or widening of the distance between the first and second metatarsal bases should suggest early neuropathic disease in the diabetic patient. Radiographic findings of early neuropathic osteoarthropathy manifested by subluxation or malalignment may be very subtle, and if there is clinical or radiographic suspicion of this, computed tomography or contralateral comparison radiographs may be helpful. In subacute stages of disease, radiographs may demonstrate the collapse and fragmentation of the articular surface, subchondral cysts, and marginal erosions (Fig. 14.9) (Allman et al. 1988). However, the bone density is generally preserved; in fact, the bones may demonstrate proliferation manifested by increased density. As the disease progresses, more significant subluxation occurs, the joint surfaces become more incongruous, and osteoarticular destruction becomes more severe.

On MR images of acute neuropathic osteoarthropathy, there is diffuse soft-tissue edema (Marcus et al. 1996). In the earliest stages of Lisfranc joint disease, axial MR images may be useful to detect disruption of the Lisfranc ligament that stretches from the medial cuneiform to the second metatarsal base. This ligament is essential for the stability of the midfoot and is readily observed on routine MR images. The involved joint or joints in this early stage of the disease often show little deformity or malalignment. Joint effusion is common, with prominent subchondral edema that

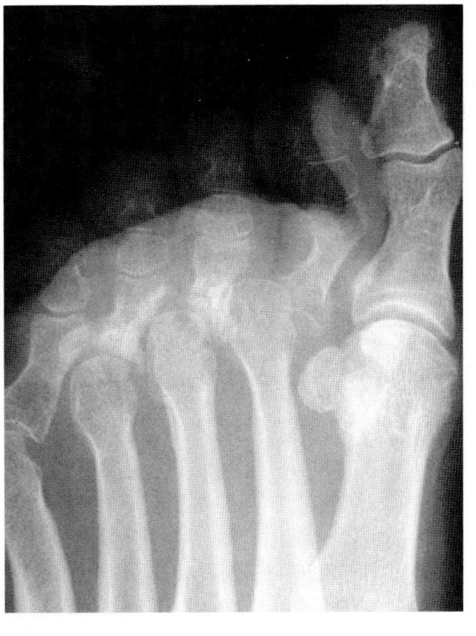

Fig. 14.9. Subacute neuropathic osteoarthritis of the 2nd to 4th MTP joints with dorsal subluxation and destruction of the bases of the proximal phalanges

may extend far into the medullary cavity. Signal intensity changes in the bone marrow, consisting of low signal intensity on T1-weighted images and high signal on T2-weighted images, may be identical to those observed in osteomyelitis (Table 14.1) (Fig. 14.10). Erosions may be seen at the margins of the joint. On gadolinium-enhanced images, marrow enhancement is typically present, with predominantly subchondral distribution (Yu 1998). Periarticular soft-tissue enhancement may also be seen. In advanced acute or subacute neuropathic osteoarthropathy, destruction of joints with cyst formation, erosions, and bony fragmentation can be observed (Fig. 14.11). Recent fractures related to neuropathic osteoarthropathy may contribute to signal intensity changes in the marrow and cortex of bones, which lead to potential diagnostic pitfalls (Marcus et al. 1996; Moore et al. 1991).

Bone scintigraphy, mostly performed as a three-phase study, has been shown to demonstrate high

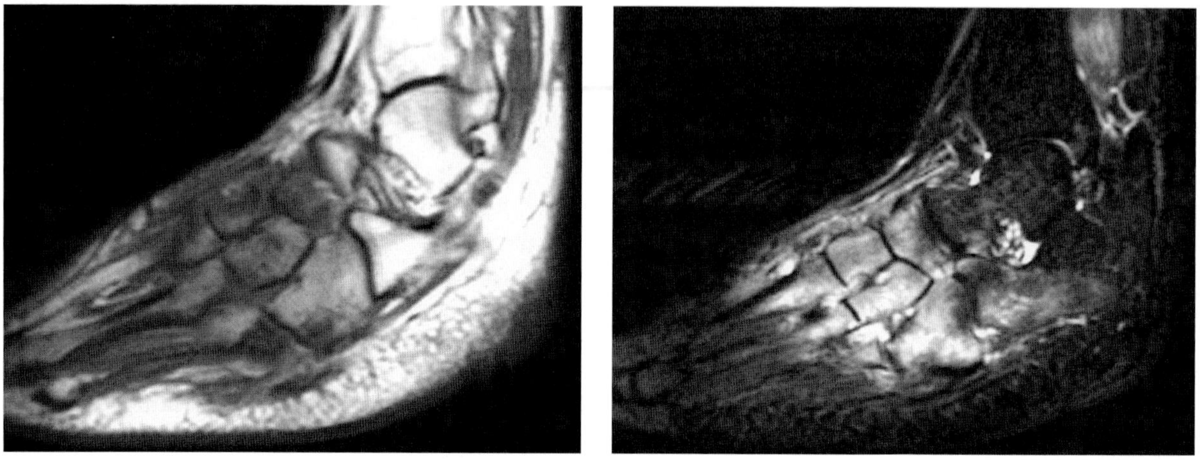

a b

Fig. 14.10a,b. Acute neuropathic osteoarthropathy of the midfoot. **a** T1-weighted image reveals diffuse decrease of fat signal in the bone marrow of the midfoot. Note absence of joint destruction in the acute phase. **b** T2-weighted image with fat suppression reveals diffuse bone marrow edema in the midfoot

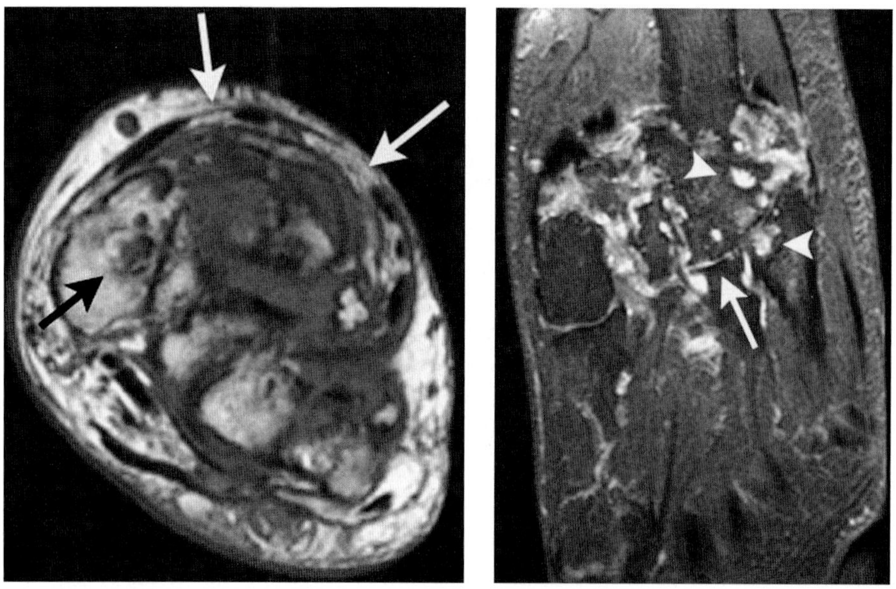

a b

Fig. 14.11a,b. Subacute neuropathic arthropathy of the Lisfranc joint and the intertarsal joints. **a** Coronal T1-weighted image reveals destruction of the articular surfaces of the midfoot with cysts (*black arrow*) and erosions. Note hypointense synovial proliferation and joint effusion (*white arrows*). **b** Axial contrast-enhanced fat-suppressed image reveals diffuse enhancement of the hypertrophied synovium, progressive destruction of the Lisfranc joint (*arrow*), and multiple cysts (*arrowheads*) tracer uptake in acute and subacute forms of neuropathic osteoarthopathy (Fig. 14.12) (Eymontt et al. 1981; Schauwecker 1995). Some reports suggest that In-111-labeled WBC scintigraphy may be superior to MRI in correctly identifying a Charcot joint and in diagnosing superimposed infection (Lipman et al. 1998; Schauwecker 1995). It has been shown, however, that In-111-labeled WBC scans can be positive in noninfected neuropathic joints with rapid destruction (Seabold et al. 1990).

14.3.5.2 *Chronic Neuropathic Osteoarthropathy*

Radiographically, chronic neuropathic osteoarthropathy results in joint subluxation and dislocation (Fig. 14.13), as well as the destruction and fragmentation of juxta-articular bone. In later stages of the disease, adjacent bones can become necrotic and collapse (Fig. 14.14) (Clouse et al. 1974). The classic radiographic appearance of chronic neuropathic

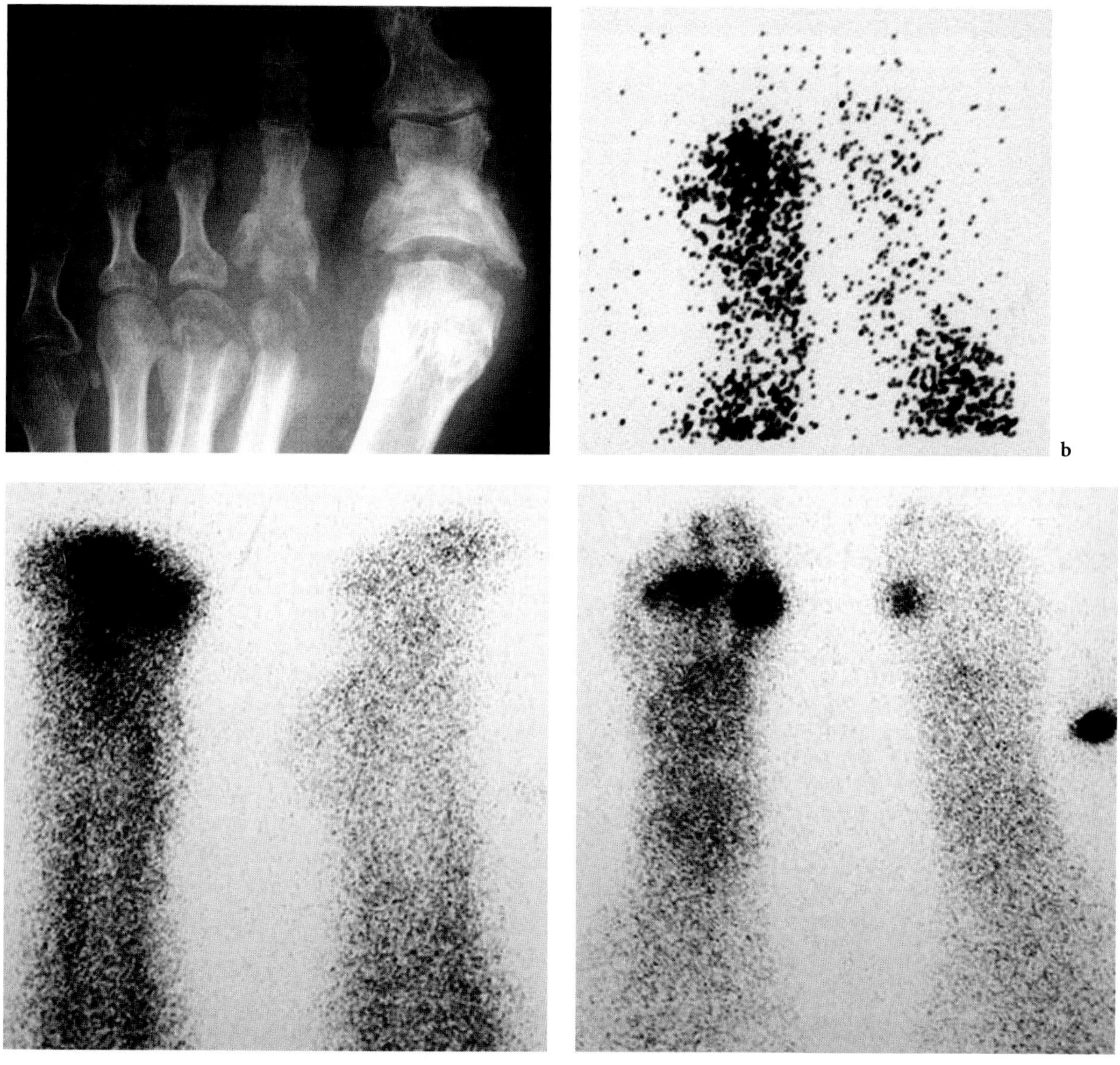

a b c d

Fig. 14.12a–d. Subacute neuropathic osteoarthropathy of the 1st to 4th MTP joints. **a** Conventional radiograph reveals extensive destruction of the second MTP joint and the third metatarsal head with soft-tissue swelling. The first proximal phalanx is fractured, and there is bony debris in the first MTP joint. **b** Blood flow phase of the Tc-99m methylene diphosphonate (MDP) bone scan reveals hyperemia in the left forefoot. **c** Blood-pool image demonstrates asymmetric tracer accumulation in the left forefoot. **d** Late-phase scintigraphy confirms increased tracer uptake in the first four MT joints compatible with neuropathic osteoarthropathy

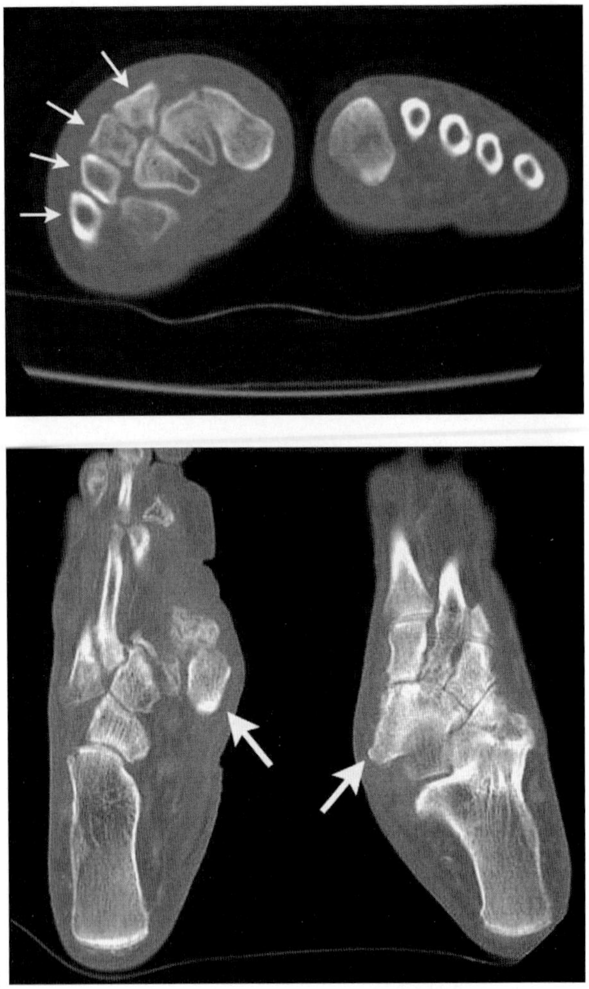

a

b

Fig. 14.13a,b. Chronic neuropathic osteoarthropathy of the right foot in a diabetic patient with total dorsolateral dislocation of the Lisfranc joint. **a** CT exam reveals total dorsolateral dislocation of the 2nd to 5th metatarsal bases (*arrows*) at the right Lisfranc joint. **b** Total collapse of the medial arch of both feet with medial prominence of the midfoot (*arrows*) (so-called rocker bottom deformity) bilaterally. Note preserved bone density, multiple small intraosseous cysts, and degenerative changes in the joints of the midfoot

osteoarthropathy has been characterized by words beginning with 'D', including destruction, dislocation, debris, disorganization, and preservation of bone density. Collapse, sclerosis, and fragmentation of the metatarsal heads may resemble changes of Freiberg's infarction (Nguyen et al. 1991), but are more aggressive and extensive. Broadening of the bases of phalanges may lead to a cupped appearance (Schwarz et al. 1969). Occasionally, shortening and resorption of the ends of the metatarsals and phalanges occur (Zlatkin et al. 1987). Bony ankylosis represents the end-stage of joint destruction

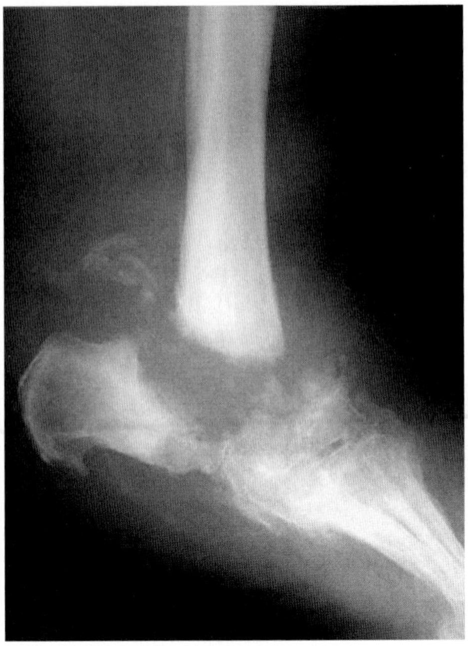

Fig. 14.14. Total destruction of the ankle joint in a patient with neuropathic osteoarthropathy and long-term diabetes

(Clouse et al. 1974) but is uncommon (Fig. 14.15) (Sella and Barrette 1999). Asymptomatic fractures can be discovered in 22% of diabetic patients with neuropathy (Cavanagh et al. 1994). Calcaneal fractures are common and avulsion by the Achilles tendon may be the first radiographic abnormality at the time of presentation (El Khoury and Kathol 1980; Kathol et al. 1991).

On MR images, edema and enhancement are absent or less prominent in the chronic form of neuropathic osteoarthropathy (Beltran et al. 1990; Marcus et al. 1996). Subchondral cysts present as well marginated foci of low signal intensity on T1-weighted images and high signal intensity on T2-weighted images. Bone proliferation is present, with 'debris' or intraarticular bodies (Sella and Barrette 1999). Typically, chronic neuropathic osteoarthropathy appears as a decreased signal intensity, consistent with osteosclerosis on all sequences (Fig. 14.16). Joint deformity is common, with subluxation or dislocation (Cofield et al. 1983; Sella and Barrette 1999). Neuropathic disease of the Lisfranc joint typically results in superior and lateral subluxation of the metatarsals, leading to a 'rocker-bottom' type of deformity (Fig. 14.17) (Nguyen 1992; Schon et al. 1998), with increased weight-bearing stress on the cuboid. In this setting, callus and ulcer formation beneath the cuboid is common; ulcers may also form dorsally, over the superiorly subluxed metatarsals.

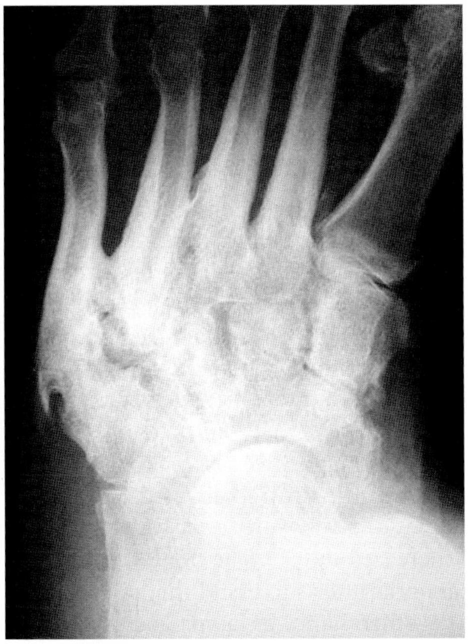

Fig. 14.15. Ankylosis of the Lisfranc joint and of the joints of the midfoot in a patient with chronic neuropathic osteoarthropathy

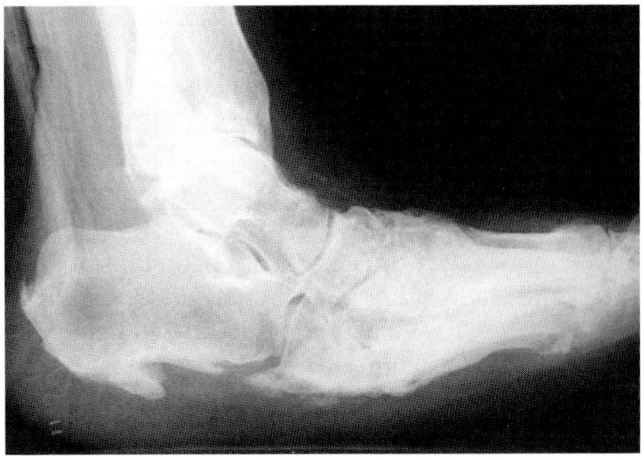

Fig. 14.17. Rocker-bottom deformity of the foot

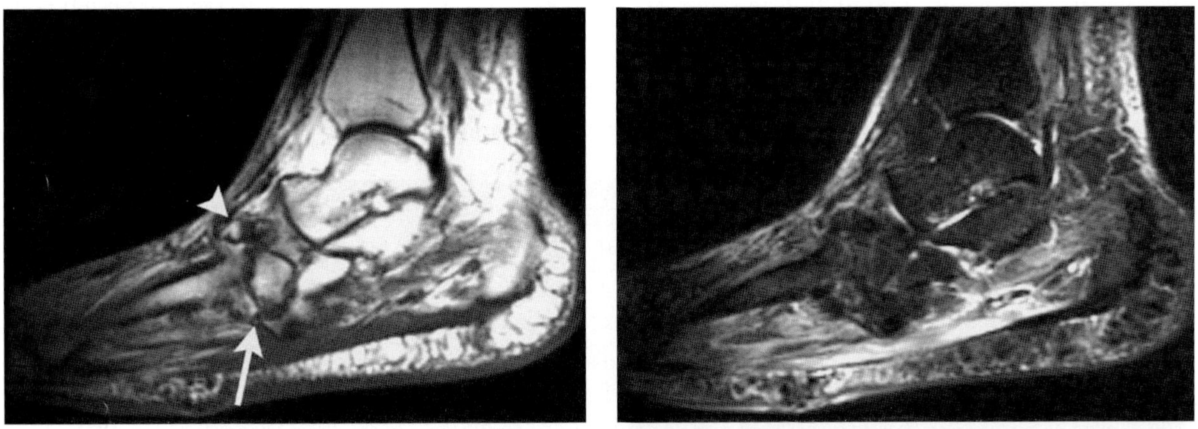

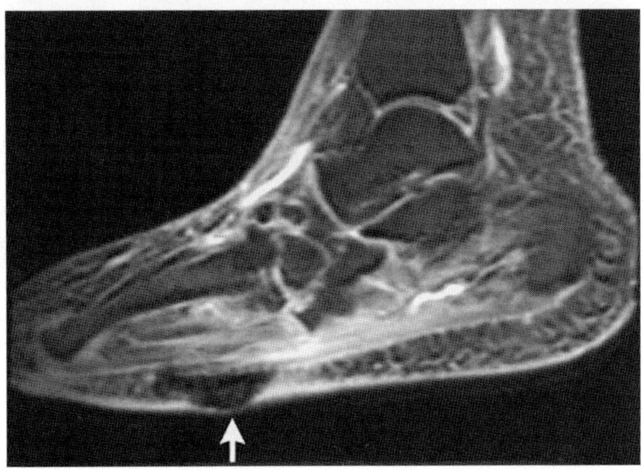

Fig. 14.16a–c. MR signal characteristics of chronic neuropathic osteoarthropathy. **a** T1-weighted image reveals destruction of the Lisfranc and midfoot joints (*arrow*) with malalignment and bone fragmentation (*arrowhead*). **b** T2-weighted fat-suppressed image confirms absence of marrow edema around the Lisfranc joint and the midfoot. **c** Contrast-enhanced fat-suppressed image with normal marrow signal confirming chronic neuropathic osteoarthropathy. Note gas inclusion (*arrow*) in the subcutaneous tissue from an adjacent ulcer

14.3.6 Osteomyelitis

The typical findings of pedal osteomyelitis have been discussed in Chapter 13. However, underlying peripheral vascular disease and neuropathic osteoarthropathy can modify the appearance of bone infection. In the ischemic foot, bone resorption, periosteal new bone formation, and healing are inhibited. Severe pedal ischemia may furthermore result in lack of contrast enhancement on MR imaging and lack of radiotracer uptake on scintigraphy (Park et al. 1982). Chronicity of diabetic foot infection combined with absence of pain and proprioceptive sensation can lead to bone sclerosis (Fig. 14.18), pathological fractures, and subluxation (Gold et al. 1995). MR findings of acute Charcot arthropathy can be identical to the findings of osteomyelitis (Fig. 14.19).

The distinction between neuropathic osteoarthropathy and infection may be facilitated by considering these general principles that are also summarized in Table 14.2. First, the vast majority of cases of osteomyelitis in diabetic feet occur via contiguous spread related to ulceration and cellulitis. Therefore, a bone marrow abnormality without contiguous soft-tissue infection or nearby skin ulceration favors diagnoses other than infection. Also, neuropathic osteoarthropathy is primarily an articular disease; marrow abnormalities centered in a subarticular location favor such an articular disorder. The distribution of osteomyelitis mirrors that of ulceration, which is most common at the toes, metatarsal heads, calcaneus, and malleoli, whereas neuropathic arthropathy is most common at the Lisfranc and Chopart joints. Finally, neuropathic arthropathy tends to involve a number of joints in a region, whereas infection tends to remain localized or spread contiguously. To summarize, location in the midfoot, polyarticular involvement, predominant subarticular changes, and absence of or large distance from soft-tissue infection or ulceration favor the diagnosis of acute, evolving neuropathic osteoarthropathy rather than infection (Marcus et al. 1996).

Three-phase technetium-99 methylene diphosphonate scan has a high sensitivity for osteomyelitis but also a high rate of false-positive results in the diabetic foot, since neuropathic arthropathy, fractures, periosteal inflammation, and soft-tissue infection may also lead to increased uptake. The bone scan may be positive for months after successful therapy (Becker 1999). On the other hand, ischemia may lead to a false-negative test (Park et al. 1982). The indium-111-labeled white blood cell scan has the highest specificity of all radionuclide studies for osteomyelitis in the diabetic foot (Crim and Seeger 1994; Keenan et al. 1989; Larcos et al. 1991; Maurer et al. 1986; Newman et al. 1991; Schauwecker et al. 1988; Seabold et al. 1990). However, it has been shown that up to 31% of In-111-labeled WBC scans are positive in noninfected neuropathic joints, especially those in which destruction is rapidly progressive (Seabold et al. 1990).

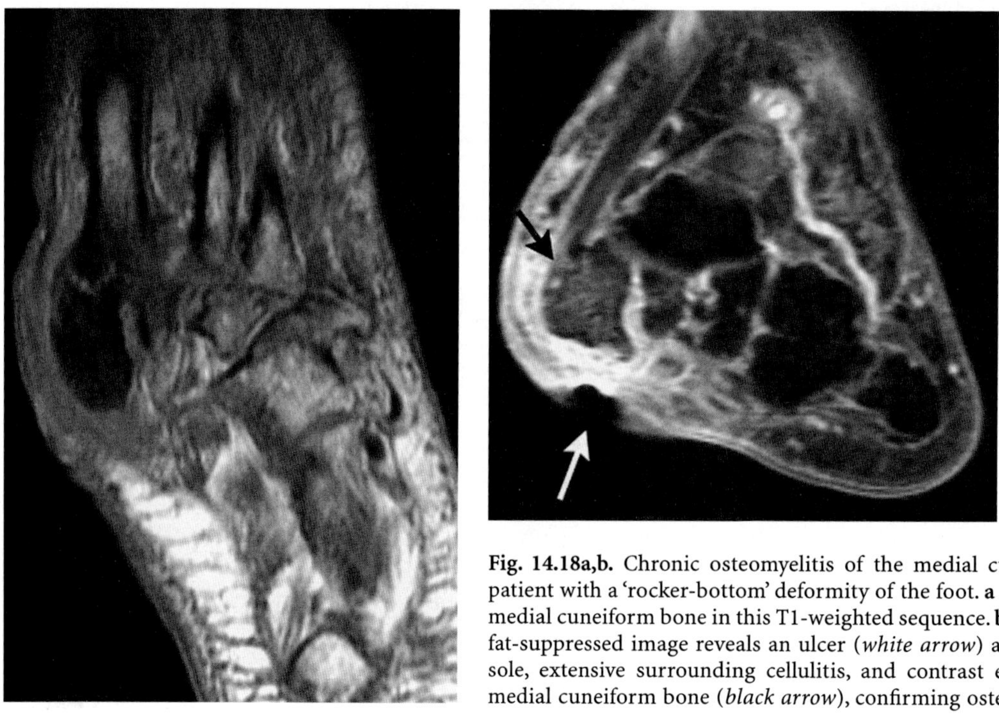

a b

Fig. 14.18a,b. Chronic osteomyelitis of the medial cuneiform bone in a patient with a 'rocker-bottom' deformity of the foot. **a** Note sclerosis of the medial cuneiform bone in this T1-weighted sequence. **b** Contrast-enhanced fat-suppressed image reveals an ulcer (*white arrow*) at the medial plantar sole, extensive surrounding cellulitis, and contrast enhancement of the medial cuneiform bone (*black arrow*), confirming osteomyelitis

Table 14.2. Differentiation of osteomyelitis from neuropathic osteoarthropathy

	Osteomyelitis	Neuropathic osteo-arthropathy	Comments
Typical location	Toes (tips, dorsum)	Lisfranc joint	In the setting of foot deformity, osteomyelitis can occur at atypical locations
	Metatarsal heads (esp. 1st, 5th)	Chopart joint	
	Calcaneus		
	Malleoli		
Distribution	Focal, local, centripetal spread	Multiple joints in a region	
Pattern of edema/enhancement	Predominant involvement of one bone	Epicenter in joint and subchondral bone	
Deformity	Uncommon (unless there is underlying neuropathic disease)	Common	
Soft tissues	Adjacent ulcer, cellulitis, sinus tract	Enhancement limited to juxtaarticular soft tissues; skin, subcutaneous tissues intact	Diffuse subcutanoeus edema is typical in diabetic feet

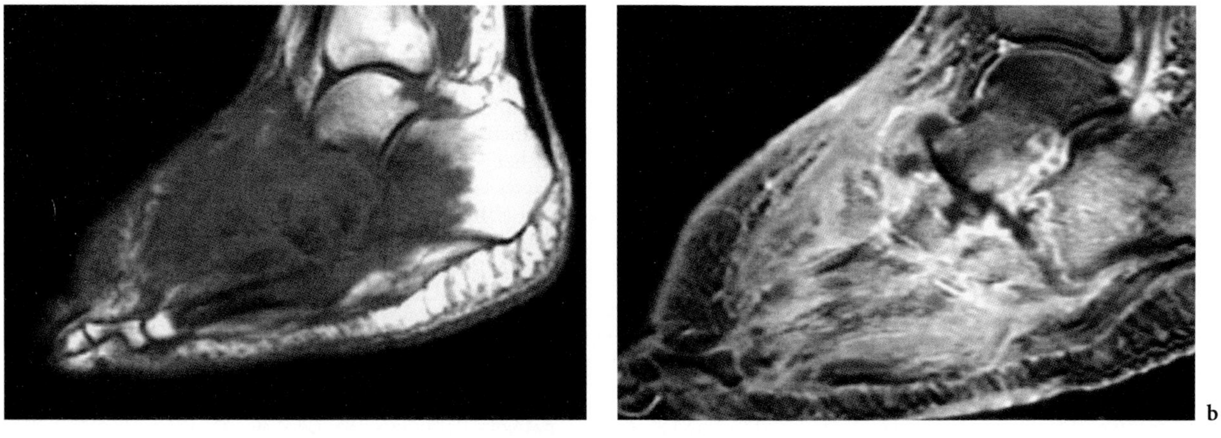

a b

Fig. 14.19a,b. Simultaneous occurrence of acute neuroarthropathy of the forefoot and histologically proven osteomyelitis of the anterior aspect of the calcaneus due to a medial hindfoot ulceration. **a** Note identical hypointense signal in the forefoot (acute neuroarthropathy) and calcaneus (osteomyelitis) on this T1-weighted image. **b** Contrast-enhanced fat-suppressed image with enhancement in the region of neuropathic osteoarthropathy (forefoot) and osteomyelitis (calcaneus)

References

Abbott CA, Vileikyte L, Williamson S et al (1998) Multicenter study of the incidence of and predictive risk factors for diabetic neuropathic foot ulceration. Diabetes Care 21: 1071–1075

Allman RM, Brower AC, Kotlyarov EB (1988) Neuropathic bone and joint disease. Radiol Clin North Am 26:1373–1381

Alson MD, Lang EV, Kaufman JA (1997) Pedal arterial imaging. J Vasc Intervent Radiol 8:9–18

Apelqvist J, Ragnarson-Tennvall G, Persson U et al (1994) Diabetic foot ulcers in a multidisciplinary setting. An economic analysis of primary healing and healing with amputation. J Intern Med 235:463–471

Archer AG, Roberts VC, Watkins PJ (1984) Blood flow patterns in painful diabetic neuropathy. Diabetologia 27: 563–567

Armstrong DG, Lavery LA (1998) Elevated peak plantar pres-

sures in patients who have Charcot arthropathy. J Bone Joint Surg Am 80:365–369
Armstrong DG, Todd WF, Lavery LA et al (1997) The natural history of acute Charcot's arthropathy in a diabetic foot specialty clinic. Diabet Med 87:357–363
Armstrong DG, Peters EJ, Athanasiou KA et al (1998) Is there a critical level of plantar foot pressure to identify patients at risk for neuropathic foot ulceration? J Foot Ankle Surg 37:303–307
Armstrong DG, Stacpoole-Shea S, Nguyen H et al (1999) Lengthening of the Achilles tendon in diabetic patients who are at high risk for ulceration of the foot. J Bone Joint Surg Am 81:535–538
Bamberger DM, Daus GP, Gerding DN (1987) Osteomyelitis in the feet of diabetic patients. Long-term results, prognostic factors, and the role of antimicrobial and surgical therapy. Am J Med 83:653–660
Baum RA, Rutter CM, Sunshine JH et al (1995) Multicenter trial to evaluate vascular magnetic resonance angiography of the lower extremity. American College of Radiology Rapid Technology Assessment Group. JAMA 274:875–880
Becker W (1999) Imaging osteomyelitis and the diabetic foot. Q J Nucl Med 43:9–20
Beltran J, Campanini DS, Knight C et al (1990) The diabetic foot: magnetic resonance imaging evaluation. Skeletal Radiol 19:37–41
Bild DE, Selby JV, Sinnock P et al (1989) Lower-extremity amputation in people with diabetes. Epidemiology and prevention. Diabetes Care 12:24–31
Birke JA, Franks BD, Foto JG (1995) First ray joint limitation, pressure, and ulceration of the first metatarsal head in diabetes mellitus. Foot Ankle Int 16:277–284
Boulton AJ (1996) The pathogenesis of diabetic foot problems: an overview. Diabet Med 13 [Suppl 1]:S12–S16
Boulton AJ, Vileikyte L (2000) The diabetic foot. The scope of the problem. J Fam Pract 49 [Suppl 119:S3–S8
Boutin RD, Brossmann J, Sartoris DJ et al (1998) Update on imaging of orthopedic infections. Orthop Clin North Am 29:41–66
Brower AC, Allman RM (1981) Pathogenesis of the neurotrophic joint: neurotraumatic vs. neurovascular. Radiology 139:349–354
Caputo GM, Cavanagh PR, Ulbrecht JS et al (1994) Assessment and management of foot disease in patients with diabetes. N Engl J Med 331:854–860
Carpenter JP, Golden MA, Barker CF et al (1996) The fate of bypass grafts to angiographically occult runoff vessels detected by magnetic resonance angiography. J Vasc Surg 23:483–489
Cavanagh PR, Young MJ, Adams JE et al (1994) Radiographic abnormalities in the feet of patients with diabetic neuropathy. Diabetes Care 17:201–209
Cavanagh PR, Ulbrecht JS, Caputo GM (1996) Biomechanical aspects of diabetic foot disease: aetiology, treatment, and prevention. Diabet Med 13 [Suppl 1]:S17–S22
Cicchinelli LD, Corey SV (1993) 1993 William J. Stickel Bronze Award. Imaging of the infected foot. Fact or fancy? J Am Podiatr Med Assoc 83:576–594
Clouse ME, Gramm HF, Legg M et al (1974) Diabetic osteoarthropathy. Clinical and roentgenographic observations in 90 cases. Am J Roentgenol Radium Ther Nucl Med 121:22–34
Cofield RH, Morrison MJ, Beabout JW (1983) Diabetic neuroarthropathy in the foot: patient characteristics and patterns of radiographic change. Foot Ankle 4:15–22
Crim JR, Seeger LL (1994) Imaging evaluation of osteomyelitis. Crit Rev Diagn Imaging 35:201–256
Criqui MH, Langer RD, Fronek A et al (1992) Mortality over a period of 10 years in patients with peripheral arterial disease. N Engl J Med 326:381–386
Cundy TF, Edmonds ME, Watkins PJ (1985) Osteopenia and metatarsal fractures in diabetic neuropathy. Diabet Med 2:461–464
Deanfield JE, Daggett PR, Harrison MJ (1980) The role of autonomic neuropathy in diabetic foot ulceration. J Neurol Sci 47:203–210
Durham JR, Lukens ML, Campanini DS et al (1991) Impact of magnetic resonance imaging on the management of diabetic foot infections. Am J Surg 162:150–153
Edelman SV, Kosofsky EM, Paul RA et al (1987) Neuro-osteoarthropathy (Charcot's joint) in diabetes mellitus following revascularization surgery. Three case reports and a review of the literature. Arch Intern Med 147:1504–1508
Edmonds ME (1986) The neuropathic foot in diabetes, part I. Blood flow. Diabet Med 3:111–115
Edmonds ME (2000) Medial arterial calcification and diabetes mellitus. Z Kardiol 89 [Suppl 2]:101–104
Edmonds ME, Clarke MB, Newton S et al (1985) Increased uptake of bone radiopharmaceutical in diabetic neuropathy. Q J Med 57:843–855
El Khoury GY, Kathol MH (1980) Neuropathic fractures in patients with diabetes mellitus. Radiology 134:313–316
Eymontt MJ, Alavi A, Dalinka MK et al (1981) Bone scintigraphy in diabetic osteoarthropathy. Radiology 140:475–477
Fry DE, Marek JM, Langsfeld M (1998) Infection in the ischemic lower extremity. Surg Clin North Am 78:465–479
Frykberg RG, Lavery LA, Pham H et al (1998) Role of neuropathy and high foot pressures in diabetic foot ulceration. Diabetes Care 21:1714–1719
Gallacher SJ, Thomson G, Fraser WD et al (1995) Neutrophil bactericidal function in diabetes mellitus: evidence for association with blood glucose control. Diabet Med 12: 916–920
Gold RH, Tong DJ, Crim JR et al (1995) Imaging the diabetic foot. Skeletal Radiol 24:563–571
Goldner MG (1960) The fate of the second leg in the diabetic amputee. Diabetes 9:100–103
Goodwin DW, Salonen DC, Yu JS et al (1995) Plantar compartments of the foot: MR appearance in cadavers and diabetic patients. Radiology 196:623–630
Green DR, Brekke M (1996) Anatomy, biomechanics, and pathomechanics of lesser digital deformities. Clin Podiatr Med Surg 13:179–200
Grumbine NA, King GA (1996) Clawfoot deformity: an analysis of the causes and surgical treatment using a modification of the Jones suspension procedure. Clin Podiatr Med Surg 13:221–238
Hill SL, Holtzman GI, Buse R (1999) The effects of peripheral vascular disease with osteomyelitis in the diabetic foot. Am J Surg 177:282–286
Hoar CS, Torres J (1962) Evaluation of below-the-knee amputation in the treatment of diabetic gangrene. N Engl J Med 266:440–443
Holmes GB Jr, Mann RA (1992) Possible epidemiological factors associated with rupture of the posterior tibial tendon. Foot Ankle 13:70–79
Holstein PE, Sorensen S (1999) Limb salvage experience in

a multidisciplinary diabetic foot unit. Diabetes Care 22 [Suppl 2]:B97–B103
Horowitz JD, Durham JR, Nease DB et al (1993) Prospective evaluation of magnetic resonance imaging in the management of acute diabetic foot infections. Ann Vasc Surg 7: 44–50
Humphrey LL, Palumbo PJ, Butters MA et al (1994) The contribution of non-insulin-dependent diabetes to lower-extremity amputation in the community. Arch Intern Med 154:885–892
Jeffcoate W, Lima J, Nobrega L (2000) The Charcot foot. Diabet Med 17:253–258
Johnson JT (1967) Neuropathic fractures and joint injuries. Pathogenesis and rationale of prevention and treatment. J Bone Joint Surg 49A:1–30
Joshi N, Caputo GM, Weitekamp MR et al (1999) Infections in patients with diabetes mellitus. N Engl J Med 341: 1906–1912
Karchmer AW, Gibbons GW (1994) Foot infections in diabetes: evaluation and management. Curr Clin Top Infect Dis 14: 1–22
Kathol MH, el Khoury GY, Moore TE et al (1991) Calcaneal insufficiency avulsion fractures in patients with diabetes mellitus. Radiology 180:725–729
Katz I, Rabinovitz JG, Dziadiw R (1961) Early changes in Charcot's joints. AJR 86:965–974
Keenan AM, Tindel NL, Alavi A (1989) Diagnosis of pedal osteomyelitis in diabetic patients using current scintigraphic techniques. Arch Intern Med 149:2262–2266
King H, Aubert RE, Herman WH (1998) Global burden of diabetes, 1995–2025: prevalence, numerical estimates, and projections. Diabetes Care 21:1414–1431
Kreitner KF, Kalden P, Neufang A et al (2000) Diabetes and peripheral arterial occlusive disease: prospective comparison of contrast-enhanced three-dimensional MR angiography with conventional digital subtraction angiography. AJR 174:171–179
Larcos G, Brown ML, Sutton RT (1991) Diagnosis of osteomyelitis of the foot in diabetic patients: value of 111In-leukocyte scintigraphy. AJR 157:527–531
Lavery LA, Gazewood JD (2000) Assessing the feet of patients with diabetes. J Fam Pract 49 [Suppl 11]:S9–S16
Lavery LA, Lavery DC, Quebedeax-Farnham TL (1995) Increased foot pressures after great toe amputation in diabetes. Diabetes Care 18:1460–1462
Lavery LA, Armstrong DG, Vela SA et al (1998) Practical criteria for screening patients at high risk for diabetic foot ulceration. Arch Intern Med 26:157–162
Ledermann HP, Morrison WB, Schweitzer ME (2002a) MR image analysis of pedal osteomyelitis: distribution, patterns of spread, and frequency of associated ulceration and septic arthritis. Radiology 223:747–755
Ledermann HP, Schweitzer ME, Morrison WB (2002b) Nonenhancing tissue on MR imaging of pedal infection: characterization of necrotic tissue and associated limitations for diagnosis of osteomyelitis and abscess. AJR Am J Roentgenol 178:215–222
Lee HM, Wang Y, Sostman HD et al (1998) Distal lower extremity arteries: evaluation with two-dimensional MR digital subtraction angiography. Radiology 207:505–512
Levin ME (1995) Preventing amputation in the patient with diabetes. Diabetes Care 18:1383–1394
Lipman BT, Collier BD, Carrera GF et al (1998) Detection of osteomyelitis in the neuropathic foot: nuclear medicine, MRI and conventional radiography. Clin Nucl Med 23: 77–82
Lower RF, Kenzora JE (1994) The diabetic neuropathic foot: a triple crush syndrome – measurement of compartmental pressures of normal and diabetic feet. Orthopedics 17: 241–248
Marcus CD, Ladam-Marcus VJ, Leone J et al (1996) MR imaging of osteomyelitis and neuropathic osteoarthropathy in the feet of diabetics. Radiographics 16:1337–1348
Maurer AH, Millmond SH, Knight LC et al (1986) Infection in diabetic osteoarthropathy: use of indium-labeled leukocytes for diagnosis. Radiology 161:221–225
Mayfield JA, Reiber GE, Sanders LJ et al (1998) Preventive foot care in people with diabetes. Diabetes Care 21:2161–2177
Mitchell DG, Joseph PM, Fallon M et al (1987) Chemical-shift MR imaging of the femoral head: an in vitro study of normal hips and hips with avascular necrosis. AJR 148: 1159–1164
Moore TE, Yuh WT, Kathol MH et al (1991) Abnormalities of the foot in patients with diabetes mellitus: findings on MR imaging. AJR 157:813–816
Moore TE, Yuh WT, el Khoury GY (1996) Plantar compartments of the foot: MR appearance in cadavers and diabetic patients. Radiology 198:909
Morrison WB, Schweitzer ME, Wapner KL et al (1995) Osteomyelitis in feet of diabetics: clinical accuracy, surgical utility, and cost-effectiveness of MR imaging. Radiology 196:557–564
Morrison WB, Schweitzer ME, Batte WG et al (1998) Osteomyelitis of the foot: relative importance of primary and secondary MR imaging signs. Radiology 207:625–632
Most RS, Sinnock P (1983) The epidemiology of lower extremity amputations in diabetic individuals. Diabetes Care 6: 87–91
Mozes G, Keresztury G, Kadar A et al (1998) Atherosclerosis in amputated legs of patients with and without diabetes mellitus. Int Angiol 17:282–286
Muchova J, Liptakova A, Orszaghova Z et al (1999) Antioxidant systems in polymorphonuclear leucocytes of Type 2 diabetes mellitus. Diabet Med 16:74–78
Mueller MJ, Diamond JE, Delitto A et al (1989) Insensitivity, limited joint mobility, and plantar ulcers in patients with diabetes mellitus. Phys Ther 69:453–459
Mueller MJ, Minor SD, Diamond JE et al (1990) Relationship of foot deformity to ulcer location in patients with diabetes mellitus. Phys Ther 70:356–362
Munk PL, Helms CA, Holt RG (1989) Immature bone infarcts: findings on plain radiographs and MR scans. AJR 152: 547–549
Myerson MS (2000) Diabetic neuroarthropathy. In: Myerson MS (ed) Foot and ankle disorders. Saunders, Philadelphia, pp 439–465
Newman AB, Sutton-Tyrrell K, Vogt MT et al (1993) Morbidity and mortality in hypertensive adults with a low ankle/arm blood pressure index. JAMA 270:487–489
Newman JH (1979) Spontaneous dislocation in diabetic neuropathy. A report of six cases. J Bone Joint Surg [Br] 61B: 484–488
Newman LG, Waller J, Palestro CJ et al (1991) Unsuspected osteomyelitis in diabetic foot ulcers. Diagnosis and monitoring by leukocyte scanning with indium in 111 oxyquinoline. JAMA 266:1246–1251

Nguyen VD (1992) The radiologic spectrum of abnormalities of the foot in diabetic patients. Can Assoc Radiol J 43:333–339

Nguyen VD, Keh RA, Daehler RW (1991) Freiberg's disease in diabetes mellitus. Skeletal Radiol 20:425–428

Nigro ND, Bartynski WS, Grossman SJ et al (1992) Clinical impact of magnetic resonance imaging in foot osteomyelitis. J Am Podiatr Med Assoc 82:603–615

Oser RF, Picus D, Hicks ME et al (1995) Accuracy of DSA in the evaluation of patency of infrapopliteal vessels. J Vasc Intervent Radiol 6:589–594

Owen RS, Carpenter JP, Baum RA et al (1992) Magnetic resonance imaging of angiographically occult runoff vessels in peripheral arterial occlusive disease. N Engl J Med 326: 1577–1581

Park HM, Wheat LJ, Siddiqui AR et al (1982) Scintigraphic evaluation of diabetic osteomyelitis: concise communication. J Nucl Med 23:569–573

Pell JP, Donnan PT, Fowkes FG et al (1993) Quality of life following lower limb amputation for peripheral arterial disease. Eur J Vasc Surg 7:448–451

Pinzur MS (1999) Benchmark analysis of diabetic patients with neuropathic (Charcot) foot deformity. Foot Ankle Int 20:564–567

Pitei DL, Foster A, Edmonds M (1999) The effect of regular callus removal on foot pressures. J Foot Ankle Surg 38:251–255

Pomposelli FB Jr, Marcaccio EJ, Gibbons GW et al (1995) Dorsalis pedis arterial bypass: durable limb salvage for foot ischemia in patients with diabetes mellitus. J Vasc Surg 21:375–384

Ramsey SD, Newton K, Blough D et al (1999) Incidence, outcomes, and cost of foot ulcers in patients with diabetes. Diabetes Care 22:382–387

Rassias AJ, Marrin CA, Arruda J et al (1999) Insulin infusion improves neutrophil function in diabetic cardiac surgery patients. Anesth Analg 88:1011–1016

Reiber GE (1992) Diabetic foot care. Financial implications and practice guidelines. Diabetes Care 15 [Suppl 1]:29–31

Reiber GE, Lipsky BA, Gibbons GW (1998) The burden of diabetic foot ulcers. Am J Surg 176 [2A Suppl]:5S–10S

Reiber GE, Vileikyte L, Boyko EJ et al (1999) Causal pathways for incident lower-extremity ulcers in patients with diabetes from two settings. Diabetes Care 22:157–162

Resnick D (1995) Neuropathic Osteoarthropathy. In: Resnick D (ed) Diagnosis of bone and joint disorders. Saunders, Philadelphia, pp 3413–3442

Rosenbloom MS, Flanigan DP, Schuler JJ et al (1988) Risk factors affecting the natural history of intermittent claudication. Arch Surg 123:867–870

Schauwecker DS (1995) Differentiation of infected from non-infected rapidly progressive neuropathic osteoarthropathy. J Nucl Med 36:1427–1428

Schauwecker DS, Park HM, Burt RW et al (1988) Combined bone scintigraphy and indium-111 leukocyte scans in neuropathic foot disease. J Nucl Med 29:1651–1655

Schon LC, Easley ME, Weinfeld SB (1998) Charcot neuroarthropathy of the foot and ankle. Clin Orthop 349:116–131

Schwarz GS, Berenyi MR, Siegel MW (1969) Atrophic arthropathy and diabetic neuritis. Am J Roentgenol Radium Ther Nucl Med 106:523–529

Schweitzer ME, Karasick D (2000) MR imaging of disorders of the posterior tibialis tendon. AJR 175:627–635

Schweitzer ME, Caccese R, Karasick D et al (1993) Posterior tibial tendon tears: utility of secondary signs for MR imaging diagnosis. Radiology 188:655–659

Seabold JE, Flickinger FW, Kao SC et al (1990) Indium-111-leukocyte/technetium-99m-MDP bone and magnetic resonance imaging: difficulty of diagnosing osteomyelitis in patients with neuropathic osteoarthropathy. J Nucl Med 31:549–556

Sella EJ, Barrette C (1999) Staging of Charcot neuroarthropathy along the medial column of the foot in the diabetic patient. J Foot Ankle Surg 38:34–40

Siperstein MD, Unger RH, Madison LL (1968) Studies of muscle capillary basement membranes in normal subjects, diabetic, and prediabetic patients. J Clin Invest 47: 1973–1999

Smith DM, Weinberger M, Katz BP (1987) A controlled trial to increase office visits and reduce hospitalizations of diabetic patients. J Gen Intern Med 2:232–238

Stadelmann WK, Digenis AG, Tobin GR (1998) Impediments to wound healing. Am J Surg 176 [2A Suppl]:39–47

Sumpio BE (2000) Foot ulcers. N Engl J Med 343:787–793

Tan JS, Friedman NM, Hazelton-Miller C et al (1996) Can aggressive treatment of diabetic foot infections reduce the need for above-ankle amputation? Clin Infect Dis 23: 286–291

Thomasson JL, Sundaram M (1985) The diabetic foot–radiographic appearances. Orthopedics 8:668–677

Thornton GF (1971) Infections and diabetes. Med Clin North Am 55:931–938

Tooke JE (1995) Microvascular function in human diabetes. A physiological perspective. Diabetes 12:721–726

Umans H, Haramati N, Flusser G (2000) The diagnostic role of gadolinium enhanced MRI in distinguishing between acute medullary bone infarct and osteomyelitis. Magn Reson Imaging 18:255–262

Ward JD (1982) The diabetic leg. Diabetologia 22:141–147

Wheat LJ (1980) Infection and diabetes mellitus. Diabetes Care 3:187–197

Young MJ, Breddy JL, Veves A et al (1994) The prediction of diabetic neuropathic foot ulceration using vibration perception thresholds. A prospective study. Diabetes Care 17: 557–560

Young MJ, Marshall A, Adams JE et al (1995) Osteopenia, neurological dysfunction, and the development of Charcot neuroarthropathy. Diabetes Care 18:34–38

Younger DS, Bronfin L (1996) Overview of diabetic neuropathy. Semin Neurol 16:107–113

Yu JS (1998) Diabetic foot and neuroarthropathy: magnetic resonance imaging evaluation. Top.Magn Reson.Imaging 9:295–310

Zlatkin MB, Pathria M, Sartoris DJ et al (1987) The diabetic foot. Radiol Clin North Am 25:1095–1105

15 Arthritis

M. Cobby and I. Watt

CONTENTS

15.1 Introduction

This chapter is concerned primarily with the conventional radiographic appearances of arthritis, illustrating the various common and less common patterns of disease. It is divided into two sections. In the first part a general approach to the diagnosis of joint disease is described and in the second follows a brief description of the most pertinent features of those arthritides that affect the foot and ankle. It should be remembered, however, that imaging studies may be performed for a variety of reasons other than making or establishing a diagnosis (Table 15.1). Some of these require adaptations to the usual radiographic technique. For example, weight-bearing standing views in both the dorsoplantar and lateral projections are necessary to adequately demonstrate structural changes of the midfoot and hindfoot. Such changes include hindfoot varus or valgus abnormalities and the evaluation of patients for surgical correction of deforming foot diseases such as hallux valgus or congenital equinovarus.

The differential diagnosis of arthritis is most easily accomplished by considering a combination of which joint is involved and what component of the joint is primarily affected (Watt 1997). An example of the importance of the location is the finding of osteoarthritis of the ankle joint. This is rarely seen in the absence of previous severe trauma and joint instability, whereas it is a classical site for involvement in haemophilia or haemochromatosis. A number of components within the joint should be scrutinised when attempting to determine which tissue is principally involved, although it must be remembered that no individual component exists in isolation. These include the joint capsule, synovium, cartilage, subchondral bone, entheses and joint fluid (Fig. 15.1). By analysing what area the disease primarily affects within a joint, it is possible to suggest what tissue is mainly implicated.

Table 15.1. Reasons for imaging studies in arthritis

Establishing or confirming a diagnosis
Determining the extent of disease
Monitoring change and disease activity
Determining appropriate drug therapy
Selecting patients for surgery
Identifying complications
- of the disease
- of the treatment
- of surgery
For outcome assessment of new treatments
For research

M. Cobby, MD
Department of Radiology, Frenchay Hospital, Bristol BS16 1LE, UK
I. Watt, MD
Department of Clinical Radiology, Bristol Royal Infirmary, Bristol BS2 8HW, UK

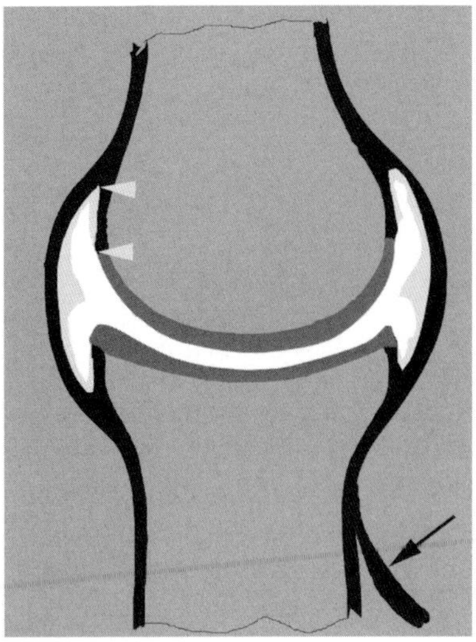

Fig. 15.1. Diagram of a synovial joint illustrating the joint capsule, synovium and hyaline cartilage. The so-called bare area is located between the two *arrowheads* where the synovium directly contacts the bone. The entheses include capsular and tendon attachments (*arrow*)

On a conventional radiograph, three locations can be identified. The first is where the synovium directly contacts bone at the so-called bare area, where no hyaline cartilage interposes between the synovium and the cortical bone (Martel et al. 1980). Here, invading pannus (see synovial diseases below) erodes the bone first. The second location is hyaline cartilage and the immediate subchondral bone, and involvement at this site can be considered as primarily due to cartilage disease. The last location is the enthesis, i.e. those places where the capsule, ligament or tendons are inserted into bone. The entheseal diseases include ankylosing spondylitis, psoriatic arthritis and Reiter's disease, where associated erosions are classically seen, and Forestier's disease or diffuse idiopathic skeletal hyperostosis (DISH), fluorosis and other related diseases, where they are not.

It is often much easier to diagnose an arthritis early in its course than when it is more radiologically advanced as end-stage changes of several arthropathies may look very similar. As some of these arthropathies are fairly common, not infrequently more than one disease may be present or be superimposed upon another. For reasons that are not clear, however, it is extremely uncommon to see gout in the presence of rheumatoid arthritis (Rizzoli et al. 1980). Indeed, the deposition of calcium pyrophosphate crystals is rare also in conjunction with rheumatoid disease (Doherty et al. 1984).

15.2 Synovial Diseases

The radiological features of synovial disease include soft-tissue swelling, due either to synovial proliferation and thickening, a joint effusion or both. For many joints within the foot, this is difficult to determine, although an effusion at the ankle joint can be reliably determined from the lateral examination. Other investigations such as ultrasound or MRI are required to differentiate synovial thickening from a joint effusion. The transition from inflammatory synovitis to invasive pannus marks an important step in the disease evolution, although only MRI can reliably differentiate the two.

Ill-definition of the soft-tissue swelling indicates that an inflammatory or infectious cause is most likely. Occasionally, the synovium may appear diffusely opaque or unusually radiodense due to haemosiderin deposition from repeated intra-articular haemorrhage, as is seen commonly in bleeding disorders such as haemophilia or Von Willebrand's disease.

Numerous ring-like areas of calcification within the synovium typically occur in synovial chondromatosis (Fig. 15.2). This has to be differentiated

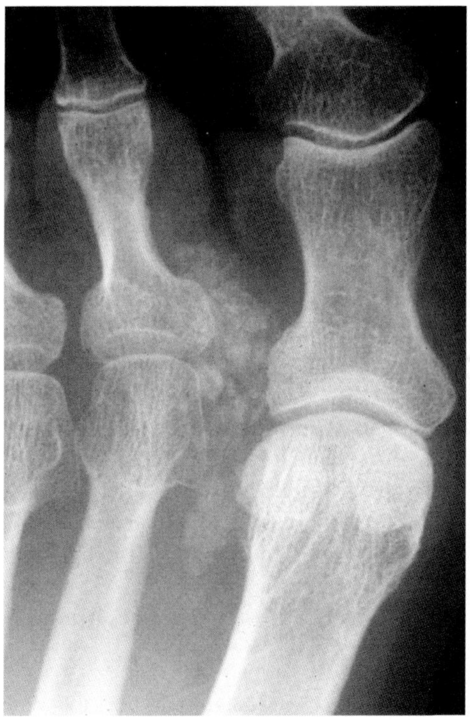

Fig. 15.2. Synovial osteochondromatosis in second toe metatarsophalangeal joint. Note the numerous ring-like areas of calcification

from the coarser soft-tissue calcification that results from the heavy deposition of calcium pyrophosphate dihydrate crystals within the synovium or joint capsule often seen in association with linear deposits in hyaline cartilage or fibrocartilage in areas outside of the foot or ankle.

Metallic or cement debris from the disintegration of a failed prosthetic joint may become lodged within the synovium. Alternatively, modestly radiodense debris can be seen in silicone synovitis if one of these implants has failed, together with soft-tissue swelling and subchondral lucencies (Fig. 15.3).

Fusiform soft-tissue swelling of the joint on its own is a non-specific feature, but asymmetric soft-tissue swelling indicates the presence of a depositional disease or other synovial mass lesion. These eccentric areas of soft-tissue swelling are frequently associated with 'pressure' erosions of the joint and adjacent bone. When only one or two such lesions are shown in several joints, then diseases such as rheumatoid nodules, gouty tophi, xanthomata and amyloidosis should be considered. Those diseases confined to single joints, such as synovial chondromatosis and pigmented villonodular synovitis (PVNS), are usually associated with multiple well-defined erosions generally affecting both sides of the joint involved.

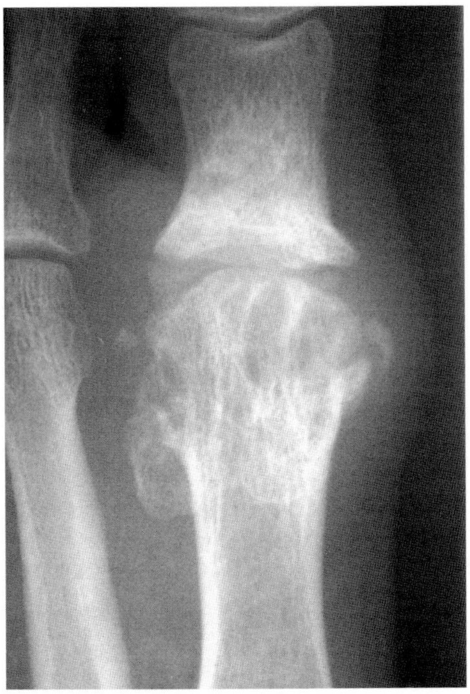

Fig. 15.3. Silicone synovitis. Failure of the implant at the great toe metatarsophalangeal joint is associated with soft-tissue swelling, partial disintegration of the prosthesis and well-defined subchondral lucencies

15.2.1 Erosions

15.2.1.1 Ill-Defined Erosions

Ill-defined erosions imply active invasive disease and are characterised by the absence of a cortical or sclerotic margin. They can be further subdivided into proliferative and non-proliferative erosions. Proliferative erosions are associated with new bone formation either within, adjacent to or near the erosion (Fig. 15.4). The new bone formation is characteristic of the seronegative arthropathies including psoriasis and Reiter's syndrome. Medullary sclerosis frequently accompanies these proliferative erosions and, when seen in a toe, can result in the typical 'ivory phalanges'. Non-proliferative erosions, where no new bone formation is evident and involving more than one joint, are most likely due to rheumatoid arthritis. Here, in contradistinction to psoriatic joint disease, bony sclerosis is rare. If only a single joint is involved, particularly when juxta-articular osteopenia and joint space narrowing are prominent, this should suggest a septic arthritis. Early and rapid chondrolysis together with loss of the cortical margins of the articular surface are virtually diagnostic of sepsis.

Early erosions, especially those encountered in rheumatoid arthritis, typically occur on the tibial aspects of the metatarsal heads and on the fibular aspect of the

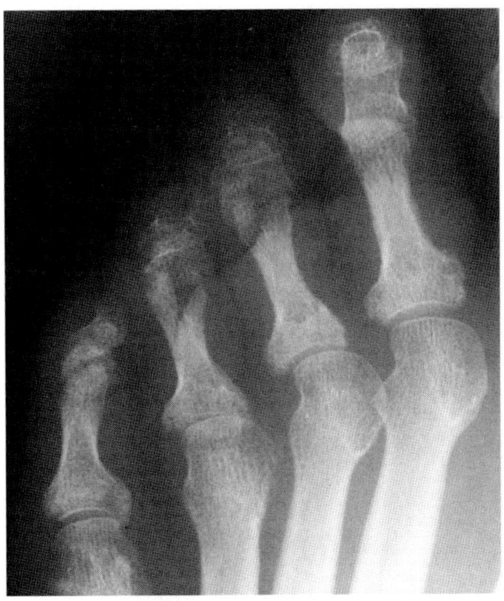

Fig. 15.4. Psoriatic arthritis. Numerous marginal erosions are shown at the metatarsophalangeal and interphalangeal joints. These show characteristic ill-defined proliferative changes most notable around the bases of the proximal phalanges where accompanying new bone formation is observed

head of the little toe metatarsal (Fig. 15.5). The erosions are first identified as focal areas of osteopenia with subsequent interruption of the subchondral bone plate, resulting in a dot-dash appearance. Deeper areas of bone loss then develop with ill-defined margins. These may progress to severe panarticular damage and finally ankylosis or may become static and 'heal', developing a sclerotic margin. Soft-tissue swelling, joint space narrowing and juxta-articular or regional osteopenia are typical accompanying features. Fluffy margins to the erosions resulting from proliferative new bone formation are a feature of the seronegative spondyloarthropathies.

The metatarsal heads have relatively large bare areas, making them susceptible to bony destruction by proliferating synovial pannus. Similarly, the joint capsule extends for some distance over the head of the proximal phalanx at the proximal interphalangeal joint, producing a large bare area, whereas on the other side of the joint, the capsule inserts near to the margin of the base of the phalanx, so that the erosions on this side are small and more difficult to detect.

Although non-proliferative marginal erosions are a characteristic feature of rheumatoid arthritis, destruction of cartilage, with concentric joint space narrowing and other atrophic changes, such as regional osteopenia and osteolysis, may be the dominant or only findings. Such findings, along with subtle periosteal new bone formation, should suggest Reiter's syndrome, however.

15.2.1.2 Well-Defined Erosions

These erosions are demarcated by a line of cortical bone or sclerosis and usually correspond to relatively inert, slow-growing or contained disease. Conditions in which these are commonly seen include well established rheumatoid arthritis (these erosions probably indicate biologically inert disease) and gout, typically involving the great toe metatarsophalangeal joint and not uncommonly associated with peripheral, deforming, soft-tissue masses (Fig. 15.6). Less common causes include xanthomatous deposits either as solitary focal lesions or as part of a generalised disease such as multicentric reticulohistiocytosis. As described earlier, solitary synovial diseases such as synovial chondromatosis or PVNS may produce multiple 'pressure-like', well-defined erosions of the involved joint, and synovial opacification, when present, should confirm the diagnosis.

15.3 Cartilage Disease

In the absence of contrast medium, it is clearly impossible to see the cartilage thickness directly on conventional radiographs. Thickness is inferred by the width of the joint space taken as the distance between the two opposing subchondral bony surfaces. Direct

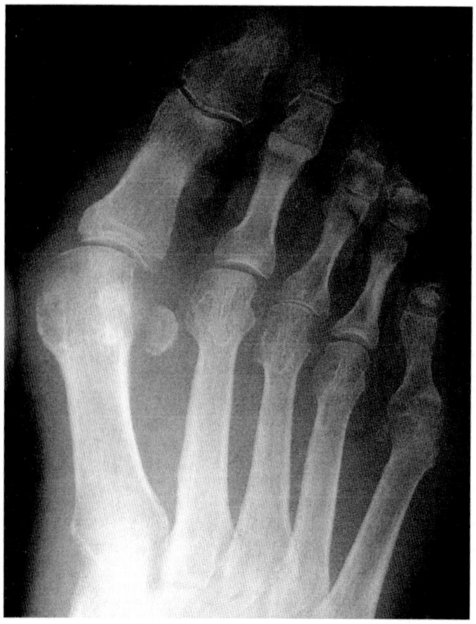

Fig. 15.5. Rheumatoid arthritis. Numerous erosions are shown in various states of evolution with variable joint space loss and joint subluxation

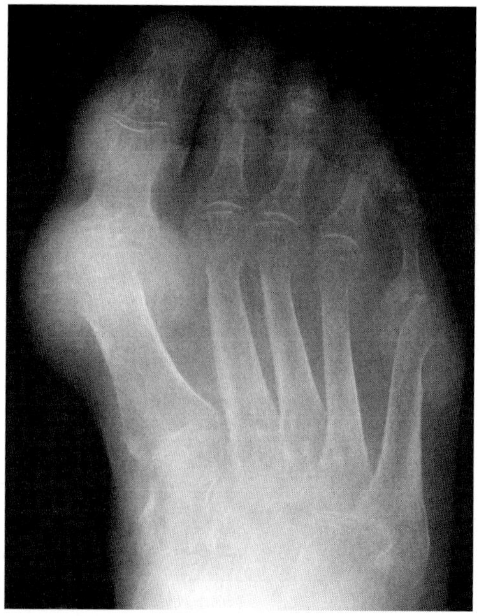

Fig. 15.6. Gout. Multiple eccentric soft-tissue masses and well-defined erosions are shown. A punched-out erosion with overhanging margins is seen at the great toe tarsometatarsal joint

imaging of the cartilage is possible, of course, with MRI or invasively by arthrography. Most articular disorders are associated with the loss of hyaline cartilage, but thickening of the articular cartilage with widening of the joint space is seen in acromegaly where it may be the first clue to such a diagnosis. Preservation of joint space often until late in the course of the disease is typically seen in the depositional diseases such as gout and multicentric reticulohistiocytosis and in PVNS.

Thinning and loss of hyaline cartilage occur in many disease processes. This occurs rapidly in infectious arthritis when concentric joint space narrowing is soon followed by destruction of the subchondral bone plate (Fig. 15.7). Similarly, inflammatory mediators within the joint fluid of many of the inflammatory arthropathies, such as rheumatoid arthritis or psoriatic arthritis, result in destruction of hyaline cartilage with concentric joint space narrowing. Synovial-based erosions may or may not be part of this process. With rheumatoid involvement, this is frequently accompanied by juxta-articular demineralisation. In juvenile idiopathic arthritis, erosions are infrequent, but joint space narrowing with osteopenia and epiphyseal overgrowth secondary to hyperaemia are typical findings. Asymmetric joint space narrowing with accompanying marginal osteophytes and subchondral sclerosis are, of course, the hallmark of osteoarthritis.

15.4 Entheseal Disease

The seronegative spondyloarthropathies, including ankylosing spondylitis, Reiter's syndrome and psoriatic arthritis, result in an erosive enthesitis commonly involving the plantar aponeurosis at its origin from the posterior tuberosity of the calcaneum, where there may be associated erosive and proliferative changes, to a calcaneal spur. The Achilles tendon insertion is another obvious site of involvement for either a local or systemic enthesopathy (Fig. 15.8). In systemic diseases such as the seronegative spondyloarthropathies or rheumatoid arthritis, this is frequently associated with prominent distension of the retrocalcaneal pre-Achilles bursa. Tendinous ossification and calcification can also be seen in the non-erosive entheseal diseases, most commonly due to diffuse idiopathic skeletal hyperostosis (DISH), although other causes include fluorosis and metabolic disorders such as gout. By definition, the absence of erosions distinguishes these changes from the seronegative spondyloarthropathies.

Distinguishing between the various seronegative spondyloarthropathies is difficult, although prominent peripheral involvement of the foot and ankle in ankylosing spondylitis is less common than in Reiter's syndrome or psoriasis.

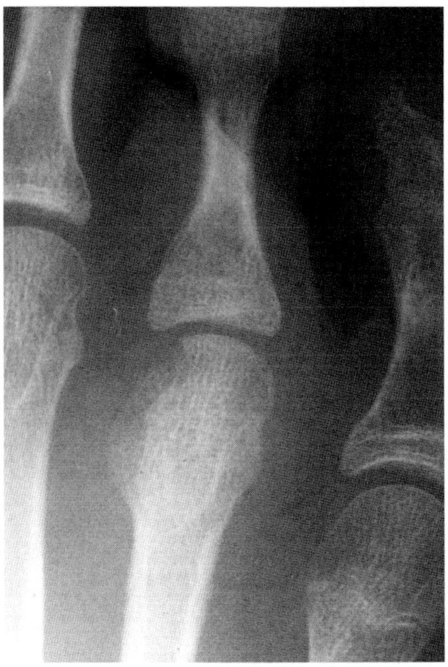

Fig. 15.7. Septic arthritis. Soft-tissue swelling, concentric joint space narrowing, marginal erosions and subtle loss of the subchondral bone plate are seen in association with metaphyseal periosteal new bone formation

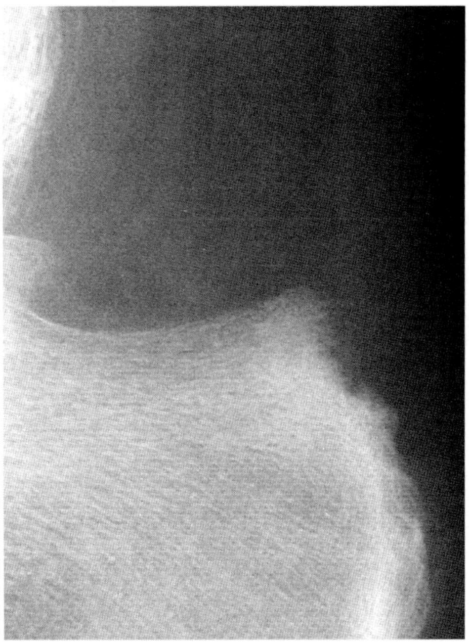

Fig. 15.8. Psoriatic arthritis. Ill-defined proliferative erosion of the calcaneal tuberosity adjacent to the insertion of the Achilles tendon

15.5 Rheumatoid Arthritis

15.5.1 Hindfoot

Clinical involvement of the ankle and hindfoot is common in rheumatoid arthritis, although less frequent than involvement of the hand, wrist, foot and knee. Synovial hypertrophy or effusions of the ankle joint can be seen radiographically as soft-tissue masses displacing the adjacent fat planes anterior and posterior to the joint margin. Massive synovial hypertrophy will also present lateral to the joint line. Marginal erosions are uncommonly seen at these sites, but with long-standing disease progressive joint space narrowing, subluxation and secondary osteoarthritis are frequent findings.

A retrocalcaneal bursitis is often observed and may be associated with erosion of the adjacent superior part of the posterior tuberosity of the calcaneum. Rheumatoid nodules are typically located superficial to the Achilles tendon (Fig. 15.9).

15.5.2 Midfoot

Postural deformities, most frequently planovalgus, are commonly seen. It is often associated with inflammation or rupture of the posterior tibial tendon. With conventional radiographs, these deformities may be evident only on standing films. Uniform joint space narrowing of the midfoot articulations is often seen and not infrequently progresses to bony ankylosis. Involvement of the midfoot and wrists with complete or relative sparing of the hands and forefoot is a pattern of rheumatoid involvement quite often recognised.

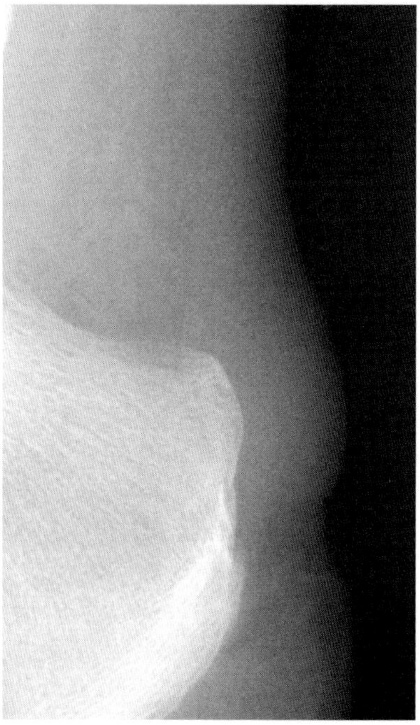

Fig. 15.9. Rheumatoid nodule superficial to the insertion of the Achilles tendon

15.5.3 Forefoot

The metatarsophalangeal joints of the lateral toes are most frequently affected, particularly the 5th. Erosions are usually located on the tibial aspect of the metatarsal head, but an early, and often the first, erosion may be seen on the fibula aspect of the 5th metatarsal head associated with adjacent soft-tissue swelling. This is a common, early and not infrequently initial manifestation of rheumatoid involvement, often predating changes in the hands and wrists. A further frequent and characteristic site of involvement is the great toe interphalangeal joint. The remaining interphalangeal joints are more seldom implicated. Erosions are almost always larger on the metatarsal side of the metatarsophalangeal joints and on the proximal side of the great toe interphalangeal joint due to the more proximal insertion of the joint capsule around these sites and the larger associated bare areas (Fig. 15.5).

Insufficiency fractures of the calcaneum (Fig. 15.10), distal fibula (Fig. 15.11) and metatarsals are quite commonly seen accompanying the regional osteopenia, joint subluxation and postural deformities that result from a combination of joint laxity and tendon abnormalities.

15.6 Juvenile Idiopathic Arthritis

This is a generic term for a heterogeneous group of articular disorders whose classification is based on clinical, laboratory and radiological findings. Many of the radiological changes are non-specific and relate to disordered growth and extra-articular manifestations. By definition, it is a disease that begins before the age of 16 years and has a duration lasting longer than 6 weeks. Classification is made 6 months after onset into one of the following groups: systemic

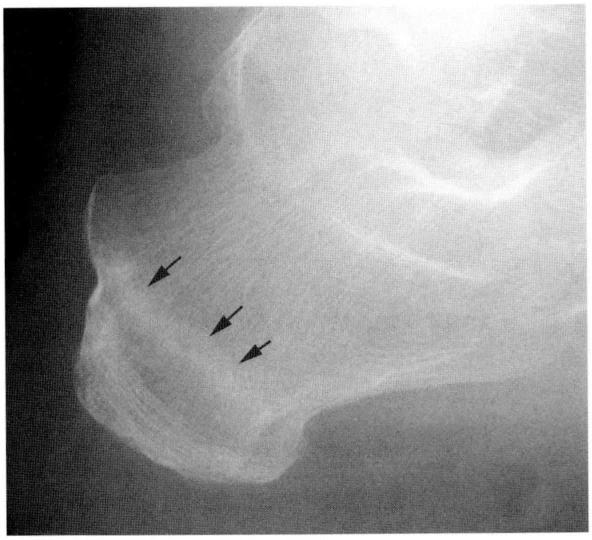

Fig. 15.10. Insufficiency fracture (*arrows*) of the calcaneum in rheumatoid arthritis

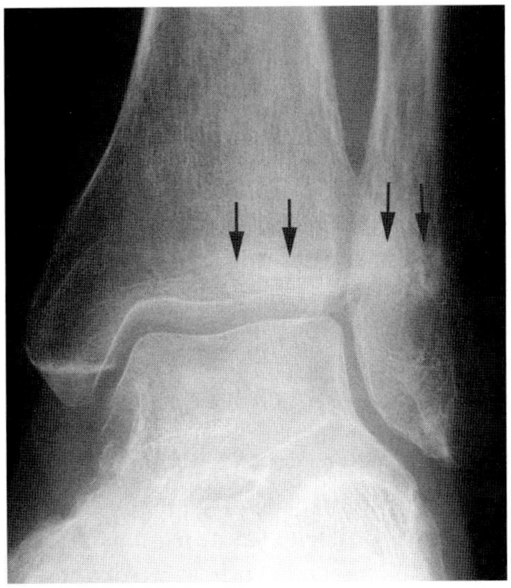

Fig. 15.11. Rheumatoid arthritis. Insufficiency fractures of the distal tibia and fibula (*arrows*)

arthritis, polyarthritis (rheumatoid factor positive or rheumatoid factor negative), oligoarthritis, extended oligoarthritis, enthesitis-related arthritis or psoriatic arthritis (PETTY 2001).

15.6.1
Ankle Joint

Growth disturbances may be seen accompanied by soft-tissue swelling and regional osteoporosis. With more severe involvement, joint space narrowing and subchondral irregularity may occur. Radiographically, if this is the only joint involved, then the changes can be difficult to distinguish from haemophiliac arthropathy. The latter may be associated, however, with radiodense joint effusions due to chronic intra-articular haemarthrosis. In addition, multiple subchondral cysts are seen more frequently than in juvenile idiopathic arthritis.

15.6.2
Foot

Involvement of the metatarsophalangeal and interphalangeal joints of the foot is usual in polyarticular disease and may be associated with a severe, destructive arthritis and joint fusion (Fig. 15.12). Soft-tissue swelling, juxta-articular osteoporosis and periosteal new bone formation around the metatarsals and phalanges occur commonly. Growth disturbances are

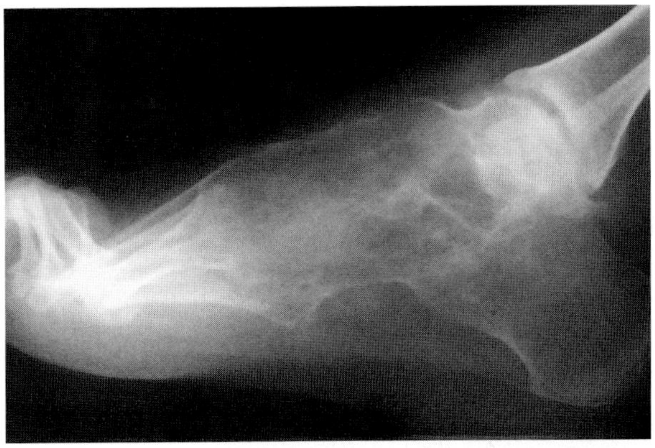

Fig. 15.12. Juvenile idiopathic arthritis. Extensive hindfoot and midfoot fusion with regions of undergrowth and overgrowth of involved bones

frequent, resulting in a balloon-like appearance to the epiphyses and variable overgrowth or undergrowth of the length of the involved bones depending on the duration of the disease and the state of the epiphyseal plate at the time of the joint involvement. Joint space narrowing and marginal erosions usually occur late in the course of the disease.

15.7
Seronegative Spondyloarthritides

This group of conditions is associated with prominent findings in synovial articulations, cartilaginous joints and the entheses. Ankylosing spondylitis shows a predilection for the axial skeleton with less frequent appendicular involvement, whereas psoriatic arthritis has a variable manifestation frequently involving the distal interphalangeal joints and the tufts of the terminal phalanges (Fig. 15.13). Reiter's syndrome commonly presents as an asymmetric arthritis of the lower extremity with or without spinal and sacroiliac involvement. In the early part of this disease, the radiographs are usually normal, but with repeated episodes of arthritis, permanent radiographic abnormalities become common. These typically have an asymmetric distribution, particularly involving the lower extremity (as opposed to psoriatic arthritis where coexistent hand and foot involvement is frequently found). Involvement of the posterior and plantar aspects of the calcaneum is frequent with a retrocalcaneal bursitis and poorly defined calcaneal erosions (Fig. 15.14). Within the foot, asymmetric involvement of the metatarsophalangeal and interphalangeal joints is relatively common, particularly of the great toe. Psoriatic arthritis may involve multiple interphalangeal and metatarsophalangeal joints often in association with erosions of the posterior tuberosity of the calcaneum. This may lead to a severe deforming arthritis with or without ankylosis of the involved joints (Fig. 15.15).

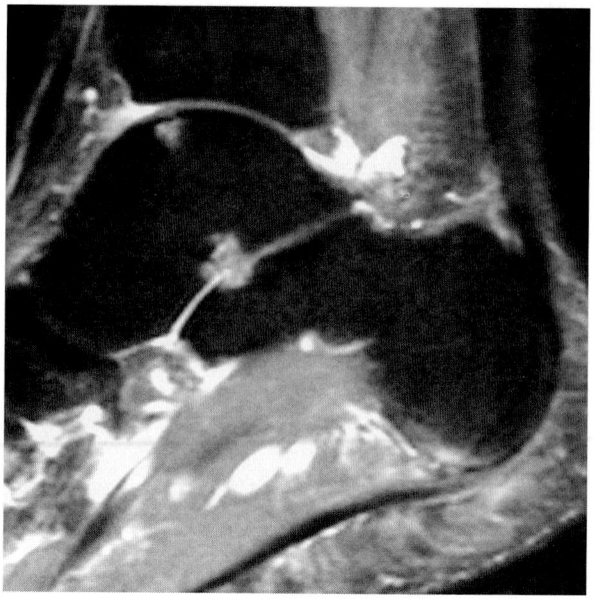

Fig. 15.14. Reiter's syndrome. Sagittal STIR image showing inflammation in the retrocalcaneal pre-Achilles bursa and an inflammatory enthesitis around the origin of the planter aponeurosis. Note the adjacent inflammatory changes in the plantar aspect of the calcaneal tuberosity

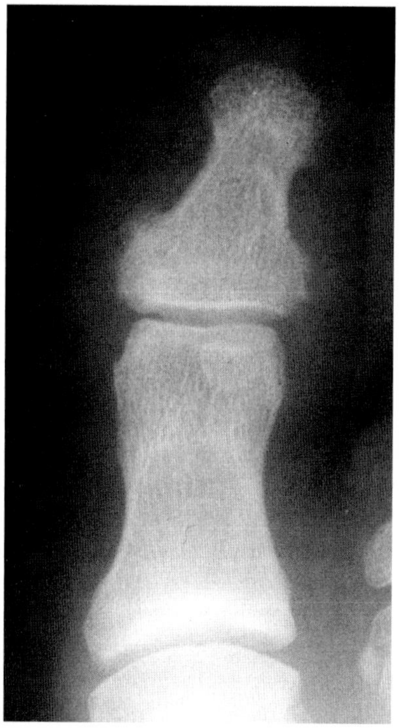

Fig. 15.13. Psoriatic arthritis of the great toe interphalangeal joint showing ill-defined marginal erosions and modest proliferative changes. Some early resorption of the tuft of the terminal phalanx is present

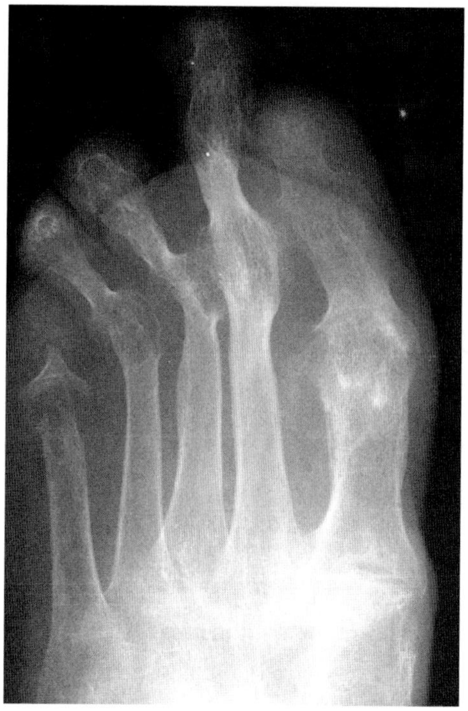

Fig. 15.15. Psoriatic arthritis. Severe deforming arthritis involving multiple interphalangeal, metatarsophalangeal and midfoot articulations with arthrodesis of many of these joints

Alternatively and characteristically, a single ray of the foot may be involved, resulting in a 'sausage' digit, frequently accompanied by endosteal sclerosis. The inflammatory bowel disease-associated arthropathies are indistinguishable from ankylosing spondylitis.

15.8 Depositional Diseases

Gout is the most common of the depositional diseases to involve the foot and results from the deposition of monosodium monourate crystals in the soft tissues, joint structure and synovial fluid. The erosions associated with this disease are eccentrically located, may be intra- or extra-articular, and characteristically have well-defined, punched-out, sclerotic margins with overhanging edges (Martel 1968) (Figs. 15.6, 15.16). Intraosseous deposits of urate occasionally may result in subchondral or metaphyseal bone destruction with multiloculated expanded areas of bone damage with or without calcification. Eccentric soft-tissue swelling, often with preservation of the joint space and normal bone density, is typical. The great toe metatarsophalangeal joint is the most common joint to be involved. The remaining joints of the first ray and the tarsometatarsal joints are further characteristic sites, although any joint within the foot may be affected.

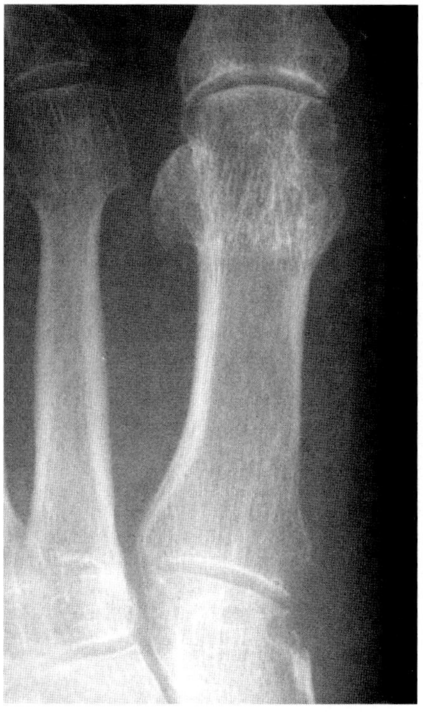

Fig. 15.16. Gout. Well-defined erosions are shown around the great toe metatarsophalangeal and tarsometatarsal joints with some accompanying eccentric soft-tissue swelling

Multicentric reticulohistiocytosis results in histiocytic proliferation in the skin, subcutaneous tissues and synovium and most frequently presents as a symmetrical polyarthritis with a predilection for the distal interphalangeal joints of the hand. Skin nodules and xanthomata from associated hypercholesterolaemia are common. In the feet, symmetrical involvement of the interphalangeal and metatarsophalangeal joints is seen. The erosions are usually marginally located but can involve the subchondral region. They are well-defined with sclerotic margins, and the joint space may or may not be preserved. The bone density is normal, and soft-tissue nodules are seen often. Progressive destructive disease can lead to arthritis mutilans.

Primary or secondary amyloidosis with deposition in the synovium, joint capsule and subchondral bone can result in soft-tissue masses and joint erosions indistinguishable from gout.

15.9 Osteoarthritis and Variants

Typically, 'primary' osteoarthritis affects the great toe metatarsal phalangeal joint. Usually of a hypertrophic type, it is characterised by osteophytosis, especially on the dorsal surface of the metatarsal head, and joint space narrowing (Fig. 15.17). Osteoarthritis also involves the articulations between the great toe metatarsal head and the underlying sesamoid bones. This latter site may be the cause of considerable symptomatology, often characterised by multiple subchondral radiolucencies rather than osteophytosis. Osteoarthritis rarely occurs in the other metatarsophalangeal or interphalangeal joints, although the first tarsometatarsal joint is an underdiagnosed site (Fig. 15.18).

'Secondary' osteoarthritis occurs in the mid-tarsal joint in patients with hindfoot deformities especially, and in the subtalar joints following trauma to the hindfoot.

Disease modification in association with crystal deposition is not a major finding in the foot, as opposed to the knee or hip (Watt and Dieppe 1990). Apatite-associated destructive osteoarthritis involves

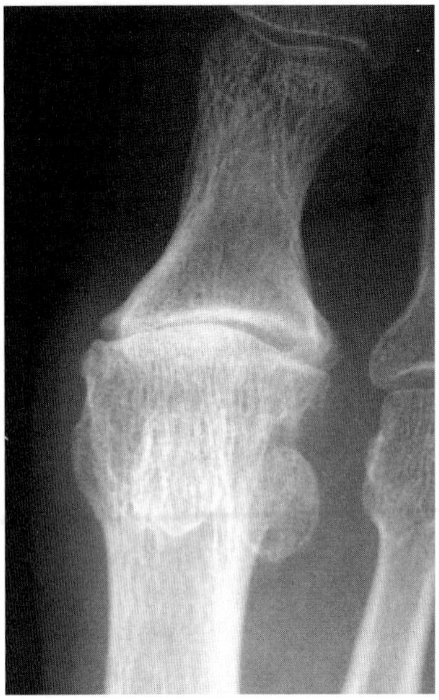

Fig. 15.17. Hallux rigidus. Osteoarthritis of the great toe interphalangeal joint showing eccentric joint space narrowing, subchondral cysts and sclerosis with marginal osteophytes

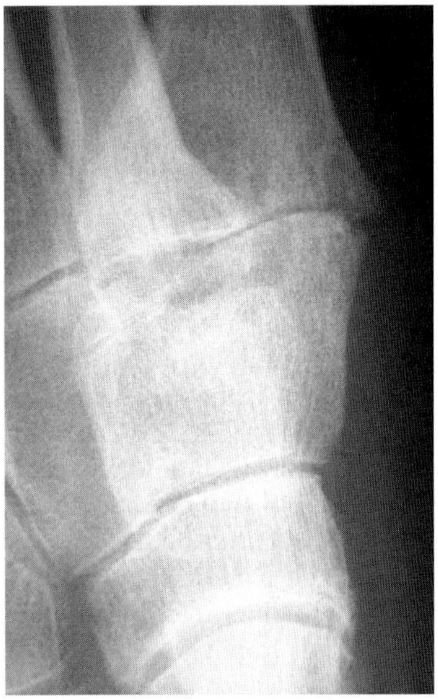

Fig. 15.18. Osteoarthritis of the first tarsometatarsal joint. An under-recognised location that is commonly overlooked

the shoulder, knee and hip. Similarly, hypertrophic osteoarthritis in association with calcium pyrophosphate dihydrate affects predominantly those joints within which fibrocartilage occurs with hyaline cartilage, thereby excluding the foot. However, chondrocalcinosis (due to calcium pyrophosphate) may occur, especially at the great toe metatarsal head, and periarticular soft-tissue deposition of both hydroxyapatite and calcium pyrophosphate crystals is not rare. The former occurs as acute periarthritis, similar to that seen in the shoulder, usually adjacent to the great toe metatarsal head; the latter is more randomly positioned and may appear tumoral.

Diabetic osteoarthropathy (see Chapter 14) is a very important differential diagnosis to 'simple' osteoarthritis. The diagnosis is crucial if significant deformity and/or loss of limb are to be prevented (Fig. 15.19). The distinction between diabetic osteoarthropathy and infectious disease presents a major radiological challenge. Other forms of Charcot or neuropathic arthropathy are rare in the foot, usually due to congenital indifference to pain (Fig. 15.20) or acquired nerve injury.

15.10 Monoarticular Disease

Whilst any generalised arthropathy may present or continue to manifest as single joint involvement, a single abnormal joint should suggest one of the following diseases.

15.10.1 Pigmented Villonodular Synovitis

Although almost any joint may be involved by this synovial proliferative disorder, large joints, including the ankle, are the ones most commonly affected. Initially, soft-tissue swelling and a joint effusion with preservation of the joint space may be the only findings, but in the ankle and foot, pressure erosions and subchondral cysts are frequently seen at presentation (Fig. 15.21). Involvement of tendon sheaths or bursae results in either diffuse or localised soft-tissue masses that may be accompanied by well-defined erosion of adjacent bone. A localised intra-articular form of the disease usually produces no detectable abnormality on conventional radiographs but can be demonstrated with MR imaging.

15.10.2 Synovial Osteochondromatosis

This disease is generally thought to be due to villous hyperplasia of the synovium with cartilage metaplaa

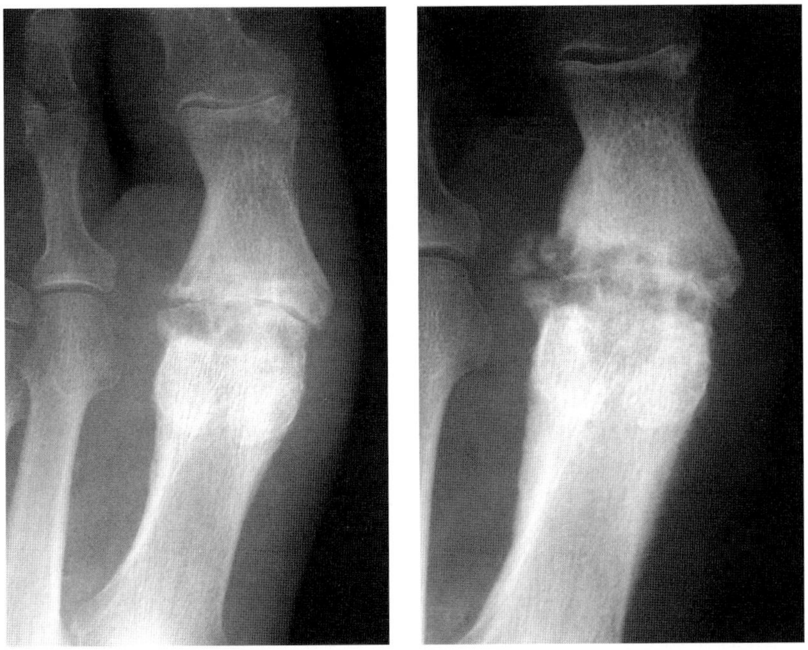

b

Fig. 15.19a. Diabetic arthropathy. At presentation, features mimicking osteoarthritis are shown. **b** Nine months later, further subchondral bone destruction has occurred, but with extensive organised new bone formation and relative preservation of the articular cortices

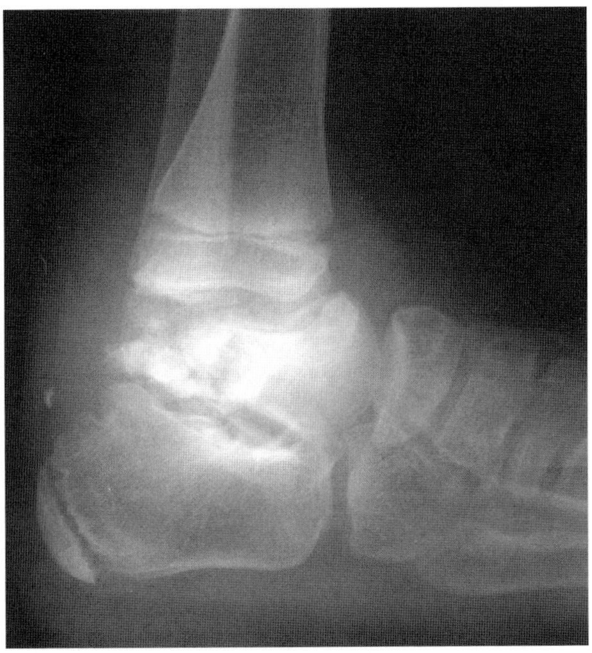

Fig. 15.20. Congenital indifference to pain. A hypertrophic neuropathic arthropathy is shown involving the hindfoot

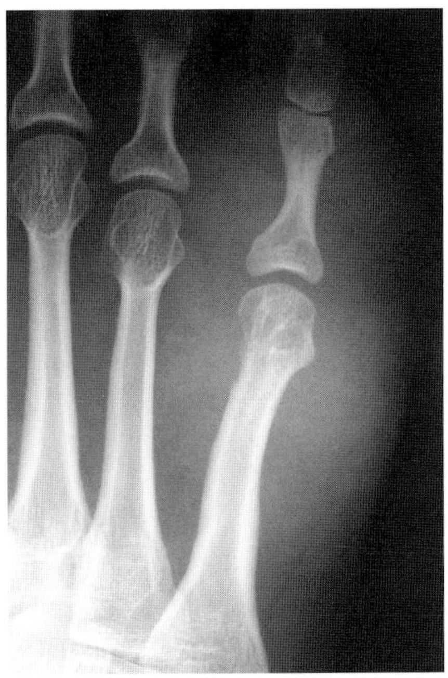

Fig. 15.21. Pigmented villonodular synovitis of the little toe metatarsophalangeal joint. Massive eccentric soft-tissue swelling and well-defined pressure erosions on the medial aspect of the head and neck of the metatarsal are evident. The joint space and bone density are preserved

sia. It results in radiological findings indistinguishable from PVNS except when the cartilaginous nodules become calcified. Often, innumerable calcified nodules can then be seen ranging in size from a few millimetres to osteochondral bodies measuring several centimetres in diameter (Fig. 15.2).

References

Doherty M, Dieppe P, Watt I (1984) Low incidence of calcium pyrophosphate dihydrate crystal deposition in rheumatoid arthritis, with modification of radiographic features in coexistent disease. Arthritis Rheum 27:1002–1009

Martel W (1968) The overhanging margin of bone: a roentgenologic manifestation of gout. Radiology 91: 755–756

Martel W, Stuck KJ, Dworin AM, Hylland RG (1980) Erosive osteoarthritis and psoriatic arthritis: a radiologic comparison in the hand, wrist, and foot. AJR Am J Roentgenol 134:125–135

Petty RE (2001) Growing pains: the ILAR classification of juvenile idiopathic arthritis. J Rheumatol 28:927–928

Rizzoli AJ, Trujeque L, Bankhurst AD (1980) The coexistence of gout and rheumatoid arthritis: case reports and a review of the literature. J Rheumatol 7:316–324

Watt I (1997) Basic differential diagnosis of arthritis. Eur Radiol 7:344–351

Watt I, Dieppe P (1990) Osteoarthritis revisited. Skeletal Radiol 19:1–3

16 Metabolic Bone Disease

A. J. Grainger, J. M. Elliott, and H. K. Genant

CONTENTS

A.J. Grainger, MRCP FRCR
Consultant Musculoskeletal Radiologist, Freeman Hospital, Newcastle upon Tyne NE7 7DN, UK
J.M. Elliott, MRCPI, FRCR
Consultant Radiologist, Department of Radiology, Musgrave Park Hospital, Stockman's Lane, Belfast BT9 7JB, UK
H.K. Genant, MD
Professor of Radiology, Medicine, Epidemiology and Orthopaedic Surgery, University of California San Francisco, San Francisco, CA 94143-0628, USA

16.1 Introduction

By their nature, the metabolic bone diseases have their effect throughout the skeleton, and changes observed in the foot and ankle will usually be accompanied by changes elsewhere in the skeleton which may be more significant. However, since the findings associated with metabolic bone disease may be incidental or unexpected, it is important to be aware of the spectrum of such disease when undertaking a radiological assessment of the foot and ankle. In this chapter, we have emphasised the changes seen in metabolic bone diseases as they apply to the foot and ankle. The reader is referred to the many excellent, more general texts for further discussion of changes seen elsewhere in the skeleton and more thorough discussion of the pathophysiology of metabolic bone disease.

16.2 Pathophysiology of Bone Remodelling

The skeleton changes throughout life, being subject to growth, modelling and remodelling. In the normal remodelling process, the synthesis of new bone by osteoblasts and the removal of old bone by osteoclasts are closely linked so that a balance is maintained. However, with increasing age, resorption tends to exceed formation. This age-related bone loss occurs irrespective of sex, race or geographical location (Parfitt 1988). The remodelling process also occurs more rapidly in trabecular bone than in cortical bone, and trabecular bone loss leads to decreased connectivity between trabeculae in the weight-bearing skeleton.

As a result of faster bone loss in trabecular bone and in oestrogen-deficient states, fractures may occur, often related to minimal trauma. Cortical bone is lost primarily from the endosteal surface, allowing the marrow space to expand and leading to decreased cortical thickness (Kalender et al. 1989). Higher trabecular bone densities are found in black people than white people, and although white women have more rapid bone loss in the spine and radius at the menopause than black women, the cortical bone loss is similar (Han et al. 1996). The differences between the two groups remain similar with increasing age and would appear to relate to peak adult bone mass rather than rates of bone loss.

16.2.1 Osteoporosis

Osteoporosis may be considered a generalised or a regional abnormality. Regional or localised osteoporosis usually relates to injury, surgery or infection, and a period of disuse, although it may represent conditions such as transient bone marrow oedema of the hip or reflex sympathetic dystrophy.

16.2.2 Generalised Osteoporosis

In view of the potential for fracture with increasing bone loss, the identification of at-risk groups has been of interest. In defining osteoporosis, attempts have been made to determine the transition from acceptable bone loss to the pathological state in this spectrum of bone physiology.

16.2.2.1 Definition

As described by the Consensus Development Conference, osteoporosis is "a disease characterised by low bone mass and microarchitectural deterioration of bone tissue, leading to enhanced bone fragility and a consequent increase in fracture risk" (WHO 1994). This definition describes the functional importance of the abnormality but lacks any objective measure. The World Health Organization (WHO) has defined osteoporosis in terms of bone mineral concentration (BMC) or bone mineral density (BMD) values obtained from dual-energy X-ray absorptiometry (DXA) measurements such that a BMC or BMD more than 2.5 standard deviations below peak bone mass represents osteoporosis (referred to as T score <--2.5) (WHO 1994). BMD is normally distributed in the population, and criteria have been proposed to categorise results, although in view of the overlap between normal patients and those with fractures, these should be considered guidelines in the management of osteoporosis (Table 16.1).

This has proved a useful definition based on objective measures, although 'peak bone mass' cannot be applied consistently for all ages and all bone sites. Application of the female 'normal' values to a male population may give spurious results, and application across different racial groups is also questionable. Its use has become established, and the bone mass has been shown to correlate with bone strength (Hodgskinson et al. 1997). The WHO definition is limited by its objectivity and does not consider issues of bone quality and those factors that contribute to it such as the geometric arrangement of trabeculae.

Generalised osteoporosis may be idiopathic or may occur as a result of various risk factors and medical conditions. In addition to genetic and lifestyle factors, chronic diseases of the gastrointestinal or urinary tracts that interfere with calcium and vitamin D metabolism may be responsible. Endocrine disorders such as hyperthyroidism and hyperparathyroidism and prolonged treatment with corticosteroids and anticoagulants have also been implicated.

In the individual patient it was often the clinical end-point of a fracture (particularly hip, spine and forearm) that led to the diagnosis of osteoporosis. The associated morbidity and mortality of such complications remain considerable, and the health care costs involved in treatment are escalating as the older population increases. Despite the limitations of the WHO criteria, a greater awareness of the disease and those at risk now means that treatment can be implemented prior to end-stage disease.

16.2.2.2 Bone Mineral Density and Its Measurement

The radiological changes of osteoporosis reflect the underlying pathology. Radiographs show a reduction in bone density in keeping with osteopaenia. The dis-

Table 16.1. WHO definitions of osteoporosis based on bone mineral density (BMD) or bone mineral concentration (BMC)

Normal	BMC/BMD more than 1 SD below average young adult (T<–1)
Osteopaenia	BMC/BMD more than 1 SD below average young adult but not more than 2.5 SD below (–2.5<T<–1)
Osteoporosis	BMC/BMD more than 2.5 SD below young adult (T<–2.5)
Established osteoporosis	BMC/BMD more than 2.5 SD below the young adult average and one or more osteoporotic fractures

tinction between the different causes of osteopaenia, which include osteoporosis, is generally not possible on conventional radiographs.

Accurate quantification of bone loss from conventional radiographs is not possible. In the foot, attempts have been made to quantify bone loss by analysis of the trabecular pattern of the calcaneus (AGGARWAL et al. 1986). However, correlation with bone density measurement elsewhere is poor (COCKSHOTT et al. 1984).

Several techniques are available for the non-invasive quantitative assessment of BMD including photon and X-ray absorptiometry (single and dual), quantitative CT (spinal and peripheral) and quantitative ultrasound (GENANT 1997). If density is considered to be 'mass per unit volume', then the only true volumetric measure of bone density is provided by quantitative CT. In this method volumetric data are acquired, and regions of interest placed selectively around cortical or trabecular bone. Comparison with phantom standards allows BMD to be calculated. Traditionally, however, BMD can also be considered as an 'amount per unit area measure' and is given in the form gcm^{-2} (mass per unit area) when estimated by X-ray absorptiometry.

16.2.2.3
Dual X-ray Absorptiometry

Dual X-ray absorptiometry (DXA) is probably the most widely used method of bone density measurement. It is readily available, reproducible and accurate and delivers a low ionising radiation dose. Two distinct energy X-ray beams are used with bone and soft-tissue standards for calibration. Pencil and fan-beam X-ray sources and single and multiple detector arrays are available, and while there is less radiation with the pencil beam types, examination times are shorter with the fan-beam type, and soft-tissue and bone composition can be estimated (MAZESS et al. 1992). The preferred anatomical sites are the lumbar spine and proximal femur, but peripheral sites can be examined (Fig. 16.1). In fact, dedicated peripheral extremity scanners (pDXA) are available which utilise the high trabecular bone arrangement in

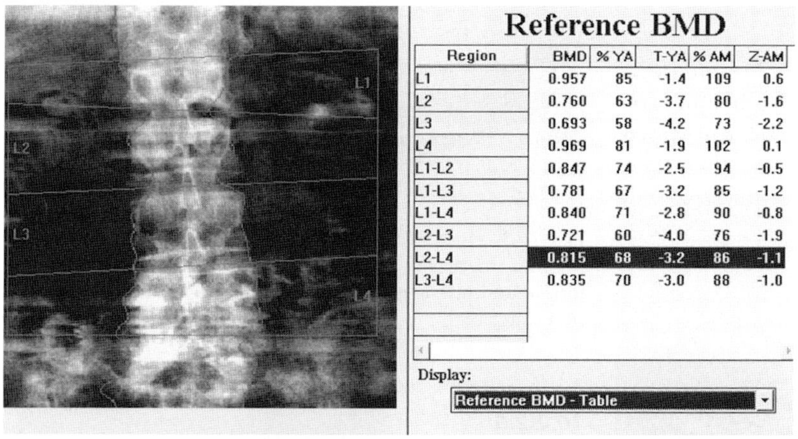

Region	BMD	% YA	T-YA	% AM	Z-AM
L1	0.957	85	-1.4	109	0.6
L2	0.760	63	-3.7	80	-1.6
L3	0.693	58	-4.2	73	-2.2
L4	0.969	81	-1.9	102	0.1
L1-L2	0.847	74	-2.5	94	-0.5
L1-L3	0.781	67	-3.2	85	-1.2
L1-L4	0.840	71	-2.8	90	-0.8
L2-L3	0.721	60	-4.0	76	-1.9
L2-L4	0.815	68	-3.2	86	-1.1
L3-L4	0.835	70	-3.0	88	-1.0

a

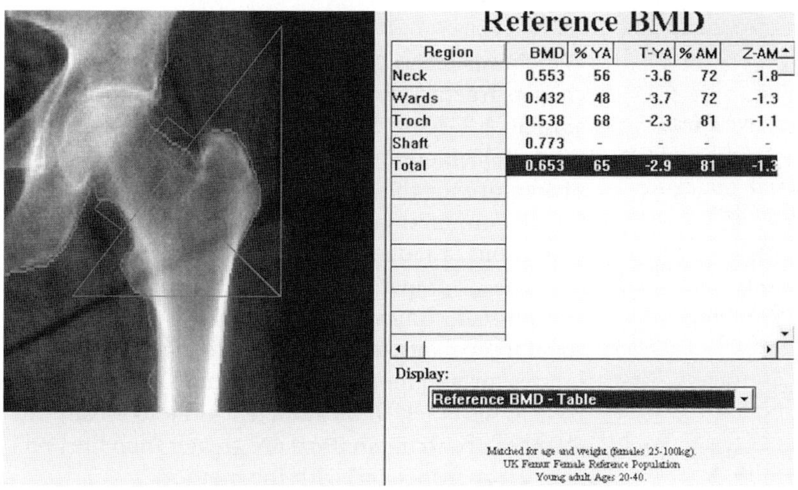

Region	BMD	% YA	T-YA	% AM	Z-AM
Neck	0.553	56	-3.6	72	-1.8
Wards	0.432	48	-3.7	72	-1.3
Troch	0.538	68	-2.3	81	-1.1
Shaft	0.773	-	-	-	-
Total	0.653	65	-2.9	81	-1.3

b

Fig. 16.1a,b. Dual-energy X-ray absorptiometry (DXA) images of the lumbar spine and proximal femur demonstrating positioning of the regions of interest and the bone mineral density (BMD) calculations in this female patient with osteoporosis. Note also the wedge fracture of L1 the calcaneus for measurement. These have the advantage of being small and hence portable and inexpensive (Fig. 16.2).Generally, examination of the spine is performed in a posteroanterior direction, but in the older population, the presence of aortic calcification, degenerative disc disease and osteophyte formation may lead to an erroneous increase in the measured bone density. Lateral examination reduces such error, but the method is less reproducible. It is important to note that with DXA methods of BMD assessment, comparison of results is not possible across equipment from different manufacturers without careful cross-calibration. This has implications for serial measurements in the follow-up of patients or in clinical trials.

Such methods allow a measure of bone quantity to be determined, but quality factors like trabecular orientation and connectivity do not influence the result. However, as noted in the earlier definitions of osteoporosis, consideration of the microarchitecture of the bone was deemed important: a factor that cannot be evaluated by standard X-ray or CT methods.

16.2.2.4 Quantitative Ultrasound

Quantitative ultrasound (QUS) is a more recent innovation that evaluates bone mass and other parameters and hence potentially provides more qualitative information (Jergas and Schmid 1999). The two principal parameters are the speed of sound (SOS) in bone and broadband ultrasound attenuation (BUA). These are altered in osteoporotic bone compared with normal bone. The various manufacturers have further derived other factors to simplify the interpretation such as 'stiffness' (Lunar Corp., Madison, WI, USA), 'quantitative ultrasound index' (QUI) (Hologic Inc., Bedford, MA, USA), 'strength index' (SI) (DMS SA, Montpellier, France) and 'soundness' (Norland Inc., Fort Atkinson, WI, USA).

The current devices are used in the calcaneus, patella, tibia, radius and phalanges, but as with DXA, comparison between manufacturers is difficult (Fig. 16.3).

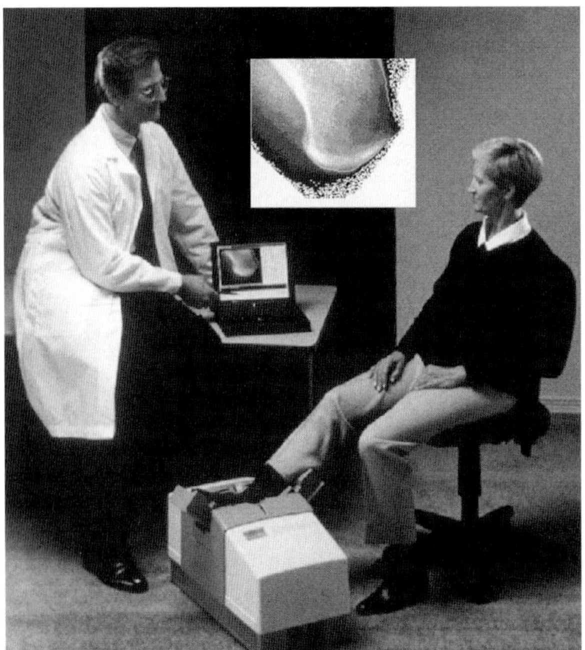

Fig. 16.2. Peripheral bone density measurement using pDXA, which estimates BMD in the calcaneus

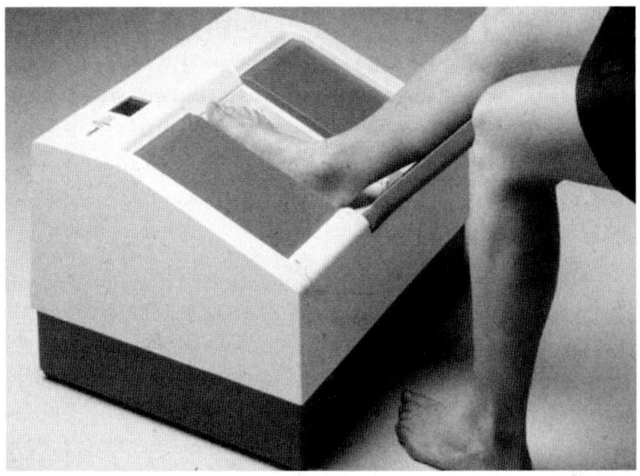

Fig. 16.3. Quantitative ultrasound (QUS) of the heel. This scanner measures speed of sound (SOS) and broadband ultrasound attenuation (BUA) at the calcaneus with the heel in a water bath

16.2.2.5 Fracture Risk

Whichever technique of bone density assessment is chosen, fracture risk prediction for that population is similar. A T-score of less than –2.5 is associated with a two-fold increase in the risk of fracture. The risk of fracture for the individual cannot be determined, but in conjunction with other lifestyle and medical conditions, a judgement can be made on the appropriateness of instituting therapy. Unless there are exceptional clinical reasons (e.g. corticosteroids or renal transplant), follow-up in osteoporosis is usually not performed more frequently than on a two-yearly basis. This is felt to be sufficient time to ensure that changes occurring in BMD are greater than the precision error associated with the method.

16.3 Regional Osteoporosis

16.3.1 Reflex Sympathetic Dystrophy Syndrome

16.3.1.1 Aetiology and Pathogenesis

The aetiology of reflex sympathetic dystrophy or Sudeck's atrophy remains obscure, as suggested by the variety of synonyms that have been applied (Atkins and Duthie 1987). The traditional understanding has been of an alteration in the vasomotor status due to a sympathetic reflex following a local insult. Increased osteoclastic activity occurs as a result of acidic metabolites. The abnormal sympathetic response has also been considered at the spinal cord or even cerebral cortical level. A more recent study found that signs of sympathetic response were infrequent and that early symptoms were more suggestive of an exaggerated inflammatory reaction (Veldman et al. 1993).

A number of diagnostic factors have been described, including pain and tenderness, soft-tissue swelling, diminished motor function, trophic skin changes, vasomotor instability and patchy osteoporosis (Genant et al. 1975; Kozin et al. 1976b).

The vasomotor instability may progress from an early 'warm phase' lasting days to weeks in which the skin is warm, red and swollen to a 'cold phase' where the skin is cool, clammy and cyanosed.

16.3.1.2 Radiological Appearances

Radiological features include endosteal and intracortical excavation and subperiosteal and patchy trabecular bone resorption (Fig. 16.4). Juxta-articular and subchondral bone erosions may also be present, and there is increased tracer uptake on bone scintigraphy (Kozin et al. 1976a). More recently, the role of MR imaging has been examined. While one study suggested that it was of little value; a larger study demonstrated that fat-suppressed T2-weighted or STIR images were helpful in identifying those patients with the warm form of the process. Its use in the cold form of the condition was primarily to exclude other causes for the symptoms (Darbois et al. 1999; Koch et al. 1991). Quantitative ultrasound has been evaluated in the diagnosis and monitoring of response to calcitonin in the feet and was found to be a sensitive tool, particularly when BUA and 'stiffness' were considered (Cepollaro et al. 1998). The final diagnosis can only be made on the clinical course by regression of findings or the development of aponeurotic and tendinous retractions with bony sclerosis over many months to years.

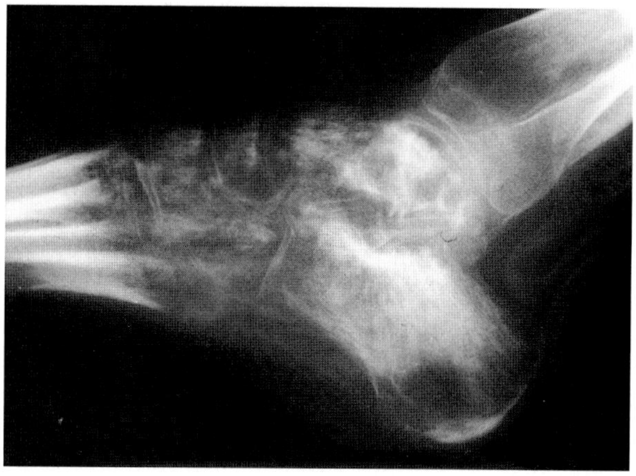

Fig. 16.4. Radiographic features of reflex sympathetic dystrophy syndrome (RSDS). Striking, patchy osteopaenia, resorption noted in the foot

It should be remembered that the error in judging osteopaenia based on conventional radiographic appearances has been estimated at 30%–50%. Whilst in most cases osteopaenia seen on radiographs of the foot and ankle is likely to be self-limiting and related to the primary pathology and disuse, it may also be the manifestation of an underlying generalised osteoporosis or an indicator of an abnormal response to injury such as RSDS.

16.3.2 Rickets/Osteomalacia

In contrast to osteoporosis, where there is a reduction in bone mass, osteomalacia and rickets are the result of inadequate mineralisation of the osteoid bone matrix. The term rickets is applied to the condition when seen in children, while osteomalacia is the adult form of the disease.

16.3.2.1 Aetiology and Pathogenesis

There are many causes of osteomalacia and rickets, but the underlying aetiology usually results in a deficiency of the active (dihydroxy) form of vitamin D, 1,25-$(OH)_2$-cholecalciferol. Vitamin D is synthesised in the skin by the action of sunlight and is obtained from the diet. The initial hydroxylation of the vitamin occurs in the liver, but a second hydroxylation is required to produce the active form of the hormone. This final step occurs in the kidney. As a consequence, deficiency may be the result of dietary insufficiency or inadequate sunlight exposure. However, more common causes relate to malabsorption of the vitamin from the gut or the presence of renal disease resulting in inadequate hydroxylation of the 25-OH-vitamin D molecule to active 1,25-$(OH)_2$-cholecalciferol. Less commonly, osteomalacia and rickets result from liver failure (inadequate primary hydroxylation of vitamin D) or interference in the metabolism of vitamin D by drugs. In some cases the condition results from phosphate deficiency, usually due to renal tubular disorders.

16.3.2.2 Radiological Appearances

Although rickets and osteomalacia share a common aetiology, they have different radiological manifestations. Rickets affects the immature skeleton and primarily affects the site of bone growth at the cartilaginous growth plate. In contrast, osteomalacia has its effects on the mature bone.

16.3.2.2.1 Rickets

The generalised, non-specific skeletal effects of rickets include retarded bone growth and osteopaenia. However, more specific findings are growth plate widening (due to the failure of mineralisation of the proliferating cartilage) and increasing irregularity at the interface between the growth plate and metaphysis (Pitt 1991). In more advanced cases the metaphyses become widened and cup shaped. A further feature of rickets is a characteristic bowing seen in the long bones of the arms and legs. These features become more marked as weight-bearing begins to have an effect (Pitt 1981, 1991).The features are most marked at sites where bone growth, and therefore the requirement for mineralisation, is most rapid. In the foot, involvement of the metatarsals and phalanges is unusual and only seen in severe cases (Bhargava et al. 1983). However, typical changes may be seen in less severe cases at the distal tibial physis and metaphysis (Fig. 16.5). Furthermore, bowing deformities commonly involve the tibia and fibula and may be demonstrated on ankle radiographs (Fig. 16.6). Such a bowing deformity may persist into adulthood (Fig. 16.7).

16.3.2.2.2 Osteomalacia

As with rickets, generalised osteopaenia is a feature, albeit rather non-specific. Since osteomalacia affects the mature skeleton, the involvement of the metaphyses is not seen. The most characteristic feature of osteomalacia is the presence of pseudofractures also known as Looser zones. These characteristically occur at sites of stress where there is high bone turnover and histologically consist of unmineralised osteoid. This is deposited during the natural repair processes the bone undergoes at this site (Pitt 1981). They are often symmetrical and appear as linear radiolucencies seen perpendicular to the bone cortex. They extend into the bone, appearing as small fissures, often with sclerotic margins. Pseudofractures are seen at characteristic sites within the skeleton, particularly along the lateral borders of the scapulae and along the pubic

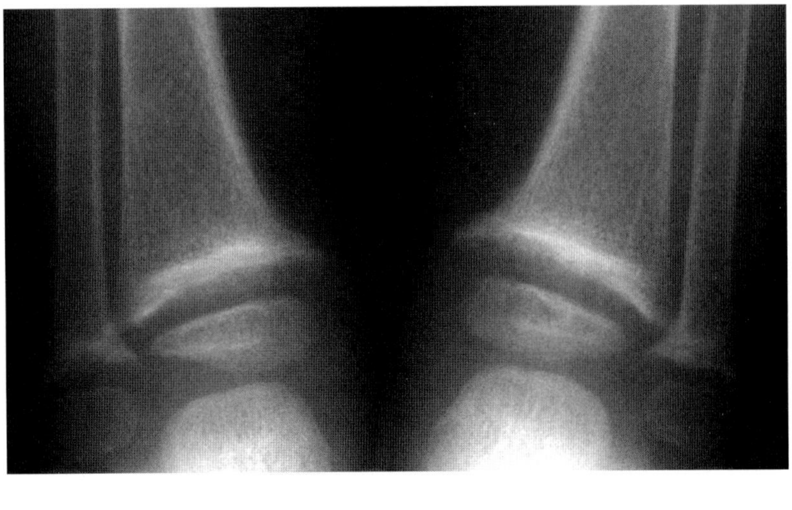

Fig. 16.5. AP view of both distal tibia and fibular metaphyses. Bilateral metaphyseal changes typical of rickets are apparent in this child who emigrated to the UK from India. There is widening and irregularity of all the metaphyses

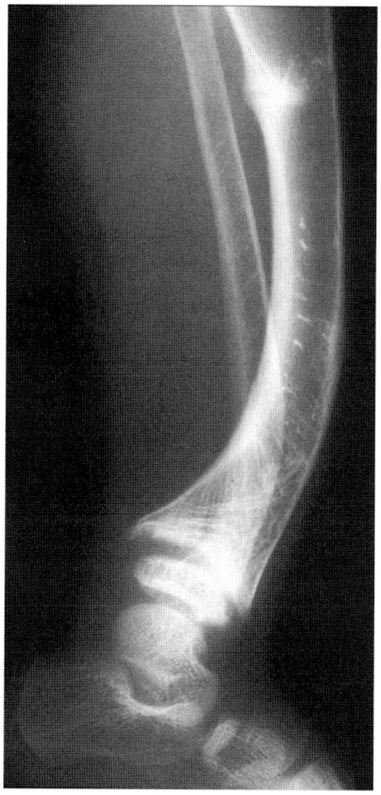

Fig. 16.6. Lateral view of the tibia and fibula. This child with advanced nutritional rickets shows bowing deformity of both the tibia and fibula. Note also the typical cupped metaphyseal changes of rickets, as well as Looser's zone in the tibial shaft

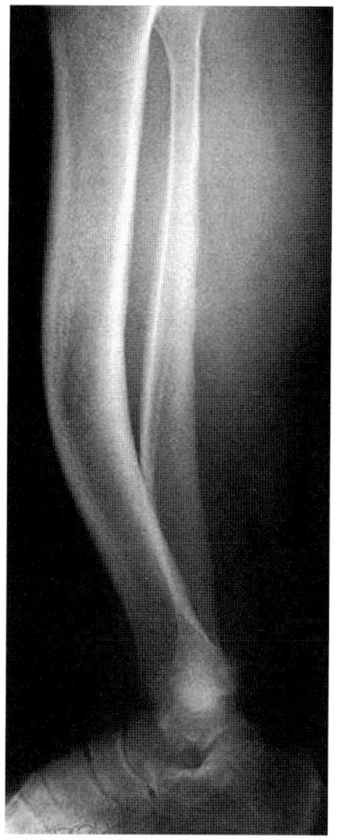

Fig. 16.7. Lateral view of tibia and fibula. This adult suffered severe rickets as a child and has a persistent bowing deformity of the tibia despite treatment

rami and medial borders of the femoral neck. They may be seen elsewhere in the long bones, including the tibia, where they may be seen during radiological review of the ankle (Fig. 16.6). However, they are only rarely seen in the bones of the foot and ankle themselves (Fig. 16.8).

Severe hypophosphataemic osteomalacia has been reported as a complication of connective tissue tumours. Crouzet et al. undertook a review of the literature of such cases and found that the underlying tumour was usually located in a limb, generally the lower limb. They themselves described a case in which the underlying tumour was a plantar neurilemmoma. It is thought that the tumour produces substances capable of blocking intracellular phosphate transfer and inhibiting renal vitamin D hydroxylation (Crouzet et al. 1995).

It would be unusual to make a diagnosis of osteomalacia or rickets on the basis of radiographs of the foot and ankle, and if these diagnoses are suspected, then confirmatory evidence from radiographs of other areas along with clinical and biochemical evidence should be sought.

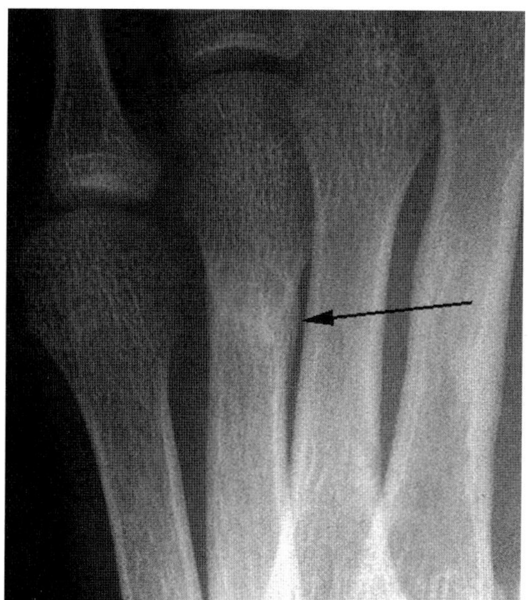

Fig. 16.8. Dorsoplantar radiograph of the foot. Looser zone (pseudofracture) in the fourth metatarsal in a patient with nutritional osteomalacia (*arrow*)

16.3.3 Hyperparathyroidism

16.3.3.1 Pathogenesis

The hyperparathyroid disorders result from overactivity of the parathyroid hormone (PTH)-producing parathyroid glands. PTH is of fundamental importance in calcium and phosphate homeostasis. It has two main target organs:

- The bones, where it stimulates osteoclastic activity, thereby releasing calcium and phosphate and bringing about bone resorption
- The kidneys, where it acts to conserve calcium and stimulates phosphate excretion.
- The net effect is to increase the serum free-ionised calcium.

Hyperparathyroidism is subdivided into three types:

1. Primary hyperparathyroidism: the overproduction of PTH due to parathyroid hyperplasia or adenoma. Rarely this can also be brought about by a parathyroid carcinoma. Occasionally, the cause lies outside the parathyroids in the form of ectopic production of PTH by non-parathyroid tumours.
2. Secondary hyperparathyroidism: this results from increased PTH production in response to persistent hypocalcaemia that fails to correct. The most common cause is chronic renal failure, but the condition is also seen in cases of prolonged vitamin D deficiency such as may be seen with inadequate intestinal absorption following gastrectomy or in cases of malnutrition.
3. Tertiary hyperparathyroidism: this usually occurs in patients receiving renal dialysis when the parathyroid gland has been in a state of prolonged positive feedback due to hypocalcaemia (secondary hyperparathyroidism) and becomes autonomous, no longer responding to the normal feedback mechanisms.

16.3.3.2 Radiological Appearances

The radiological appearances of hyperparathyroidism are the result of the process of bone resorption stimulated by the excess PTH. Typically, bone resorption is first noted radiographically in the form of subperiosteal and cortical bone resorption. Cortical bone resorption may be seen in the form of cortical tunnelling (Genant et al. 1973). Typically, these changes are noted first in the bones of the hand, but such changes may be observed in the short bones of the foot (Fig. 16.9). In severe cases hyperparathyroidism may bring about resorption of the terminal phalangeal tufts or midportion.

Resorption may also occur at the sites of tendinous and ligamentous insertion. In the foot, resorption may frequently be seen on the inferior aspect of the calcaneum, an appearance that can be confused with inflammatory arthropathies such as Reiter's disease (Hayes and Conway 1991; Resnick et al. 1981).

Brown tumours in the form of localised areas of bone lysis may also be observed, although these are not typically found in the feet.

In hyperparathyroidism the bones will characteristically show generalised osteopaenia. The weakened bone may be subject to stress fractures, and this has been described as a complication of hyperparathyroidism in the os calcis (Fishco and Stiles 1999). Fractures of the metatarsals may also be seen (Fig. 16.10).

In addition to the bone changes seen in hyperparathyroidism, soft-tissue changes may be observed. These include vascular and periarticular calcification (Hamilton 1972). Vascular calcification is particularly a feature of secondary hyperparathyroidism.

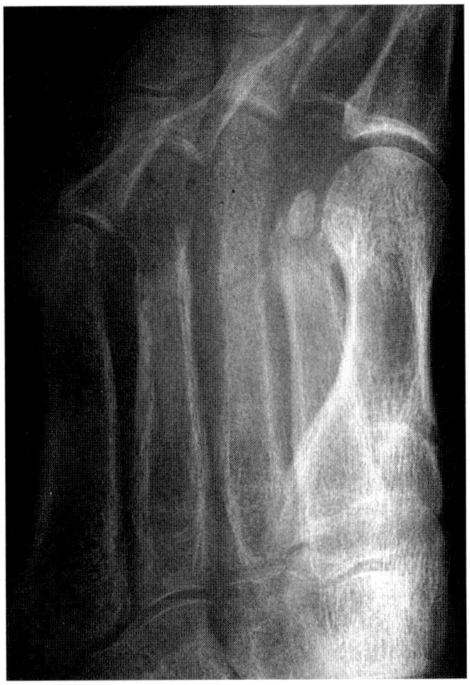

Fig. 16.9. Dorsoplantar oblique view of the foot. This patient has severe primary hyperparathyroidism. There is marked cortical bone resorption and focal destruction characteristic of brown tumour in the metatarsals. Both subperiosteal resorption and intracortical tunnelling can be seen

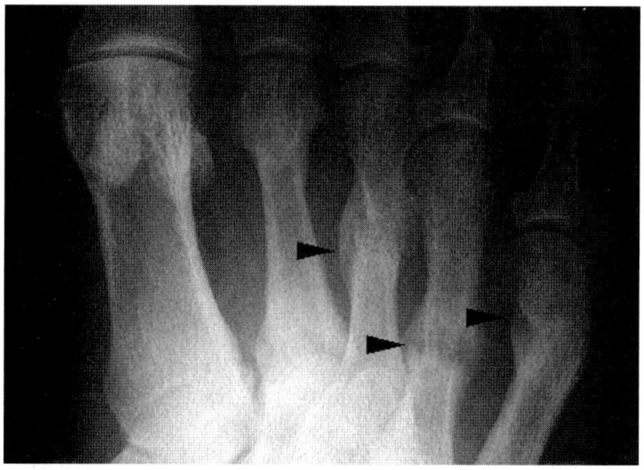

Fig. 16.10. Dorsoplantar view of foot. There are insufficiency fractures in the 3rd, 4th and 5th metatarsals in this patient with primary hyperparathyroidism (*arrowheads*). Cortical resorption is also noted

16.3.4 Renal Osteodystrophy

16.3.4.1 Pathogenesis

Renal osteodystrophy has a complex pathogenesis resulting from an interplay between the metabolic pathways involved. Two main processes are involved:

Abnormal Vitamin D Metabolism. This results from insufficient active 1,25-$(OH)_2$-cholecalciferol as a consequence of inadequate secondary hydroxylation in the damaged kidney.

Secondary Hyperparathyroidism. Phosphate retention by the damaged kidney leads to hypocalcaemia, which in turn stimulates PTH production by the pituitary gland. PTH secretion attempts to restore the serum calcium. With time, the action of PTH produces characteristic changes in the skeleton with features of both skeletal decalcification and osteosclerosis.

These two processes both play a role in bringing about the radiological appearances seen in renal osteodystrophy. However, the contribution each makes varies, and this results in a spectrum of appearances seen radiologically.

16.3.4.2 Radiological Appearances

The features of osteomalacia are seen in renal osteodystrophy in the form of reduced bone density and findings of rickets in children. However, Looser zones are rare. The features of secondary hyperparathyroidism usually predominate, with evidence of bone resorption (most usually seen in the hands). Sclerotic changes, or osteosclerosis, may also be seen (Fig. 16.11). These are most frequently seen in the axial skeleton, most typically in the spine in the form of the 'rugger jersey spine'. However, these appearances may also be seen in the metaphyses of long bones and in the tarsal bones of the foot (Garver et al. 1981).

Many patients with renal disease or with renal transplants receive steroid therapy, making them susceptible to developing avascular necrosis (AVN). The talus is a common site for this to occur. Conventional radiographs may show no abnormality in the early stages of AVN, but subsequently an area of

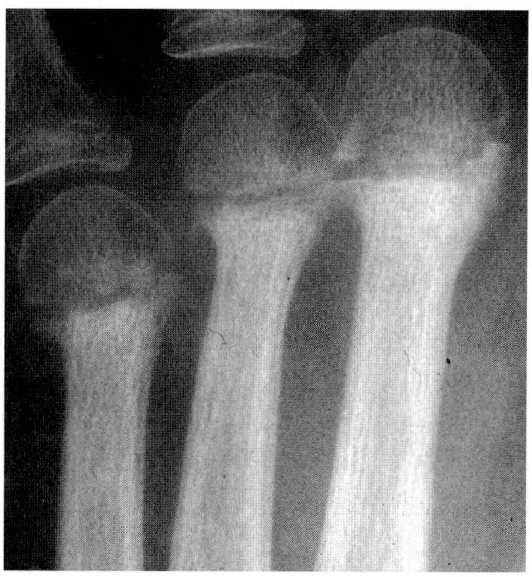

Fig. 16.11. Dorsoplantar view of the forefoot. Features of renal osteodystrophy with osteosclerosis, intracortical tunneling and metaphyseal fractures in this child with advanced renal failure

subchondral lysis may be seen which later develops into an area of subchondral sclerosis, which may be associated with subchondral collapse. The changes are more sensitively demonstrated on MR imaging, with a characteristic subchondral segmental area of signal abnormality delineated by a sclerotic band of low signal intensity on T1-weighted sequences. On T2-weighting this marginal zone classically shows an outer low signal band with an inner margin of high signal intensity representing the reactive interface between the normal marrow and the area of ischaemia.As with hyperparathyroidism, soft-tissue and vascular calcifications may be observed in the feet. Such soft-tissue calcification may present as a painful nodule, and ulceration has been described (Chalmers et al. 1998; De Palma et al. 1993; Edwards and Spinner 1994). Calcium deposition in tendons may also occur, and spontaneous tears of tendons have been described in renal osteodystrophy, including avulsion of the tendon at its bony insertion (Meneghello and Bertoli 1983). Such occurrences may be associated with the tendo Achilles (De Palma et al. 1993).

16.3.5 Hypoparathyroidism

16.3.5.1 Pathogenesis

Idiopathic hypoparathyroidism is a rare condition in which the parathyroid glands are hypoplastic and produce inadequate PTH. This condition usually presents in childhood.

A more common cause of hypoparathyroidism is the result of surgical damage to the parathyroid glands or their blood supply at the time of thyroid surgery (Sherwood 1993). The effect of the reduced PTH levels is to induce hypocalcaemia with hyperphosphataemia.

16.3.5.2 Radiological Appearances

Sclerotic change is the most frequent radiological change in hypoparathyroidism. This may be generalised or focal (Resnick and Niwayama 1995b). Other features include band-like densities in the metaphyses of long bones and premature epiphyseal closure.

16.3.6 Pseudohypoparathyroidism and Pseudopseudohypoparathyroidism

In addition to primary hypoparathyroidism, a hypoparathyroid state can result from a rare inborn error of metabolism that leads to the impaired response of the end-organs (kidneys and bone) to PTH. This condition is known as pseudohypoparathyroidism and is associated with short stature, obesity, mental retardation and a round face. The condition has several different variants depending on the precise nature of the defect in the metabolism (Levine 1993). However, the radiological features are similar in each. In addition to the changes in the skeleton seen in primary hypoparathyroidism (bone sclerosis and premature epiphyseal closure), the patients characteristically have shortened metatarsals and phalanges affecting the first and fourth digits (Resnick and Niwayama 1995b). Shortening of the metacarpals and phalanges is also seen in the hands.

Pseudopseudohypoparathyroidism is a condition in which the patients have clinical somatypic features similar to pseudohypoparathyroidism (short stature, obesity, etc.) but are normocalcaemic. The radiological features are similar to those of pseudohypoparathyroidism.

16.3.7 Thyroid Disorders

Thyroid hormones play an important part in normal growth and development. They act primarily on cartilage formation. However, they also act to stimulate bone resorption and can be a cause of secondary osteoporosis (Canalis 1993).

16.3.7.1 Hypothyroidism

Hypothyroidism can either result from a primary deficiency of the thyroid gland or be secondary to the failure of thyroid-stimulating hormone (TSH) secretion by the pituitary gland.

In adults the effect of hypothyroidism on the skeleton is mild, with a normal or mildly increased bone mass. However, soft-tissue calcific deposits and increased radiodensity of the bones have been reported (Chew 1991).

It is in children that the most significant effects of thyroid deficiency are seen radiographically. The changes are most in evidence at the physeal plates and epiphyses. There is delayed skeletal maturation, with late appearance of the secondary ossification centres, which are typically stippled or even fragmented. Delayed or even failure of physeal plate closure is also a feature.

16.3.7.2
Hyperthyroidism

Thyrotoxicosis most frequently results from Graves' disease, an autoimmune process affecting the thyroid gland and stimulating thyroid hormone production, or from the presence of solitary or multiple thyroid hormone-producing (toxic) nodules. The condition results in increased bone turnover and remodelling and may be associated with hypercalcaemia (CHEW 1991).

Bone loss results in the progressive development of osteopaenia. This is particularly marked in the appendicular skeleton where changes may be prominent in the feet, and there may be associated insufficiency fractures (CHEVROT et al. 1978). The appearance in the short tubular bones of the hands and feet is that of 'busy bone', namely increased intracortical bone resorption producing striations or tunnelling (Fig. 16.12). This finding is nonspecific and can be seen in disuse osteoporosis, reflex sympathetic dystrophy, hyperparathyroidism, and even radiation-induced osteolysis (Fig. 16.13).

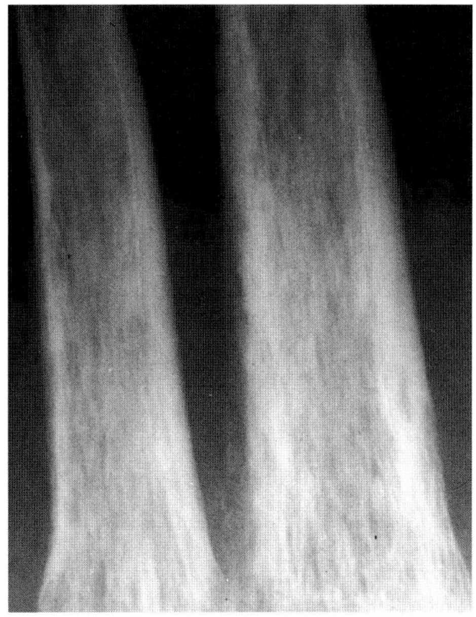

Fig. 16.12. Close-up view of the metatarsals. Marked intracortical tunnelling or 'busy bone' in a patient with advanced thyrotoxicosis

16.3.7.2.1
Thyroid Acropachy

This represents a complication of thyrotoxicosis occurring in around 1% of patients (RESNICK 1995b). Clubbing of the fingers and toes is seen. Involve-

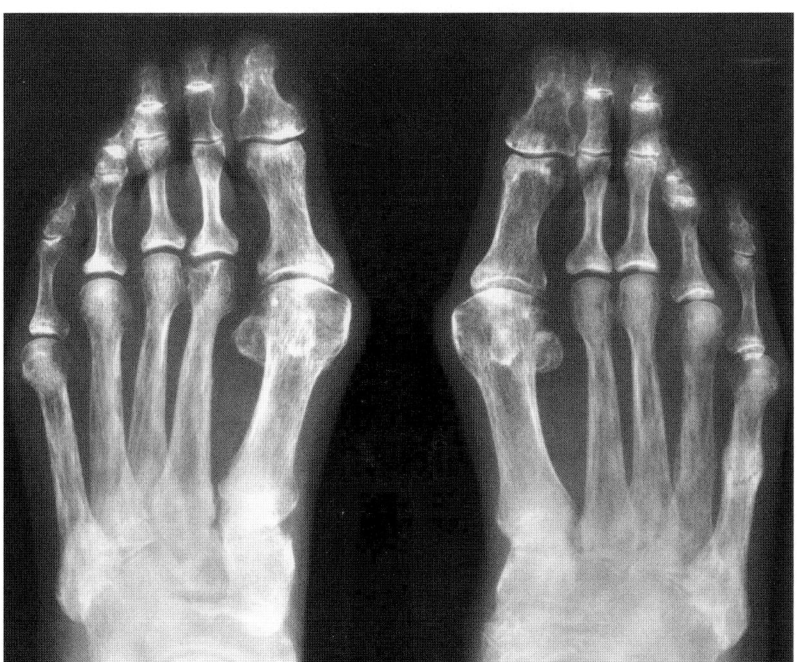

Fig. 16.13. Dorsoplantar view of the forefeet. Patchy osteolysis and sclerosis of the shafts of the tubular bones with osteonecrosis of the left 2nd metatarsal head and insufficiency fracture of the right 5th metatarsal shaft in a rare patient with radiation necrosis due to radium ingestion

ment is characteristically limited to the hands and feet where dense periosteal new bone formation is seen along the diaphyses of the metacarpals and metatarsals. There is usually overlying soft-tissue swelling, and the bone involvement may be asymmetrical (Chew 1991). This appearance may simulate the periosteal changes of pulmonary hypertrophic osteoarthropathy (Fig. 16.14).

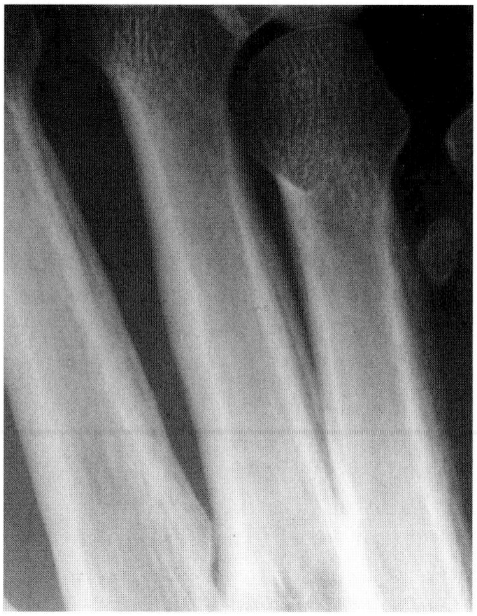

Fig. 16.14. Dorsoplantar view of the forefoot. Striking periosteal reaction along the metatarsal shafts related to hypertrophic pulmonary osteoarthropathy

16.3.8 Acromegaly

16.3.8.1 Pathogenesis

Acromegaly results from the inappropriate secretion of growth hormone by the pituitary gland. The action of growth hormone is to promote skeletal growth. Prior to skeletal maturity, such secretion results in gigantism. However, once the growth plates have closed, the action of the growth hormone results in acromegaly. In the majority of cases, the cause is a secreting pituitary adenoma. Other less common causes include ectopic production of growth hormone by non-pituitary tumours. The condition is seen in both men and women with equal incidence (Chew 1991).

16.3.8.2 Radiological Appearances

16.3.8.2.1 Soft-Tissue Changes

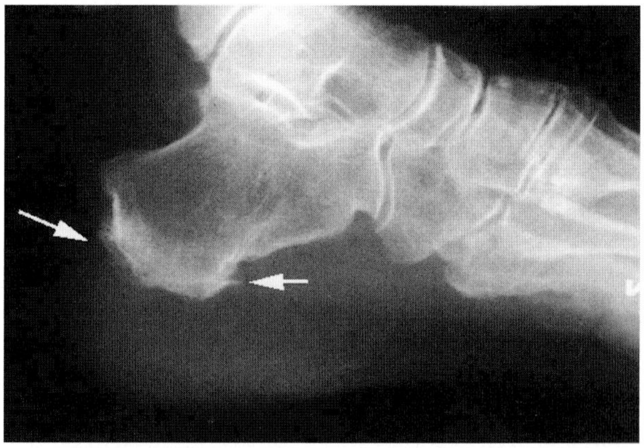

Fig. 16.15. Lateral radiograph of the calcaneus. There is thickening of the heel pad in this woman with acromegaly. The heel pad was measured at 31 mm. Note also the bone proliferation at the enthesis sites (*arrows*)

Acromegaly induces thickening of the soft tissues. Clinically, this is manifest in the coarsened facies characteristic of acromegaly along with thickened oily skin. Radiologically, the soft-tissue thickening can be detected, and this is seen characteristically over the calcaneus (Fig. 16.15). Heel pad thickness has been considered a useful diagnostic tool for acromegaly. However, there has been and still is considerable debate in the literature as to the upper limit of normal heel pad thickness (Gonticas et al. 1969; MacSweeney et al. 1990; Paisey et al. 1984; Puckette and Seymour 1967). Attempts have been made to relate the measurement to body weight (Gonticas et al. 1969), and the measurement is also shown to vary with race (Mittal et al. 1983). For practical purposes, values of heel pad thickness over 23 mm in men and 21.5 mm in women are suggestive of the diagnosis of acromegaly if local causes of skin thickening are excluded (Resnick 1995a). The use of ultrasound in the measurement of heel pad thickness has also been described (Gooding et al. 1985). However, radiological morphometry now has little role to play in the diagnosis and monitoring of acromegaly given the ready availability of accurate and sensitive biochemical assays for growth hormone.

16.3.8.2.2
Bone Changes

Acromegaly brings about many well-recognised radiological changes in the skeleton as a result of the effect of growth hormone in stimulating bone proliferation. The feet are commonly affected by the disease. The changes seen include enlargement of the tufts and bases of the terminal phalanges, overgrowth of the metatarsal heads, often with hypertrophic beaking, and increase in the joint space, seen particularly at the metatarsal phalangeal joints (Fig. 16.16). In addition, there is enlargement of the sesamoid bones, and bone proliferation is seen at enthesis sites of tendinous and ligamentous attachments (Fig. 16.15). Ultrasound has been successfully used to monitor joint and soft-tissue changes, including tendon thickness, in acromegaly (Colao et al. 1998, 1999). Despite the general picture of bone proliferation in acromegaly, the tubular bones in the foot may show thinning or pencilling. This may be seen particularly in the shafts of the distal metatarsals and the phalanges. Doppman and colleagues have proposed that this is the result of remodelling along the plantar aspect of the metatarsals as a response to the thickened soft tissues overlying the bones during weight-bearing (Doppman et al. 1988).

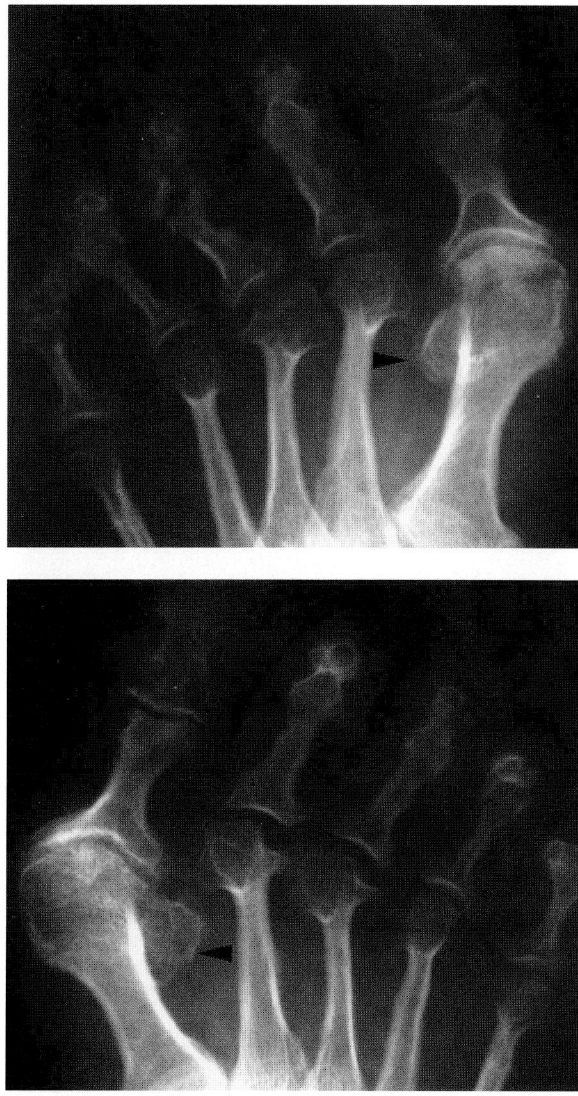

a

b

Fig. 16.16a,b. Dorsoplantar views of left (**a**) and right (**b**) feet. The typical features of acromegaly are shown. There is widening of the metatarsophalangeal joint spaces, with overgrowth of the metatarsal heads and hypertrophic beaking. There is also enlargement of the sesamoid bones (*arrowheads*) and proliferation of the terminal phalangeal tufts and bases

16.3.9
Paget Disease

Paget disease is a common disease of unknown aetiology. It is characterised by a combination of bone resorption and formation, resulting in disordered bone remodelling. The condition has a predilection for the axial skeleton and long bones of the leg (Guyer et al. 1981; Resnick and Niwayama 1995a) but can be seen in the small bones of the foot. It may affect one bone in isolation or show widespread bone involvement.

The radiological features reflect the pathophysiology of the disease, with distinct phases of the disease demonstrated radiologically. During the early osteolytic (hot) phase of the disease, the affected bone undergoes a process where resorption predominates, and bone lysis is seen radiologically. The mixed phase of Paget disease involves processes of both resorption and proliferation occurring together. During this stage remodelling of the bone occurs, and the radiological picture is characterised by coarsening of the bone trabeculae and cortical thickening. In its sclerotic (cool) phase there is a diffuse increase in bone density with further cortical thickening and widening of the bone.

A number of complications of Paget disease exist. The most serious one is the development of sarcoma within the pagetic bone. Fortunately, this is rare, the most common sarcoma to develop being osteosarcoma. More commonly, pathological fractures are seen, particularly in the long bones where they often appear as stress fractures.

Involvement of Paget disease in the foot is relatively unusual, although when seen, it seems to have a predilection for the os calcis (Fig. 16.17) (Korber et al. 1993; Resnick and Niwayama 1995a; Rubin et al. 1983). However, it may also be seen in the short bones of the foot (Fig. 16.18). The tibia is more commonly affected, and where it involves the distal tibia, the patient may present with chronic ankle pain (Neylon 1995).

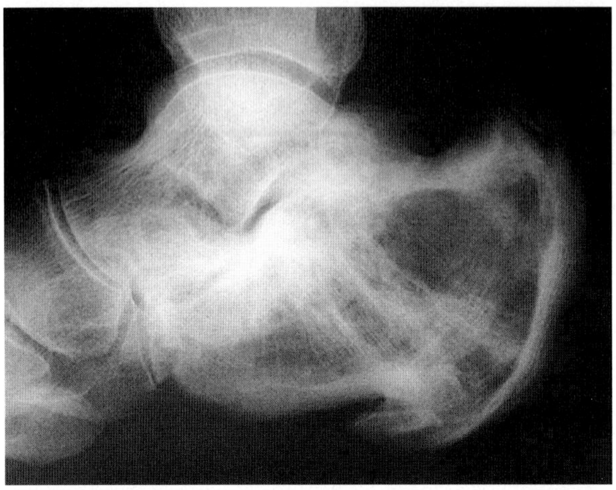

Fig. 16.17. Lateral radiograph of the calcaneus. There is coarsening of the trabecular pattern with bony expansion and cortical thickening. The appearance is that of Paget disease

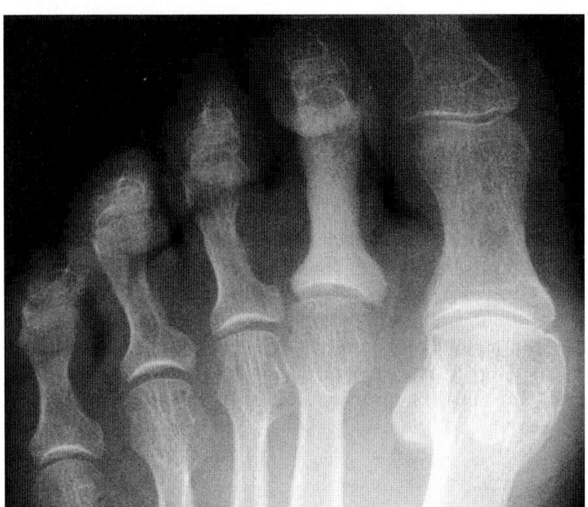

Fig. 16.18. Dorsoplantar radiograph of left foot. Paget disease of the 2nd proximal phalanx seen as sclerosis and mild expansion

References

Aggarwal ND, Singh GD, Aggarwal R et al (1986) A survey of osteoporosis using the calcaneum as an index. Int Orthop 10:147–153

Atkins RM, Duthie RB (1987) Algodystrophy (reflex sympathetic dystrophy or Sudeck's atrophy). In: Weatherall DJ, Ledingham JGG, Warrell DA (eds) Oxford textbook of medicine. Oxford University Press, pp 16.89–16.91

Bhargava SK, Gupta R, Lohchab VS et al (1983) Unusual radiological changes in metacarpals, metatarsals and phalanges in rickets. J Indian Med Assoc 81:175–179

Canalis E (1993) Regulation of bone remodeling. In: Favus MJ (ed) Primer on the metabolic bone diseases and disorders of mineral metabolism. Raven, New York, pp 33–37

Cepollaro C, Gonnelli S, Pondrelli C et al (1998) Usefulness of ultrasound in Sudeck's atrophy of the foot. Calcif Tissue Int 62:538–541

Chalmers GW, Brown WR, Stienstra JJ (1998) Tumoral calcinosis-like lesion of the foot. A case report. J Am Podiatr Med Assoc 88:87–91

Chevrot A, Pallardy G, Ledoux-Lebard G (1978) Skeletal manifestations of hyperthyroidism (author's translation). J Radiol Electrol Med Nucl 59:167–173

Chew FS (1991) Radiologic manifestations in the musculoskeletal system of miscellaneous endocrine disorders. Radiol Clin North Am 29:135–147

Cockshott WP, Occleshaw CJ, Webber C et al (1984) Can a calcaneal morphologic index determine the degree of osteoporosis? Skeletal Radiol 12:119–122

Colao A, Marzullo P, Vallone G et al (1998) Reversibility of joint thickening in acromegalic patients:an ultrasonography study. J Clin Endocrinol Metab 83:2121–2125

Colao A, Marzullo P, Vallone G et al (1999) Ultrasonographic evidence of joint thickening reversibility in acromegalic patients treated with lanreotide for 12 months. Clin Endocrinol (Oxf) 51:611–618

Crouzet J, Mimoune H, Beraneck L et al (1995) Hypophosphatemic osteomalacia with plantar neurilemoma. A review of the literature (100 cases). Rev Rhum Engl Ed 62:463–466

Darbois H, Boyer B, Dubayle P et al (1999) MRI symptomology in reflex sympathetic dystrophy of the foot. J Radiol 80:849–854

De Palma L, Serra F, Coletti V et al (1993) Foot alterations in the hemodialyzed patient. J Foot Ankle Surg 32:526–529

Doppman JL, Sharon M, Gorden P (1988) Metatarsal penciling in acromegaly:a proposed mechanism based on CT findings. J Comput Assist Tomogr 12:708–709

Edwards MC Jr, Spinner S (1994) Renal osteodystrophy with pedal involvement. J Am Podiatr Med Assoc 84:26–29

Fishco WD, Stiles RG (1999) Atypical heel pain. Hyperparathyroidism-induced stress fracture of the calcaneus. J Am Podiatr Med Assoc 89:413–418

Garver P, Resnick D, Niwayama G et al (1981) Epiphyseal sclerosis in renal osteodystrophy simulating osteonecrosis. AJR Am J Roentgenol 136:1239–1241

Genant HK (1997) Interpretation of bone densitometry. Rev Rhum Engl Ed 64 [6 Suppl]:20S–25S

Genant HK, Heck LL, Lanzl LH et al (1973) Primary hyperparathyroidism. A comprehensive study of clinical, biochemical and radiographic manifestations. Radiology 109: 513–524

Genant HK, Kozin F, Bekerman C et al (1975) The reflex sympathetic dystrophy syndrome. A comprehensive analysis using fine-detail radiography, photon absorptiometry, and bone and joint scintigraphy. Radiology 117:21–32

Gonticas SK, Ikkos DG, Stergiou LH (1969) Evaluation of the diagnostic value of heel-pad thickness in acromegaly. Radiology 92:304–307

Gooding GA, Stress RM, Graf PM et al (1985) Heel pad thickness: determination by high-resolution ultrasonography. J Ultrasound Med 4:173–174

Guyer PB, Chamberlain AT, Ackery DM et al (1981) The anatomic distribution of osteitis deformans. Clin Orthop 156: 141–144

Hamilton EB (1972) Hyperparathyroidism with chondrocalcinosis and periarticular calcification. Proc R Soc Med 65: 1013

Han ZH, Palnitkar S, Rao DS et al (1996) Effect of ethnicity and age or menopause on the structure and geometry of iliac bone. J Bone Miner Res 11:1967–1975

Hayes CW, Conway WF (1991) Hyperparathyroidism. Radiol Clin North Am 29:85–96

Hodgskinson R, Njeh CF, Currey JD et al (1997) The ability of ultrasound velocity to predict the stiffness of cancellous bone in vitro. Bone 21:183–190

Jergas M, Schmid G (1999) The role of quantitative ultrasound versus other techniques in osteoporosis assessment. In: Njeh CF, Hans D, Fuerst T, Gluer C, Genant HK (eds) Quantitative ultrasound: assessment of osteoporosis and bone status. Dunitz, London, pp 245–281

Kalender WA, Felsenberg D, Louis O et al (1989) Reference values for trabecular and cortical vertebral bone density in single and dual-energy quantitative computed tomography. Eur J Radiol 9:75–80

Koch E, Hofer HO, Sialer G et al (1991) Failure of MR imaging to detect reflex sympathetic dystrophy of the extremities. AJR Am J Roentgenol 156:113–115

Korber J, McCarthy S, Marsden W (1993) Case report 782. Predominantly osteolytic Paget's disease of the calcaneus. Skeletal Radiol 22:222–225

Kozin F, Genant HK, Bekerman C et al (1976a) The reflex sympathetic dystrophy syndrome. II. Roentgenographic and scintigraphic evidence of bilaterality and of periarticular accentuation. Am J Med 60:332–338

Kozin F, McCarty DJ, Sims J et al (1976b) The reflex sympathetic dystrophy syndrome. I. Clinical and histologic studies: evidence for bilaterality, response to corticosteroids and articular involvement. Am J Med 60:321–331

Levine MA (1993) Parathyroid hormone resistance syndromes. In: Favus MJ (ed) Primer on the metabolic bone diseases and disorders of mineral metabolism. Raven, New York, pp 194–200

MacSweeney JE, Baxter MA, Joplin GF (1990) Heel pad thickness is an insensitive index of biochemical remission in acromegaly. Clin Radiol 42:348–350

Mazess R, Chesnut CH III, McClung M et al (1992) Enhanced precision with dual-energy X-ray absorptiometry. Calcif Tissue Int 51:14–17

Meneghello A, Bertoli M (1983) Tendon disease and adjacent bone erosion in dialysis patients. Br J Radiol 56:915–920

Mittal RK, Ahuja IS, Ahuja GK (1983) Heel pad thickness in normal Nigerians and patients with acromegaly. East Afr Med J 60:156–159

Neylon TA (1995) Paget's disease of bone presenting as chronic ankle pain. J Am Podiatr Med Assoc 85:556–559

Paisey R, Jeans WD, Hartog M (1984) Is soft tissue radiology useful in acromegaly? Br J Radiol 57:561–564

Parfitt AM (1988) Bone remodeling: relationship to the amount and structure of bone, and the pathogenesis and prevention of fractures. In: Riggs BL, Melton LJ III (eds) Osteoporosis: etiology, diagnosis and management. Raven, New York, pp 45–93

Pitt MJ (1981) Rachitic and osteomalacic syndromes. Radiol Clin North Am 19:581–599

Pitt MJ (1991) Rickets and osteomalacia are still around. Radiol Clin North Am 29:97–118

Puckette SE Jr, Seymour EQ (1967) Fallibility of the heel-pad thickness in the diagnosis of acromegaly. Radiology 88: 982–983

Resnick D (1995a) Pituitary disorders. In: Resnick D (ed) Diagnosis of bone and joint disorders. Saunders, Philadelphia, pp 1971–1994

Resnick D (1995b) Thyroid disorders. In: Resnick D (ed) Diagnosis of bone and joint disorders. Saunders, Philadelphia, pp 1995–2011

Resnick D, Niwayama G (1995a) Paget's disease. In: Resnick D (ed) Diagnosis of bone and joint disorders. Saunders, Philadelphia, pp 1923–1968

Resnick D, Niwayama G (1995b) Parathyroid disorders and renal osteodystrophy. In: Resnick D (ed) Diagnosis of bone and joint disorders. Saunders, Philadelphia, pp 2012–2075

Resnick D, Deftos LJ, Parthemore JG (1981) Renal osteodystrophy:magnification radiography of target sites of absorption. AJR Am J Roentgenol 136:711–714

Rubin RP, Adler JJ, Adler DP (1983) Paget's disease of the calcaneus. J Am Podiatry Assoc 73:263–267

Sherwood LM (1993) Hypoparathyroidism. In: Favus MJ (ed) Primer on the metabolic bone diseases and disorders of mineral metabolism. Raven, New York, pp 191–193

Veldman PH, Reynen HM, Arntz IE et al (1993) Signs and symptoms of reflex sympathetic dystrophy:prospective study of 829 patients. Lancet 342:1012–1016

WHO (1994) Assessment of fracture risk and its application to screening for postmenopausal osteoporosis. WHO Tech Rep Ser 843:1–129

17 Osteonecrosis and Osteochondritis

J. Kramer, S. Hofmann, and M. Recht

CONTENTS

17.1 Osteonecrosis

17.1.1 Introduction

Osteonecrosis (ON) is a disease caused by ischemic death of the bony and marrow tissues (Jones 1994). Avascular necrosis is a term applied to ischemic necrosis involving the epiphyseal region, while ON of the metadiaphysis is referred to as bone infarction (Sweet and Madewell 1995). ON most commonly affects the femoral head, but it can also affect other epiphyseal areas including the knee, shoulder, and bones of the ankle joint as well as other locations on rare occasions (Mankin 1992; Jacobs et al. 1989; Mont et al. 1996; Urquart et al. 1996). The keys to treating this condition lie in understanding the pathologic process. Although it is possible to point to specific groups of patients that seem to be at risk, it is very difficult to assess the true incidence of ON because of the asymptomatic nature of the early stages of the disease. It is unclear how long the early stages of the disease are actually present in a bone before becoming symptomatic. The different imaging modalities reflect divergent information concerning the mineralized and nonmineralized parts of the bone. The clinical presentation, imaging, and prognosis of ON depend on the etiology (traumatic or nontraumatic), location (classical epiphyseal ON or metadiaphyseal bone marrow infarction), and the repair capacity (sufficient repair in the child with open growth plate, limited or insufficient repair in the adolescent, adult, or old patient with or without systemic diseases or risk factors) (Hofmann et al. 1994a). Although specific changes depend on these several factors, the morphological and imaging findings are remarkably similar in all locations (Resnick and Niwayama 1995). The early diagnosis and proper staging of ON are important to define the treatment and predict the clinical outcome (Mont and Hungerford 1995; Steinberg et al. 1995; Stulberg et al. 1989).

17.1.2 Etiology

The etiology of ON is frequently unclear. However, all etiologies are felt to result in interruption of the blood flow. The vascular supply to a region may be reduced by traumatic disruption of the blood supply, vascular occlusion (thrombosis or sludging), vascular compression, or prolonged vasospasm (Bluemke and Zerhouni 1996; Hofmann et al. 1996; Imhof et al. 1997; Lecouvet et al. 1998). The type of vessel

J. Kramer, MD, PhD
Institute for CT & MRI Diagnosis –Am Schillerpark, Rainerstr. 6-8, 4020 Linz, Austria
S. Hofmann, MD
Orthopedic Hospital Stolzalpe, 8852 Stolzalpe, Austria
M. Recht, MD
Cleveland Clinic Foundation, Diagnostic Radiology, Musculoskeletal Section, 9500 Euclid Avenue, Cleveland, Ohio 44195-5145, USA

involved and the anatomic site (epiphysis, metaphysis, or diaphysis) are important. Arterial collateral vessels serve a protective function, whereas sinusoids are more susceptible to occlusion, especially in patients with sickle-cell disease or other hemoglobinopathies. The epiphyses have fewer collaterals, especially before growth plate closure. The incidence of traumatic ON varies with the location of the injury, severity of injury, type of treatment, timing of treatment, and associated injuries (HERNDON and AUFRANC 1972; HOUGARD and THOMSEN 1986; HALIBURTON et al. 1958; KRUCZYNSKI 1996). Although the hip is the most common anatomic location for the development of ON after trauma, other bones, such as the proximal humerus and the talus, are also vulnerable. ON is not common after nondisplaced talar neck fractures, but it is a well-recognized complication of severe ankle trauma, with an incidence ranging between 40% and 50% in patients following a fracture-dislocation (HAWKINS 1970; MINDELL et al. 1963; BLAIR 1943; DENNIS and TULLOS 1980).

Approximately two-thirds of nontraumatic ON is related to hypercortisonism, hyperlipidemia, and/or increased alcohol intake. The other third includes hemoglobinopathies, pregnancy, familial thrombophylia, and other coagulopathies (JONES 1994). ON is also increased in patients with organ transplants, inflammatory bowel disease, systemic lupus erythematosus (SLE), sickle-cell hemoglobinopathies, and dysbaric trauma (HARRIS and SILVER 1973; HUNGERFORD and ZIZIC 1978; CRUESS 1981; ADLEBERG and SMITH 1991; DALL and MACNAB 1970; LANGEVITZ et al. 1990; MISKEW and GOLDFLIES 1980; BARON et al. 1984). Dysbaric ON occurs because of rapid changes in pressure resulting in the release of gases, primarily nitrogen, into the blood and soft tissue. Disruption of fat cells with associated fat emboli has also been implicated (ELLIOT and HARRISON 1970; FICAT and ARLET 1980; FICAT 1985; TEGETMEYER et al. 1997). The fatty marrow may be especially vulnerable to infarction, particularly in the presence of repeated and sustained gas emboli, because it has an inadequate collateral circulation (AMAKO et al. 1974; GREGG and WALDER 1986). The incidence of dysbaric ON is higher in obese patients. The most common sites of dysbaric ON are the humerus and femur.

ON of the foot and ankle is relatively uncommon (CONI 1983; ELLIOT and HARRISON 1970; PETERSON and GOLDIE 1975). ON of the the tarsal navicular bone can occur in children (Köhler's disease) and manifests radiologically as sclerosis, irregularity, and fragmentation of the bone (KÖHLER 1908) (Fig. 17.1). A form of ON of the tarsal navicular bone has also been described in adults (Mueller-Weiss syndrome). ON of the foot region is also frequently noted in the second metatarsal head (Freiberg's disease), with flattening and sclerosis of the metatarsal head seen on conventional radiography (FREIBERG 1914, 1926) (Fig. 17.2).

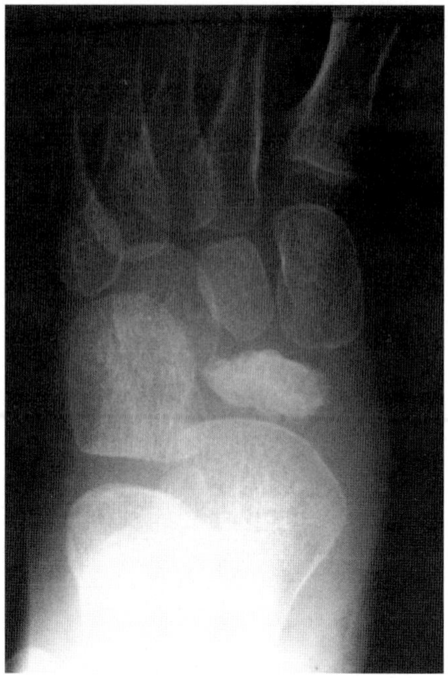

Fig. 17.1. AP radiograph demonstrates a compressed navicular with increased density (Köhler's disease). The space by the navicular appears almost normal, indicating an intact cartilage model

17.1.3 Imaging Techniques

17.1.3.1 Radiography

The plain film findings in late-stage ON are often pathognomonic (MONT and HUNGERFORD 1995; RESNICK and NIWAYAMA 1995). Typical radiographic signs of ON include subchondral patchy radiolucent regions, sclerosis, radiolucent areas with a peripheral sclerotic rim, osseous or osteochondral collapse, and degenerative changes with deformation in late-stage ON. Rarely, a mixture of the above-mentioned findings may simulate the aggressive pattern of bone destruction of malignant tumors as well as osteomyelitis. In rare cases, conventional tomography may be indicated for the accurate diagnosis of ON. As opposed to the situation with late-stage ON, the

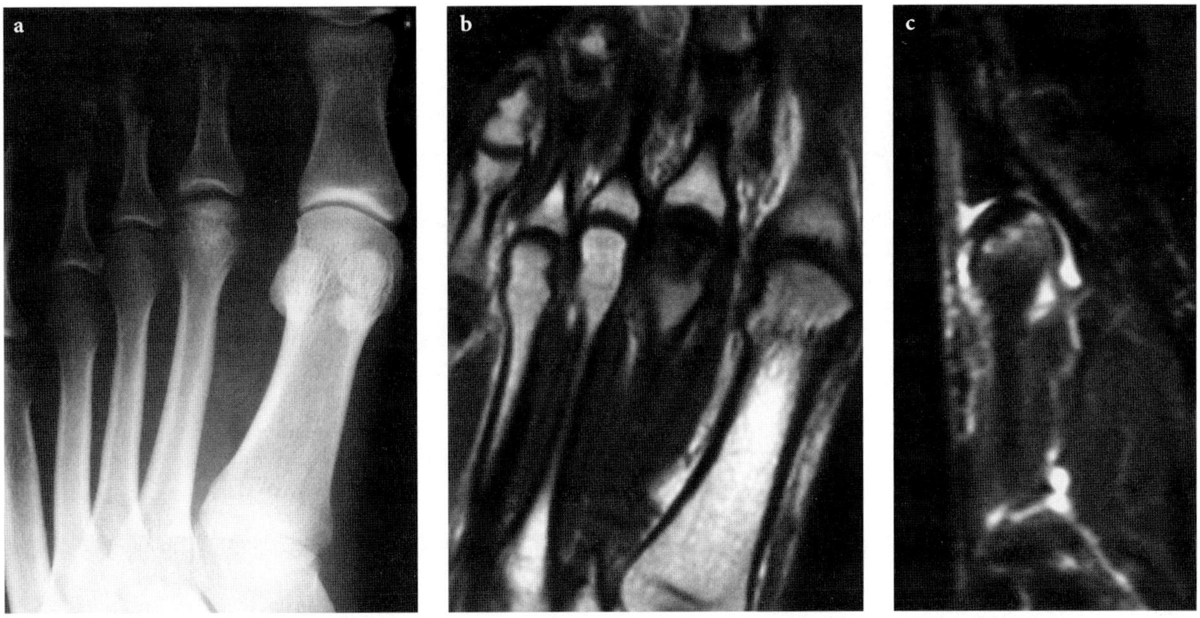

Fig. 17.2a–c. Plain radiograph (AP view) of the forefoot (**a**), paracoronal T1-weighted spin-echo (SE) image (**b**), and sagittal STIR image (2nd metatarsal) (**c**). **a** The head of the second metatarsal is slightly depressed and demonstrates increased density (avascular necrosis – Freiberg's disease). **b** Most of the metatarsal head shows low signal intensity. **c** On the fat-suppressed image, the subchondral area of low signal intensity corresponds to the region of increased density on the plain film. Adjacent to this alteration, edematous marrow changes and a joint effusion are visible

early stages of ONare often difficult to diagnose and grade with plain-film radiography. Despite this limitation for the diagnosis of ON, plain-film radiographs remain the first imaging step in the evaluation of hip pain.

17.1.3.2 Computed Tomography

The value of CT in the detection of ON is limited. Although CT enables the delineation of subtle alterations of bone necrosis before plain radiographs become positive, MR imaging has largely replaced it as the imaging modality of choice for the detection of early ON (Hofmann et al. 1995). Characteristic findings of ON on CT are a rim of increased attenuation surrounding a subchondral region of decreased attenuation (Magid et al. 1985). The standard CT technique includes high-resolution scans with contiguous axial slices enabling two-dimensional reconstructions in the coronal and/or sagittal plans, which may be helpful for correct staging. Reconstructions have been improved during the past few years due to the use of multislice CT scans providing thin slices in a reasonable examination time. The main advantage of CT is the accurate detection of a subchondral fracture or early collapse (Kramer et al. 1994). The disadvantage of this method is that small lesions might be overlooked because of partial volume effects.

17.1.3.3 Magnetic Resonance Imaging

MR imaging is the most accurate imaging modality for the diagnosis of ON, especially in the early phases. Signal abnormalities depend on alterations of the fat cells in the bone marrow (Mitchell et al. 1989). Ischemic changes first become evident in the hematopoetic cells 6–12 h after an ischemic event. Fat cells are more resistent to ischemia, surviving for 2–5 days after the insult. An inflammatory and hyperemic response in viable tissue adjacent to the devascularized regions produces a reactive interface about the osteonecrotic areas that is associated with increased vascularity, inflammation, granulation tissue, and new bone formation. MR imaging is sensitive to the presence of this reactive interface. Chracteristic MR signal changes of ON were described by Mitchell (Mitchell et al. 1989) (Figs. 17.3–17.5). The MR appearance of the necrotic area is classified into four types on the basis of the signal intensities of both T1-weighted and T2-weighted spin-echo images. In the type A pattern, the signal changes are of increased intensity on T1-weighted images and intermediate a 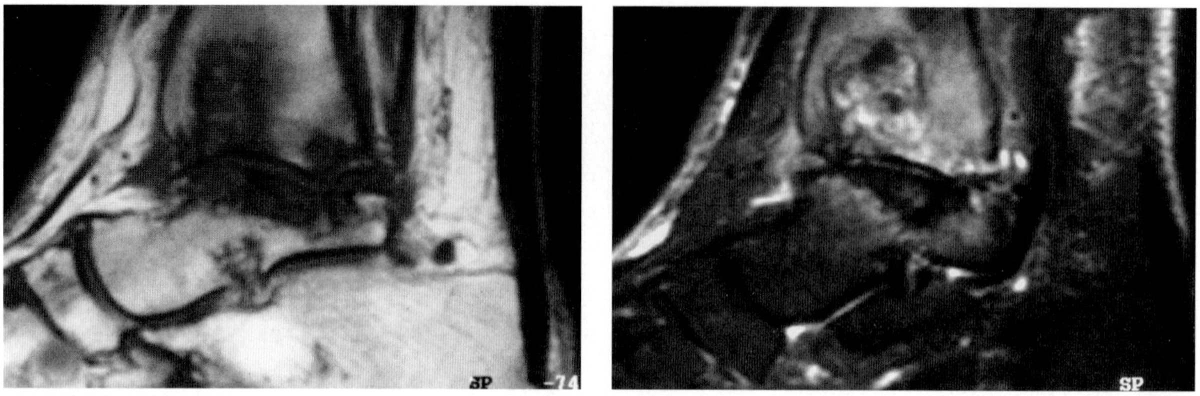 b

Fig. 17.3a,b. Sagittal T1-weighted SE (**a**) and STIR image (**b**). Patient suffered a motor vehicle accident 2 years prior to this MR examination. **a** Depression of the talar dome with a broad subchondral necrotic region as well as a necrotic area in the distal talus outlined by a sclerotic rim and a subtle concomitant edema are visible

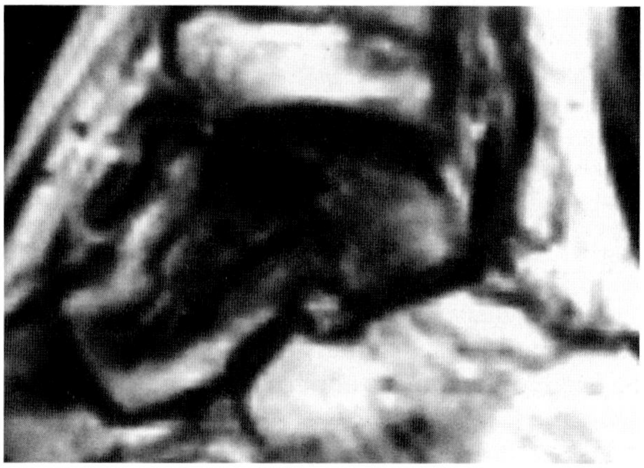

Fig. 17.4. Sagittal T1-weighted SE image demonstrates avascular necrosis of the talus. The necrotic zone has mixed signal intensity. The hypointense border is characteristic for the sclerotic interface. In the talar head, the lesion is surrounded by edematous changes. No definite deformity can be observed

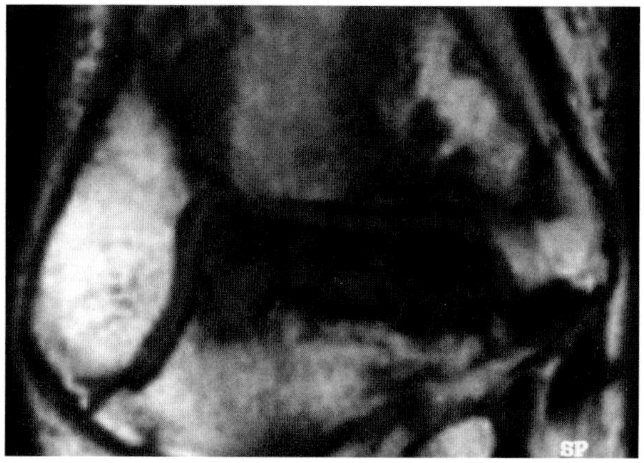

Fig. 17.5. Coronal T1-weighted SE image. Patient had received steroid therapy (renal transplantation). The cortical suface of the tibia and talus is preserved. In the medial aspect of the tibia, an osteonecrotic lesion is visible. The necrotic zone has a signal intensity similar to fat, surrounded by a low intensity margin (sclerosis). The necrosis in the subtalar region shows a slightly inhomogenous hypointense signal. The border of the lesion to the remaining talar bone is formed by the sclerotic rim (interface)

signal intensity on T2-weighted images (fat-like). This stage has been postulated to represent an early phase of the disease. The type B pattern is characterized by high signal intensity on both T1-weighted and T2-weighted images, analogous to the appearance of blood. In type C, there is low signal intensity on T1-weighted images and high signal intensity on T2-weighted images, a pattern consistent with the presence of fluid. The type D pattern shows low signal intensity on both T1-weighted and T2-weighted images, representing the presence of fibrous tissue and sclerosis. However, this classification has been found to have no prognostic impact on the clinical outcome, and therefore, it is not included in clinical staging systems (Hofmann et al. 1994b). These signal changes within the necrotic area are surrounded by a band of low signal intensity on T1-weighted images, which represents fibrous tissue and new bone formation in the reactive interface. In most patients, a high signal line central to the low signal rim can be observed in the reactive interface on T2-weighted images, indicating the well-vascularized granulation tissue. This so-called 'double line sign' represents the sclerotic rim (outer dark line) and the hypervascularity of the repair zone (inner high signal line) and not a chemical shift artifact (Mitchell et al. 1989). The reactive interface and the double line sign have been considered to be pathognomonic of ON. The use of an intravenous MR contrast agent will help distinguish between vascularized and nonvascularized tissue (VAN DE BERG et al. 1992; LANG et al. 1993). Some investigators have demonstrated a correlation between enhanced areas and sites of viable tissue, whereas nonenhanced regions correspond to necrotic tissue. It is important to realize that the enhancement of the necrotic lesion by a contrast agent is only an indirect indicator of bone viability, because necrotic bone and marrow can be infiltrated by vascularized granulation tissue without the instigation of a sufficient repair process. An additional finding seen in ON is joint effusion, which is frequently secondary to mechanical failure (subchondral or osteochondral fracture) or concomitant bone marrow edema (FICAT 1985; HAUZEUR et al. 1989; HUNGERFORD and JONES 1993).

17.1.3.4 Bone Scintigraphy

Bone scintigraphy has been shown to be an accurate technique for the early diagnosis of ON (D'AMBROSIA et al. 1975; RESNICK and NIWAYAMA 1995). The standard technique should include three-phase scintigraphy with ^{99m}Tc-methylene diethylenetriamine penta-acetic acid (MDTP). This method allows visualization of the regional blood flow. Interruption of the blood supply, detected as a cold spot, is a nonspecific pattern and can be observed in a variation of conditions (infection, plasma cell myeloma, metastasis, hemangioma, etc.). The repair process, detected as a hot spot, is the most common finding in ON, but it is also not specific. Only the combination of a cold spot within a hot spot represents a diagnostic pattern of ON. Bone scintigraphy is not specific and must be interpreted with the knowledge gained from the radiographic and clinical findings. Therefore, bone scans are highly sensitive for the detection of early ON, but their specificity is unacceptable for the definitive diagnosis of an ON lesion (KRAMER et al. 1994). Bone scintigraphy should be performed for screening in patients at risk of multifocal lesions when MR imaging is not available or for patients at high risk for ON when the MR imaging is negative.

17.1.4 Staging

Most knowledge about ON is based on histologic studies of the hip, but the changes are similar in all anatomic locations (BERQUIST et al. 2000). Several radiological classification systems exist. However, the ARCO (Association Research Circulation Osseous) staging system which has been used primarily for avascular necrosis of the femoral head (GARDENIERS 1993; RUTISHAUSER et al. 1960; HUNGERFORD and JONES 1993) will be described. This system includes radiological findings, clinical signs, and pathomorphologic changes. Based on imaging studies, talar ON progresses through sequential stages similar to those of femoral head lesions (MONT et al. 1993; JONES 1993).

Stage 0. The patient has no symptoms, and plain film, CT, and conventional MR imaging demonstrate no abnormal findings. The ischemic zone might be detected as a 'cold spot' with focal decreased tracer uptake in the bone scan (JONES 1994) and reduced contrast enhancement in dynamic contrast-enhanced MR imaging studies (CONWAY et al. 1993), but these imaging patterns are nonspecific for ON. In clinical practice, this stage 0 will not normally be seen, as the patient has no definite pain and/or the pain lasts for only several days. If the ischemia does not persist, the morphological changes in stage 0 are reversible.

Stage I. Normally, the patient is asymptomatic, and radiographs and CT examinations are still normal. Bone scans show a 'hot spot' indicating the high vascularity of the repair process. On MR imaging, the subchondral necrotic defect may show the typical pattern of bone marrow edema with low signal on T1-weighted images and high signal intensity on T2-weighted images (HOFMANN et al. 1994).

On histology, the bone marrow is necrotic as a result of prolonged ischemia. If the blood supply is restored at this point, the necrotic damage is reversible. Vascularized granulation tissue replaces the necrotic bone marrow, and new bone formation and resorption of necrotic trabeculae occur (RUTISHAUSER et al. 1960). This process is called creeping substitution.

Stage II. In most cases, the patient is usually still asymptomatic. Plain films show only nonspecific changes. However, pathognomonic findings for ON can be observed on CT, bone scans, and MR imaging. Plain radiographs allow the detection of a sclerotic rim surrounding the lesion, but in early stage II, it is usually seen only on CT. On bone scan, an area of decreased tracer uptake will be surrounded by increased tracer accumulation in the periphery. This 'cold in hot spot' is pathognomonic of ON. On MR imaging, the necrotic region shows different signal alterations (type A to D according to MITCHELL et al. 1989) which are surrounded by the 'double line sign'. The reactive interface and the double line sign have been considered to be pathognomonic of ON.

The imaging findings are the result of an insufficient repair process that produces a thin band of increased vascularity, granulation tissue, and new bone formation at the periphery of the necrotic lesion. This 'reactive interface' between living and dead bone represents the unsuccessful attempt of the viable tissue to repair the dead marrow and trabeculae from the periphery to the central parts of the necrotic area. As a consequence of the insufficient repair, ON becomes irreversible. However, some investigators (VANDE BERG 1992; KOPECKY et al. 1991) have reported follow-up MR imaging studies of ON of the femoral head that showed apparent healing of lesions in high-risk patients. At least some of these cases included signal alterations without a reactive interface, representing nonspecific changes that are not diagnostic for irreversible ON. But it seems that rarely in early stage II disease, the lesion may be reversible.

Stage III. Acute onset of joint pain, usually aggravated by weight-bearing and relieved by rest, is the clinical sign of stage III. Pathognomonic changes for stage III on radiographs and CT can be identified, whereas only indirect findings differentiating stage II from stage III can be found on bone scans and MR imaging. The histology of stage III lesions shows a subchondral fracture. The combination of osteoclastic resorption induced by the repair process and microfractures induced by shear forces at the chondro-osseous junction is the cause of this subchondral fracture (GARDENIERS 1993). Fibrocartilaginous metaplasia often occurs surrounding the fracture line, blocking further revascularization. The pathognomonic fracture line is identified on CT with higher accuracy than on plain film.

Stage IV. Patients suffer continuously from progressive joint pain. With stage IV, nonspecific secondary osteoarthritic changes can be identified on all imaging modalities. Macroscopically, a collapse of the affected bone and secondary osteoarthritic joint destruction with subchondral cysts are visible. The fracture, the collapse, and the secondary osteoarthritic changes can be identified on plain radiographs as well as CT. In late ON stages with severe degenerative changes, the differential diagnosis of osteoarthritis can be difficult. Bone scans show the mechanical effect of the collapse and the hypervascularization at the chondro-osseous junction of the collapse as a 'hot in hot' spot.

17.1.5 Conclusions

ON represents a bone disease caused by ischemic death of the bony and marrow tissues. For the clinical practice, early diagnosis and proper staging of ON are important for the treatment strategies and the clinical outcome since the prognosis and the success of the different treatment modalities are clearly related to the stage of the disease. Plain radiographs remain the first diagnostic step because they permit the exclusion of several pathologies other than ON. MR imaging is best suited for the detection of early lesions. Careful assessment of MR imaging changes occurring in the subchondral area can enable confident differentiation between transient lesions and early irreversible necrosis. Furthermore, MR imaging allows an exact identification and assessment of the location and the extent of the necrotic area and provides valuable information for therapeutic management planning.

17.2 Osteochondritis Dissecans

17.2.1 Introduction

In 1888, osteochdondrosis dissecans (OCD) was named by KOENIG, who emphasized its spontaneous nature (KÖNIG 1888). However, in 1870, PAGET had already considered trauma-induced necrosis as a cause of free intra-articular bodies (PAGET 1870). OCD indicates fragmentation and possible separation of an osteochondral portion of the articular suface. The clinical manifestations are variable, related to the specific site of involvement. OCD of the ankle is often associated with ligamentous injury (NISHIMURA et al. 1996). Definitive knowledge of the course of OCD in vivo and its pathologic-anatomic correlation does not exist. In particular, histologic observations of early forms of OCD are missing (BOHNDORF 1998).

17.2.2 Etiology

The etiology of OCD lesions is controversial. Several theories have been proposed. Today, it is widely accepted that focal stress, ischemia, abnormal ossification within the epiphysis, or a combination of these factors is responsible for the osteochondral damage

(Clanton and De Lee 1982; Langer and Percy 1971). The most commonly accepted theory is that OCD lesions are posttraumatic, resulting from either shearing or impaction forces. Evidence to support this opinion includes a higher prevalence of OCD in athletically active children and the strong association of OCD lesions of the talus with recent ankle trauma. Abnormal alignment or ligamentous laxity predisposes the ankle to excessive shearing forces. Because of the subchondral bone's relative insensitivity to pain and the often resultant lack of symptoms, it is not always possible to define the exact time and mechanism of the injury or even to determine if more than one injury has occurred, nor is it possible to exclude the etiologic contributions of nontraumatic factors (Morris 1974). Classic OCD is a lesion found in adolescence and adulthood, with men affected more frequently than women (Magee and Hinson 1998; Schoenberg and Lehmann 1994). Although in some patients OCD may not become symptomatic until late in life, this disease should not be confused with spontaneous ON, which was described as a different syndrome of subchondral bone necrosis of the distal femur (Ahlbäck et al. 1968). The classic finding of OCD of the talus consists of a medial lesion close to the margin and exhibits a round, 'deep' character. The OCD fragment itself can be round, oval, or fragmented. In contrast, the acute, mostly laterally located osteochondral fractures are sharply demarcated and produce a rather flat fragment. Differentiation of OCD from old traumatic lesions may be very difficult or even impossible. OCD most commonly involves the talar dome, typically its medial or lateral corner (Schoenberg and Lehmann 1994; Horton 1997; Morscher 1971). The medial lesion is typically larger, is more cup-shaped, and extends more deeply into the body of the talus. OCD lesions rarely occur in the tibial plafond. There are several potential explanations for the higher occurrence of OCD in the talus than in the tibiofibular planfond. Osteochondral lesions are more commonly observed at the convex surface of a joint, whereas the concave surface is generally spared. The convex surface is believed to transmit the convergence forces toward a central focus, whereas a concave surface dissipates the forces. As a result, the convex joint surface, such as that of the talus, is likely to be more severely damaged by trauma than the tibial plafond (Camasta et al. 1994). Furthermore, the cartilage of the tibia is stiffer than of the talus because of differences in composition (Athanasiou et al. 1995). Lastly, in some cases, the lesion may not be visible on conventional radiographs or radiogists may not be aware of this entity and may not recognize the lesion on conventional radiographs (Bui-Mansfield et al. 2000a,b).

17.2.3 Imaging Methods

17.2.3.1 Radiography, CT, and Scintigraphy

Conventional roentgenography, high resolution CT, and bone scintigraphy have been used for the radiographic evaluation of osteochondral lesions, although none of these modalities is suitable to assess the integrity of the articular cartilage (Yulish et al. 1987) (Figs. 17.6–17.8). Double-contrast arthrography has also been proposed and allows only incomplete (surface) assessment of intraarticular structures. Arthography and conventional or computed arthrotomography are indicated in some cases to delineate the lesion site better, define the condition of the overlying cartilage, and detect intraarticular osseous and cartilaginous bodies. However, none of these methods is suitable to assess subtle changes of the articular cartilage.

17.2.3.2 MR Imaging

MR imaging has been shown to be very useful to define the site and the extent of the lesion (Nelson et al. 1990). Precise identification of the location and the extent of the lesion, correct assessment of the overlying articular cartilage, and determination of fragment stability are important in determining the need for surgery and the specific surgical approach that must be used (Bauer et al. 1987; Bloem et al. 1990). The accuracy of MR imaging in assessing cartilage lesions is said to improve with the presence of joint effusions, because of the arthrographic effect of free joint fluid on T2-weighted sequences. High spatial resolution is indispensable for the delineation of small cartilage lesions. Three-dimensional (3D) gradient-echo (GE) sequences have been advocated for the evaluation of OCD lesions because of their ability to acquire thin contiguous slices with minimal volume averaging artifacts (Tyrrell et al. 1988). With T2*-weighted or fat-suppressed T1-weighted GE sequences, the cartilaginous surface can usually be clearly differentiated from intraarticular fluid, because the contrast difference cartilage/fluid is even greater than with SE T2-weighted sequences (Adam et al. 1988). With the intraarticular injection of a

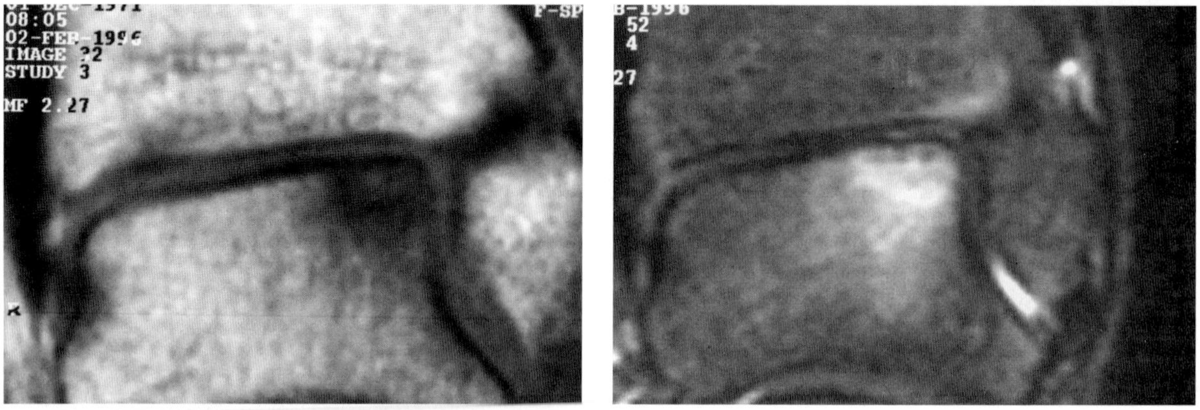

a b

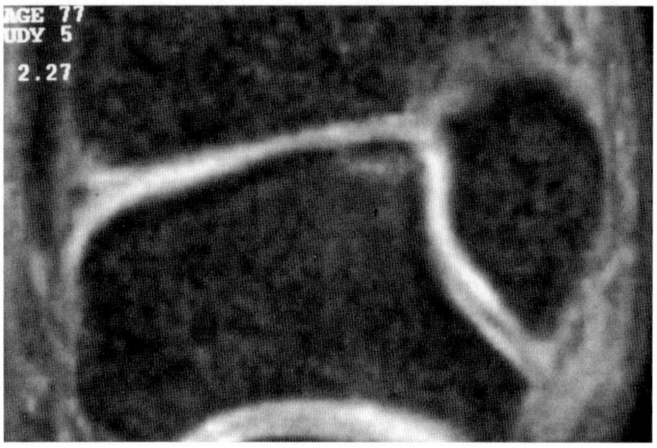

c

Fig. 17.6a–c. Osteochondritis dissecans of the talus. The patient cannot remember a trauma during the last month. Coronal T1-weighted SE (**a**), fat-saturated turbo T2-weighted SE (**b**), and fat-saturated 3D GE sequence (**c**). **a,b** At the medial corner of the talar dome, a subchondral area of low signal intensity and an increase in signal intensity compared with the surrounding bone marrow can be detected. The osteochondral plate appears intact. On the T1-weighted SE image (**a**), a thin hypointense line (demarcation) is faintly visible at the periphery of the lesion. **c** GE image demonstrates the lesion involving the subchondral plate but sparing the cartilage layer

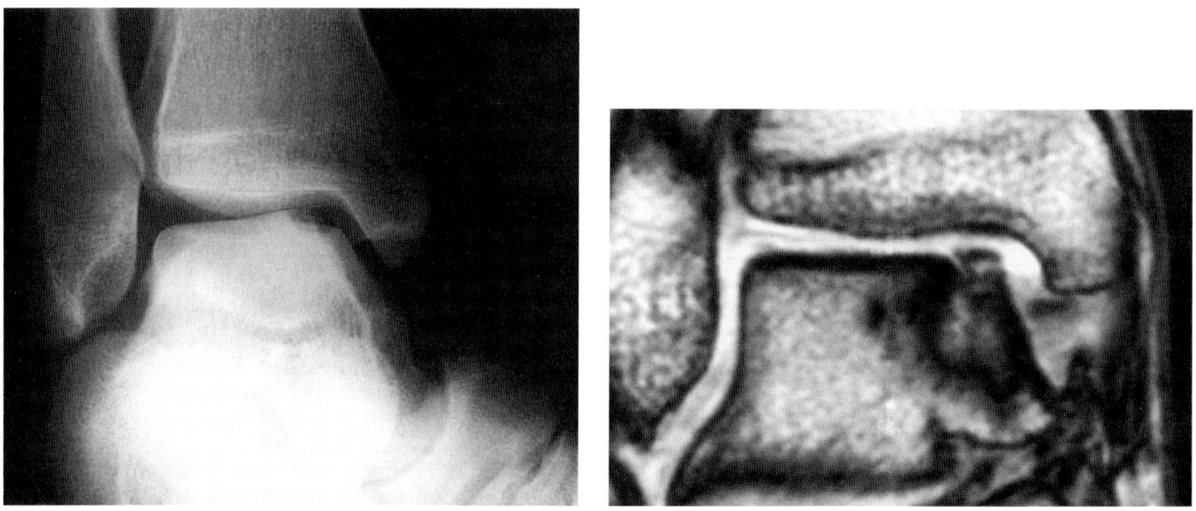

a b

Fig. 17.7a,b. Osteochondritis dissecans of the talus: AP view of the ankle (**a**) and coronal T1-weighted GE sequence (**b**). **a** A lesion at the medial aspect of the talar dome is shown. **b** GE image allows visualization of the lesion (site, size, and demarcation). However, due to the absence of any joint effusion, an exact assessment of any likely involvement of the overlying cartilage is not possible. Reactive changes of the talar bone are visible adjacent to the lesion

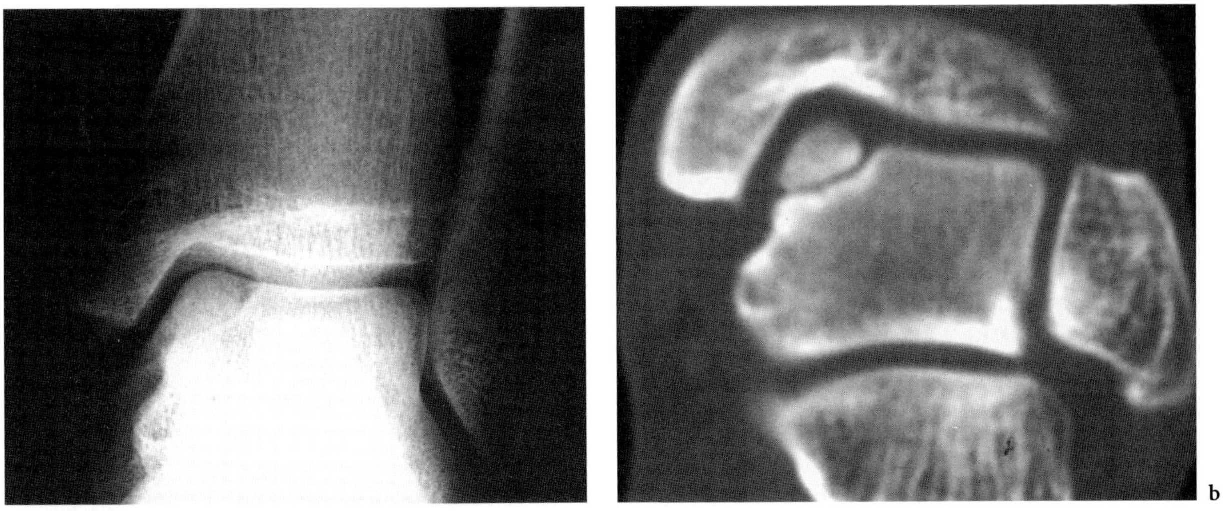

a b

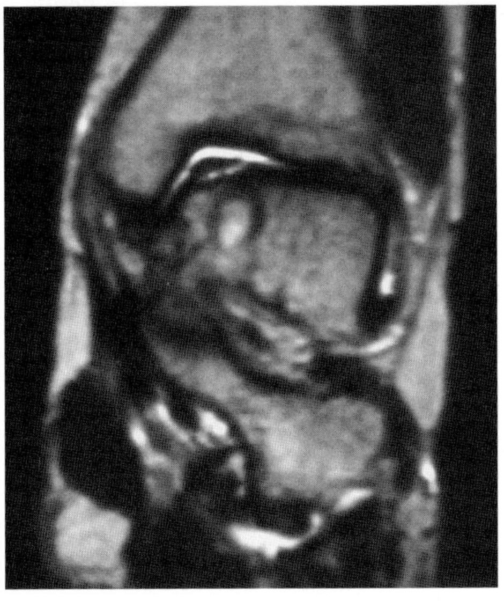

c

Fig. 17.8a–c. Three different patients with osteochondritis dissecans of the talar dome with similar findings: AP radiograph (**a**), coronal CT scan (**b**), and coronal T2-weighted SE sequence (**c**). The medial talar lesion is clearly seen in all three patients. However, only the MR image allows differentiation of demarcation from separation and demonstrates in this case the complete separation of the osteochondral lesion from the talus, since fluid can be detected between the talus and the osteochondral fragment

contrast agent, tiny superficial lesions can be visualized, and delineation of the cartilaginous articular surface is possible with excellent detail (Winalski et al. 1991; Kramer et al. 1992; Adam et al. 1994; Vahlensieck et al. 1996, 1998). The conspicuity of chondral lesions is increased with MR arthrography as there is imbibition of contrast into damaged cartilage with essentially no uptake of contrast material into the normal hyaline cartilage.

17.2.4 Staging

The Clanton DeLee classification is the most frequently used staging system. Although developed for OCD lesions of the knee, it can be applied to OCD lesions of the talus (Clanton and De Lee 1982). This scheme corresponds roughly to the classification used by Nelson et al. as well as to the arthroscopic classification proposed in the report by De Smet (Clanton and De Lee 1982; De Smet et al. 1990; Engel et al. 1990; Nelson et al. 1990).

Type I lesions have focal, irregularly outlined subchondral areas demonstrating hypointense signals on T1-weighted SE sequences and high signal intensities on long TR/TE sequences. These signal alterations are less clearly visible on GE sequences. The overlying cartilage is macroscopically intact. Those subchondral signal changes are nonspecific and may represent the initial stage of OCD, avascular necrosis, or bone marrow edema due to a bone bruise (Deutsch and Mink 1989).

In the type II lesion, areas of subchondral bone demarcated by a thin hypointense line are observed, exhibiting either normal hyperintense or hypointense signals on T1-weighted images. There are no signs of cartilage disruption. The differentiation of type II lesions from type I lesions is important since the therapeutic management changes from immobilization to surgery. MR imaging is quite helpful in this regard. The band-like, partially irregularly outlined broad zone is filled with fibrous and fibrocartilage tissue, which appears like actively formed new tissue that partially extends into the necrotic tissue. Histologically, blood-distended capillaries can be seen as well as fibrous tissue extending through the border zone into the cartilage (Bohndorf 1998). In type III lesions, a cartilage fracture and partial separation of the osteochondral fragment from the parent bone occur. In this stage, small cyst-like bone lesions may exist at the base of the lesion. Focal disruption of the overlying cartilage allows a small amount of fluid or contrast material to intrude between the nonattached part of the fragment and the subchondral bone. Progression of the process completes the demarcation of the tissue fragment beneath a thin or even edematous layer of cartilage, which not infrequently exhibits signs of degeneration. Caused by repetitive trauma or by an otherwise disturbed healing process, a zone of separation forms between the mouse bed and the OCD lesion. In this band-like area, loosely connected fibrous tissue containing many vessels, fibroblasts, and leukocytes are observed. Osteoclasts dominate toward the articular side and osteoblasts toward the osseous side. The separations in this border zone first become visible on the articular side.

Type IV lesions are characterized by complete separation of a nondisplaced osteochondral fragment from the adjacent bone with disruption of the overlying articular cartilage. On MR imaging, this is demonstrated by the contrast material or fluid penetration in the space between the fragment and the bony crater. Although surgical therapy is mandatory for all these cases, different techniques using stabilization pins, curettage of damaged cartilage, or transplantation may be necessary, depending on the size of the lesion and the status of the articular cartilage. It has been demonstrated that recognition of cartilage defects with partial (type III) or complete (type IV) separation as well as the unequivocal visualization of intact cartilage (types I and II) improve significantly after the intraarticular administration of Gd-DTPA (Kramer et al. 1992, 1995).

A type V lesion has a free intraarticular cartilaginous/osteocartilaginous fragment displaced from its donor site. The donor site demonstrates a variable appearance depending on the age of the lesion (fresh: large defect; old: smooth shallow crater).

17.2.5 Therapeutic Considerations

The management and prognosis of OCD, including planning of surgical procedures, depend to a great extent on the status of the overlying articular cartilage and the osteochondral fragments. Two important clinical features influence the prognosis of OCD lesions. Those in young patients frequently heal with protected weight-bearing, but symptomatic OCD lesions in adults rarely heal without surgical intervention. The second important feature is the size of the lesion. Lesions less than 0.2 cm^2 are more likely to heal than larger ones (De Smet et al. 1990, 1997; De Smet 1998; Mesgarzadeh et al. 1987).

Early detection of osteochondral lesions is desirable because the onset of degenerative arthritis in patients with OCD is estimated to occur about 10 years earlier than in normal individuals (Linden 1977). Patients may be entirely asymptomatic; however, pain aggravated by movement, limitation of motion, clicking, locking, and swelling may be apparent. Single or multiple sites can be affected. The precise managment of OCD is not agreed on, and the clinical manifestation, level of physical activity, as well as the specific anatomic location of the lesion and the experience and preference of the orthopedic surgeon all influence the choice of therapy. In low grade (I) OCD, conservative management may be sufficient. For stages II and III, drilling, currettage, and/or stabilization by pins is recommended. In higher stage lesions (IV, V), drilling of the base of the crater, currettage, removal of the loose body, or even osteochondral transplantation is performed. Considerable interest has developed concerning the determination of the stability of the fragment. Those fragments that are ballotable but are associated with intact overlying cartilage, sometimes referred to as loose in situ fragments, may be fixed surgically; those that are grossly loose may be removed. This has created a need for accurate noninvasive assessment of the status of the overlying articular cartilage. Early studies using MR imaging to evaluate OCD noted its value in delineating the status of the overlying cartilage (Lehner et al. 1987), and De Smet and co-workers described four MR imaging findings for predicting the stability of OCD lesions (De Smet et al. 1997; De Smet 1998). Demarcation of OCD lesions by a hyperintense linear structure as seen on proton-density and T2-weighted images has been considered a good indicator of mechanical instability of OCD lesions, although a definite explanation for this finding has not been given. It may represent fluid or granulation tissue at the base of the osteochondral fragment and suggests indirect evidence that the overlying cartilage may be weakened or even no longer intact. Similarly, the absence of a zone of high signal intensity at the interface of the fragment and the parent bone is a reliable sign of lesion stability. The presence of fluid encircling the fragment or focal cystic areas beneath the fragment are the best indicators of instability. The likelihood of fluid extending through the cartilaginous defect and into the base of the fragment depends not only on the extent of the chondral damage but also on the amount of fluid. In addition, the sensitivity of MR imaging for the detection of fluid at the interface between the fragment and the parent bone varies according to the precise methods that are employed and may be greater when volumetric acquisition and thin sections are employed. Furthermore, the differentiation of fluid and granulation tissue in this interface with MR imaging techniques may be challenging. The intravenous or intraarticular (Kramer et al. 1992; Adam et al. 1991) administration of a contrast agent has been used as a supplementary MR imaging method in the assessment of OCD. With intravenous administration, the contrast material has led to the enhancement of signal intensity in the zone between the fragment and the parent bone, which corresponds to a loose fragment and subjacent granulation tissue; the absence of such enhancement corresponded to histologic findings of a stable fragment with subjacent trabeculae and without granulation tissue. When compared to standard T1-weighted spin-echo and gradient-echo MR imaging techniques, the administration of intraarticular gadolinium contrast agent (MR arthrography) resulted in an improvement in the accurate assessment of the overlying articular cartilage. The signal intensity of the fragment itself, which usually increased on T2-weighted MR images, was not a useful indicator of the stable or unstable nature of the lesion. Bachmann et al. reported that radiographic findings corresponded with arthroscopic staging in only 56% of the patients because fibrosis may provide stability in instances of osseous sparation (Bachmann et al. 1995, 1999). However, because arthroscopy is invasive and expensive, MR imaging has become the examination of choice for noninvasively determining the stability of OCD lesions.

17.2.6 Conclusions

The etiology of OCD is most likely related to repetitive microtraumas or overuse. There is no doubt, however, that a genetic or developmental predisposition also plays a contributing though unspecified role in the development of OCD lesions. MR imaging has been proven to be of special value in the diagnostic evaluation of osteochondral lesions. If plain MR imaging does not supply the necessary information for therapeutic management, MR arthrography should be utilized. A good clinical outcome is likely in young patients, when the OCD is small, and when the lesion is stable according to MR imaging. Conversely, when a cartilage fracture or articular defect is found on MR imaging, the patient is likely to have a poor outcome.

References

Adam G, Bohndorf K, Prescher A, Krasny R, Gunther RW (1988) Der hyaline Gelenksknorpel in der MR-Tomographie des Kniegelenkes bei 1,5 T. Fortschr Geb Rontgenstr Nuklearmed Ergänzungsband 148:648–651

Adam G, Bühne M, Prescher A (1991) Stability of osteochondral fragments of the femoral condyle: magnetic resonance imaging with histhopathologic correlation in an animal model. Skeletal Radiol 20:601–606

Adam G, Neuerburg J, Peiß J, Bohndorf K, Günther WR (1994) Magnetresonanztomographie der Osteochondrosis dissecans des Kniegelenkes nach intravenöser Gadolinium-DTPA-Gabe. Fortschr Röntgenstr 160:459–464

Adleberg JS, Smith GH (1991) Corticosteroid-induced avascular necrosis of the talus. J Foot Sorg 30:66–69

Ahlbäck S, Bauer GCH, Bohne WH (1968) Spontaneous osteonecrosis of the knee. Arthritis Reheum 11:705–733

Amako T, Kawashima M, Torisu T et al (1974) Bone and joint lesions in decompression sickness. Semin Arthritis Rheum 4:151–190

Athanasiou KA, Nierderauer GG, Schenck RC Jr (1995) Biomechanical topography of human ankle cartilage. Ann Biomed Eng 23:697–704

Bachmann G., Jürgensen I, Siaplaouras J (1995) Die Stadienbestimmung der Osteochondrosis dissecans am Knie- und Sprunggelenk mit der MRT. Fortschr Röntgenstr 163:38–44

Bachmann G, Jürgensen I, Rominger M, Rau WS (1999) Die Bedeutung der Magnetresonanztomographie für die Verlaufskontrolle der Osteochondrosis dissecans am Knie- und Sprunggelenk. Fortschr Röntgenstr 171:372–379

Baron M, Paltiel H, Lander P (1984) Aseptic necrosis of the talus and calcaneal insufficiency fractures in a patient with pancreatitis, subcutaneous fat necrosis, and arthritis. Arthritis Rheum 27:1309–1313

Bauer M, Jonsson K, Linden B (1987) Osteochondritis dissecans of the ankle. J Bone Joint Surg 69B:93–96

Berquist TH, Hugh JW, Oldenburg WA (2000) Bone and soft tissue ischemia. In: Berquist TH (ed) Radiology of foot and ankle, 2nd edn. Lippincott / Williams and Wilkins, Philadelphia

Blair HC (1943) Comminuted fractures and fracture dislocations of the body of the astragalus: Operative treatment. Am J Surg 59:37–43

Bloem JL, Reiser MF, Vanel D (1990) Magnetic resonance contrast agents in the evaluation of the musculoskeletal system. Magn Reson Q 6:136–163

Bluemke DA, Zerhouni EA (1996) MRI of avascular necrosis of bone. Top Magn Reson Imaging 8:231–246

Bohndorf K (1998) Osteochondritis (osteochondrosis) dissecans: a review and new MRI classification. Eur Radiol 8:103–112

Bui-Mansfield LT, Lenchik L, Rogers LF, Chew FS, Boles CA, Kline M (2000a) Osteochondritis dissecans of the tarsal naviculare bone: imaging findings in four patients. J Comput Assist Tomogr 24:744–747

Bui-Mansfield LT, Kline M, Chew FS, Rogers LF, Lenchik L (2000b) Osteochondritis dissecans of the tibial plafond: imaging characteristics and a review of the literature. AJR: 175:1305–1308

Camasta CA, Pitts TE, Corey SV (1994) Bilateral osteochondritis dissecans of the first metatarsophalangeal joint. J Am Podiatr Med Assoc 84:297–310

Clanton TO, De Lee JC (1982) Osteochondritis dissecans: history, pathophysiology and current treatment concepts. Clin Orthop 167:50–64

Coni NK (1983) Posture and arterial pressure in the ischemic foot. Age Aging 12:151–154

Conway WF, Hayes CW, Daniel WW (1993) Bone marrow edema pattern on MR images: transient osteoporosis or early osteonecrosis of bone? In: Weissman BN (ed) Syllabus: RSNA categorial course in musculoskeletal radiology. Advanced imaging of joints: theory and practice. Radiological Society of North America, pp 341–354

Cruess RJ (1981) Steroid-induced osteonecrosis: a review. Can J Surg 24:567–571

Dall D, Macnab I (1970) Spontaneous avascular necrosis of the talus: a report of two cases. S Afr Med J 44:193–196

D'Ambrosia RJ, Riggins RS, DeNardo SJ et al (1975) Fluoride 18 scintigraphy in avascular necrotic disorders of bone. Clin Orthop 107:146–155

De Smet A (1998) Radiology of osteochondritis dissecans. In: Taveras JM, Ferrucci JT (eds) Radiology diagnosis-imaging-intervention. Lippincott-Raven, Philadelphia

De Smet AA, Fisher DR, Burstein MI, Graf BK, Lange RH (1990) Value of MR imaging in staging osteochondral lesion of the talus (osteochondritis dissecans): results in 14 patients. AJR 154:555–558

De Smet A, Ilahi O, Graf B (1997) Untreated osteochondritis dissecans of the femoral condyles: Prediction of patient outcome using radiographic and MR findings. Skeletal Radiol 26:463–467

Dennis MD, Tullos HS (1980) Blair tibiotalar arthrodesis for injuries to the talus. J Bone Joint Surg 62A:103–107

Deutsch AD, Mink JH (1989) Magnetic resonance imaging of musculoskeletal injuries. Radiol Clin North Am 27: 983–1002

Elliot DH, Harrison JAB (1970) Bone necrosis occupational hazard of diving. J R Nav Med Serv 56:140–161

Engel A, Hajek PC, Kramer J et al (1990) Magnetic resonance knee arthrography. Enhanced contrast by gadolinium complex in the rabbit and in humans. Acta Orthop Scand 61 [Suppl 240]:1–57

Ficat RP (1985) Idiopathic bone necrosis of the femoral head: early diagnosis and treatment. J Bone Joint Surg 67B:3–9

Ficat RF, Arlet J (1980) Ischemia and necrosis of bone. Williams and Wilkins, Baltimore

Freiberg AH (1914) Infraction of the second metatarsal bone; a typical injury. Surg Gynecol Obstet 19:191–197

Freiberg AH (1926) The so-called infraction of the second metatarsal bone. J Bone Joint Surg 8:257–264

Gardeniers JWM (1993) ARCO international classification of osteonecrosis. ARCO Newslett 5:79–82

Gregg PJ, Walder DN (1986) Caisson disease of bone. Clin Orthop 210:43–54

Haliburton RA, Sullivan CR, Kelly PJ et al (1958) The extraosseous and intraosseous blood supply of the talus. J Bone Joint Surg Am 40:1115–1120

Harris RD, Silver RA (1973) Atraumatic aseptic necrosis of the talus. Radiology 106:81–83

Hauzeur JP, Pasteels JL, Schoutens M, Appelboom T, Chochrad L, Perlmutter N (1989) The diagnostic value of magnetic resonance imaging in non-traumatic osteonecrosis of the femoral head. J Bone Joint Surg Am 71:641–649

Hawkins LG (1970) Fractures of the neck of the talus. J Bone Joint Surg Am 52:991–1002

Herndon JH, Aufranc OE (1972) Avascular necrosis of the femoral head in the adult: a review of its incidence in a variety of conditions. Clin Orthop 86:43–62

Hofmann S, Kramer J, Leder K, Plenk H Jr, Engel A (1994a) Die nichttraumatische Hüftkopfnekrose des Erwachsenen. Teil I. Pathophysiologie, Klinik und therapeutische Möglichkeiten. Radiologe 34:1–10 (German with English abstract)

Hofmann S, Kramer J, Plenk H Jr, Leder K, Imhof H, Engel A (1994b) MRT bei Osteonekrosen. Orthopäde 23:331–341 (German with English abstract).

Hofmann S, Kramer J, Breitenseher M, Engel A, Knahr K (1995) Early avascular necrosis of the hip: diagnostic value of clinical symptoms, radiographs, computerized tomography, scintigrams and magnetic resonance imaging, 2nd edn. Orthop Trans 19:396

Hofmann S, Fialka V, Kramer J, Leitha T, Schneider W, Engel A, Plenk H Jr (1996) The Bone Marrow Oedema Syndrome of the hip and its relationship with avascular necrosis and reflex sympathetic dystrophy. Baillieres Clin Orthop 2: 291–315

Horton MG (1997) Timins ME. MR imaging of injuries to the small joints. Radiol Clin North Am 35:671–700

Hougaard K, Thomsen PB (1986) Traumatic posterior dislocation of the hip: Prognostic factors influencing the incidence of avascular necrosis of the femoral head. Arch Orthop Traumat Surg 106:32–35

Hungerford DS, Jones LC (1993) Diagnosis of osteonecrosis of the femoral head. In: Schoutens A, Arlet J, Gardeniers JWM, Hughes SPF (eds) Bone circulation and vascularization in normal and pathological conditions. Plenum, New York, pp 265–275

Hungerford DS, Zizic TM (1978) Alcoholism associated ischemic necrosis of the femoral head: Early diagnosis and treatment. Clin Orthop 130:144–153

Imhof H, Breitenseher M, Trattnig S, Kramer J, Hoffmann S, Plenk H, Schneider W, Engel A (1997) Imaging of avascular necrosis of bone. Eur Radiol 7:180–186

Jacobs MA, Loeb PE, Hungerford DS (1989) Core decompression of the distal femur for avascular necrosis of the knee. J Bone Surg 71B:583–587

Jones JP Jr (1993) Nontraumatic osteonecrosis of the talus. ARCO News 5:92

Jones JP Jr (1994) Concepts of etiology and early pathogenesis of osteonecrosis. In: Schafer M (ed) Instructional course lectures 43. American Academy of Orthopaedic Surgeons, Rosemont, IL, pp 499–512

König F (1888) Über frei Körper in den Gelenken. Dtsch Z Chir 27:90

Köhler A (1908) Über eine häufige bisher anscheinend unbekannte Erkrankung einzelner kindlicher Knochen. Munch Med Wochenschr 55:1923

Kopecky KK, Braunstein EM, Brandt KD, Filo RS, Leapman SB, Capello WN, Klatte EC (1991) Apparent avascular necrosis of the hip: appearance and spontaneous resolution of MR findings in renal allograft recipients. Radiology 179: 523–527

Kramer J, Stiglbauer R, Engel A, Prayer L, Imhof H (1992) MR Contrast Arthrography (MRA) in osteochondrosis dissecans. J Comput Assist Tomogr 16(2):254–260

Kramer J, Hofmann S, Imhof H (1994) Die nichttraumatische Hüftkopfnekrose des Erwachsenen, Teil II. Radiologische Diagnostik and Stadieneinteilung. Radiologe 34:11–20

Kramer J, Scheurecker A, Mohr E (1995) Osteochondrale Läsion. Radiologe 35:109–116

Kruczynski J (1996) Avascular necrosis of the proximal femur in developmental dislocation of the hip: incidence, risk factors, sequelae and MR imaging for diagnosis and prognosis. Acta Orthop Scand 268 [Suppl]:1–48

Lang P, Mauz M, Schörner W et al (1993) Acute fracture of the femoral neck: assessment of femoral head perfusion with gadopentetate dimeglumine-enhanced MR imaging. AJR 160:335–341

Langer F, Percy EC (1971) Osteochondritis dissecans and anomalous centres of ossification: a review of 80 lesions in 61 patients. Can J Surg 14:208–215

Langevitz P, Buskila D, Stewart J et al (1990) Ostenecrosis in patients receiving dialysis: report of two cases and review of the literature. J Rheumatol 17:402–406

Lecouvet FE, VandeBerg BC, Maldaque BE, Lebon CJ, Jamart J, Saleh M, Nöel H, Malgehim J (1998) Early irreversible osteonecrosis versus transient lesions of the femoral condyles. Prognostic value of subchondral bone and marrow changes on MR imaging. AJR Am J Roentgenol 170:71–77

Lehner K, Heuck A, Rodhammer G et al (1987) MRI bei der Osteochondrosis dissecans. ROFO 147:191–195

Linden B (1977) Osteochondritis dissecans of the femoral condyles. A long-term-up study. J Bone Joint Surg [Am] 59:769–776

Magid D, Fishman EK, Scott WW, Brooker AF, Arnold WP, Lennox DW, Siegelman SS (1985) Femoral head avascular necrosis: CT assessement with multiplanar reconstruction. Radiology 157:751–756

Magee TH, Hinson GW (1998) Usefulness of MR imaging in the detection of talar dome injuries. AJR 170:1227–1230

Mankin HJ (1992) Nontraumatic necrosis of bone (osteonecrosis). N Engl J Med 326:1473–1479

Mesgarzadeh M, Sapega AA, Bonakdarpour A et al (1987) Osteochondrosis dissecans: analysis of mechanical stability with radiography, scintigraphy and MR imaging. Radiology 165:775–780

Mindell ER, Cisek EE, Kartalian G et al (1963) Late results of injuries to the talus: analysis of forty cases. J Bone Joint Surg 45A:221–245

Miskew DB, Goldflies ML (1980) Atraumatic avascular necrosis of the talus associated with hyperuricemia. Clin Orthop 148:156–159

Mitchell DG, Steinberg ME, Dalinka MK, Rao VM, Fallon M, Kressel HY (1989) Magnetic resonance imaging of the ischemic hip: alterations within the osteonecrotic, viable and reactive zones. Clin Orthop 244:60–77

Mont MA, Hungerford DS (1995) Current concepts review: non traumatic avascular necrosis of the femoral head. J Bone Joint Surg 77A:459–474

Mont MA, Maar DC, Urquhart MW et al (1993) Avascular necrosis of the humeral head treated by core decompression: a retrospective review. J Bone Joint Surg 75B:785–788

Mont MA, Hungerford DS, Mohan V et al (1996) Abstract: demographic characterization of avascular necrosis of the proximal humerus. ARCO Trans 8:103

Morris HD (1974) Aseptic necrosis of the talus following injury. Orthop Clin North Am 5:177–189

Morscher E (1971) Cartilage-bone lesions of the knee joint following injury. Reconstr Surg Traumatol 12:2–26

Nelson DW, Di Paola J, Colville M, Schmidgall J (1990) Osteochondritis dissecans of the talus and knee: prospective comparsion of MR and arthroscopic classifications. J Comput Assist Tomogr 14:804–808

Nishimura G, Yamato M, Togawa M (1996) Trabecular trauma of the talus and medial malleolus concurrent with lateral collateral ligamentous injuries of the ankle: evaluation with MR imaging. Skeletal Radiol 25:49–54

Paget J (1870) On the production of some of the loose bodies in joints. S Barthol Hosp Rep 6:1

Peterson L, Goldie IF (1975) The arterial supply of the talus. A study on the relationship of experimental talar fractures. Acta Orthop Scand 46:1026–1034

Resnick D, Niwayama G (eds) (1995) Diagnosis of bone and joint disorders. Saunders, Philadelphia

Rutishauser E, Rohner A, Held D (1960) Experimentelle Untersuchungen über die Wirkung der Ischämie auf den Knochen und das Mark. Virchows Arch Pathol Anat 333: 101–118

Schoenberg NY, Lehmann WB (1994) Magnetic resonance imaging of pediatric disorders of the ankle and foot. Magn Reson Imaging Clin North Am 2:109–122

Steinberg ME, Hayken GD, Steinberg DR (1995) A quantitative system for staging avascular necrosis. J Bone Joint Surg 77B:34–41

Stulberg BN, Levine M, Bauer TW, Belhobek GH, Pflanze W, Feiglin DH, Roth AI (1989) Multimodality approach to osteonecrosis of the femoral head. Clin Orthop 268: 181–193

Sweet DE, Madewell JE (1995) Osteonecrosis. Pathogenesis. In: Resnick D, Niwayama G (eds) Diagnosis of bone and joint disorders, vol 5, 3rd edn. Sanders, Philadelphia, pp 3445–3494

Tegetmeyer CJ, Spinosa DJ, Matsumoto AH (1997) Angiography of bones, joints, and soft tissues. In: Baum S (ed) Abrams´ angiographiy. Little Brown, New York, pp 1179–1821

Tyrrell RL, Gluckert K, Pathria M, Modic MT (1988) Fast threedimensional MR imaging of the knee: comparison with arthroscopy. Radiology 166:865–872

Urquart MW, Mont MA, Michelson JD et al (1996) Osteonecrosis of the talus: treatment by hindfoot fusion. Foot Ankle Int 17:275–282

Vahlensieck M, Peterfy CG, Wischer T, Sommer T, Lang P, Schlippert U, Genant HK, Schild HH (1996) Indirect MR arthrography: optimization and clinical applications. RSNA 200:249–254

Vahlensieck M, Sommer T, Textor J, Pauleit D, Lang P, Genant HK, Schild HH (1998) Indirect MR arthrography: techniques and applications. Eur Radiol 8:232–235

Vande Berg BC, Malghem J, Labaisse MA et al (1992) Avascular necrosis of the hip: comparison of contrast enhanced and nonenhanced MR imaging with histologic correlation. Radiology 182:445–450

Winalski CS, Weissmabb BS, Aliabadi P et al (1991) Intravenous Gd-DTPA enhancement joint fluid: a less invasive alternative for MR arthrography. Radiology 181 (suppl 1):304

Yulish BS, Mulopulus GP, Goodfellow DB, Bryan PJ, Modic MT, Dollinger BM (1987) MR imaging of osteochondral lesions of the talus. J Comput Assist Tomogr 11:296–301

18 Acquired Deformities of the Foot and Ankle

E. G. McNally and G. Lavis

CONTENTS

This chapter will consider soft-tissue and structural foot and ankle deformity. Whilst the most common causes by far are trauma and degenerative joint disease, these topics will be dealt with elsewhere. For convenience and in an effort to apply a systematic approach, the subject will be divided into hindfoot, midfoot and forefoot (Table 18.1). It should be emphasised that many foot and ankle conditions do inter-relate and should not be thought of in isolation when treatment strategies are being planned.

While some of the conditions may not be thought of as pure deformities, those that may present with either a clinical or radiographic deformity will be considered in this review. Ultrastructural deformity and entities regarded as variations of normal will not be considered.

18.1 Hindfoot

18.1.1 Achilles Tendinopathy

Tendon injuries of the foot and ankle are the most common of all injuries, 20% of which affect the Achilles tendon (Lipscomb and Kelly 1955). Aside from traumatic partial or complete rupture, which

Table 1. Systematic approach to structural foot and ankle deformities

Hindfoot	Focal Achilles tendinopathy
	Haglund syndrome
	Bursitis
	Anterior impingement
	Posterior impingement
	Bony spurs
	Hindfoot varus and valgus
Midfoot	Tibialis posterior tendon dysfunction
	Neuropathic osteoarthropathy
Forefoot	Hallux valgus
	Hallus rigidus
	Hammertoe
	Bunionette deformity (Tailor's bunion)
	Frieberg's infraction
	Sesamoiditis

E.G. McNally, FRCR FRCPI
Consultant Musculoskeletal Radiologist, Department of Radiology, Nuffield Orthopaedic Centre, Windmill Lane, Oxford OX3 7LD, UK
G. Lavis, BSc (Hons) FpodA FChS
Associate Specialist Podiatrist, Nuffield Orthopaedic Centre, Windmill Lane, Oxford OX3 7LD, UK

will not be dealt with here, disorders of the Achilles tendon include acute and chronic paratenonitis, paratenonitis with tendinosis, tendinosis and tendinitis. This terminology follows the histopathologic classification developed by Puddu et al. (1976) and, when correlated with the clinical presentation, can be helpful when applying a treatment strategy. In many cases of chronic tendinopathy, it is the combination of pain and a focal lump that leads the patient to seek medical attention.

Achilles tendinitis is an overuse syndrome. Three types are recognised: proximal, distal and insertional.

18.1.1.1 Proximal Achilles Tendinopathy

The most common area of the tendon affected is approximately 5 cm proximal to its insertion into the os calcis. This corresponds to the relatively avascular zone which extends from 2 to 6 cm proximal to the insertion (Haglund 1928). It is more common among runners (Deutsch et al. 1997) (professional and recreational) and is reported to have a male to female ratio of 2:1. Increased and repetitive stress applied to this area as generated in athletic activity is thought to initiate microtears and subsequent inflammatory changes. Excessive foot pronation during the running cycle has been proposed as a contributory factor in Achilles tendinitis in the athlete (Lundberg et al. 1989). Abnormal rotational force on the tendon occurs when internal tibial rotation during foot pronation is followed by external tibial rotation during foot supination to a greater level of excursion than normal. Other features include a lowered medial arch and valgus on weight-bearing. Video studies will confirm the excessive rear foot frontal (coronal) plane motion and torque of the tendon.

The diagnosis of Achilles tendinopathy is made on the basis of the patient's history and clinical examination findings. Imaging techniques are very helpful to confirm and ascertain the extent and degree of pathology. The most commonly used techniques are ultrasound and MR imaging (Jacobson 1999; Schweitzer and Karasick 1994).

18.1.1.1.1 Ultrasound

The superficial position of the Achilles tendon makes it easily amenable to ultrasound examination. The normal appearances are typical of tendons elsewhere, with a combination of linear speckles of increased reflectivity on a low reflective background (Bertolotto et al. 1995). The tendon is fairly uniform in both longitudinal and transverse diameters from origin to insertion (Fig. 18.1). The ultrasound findings in chronic tendinopathy include a focal or diffuse thickening with overall decrease in reflectivity (Kainberger et al. 1996) (Fig. 18.2). It is uncommon to see fluid surrounding the tendon due to the absence of a sheath. Reflective tissue and blurring of the tendon margin can be seen when there is associated paratenonitis. In our experience, these areas tend to be acutely tender on palpation with the probe.

18.1.1.1.2 Magnetic Resonance Imaging

MR imaging of the Achilles tendon is best carried out using the sagittal and axial planes. Sagittal T1-weighted and STIR or T2 with fat suppression are optimal. Chronic tendinopathy is seen as a diffuse swelling within the tendon with or without intrasubstance signal changes (Fig. 18.3). As with ultrasound, fluid surrounding the tendon is rare, but inflammatory changes are commonly identified within the pre-Achilles fat, though this is more common in patients with distal tendinopathy as described below.

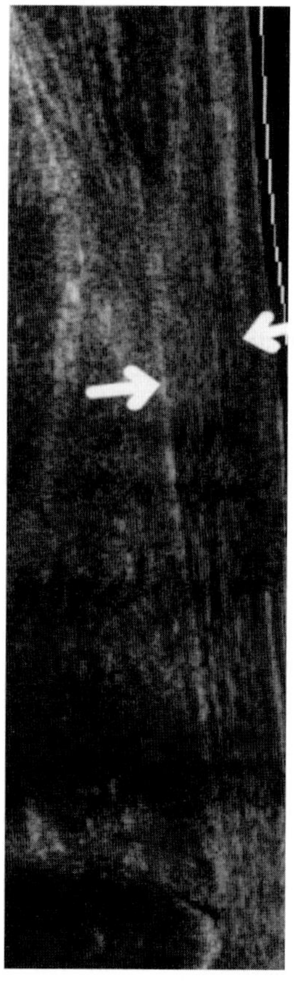

Fig. 18.1. Composite of Achilles tendon from origin to insertion in the sagittal plane. The *arrows* outline the anterior and posterior margins of the paratenon

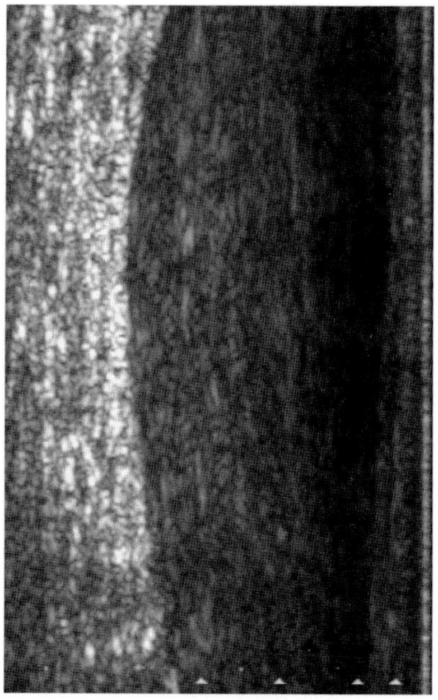

Fig. 18.2. Grossly swollen and hyporeflective tendon in Achilles tendinopathy. Compare with Fig. 18.1

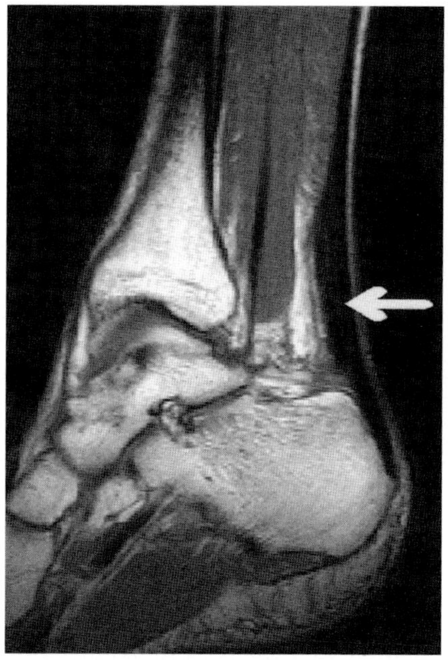

Fig. 18.3. Sagittal T1-weighted MR image showing mild swelling of the Achilles tendon with intrasubstance linear abnormal signal (*arrow*) indicating tendinopathy

18.1.1.1.3
Treatment

Where a biomechanical deformity is an aetiological factor, functional orthoses should be prescribed. In cases of refractory paratenonitis where tendon pathology per se can be excluded, injection of saline or local anaesthetic as a form of adhesiotomy may be appropriate and can be carried out under image control. Corticosteroid injections should be avoided in cases when the tendon is abnormal. Surgical debridement has been advocated in resistant cases where tendon disease is confirmed, but the results are variable.

18.1.1.2
Distal Achilles Tendinopathy, Haglund Syndrome and Bursitis

An excessive prominence of the bursal projection in the posterosuperior aspect of the calcaneus constitutes Haglund's deformity. Swelling in this area constitutes Haglund's disease and is associated with retrocalcaneal bursitis. Synonyms for this condition include winter heel and pump bump syndromes.

Haglund's syndrome is more commonly seen in the younger population (under 30 years old) and is more prevalent in women. Rigid and prominent heel counters with high heels impinge on the soft tissues overlying the prominence and give rise to symptoms of pain and swelling. In more advanced cases, the overlying skin ulcerates due to friction from footwear. Heel varus is often seen and may also be a predisposing factor in the aetiology.

Radiography in Haglund's syndrome may demonstrate a retrocalcaneal prominence first described by Haglund (1928). Large bony projections are easy to appreciate. Smaller lesions can be detected by demonstrating a superior calcaneal angle of more than 75 deg or excessive bone above the upper parallel pitch line (Fowler 1945; Stephens 1994). Lateral radiographs may not adequately assess the lateral portion of the prominence. These findings can also be appreciated on MR imaging.

Another feature of lower third achilles tendinopathy is inflammation of the anatomical bursa found between the calcaneus and the Achilles tendon. As a primary condition, Achilles bursitis is more frequently seen in the older age group and more sedentary patient population. Clinically, it presents as tenderness anterior to the tendon on lateral compression, and occasionally, a fluctuant, sometimes visible swelling may be observed either side of the tendon. Pain is often exacerbated on dorsiflexion of the ankle.

In patients with bursitis, infiltrative changes within the pre-Achilles fat triangle may be depicted on plain radiographs (Fig. 18.4). Occasionally, erosive changes are also noted, and a differential diagnosis

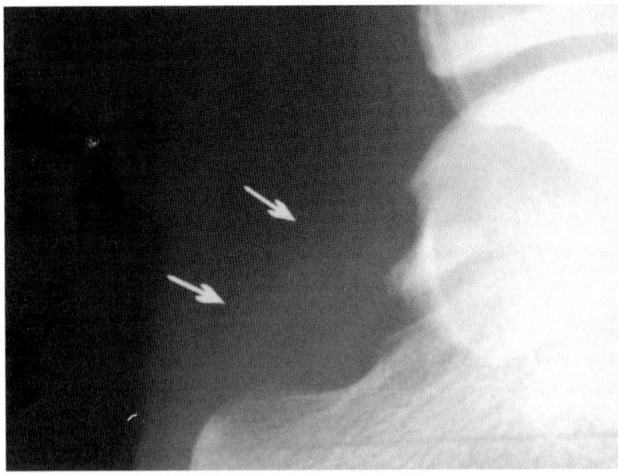

Fig. 18.4. Lateral radiograph showing soft-tissue swelling in the inferior portion of Kager's fat triangle (*arrows*). Although non-specific, bursitis is a common cause of this finding

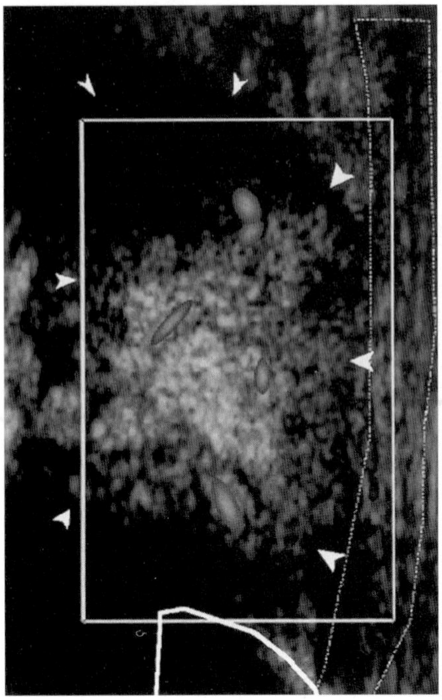

Fig. 18.5. Heterogeneous soft-tissue mass representing a distended pre-Achilles bursa (*arrowheads*). Sagittal US with *dotted lines* outlining the lower Achilles tendon and the *solid line* outlining the upper margin of the os calcis

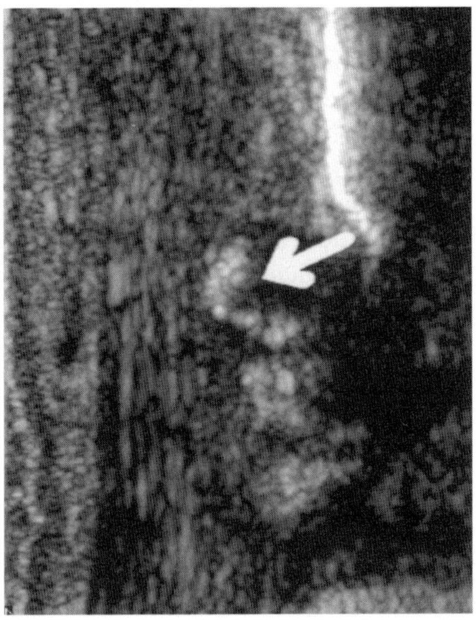

Fig. 18.6. US lobular calcification evident within the distended bursa (*arrow*)

from the arthropathies may need to be considered. Ultrasound can depict disruption of the normal fat with an increase in fluid and vessels. Increased fluid can also be demonstrated within the bursa. Occasionally, the degree of synovitis present can mimic a soft-tissue mass (Fig. 18.5). Calcification can also be demonstrated in the chronic forms (Fig. 18.6). Fat-suppressed MR sequences are sensitive to the increased fluid and surrounding oedema that occurs in bursitis (Böttger et al. 1998) (Fig. 18.7).

The treatment is similar to pre-Achilles bursitis, with conservative management employed wherever possible. In cases where heel varus is thought to be a contributing factor, an in-shoe orthosis may be appropriate to control excessive hindfoot pronation. Other measures include local protection of the retrocalcaneal tissues, heel raises, and footwear modification or change of style. Aspiration and injection of corticosteroid can be considered for some cases, and in our experience this is best achieved under image control. Surgical options are resection of the enlarged posterior tuberosity or calcaneal osteotomy (Stephens 1994; Iz 1939). The results of surgery are varied, however (Nesse and Finsen 1994; Torg and Torg 1987).

18.1.1.3
Insertional Achilles Tendonitis

Patients with this condition present with pain fairly well localised to the retrocalcaneal area and more central and distal than in Haglund's or retrocalcaneal bursitis. It is aggravated by ankle movement and again more common in recreational athletes. Pain is initiated on exercise, especially running on flat, hard surfaces.

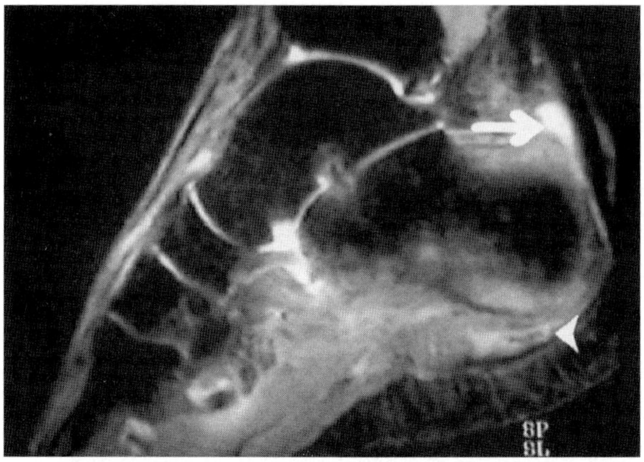

Fig. 18.7. Sagittal fat-suppressed (STIR) image of the hindfoot. The *arrow* depicts distension of the pre-Achilles bursa with fluid. The Achilles tendon is normal, but there is inflammation at the origin of the plantar fascia (*arrowhead*). There is a margin of marrow oedema around the periphery of the os calcis. The patient has Reiter's syndrome

Investigation with plain radiographs will often demonstrate areas of ossification at the insertion of the tendon. This is seen as a spur on lateral projection, but as with plantar heel 'spurs', it should be remembered that this represents a shelf of bone extending the width of the calcaneus. Ultrasound/ MRI will identify any degenerative changes in the tendon. Indeed, insertional Achilles tendinitis has been proposed as an example of paratenonitis with tendinosis by Clancy et al. (1997).

Conservative management is similar to that for other causes of posterior heel pain, i.e. physiotherapy, orthotics, night splints, and to settle acute symptoms a short period of immobilisation may be considered. Corticosteroid use is controversial, but care should be particularly taken in patients with established tendon disease and certainly should not be directly injected into the tendon. Surgery for unresponsive cases is also controversial.

Other conditions which mimic Achilles tendinopathy and bursitis include plantar fasciitis, posterior impingement syndrome and flexor tendinopathy. These diseases are dealt with elsewhere.

18.1.2 Focal Hindfoot Deformities on Plain Radiographs

There are several conditions that may present with hindfoot pain that have a radiologically evident but not clinical deformity. They include the ankle impingement syndromes (anterior, posterior and posterolateral), calcaneal spurs and fasciitis.

18.1.2.1 Posterior Impingement Syndrome

Posterior impingement syndrome is synonymous with the os trigonum or talar compression syndromes. The os trigonum is a secondary centre of ossification connected to the posterior aspect of the talus. Ossification occurs at 7–13 years, forming the Stieda process. In up to 14% of the population, fusion does not occur, and a separate ossicle remains, forming a synchondrosis with the talus (Digiovanni 1997). On plain films this can be misinterpreted as an old talar fracture in the adult foot. Symptoms may be due either to disruption of the synchondrosis, fracture of the Stieda process (Shepherd's fracture) or soft-tissue impingement.

Clinically, this cause of posterior ankle pain can be difficult to differentiate from Achilles tendinitis, flexor hallucis longus tendinitis and pre-Achilles bursitis. Indeed, some authors believe that these conditions can co-exist and may be part of the syndrome (Karasick and Schweitzer 1996; Grogan et al. 1990). Patients are often young and athletic. It is especially common in professional dancers, both ballet and modern (Wakeley et al. 1996), and may be more common when there is an associated soleus tertius (Bellemans et al. 1993). A history of a recent inversion injury is also a common feature. Posterior swelling and pain which is exacerbated by plantarfexion of the ankle are characteristic (Hendrick and McBryde 1994).

Radiographs are not sufficient to make the diagnosis as they can only demonstrate the presence of an os and not the surrounding inflammation. T1-weighted MR imaging is helpful as it clearly shows the loss of normal bright marrow signal (Karasick and Schweitzer 1996; Wakeley et al. 1996) (Fig. 18.8). Ultrasound has been used by the author, but can only demonstrate the surrounding inflammatory changes and on occasion the associated flexor hallucis tendinopathy. It is less effective at demonstrating the associated bony oedema. A normal bone scan also excludes the diagnosis.

Conservative treatment is successful in the majority of cases. Injection of the symptomatic synchondrosis under image guidance followed by 2–4 weeks of immobilisation is helpful in refractory cases.

18.1.2.2 Anterior Impingement Syndrome

True anterior impingement as opposed to anterolateral impingement (see below) is most commonly due

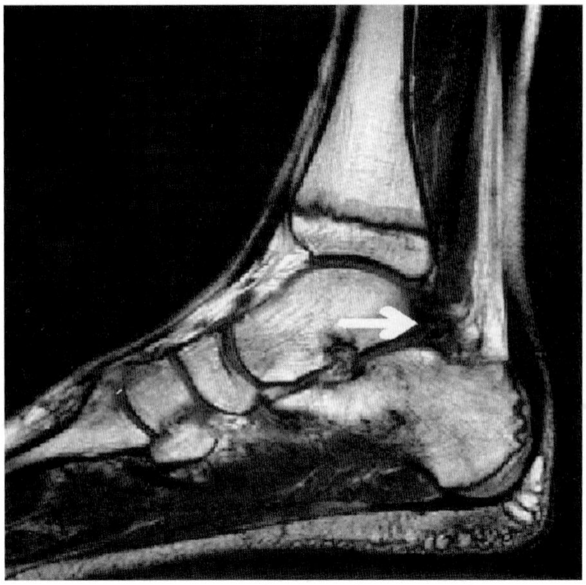

Fig. 18.8. Sagittal T1-weighted image of the hindfoot in a patient with an os trigonum (*arrow*). There is loss of the normal bright marrow signal indicating marrow oedema in the os trigonum syndrome

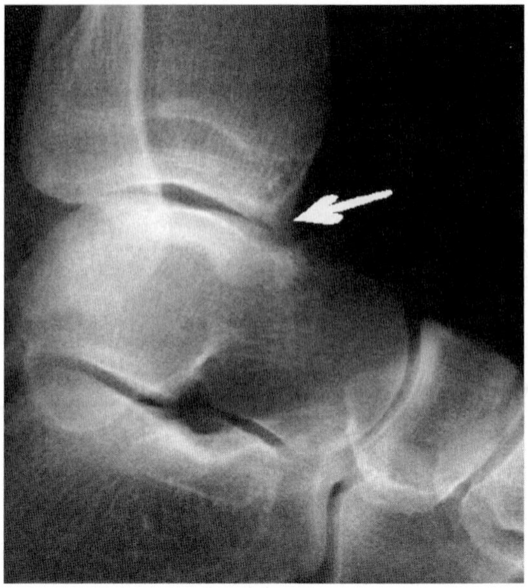

Fig. 18.9. Anterior impingement syndrome with anterior tibial osteophyte (*arrow*)

to bony impaction of an anterior tibial osteophyte against the talus. The pathogenesis of these bony outgrowths is not clear. Chronic traction on the anterior capsule has been proposed (Parkes et al. 1980), but not everyone agrees with this theory. The spurs are often accompanied by synovial hypertrophy, which can either augment a bony impingement or, in rarer cases, be the sole cause itself.

Patients complain of activity-related pain exacerbated by ankle dorsiflexion. If pain is only elicited on active ankle movement, extensor tendinopathy should also be considered in the differential diagnosis. When the impingement is of bony origin, there will be a block to ankle dorsiflexion to less than the normal of approximately 20 deg in excess of neutral. Interestingly, this group of patients often has posterior ankle symptoms in addition to localised anterior joint margin pain. This is probably due to a compensatory 'hinge opening' effect applying tensile stress to the Achilles tendon and other posterior soft tissues.

Plain radiographs are usually sufficient to confirm the diagnosis of bony anterior ankle impingement (Fig. 18.9). The angle between the bevel of the tibia and the talar neck should be more than 60 deg on a neutral film. Positional variations during routine radiography can render the interpretation difficult. In advanced cases, the tibia and talus demonstrate 'kissing' osteophytes on lateral projection. The aptly termed 'divot sign' is also occasionally seen when the tibial osteophyte has impacted into the talus (Ferkel and Fasulo 1994). MRI should be considered when plain films are normal but soft-tissue impingement is suspected (Fig. 18.10), although one study comparing clinical and MRI results demonstrated a majority of negative findings in symptomatic patients (Liu and Mirzayan 1993). The definitive diagnosis may require arthroscopy.

Where impingement is due to osteophyte development, removal by arthroscopic technique is advocated (Ogilvie Harris et al. 1993; Reynaert et al. 1994). As with any cheilectomy, where there are degenerative joint changes, increasing the range of movement may exacerbate symptoms.

18.1.2.3 Anterolateral Impingement Syndrome

Anterolateral impingement is also discussed briefly here for completeness, although it is rare for this poorly understood entity to present as either a focal clinical or radiological deformity. The impingement refers to an inflammatory mass in the anterolateral gutter that is thought to follow chronic anterior talofibular ligament sprain and has been well documented by Ferkel et al. (1991). The term 'meniscoid' lesion or Ferkel's phenomenon of the ankle has been used for this syndrome, although the occurrence of a true meniscoid lesion in this condition is rare. Anterolateral impingement commonly appears following severe ankle sprains. The patient presents

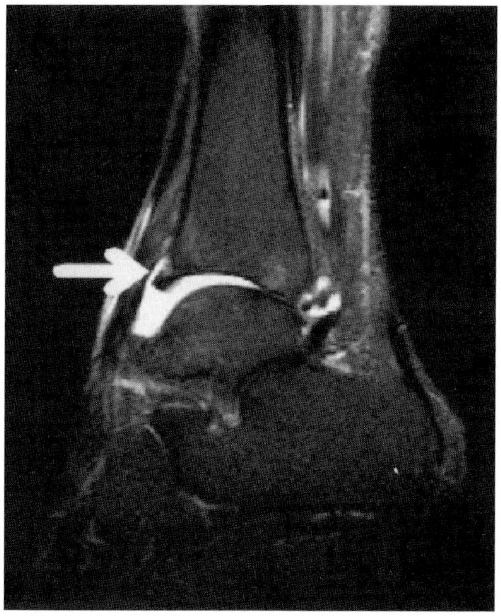

Fig. 18.10. Sagittal STIR image of anterior osteophyte (*arrow*) with thickening of the anterior capsule

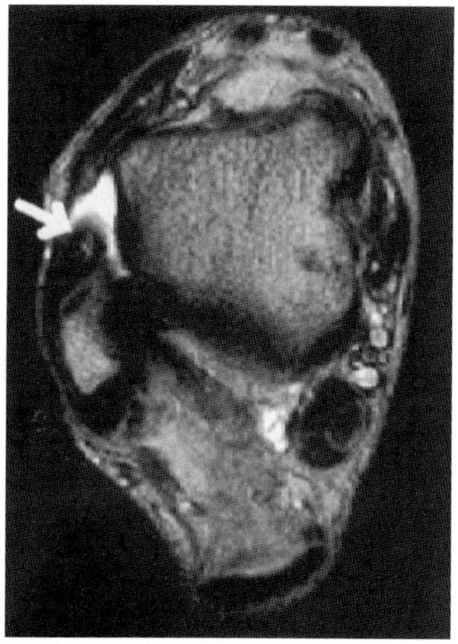

Fig. 18.11. Axial T2-weighted image of a tear of the anterior-talofibular ligament (*arrow*)

with pain on weight-bearing inferior to the tip of the fibula. The foot is often seen to be excessively pronated with a degree of hindfoot valgus. It is therefore also seen as a sequel of posterior tibial tendon dysfunction (see below). Compression of the lateral soft tissues in the lateral gutter produces synovitis and fibrosis. Lateral talar dome chondral defects are often seen at arthroscopy in severe cases.

Imaging is also an important differential diagnostic aid and will help to exclude other causes of lateral ankle pain such as sinus tarsi syndrome and peroneal pathology. Findings include absence, thickening or poor definition of the anterior talofibular ligament, indicative of a tear (Fig. 18.11). High signal inflammatory material may be noted in the gutter on plain MRI (Fig. 18.12). Sensitivity and specificity are improved when MR arthrography is used.

Treatment with conservative methods as for anterior impingement may require supplementation with synovectomy and debridement, which can be managed arthroscopically in the majority of cases (Liu et al. 1997).

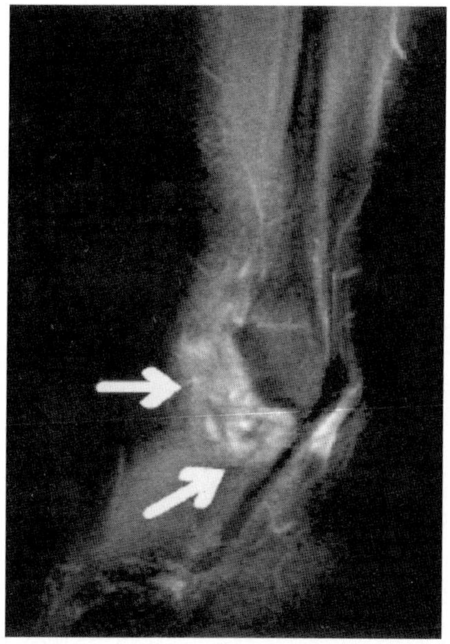

Fig. 18.12. Sagittal STIR image with poorly defined inflammatory mass anterior to fibula (*arrows*), within anterolateral gutter

18.1.3 Calcaneal Spurs

Bony spurs arising from either the dorsal or plantar surfaces of the os calcis are present in approximately 16% of the caucasian population. Plantar spurs are more common than dorsal spurs, and overall the prevalence increases with age. There is a female predominance of plantar spurs and a male predominance of dorsal spurs, which are overall slightly less common (Riepert et al. 1995).

Although spurs are present in up to 50% of patients with plantar fasciitis, the finding is nonspecific, and other diagnoses such as insertional tendinopathy need to be considered. Overall, only 10% of plantar spurs are thought to account for the symptoms (Rubin and Witton 1963). Functional ankle equinus has, however, been significantly correlated in athletes with plantar fasciitis (Berkowitz et al. 1991).

The plantar fascia is most commonly inflamed at its proximal portion. A male:female ratio of 2:1 is observed, and there is an average age of onset of 45 years. There are three bands to the plantar fascia. The central component arises from the medial calcaneal tuberosity, extending distally to insert into the five proximal phalanges. It is thicker than the medial and lateral bands, with an average of 3–4 mm at the calcaneal insertion.

Patients with plantar fasciitis present with pain which is typically worse in the morning and gradually improves as the day progresses. The location of the pain corresponds to the site of insertion of the plantar fascia into the medial tuberosity. Pain is often exacerbated when the plantar fascia is put under tension by dorsiflexion of the ankle.

The principal imaging finding in plantar fasciitis is an increase in thickness. Normal fascia measures approximately 4 mm. This can increase to an average of 7.5 mm (Berkowitz et al. 1991) with fasciitis. Ultrasound is useful in assessing the plantar fascia. The normal fascia is thin and reflective or bright (Fig. 18.13a), whereas the inflamed plantar fascia is swollen and dark (Fig. 18.13b). Features on MRI include increased signal on T2-weighted or fat-suppressed images (Fig. 18.14). Increased signal can also be seen in the os calcis at the fascial attachment and in the perifascial soft tissues.

Conservative treatment consists of physiotherapy with emphasis on calf muscle stretches and anti-inflammatory modalities, shock attenuating heel cups or custom-made in-shoe orthoses to support and reduce tension in the fascia. Strehle et al., however, did not demonstrate a significant difference between the use of customised orthoses and 'off-the-shelf' heel cups when these were incorporated into a regime of stretching exercises (Strehle 1997). The use of night splints was also reported to be beneficial in one study with a small cohort. Amelioration of an acute episode is probably the best indication for steroid injections. In 90% of patients, conservative treatment is successful (Gill and Kiebzak 1996). Surgical release of the plantar fascia, either open or endoscopically, has its protagonists, but it must be emphasised that partial or complete release of the plantar fascia can compromise the foot architecture and produce a degree of flat foot. This is reported to be a less common complication with endoscopic techniques (Harris 2000).

Treatment is directed at the underlying condition if present, for example injection of plantar fasciitis, or associated systemic condition. Surgical removal of a plantar heel spur is never indicated, although it can be difficult to convince patients that its presence is not the cause of their pain and its removal will not provide a cure.

a

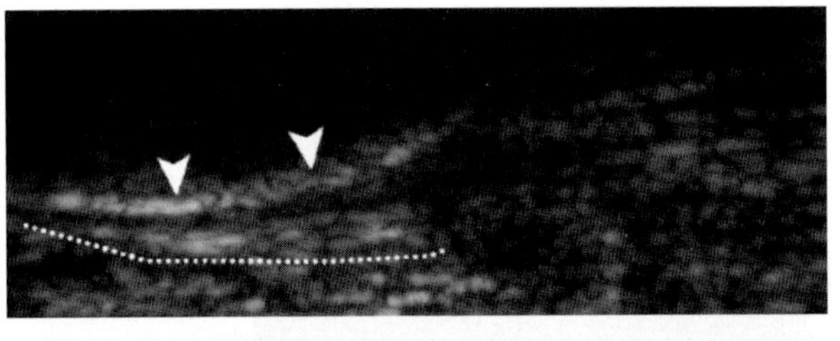

b

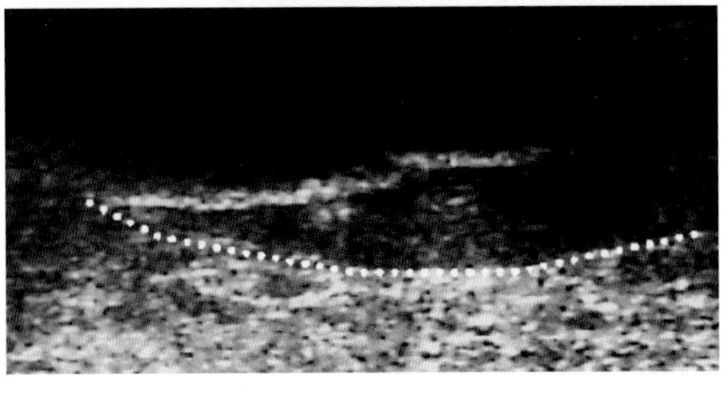

Fig. 18.13a. Sagittal US of the origin of the plantar fascia. The reflective margin of the os calcis is easily seen (*arrowheads*) and the normal bright fascia demarcated (*dotted line*). **b** Thickened and poorly reflective inflamed plantar fascia demarcated with *dotted line*

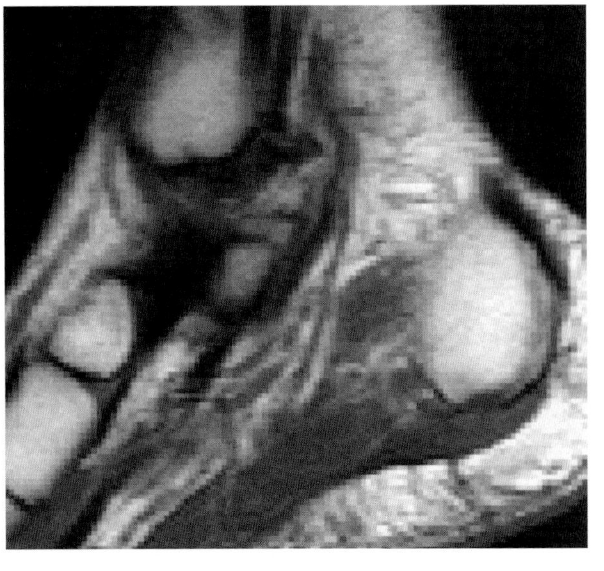

Fig. 18.14. Sagittal T1-weighted image. There is thickening and increased signal in the plantar fascia

18.1.4 Hindfoot Deformities

18.1.4.1 Hindfoot Varus

Structural deformity of the hindfoot may be the consequence of tibial, ankle, subtalar or calcaneal deformity. Hindfoot varus itself is usually a component of conditions such as talipes equino varus.

Plain radiographs are usually sufficient to assess the site and degree of the deformity. Specialist posterior hindfoot views such as the Cobey are therefore invaluable (Fig. 18.15). Stress views are necessary to detect more subtle deformities. Stress views or fluoroscopy under anaesthesia is also helpful in demonstrating instability.

18.1.4.2 Hindfoot Valgus

This deformity is common in the hyperpronated or flat foot. Minor degrees can be detected in normal individuals. Normality can be confirmed clinically by active restoration to neutral or varus when the patient stands on tiptoe. It is usually asymptomatic.

Plain films demonstrate hindfoot valgus adequately and, if part of the hyperpronated foot syndrome, will also show typical angular changes (see section on Tibialis Posterior Insufficiency). Underlying causes should be excluded, specifically osseous or non-osseous coalition. As these are congenital in aetiology, they are considered in more detail elsewhere. Degenerative arthritis, especially of the subtalar joints, can be either the cause or the consequence of hindfoot valgus. Plain films are usually sufficient to detect and classify OA if present, but MRI or spiral CT can provide a more comprehensive evaluation.

18.1.4.3 Hindfoot Equinus

As with the above hindfoot conditions, excessive plantar declination of the calcaneus in the sagittal plane (Fig. 18.16) is not usually seen as an isolated feature. It is characteristic of acquired flatfoot, vertical talus and talipes calcaneo valgus. Ankle equinus in which there is less than 10 deg of dorsiflexion is often an acquired deformity and can have soft-tissue or bony causes. Degenerative changes in particular can be associated with large anterior tibial and talar osteophytes. These effectively cause a bony block to dorsiflexion. Arthroscopic removal of these is a treatment option. Soft-tissue restriction of ankle dorsiflexion is a functional condition due to contracture or accommodative shortening of the posterior calf muscles rather than a true deformity.

18.1.4.4 Hindfoot Calcaneus

An increase in the calcaneal inclination angle above 20 deg as seen on lateral weight-bearing radiographs defines this deformity (Fig. 18.17). As in most hind-

a b

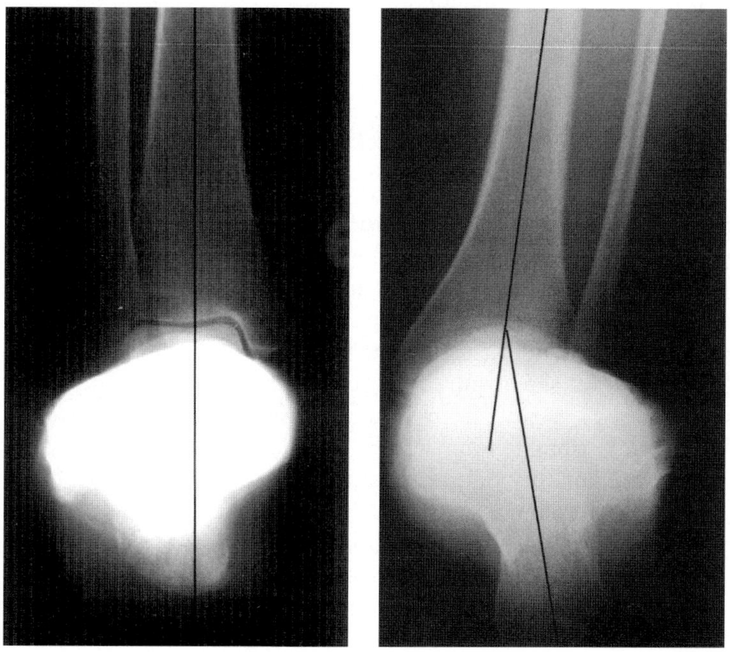

Fig. 18.15a,b. COBEY view with normal alignment between the tibia and calcaneum (**a**) and valgus hindfoot malalignment (**b**)

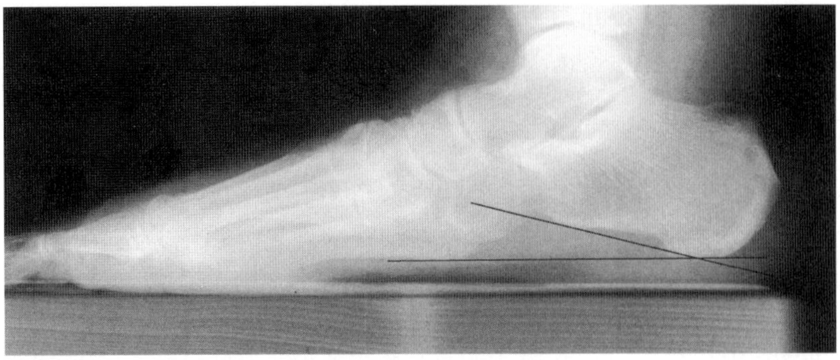

Fig. 18.16. Calcaneus hindfoot with calcaneal inclination angle less than 10 deg

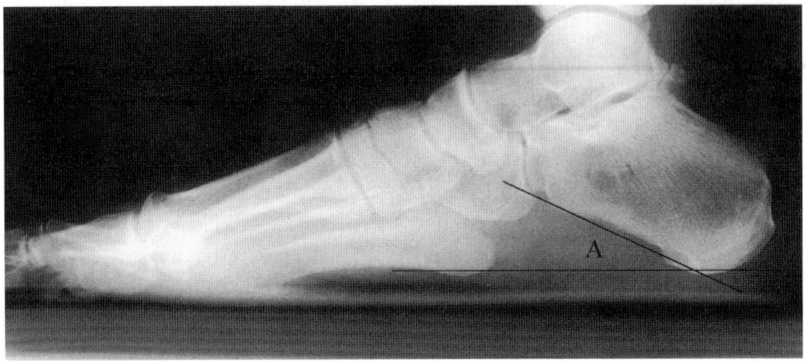

Fig. 18.17. Equinus hindfoot with increased calcaneal inclination angle (*A*)

foot deformities, it is usually seen in isolation. Hindfoot calcaneus is typically a feature of pes cavus.

18.2 Midfoot Deformities

The midfoot is generally regarded as that portion lying between the Chopart (calcaneocuboid and talonavicular) and the Lisfranc (tarsometatarsal) joints. The most common causes of focal deformity are masses, trauma and degenerative joint disease. These are dealt with elsewhere. Diffuse midfoot deformities can be due to either an increase in the arch of the foot (pes cavus) or a decrease in the plantar arch (pes planus). When pes cavus is acquired, it is usually the consequence of an underlying neurological disorder. Pes planus is more common and more often reflects local disease. The principal conditions that will be considered here are tibialis posterior tendon disease and neuropathic osteoarthropathy.

As mentioned at the beginning of this chapter, no part of the foot should be considered in isolation. This is particularly pertinent with midfoot deformities as many structural anomalies are sequelae of hindfoot instability and should be taken into consideration when the treatment of conditions such as acquired flat foot is planned. Angular/planar deformities of the midfoot which are associated with whole foot deformity can be charted on plain films. For example, on lateral projection the talocalcaneal and talometatarsal angle are both increased in the hyperpronated foot and decreased in the cavovarus foot. On anteroposterior projection the talometatarsal angle and calcaneometatarsal angles are decreased in the pronated foot and increased in the supinated/varus foot.

18.2.1 Pes Planus

18.2.1.1 Posterior Tibial Tendon Dysfunction

Tibialis posterior tendon disease can be a cause of both medial foot pain, especially where there is a pseudarthrosis at its insertion, and of a more generalised acquired flat foot in the adult.

Aside from traumatic rupture of the posterior tibial tendon, which is rare and not within the scope of this chapter, dysfunction or insufficiency of this tendon is a progressive condition commonly associated with adult flat foot. It is seen more commonly in older patients and women. Generally regarded as an overuse phenomenon, progression has been classified into three stages (Johnson 1989).

Stage 1. Clinically, there is no loss of power and usually mild tenderness along the tendon, extending distally from the medial malleolus. Symptoms are exacerbated on resisted inversion of the foot. Characteristic changes seen on MRI include tendon thickening, increased signal within the substance of the tendon on T1-weighted and T2-weighted images, and fluid within the tendon sheath (Fig. 18.18). Ultrasound can also demonstrate the internal fibre disruption and the surrounding tenosynovitis. Differential diagnosis from other causes of heel pain including flexor hallucis and digitorum longus tendinitis, tarsal tunnel and ligament tears is important. If treated at this stage, progression to structural pathology can be avoided. Treatment consists of rest and immobilisation. The patient should then be evaluated for biomechanical anomalies and an appropriate functional or accommodative foot orthosis prescribed. It is also wise to investigate possible systemic causes with blood tests for inflammatory markers such as rheumatoid factor.

Stage 2. Progression to Stage 2 may take up to 2 years from the onset of original symptoms and follows either delayed diagnosis, inappropriate treatment or lack of patient compliance. Clinically, this presents as a flexible planovalgus foot with the inability to restore the heel to neutral or maintain the medial longitudinal arch on active heel rise. The deformity is correctable passively. The 'too-many-toes' sign with the standing patient viewed from behind indicates a lateral drift of the forefoot but is only reliable if the clinician ensures that the leg is not externally rotated and that the patella is in the coronal plane. Pain is described along the course of the tendon, and there may be either nodular thickening of the tendon characteristic of tendinosis or wasting/tendon defect. Lateral ankle pain inferior to the fibula due to impingement may also be present. As stated above, this is a flexible deformity, and as such when the hindfoot is passively corrected, if a compensatory supination of the forefoot is noted, this can also be passively reduced.

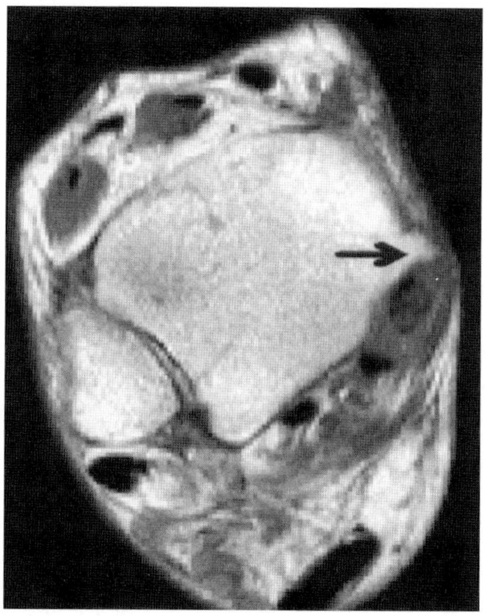

Fig. 18.18. Axial T1-weighted image of the hindfoot. The *black arrow* shows a small spur occasionally seen in combination with tibialis posterior tendinopathy. The adjacent tendon sheath is distended by fluid, and the normal dark tendon signal is replaced by poorly demarcated material of intermediate signal intensity

Radiographic evaluation of weight-bearing films will demonstrate a decrease in the calcaneal inclination angle and increase in the talocalcaneal angle on lateral projection. Karasick and Schweitzer (1996) found the calcaneal inclination angle to be the most reliable radiographic indicator in posterior tibial dysfunction. On AP views, the talus is displaced medially, and the forefoot is abducted. Hindfoot axial views (Cobey or Harris) are also helpful to evaluate leg/hindfoot alignment especially when surgery is contemplated. Plain films may also demonstrate a small bony spur arising from the posteromedial margin of the tibia. MRI is considered to be the imaging technique of choice for the assessment of tendon pathology and in stage 2 dysfunction will show typical appearances of tendinosis or partial tears. At this stage partial tears are more common. Partial tears of the tibialis posterior tendon take two forms, hypertrophic and atrophic. Hypertrophic ones are more common and, although the precise temporal relationships to the clinical stage of the disorder are incompletely worked out, probably reflect an earlier stage. Atrophic partial tears, also called type 2 partial tears, can be difficult to diagnose on MRI. The important finding is of an atrophied tendon. Atrophy is best assessed by comparing its size to the adjacent flexor digitorum. Tibialis posterior should be about twice the diameter of flexor digitorum under normal circumstances. Imaging of the spring ligament (inferior talonavicular ligament) is also advocated in these cases (Fig. 18.19) (Gazdag and Cracchiolo 1997).

Conservative treatment of stage 2 posterior tibial dysfunction should be considered for the less active/elderly patient. As the tendon is essentially nonfunctional, the foot must be support externally. Methods include thermoplastic ankle foot orthoses, shoe modifications (including callipers) and extended heel cups (UCBLs).

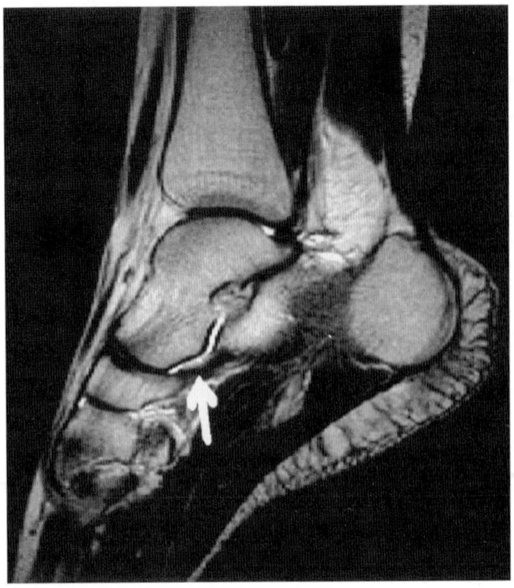

Fig. 18.19. Sagittal T2-weighted image of the normal calcaneonavicular (spring) ligament

Surgical treatment includes soft-tissue reconstruction either in isolation or in combination with bony realignment procedures. Various soft-tissue operations have been described involving tendon transfers (Helal 1990), 'turn down' techniques (Gould 1997), etc. We almost exclusively use the method advocated by Mann (1983). This is the flexor digitorum longus tendon transfer to augment tibialis posterior. We also usually include reinforcement of the spring ligament and a medial heel shift procedure. The aim of the calcaneal osteotomy is to relocate the insertion and therefore the action of the Achilles tendon more medially. Surgery is not usually an alternative to conservative management, as most patients require in-shoe orthoses in the long term.

Stage 3. In Stage 3 dysfunction the valgus deformity of the hindfoot and compensatory varus forefoot are irreducible either actively or passively. Patients complain of global hindfoot discomfort with maximum pain inferior to the tip of the fibula. They may also have associated toe deformities and pressure lesions. Radiographs show the structural changes of Stage 2 with degenerative changes in the subtalar and midtarsal joints. In severe cases, angulation of the talus in the mortise is seen on AP views of the ankle. Where this exists, Myerson (1996) has suggested an additional stage 4 to the Johnson (1989) classification.

Treatment with accommodative orthoses can be used in an attempt to arrest further deformity, but where symptoms are at unacceptable levels and the risk of ulceration and infection is high, surgery is indicated. Arthrodesis of the degenerate joints is usually required. The heel must be realigned under the tibia and the position of the forefoot evaluated intraoperatively. If the forefoot varus cannot be reduced, a triple arthrodesis will be required. Selective injection arthrograms preoperatively can of course be helpful to isolate which joints specifically are symptomatic. The structural deformity must, however, be reduced, and the extent of the surgery required to do this can often only be established intraoperatively.

18.2.1.2 Neuropathic Osteoarthropathy

Although the differential diagnosis of acquired pes planus is long, neuropathic osteoarthropathy (NOA) poses a particular diagnostic dilemma and will be dealt with here. In the early stages the diagnosis can be difficult. Later, deformity becomes more obvious, and the presence of an underlying neurological defect is detected by careful clinical examination. In many cases a prior history of diabetes will be present, though other causes of neuropathy will need to be excluded. Typically, pain is not a major feature, a further clue to the presence of the underlying nerve disease.

What may be more difficult is the differentiation between uncomplicated NOA and NOA with secondary infection. MRI can assist with the diagnosis, but no particular feature is specific. An ordered approach is necessary, with attention being paid to the soft tissues, bony cortex and medullary changes. Infection is unusual in the absence of soft-tissue involvement and equally unusual in the presence of a skin ulcer that has healed. Fragmentary cortical destruction and the presence of sharply demarcated bony margins suggest NOA. Cortical oedema and rather poorly demarcated destruction favour infection. High signal changes within the medullary cavity are common in both conditions, but their morphology may be different. Medullary abscess clearly favours infection, whereas more diffuse high signal changes may simply be reactive in nature. The site of disease can also be a valuable differentiating feature, as infection is more common in the metatarsal heads than in the midfoot. Gadolinium enhancement may be useful in the detection of both soft-tissue and bony abscess, which demonstrate rim enhancement. Additionally, the reappearance of an apparently obliterated cortex following gadolinium administration, termed the ghost sign, has been advocated as a sign of infection.

Although cross-sectional imaging is important, the complementary role of progressive changes on serial plain films should not be overlooked. Bone sclerosis, fragmentation and angular deformity on the plain radiograph favour NOA, but it is the slow rate of progression of bone destruction changes on serial films that separates NOA from infection. Much has been written about the role of scintigraphy, and some centres have achieved excellent results using a variety of isotopes including technetium and gallium. More recently, direct labelling of white blood cells and the use of subtraction techniques have improved the specificity. Scintigraphy has been criticised as being very dependent on the operator's expertise, especially in the white cell labelling process. This might explain why the excellent results reported from some centres are difficult to repeat elsewhere.

18.2.2 Pes Cavus

This is characterised by an exaggeration of the longitudinal arch of the foot which does not reduce with weight-bearing. The lateral border of the foot is included, which normally contacts the supporting surface. Pressure distribution on the plantar aspect is therefore restricted to the heel and forefoot, with typically an absence of toe function due to dorsal retraction of the toes at the metatarsophalangeal joints which also accompanies this complex disorder.

Although often idiopathic, acquired pes cavus is known to be associated with hereditary motor-sensory neuropathy (Charcot-Marie Tooth) and spinocerebellar degenerative conditions such as Friedreich's ataxia. Consequently, any patient presenting with progressive features of pes cavus should be thoroughly investigated. Where the aetiology is unclear, MRI of the spine may be indicated.

The diagnosis of pes cavus should be based on the clinical examination, but weight-bearing radiographs are helpful to evaluate the degree of deformity and aid surgical planning. Some authors differentiate between anterior and posterior pes cavus. The former has a relative increase in the plantar declination of the forefoot to the hindfoot and the latter, a higher calcaneal inclination angle and an excessive dorsiflexed position of the whole of the hindfoot relative to the forefoot. The differences are subtle, and the clinical relevance of making this distinction is in some doubt.

Treatment will depend on the patient's age, aetiology and severity of the symptoms. Generally, soft-tissue releases and tendon transfers can be performed in the skeletally immature patient with osteotomies/arthrodeses in adults. Conservative management aims to address the imbalance of pressure distribution under the foot with accommodative orthotics, with prescription footwear often being necessary to prevent pressure lesions on the dorsal aspect of the toes.

18.3 Forefoot

Acquired conditions of the forefoot are common presentations in the orthopaedic outpatient clinic. Metatarsalgia is a term used to encompass a broad range of conditions causing forefoot pain and may be associated with overuse, structural, degenerative or neurovascular pathologies. We will consider the following more commonly seen forms of metatarsalgia.

18.3.1 Hallux Valgus

Hallux valgus is a structural deformity of the first ray where the great toe is inclined towards the lateral aspect of the foot to a greater extent than normal. Associated with this is a constellation of other abnormalities of alignment including medial deviation of the first metatarsal, lateral displacement and pronation of the great toe, with lateral displacement of the sesamoids. Soft-tissue accommodative changes accompany this deformity with the formation of a medial inflammatory mass, termed a bunion. The incidence of hallux valgus in the general population varies widely, with some studies reporting variations of between 0% and 50% depending on the population under study (Gottschalk et al. 1980; Coughlin 1995). There is a prevalence among women in both shod and unshod populations (Sim-Fook and Hodgson 1958). In the UK a prevalence of 3% is generally accepted.

Footwear has traditionally been blamed as a major cause of hallux valgus, although there is no conclusive evidence to support this. It is more commonly accepted that certain styles of footwear might exacerbate a pre-existing susceptibility. This susceptibility may be due to a combination of congenital and mechanical factors. Coughlin reported maternal transmission in 72% of cases (Coughlin 1995). Metatarsophalangeal joint shape and instability are significant predictors of hallux valgus. The part played by excessive foot pronation in its development is less clear. While this deformity is rare in the high arched cavus foot (Carl and Ross 1988)], no correlation was found between arch height and hallux valgus in children (Piggott 1960). Hypermobility at the metatarsocuneiform joint predisposing to the development of primus metatarsus varus probably plays a role in the aetiology of hallux valgus in a minority of cases and may be associated with generalised joint laxity (Carl and Ross 1988). Other reported causes include amputation or dislocation of the second toe, rheumatoid arthritis, trauma, first metatarsal length and soft-tissue contractures.

Plain radiographs are important in the classification and surgical planning. Standing anteroposterior views should be used to measure the first/second intermetatarsal angle (IMA), hallux valgus angle (HVA), distal metatarsal articular angle (DMAA), joint congruency and metatarsal length (Figs. 18.20, 18.21). The sesamoid position may also be determined from the AP projection, although Talbot (1998) has suggested that axial views are more accurate.

The severity of hallux valgus has been graded according to these measured angles. In grade 1 deformities the IMA is increased up to 12 deg with a hallux valgus angle up to 20 deg. Grade 2 have IMAs up to 18 deg and HVAs up to 40 deg. The severest, grade 3, includes deformities greater than 18 deg and 40 deg, respectively. It is important to appreciate that the IMAs will be proportionately larger in patients with a coexisting metatarsus adductus.

Piggott's (1960) classification of hallux valgus is based on first metatarsophalangeal joint congruency. Three types are described: aligned, deviated and subluxed. He noted that progression of the deformity occurred only in the deviated and subluxed groups and to a proportionately lesser magnitude in the former group.

Patients with hallux valgus present with pressure symptoms related to the prominence of the

a 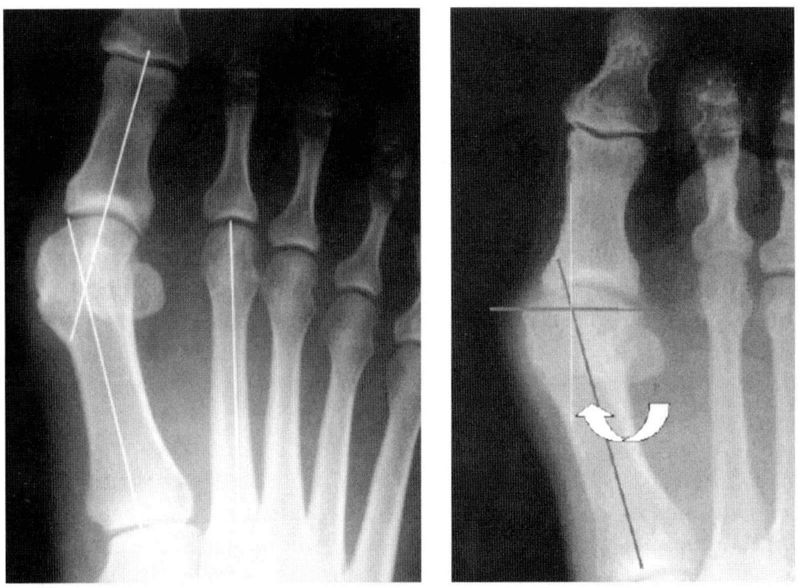 b

c 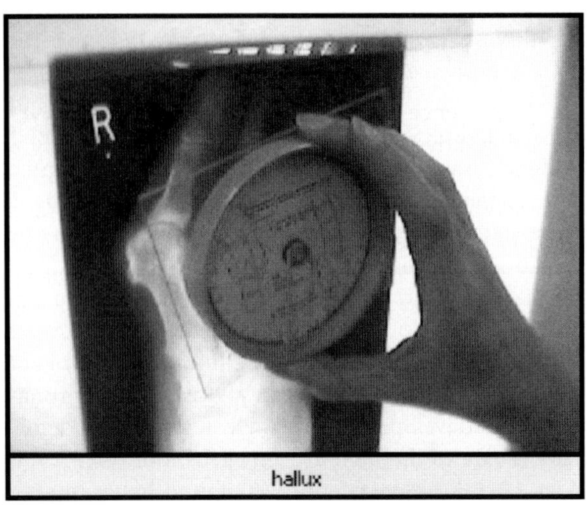

Fig. 18.20a–c. Plain radiograph of hallux valgus. **a**) Axes of the 1st and 2nd metatarsal (forming the intermetatarsal angle) with the axis of the proximal phalanx first ray (forming the hallux valgus angle). **b** The *curved arrow* indicates the distal metatarsal articular angle (DMAA). **c** Hallux valgus assessment is easily and quickly achieved with a hand-held measuring device. The type shown here is an Oxford Cobbometer

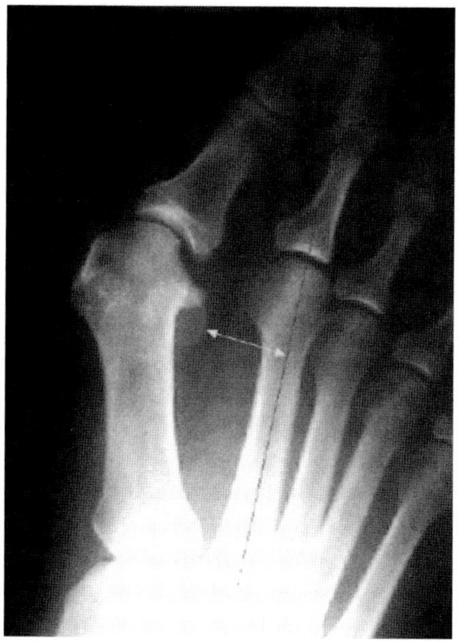

Fig. 18.21. Sesamoid position can be measured either by the proportion of the lateral sesamoid that projects lateral to the 1st metatarsal or by its distance from the axis of the second metatarsal

metatarsal head, joint pain, associated metatarsalgia and lesser toe deformities. The degree or grade of deformity is not necessarily correlated to the level of symptoms, with seemingly minor deformities being disproportionately painful.

The treatment of hallux valgus is conservative in the first instance. If there are underlying biomechanical factors such as excessive pronation or first ray hypermobility, these should be addressed with appropriate orthoses. Footwear advice and compromise by the patient are often necessary.

Surgical treatment should take into account the patient's age and activity level as well as evaluation of the pathology. Where there is little or no degenerative joint disease, the deformity should be corrected with preservation of the joint. Numerous metatarsal osteotomies have been described to correct the intermetatarsal angle. Less severe deformities can be corrected using distal or subcapital osteotomies. Deformities with an IMA of between 14 deg and 16 deg require proximal procedures.

Most osteotomies fail to address the first metatarsophalangeal joint congruency and sesamoid position, nor do they preserve the metatarsal length. These failures have been cited as the main cause of postoperative complications. For this reason, more complex surgical procedures have been proposed to address the 3D nature of severe hallux valgus. The Scarf osteotomy demonstrates versatility in correcting all the angular pathologies, including bringing about sesamoid reduction. In cases of severe articular damage, arthrodesis of the first metatarsophalangeal joint is probably still the gold standard treatment in the absence of clinically proven joint replacement. Excision arthroplasty with soft-tissue interposition remains an acceptable option in the elderly, less active patient.

18.3.2 Hallux Rigidus

Hallux rigidus is a degenerative joint disease of the first metatarsophalangeal joint. Various conditions predispose to it, including osteoarthritis, trauma, inflammatory arthropathies, and the sequelae of osteochondritis dissecans and infection. The incidence is reported to be higher in men and in the age group 31–60 years.

The early stages of hallux rigidus demonstrate a decrease in the range of movement, with end-point pain, particularly on dorsiflexion. More advanced disease results in crepitus and pain throughout all movements. Although complete loss of movement is rarely observed, there is often a functional ankylosis in advanced stages of the disease. Compensation during gait occurs by a lateral displacement of the centre of mass at toe-off. Hyperextension at the first interphalangeal joint is also a common feature.

Plain radiographs are sufficient to assess and stage this condition. In grade 1, normal or joint space narrowing is observed with mild to moderate osteophytes. Grade 2 shows joint space narrowing, subchondral sclerosis and enlargement of osteophytes. In grade 3, there is a loss of joint space with circumferential osteophyte formation. Kravitz et al. described four stages and related these to a treatment strategy (Kravitz 1994).

Stage 1 is essentially asymptomatic hallux limitus with the presence of primary aetiological factors, and only conservative treatment is advocated. Conservative measures include shoe modification, e.g. rocker soles and functional foot orthoses with Morton's extension under the great toe. Stage 2 exhibits pain at the end of the range of motion (ROM), minor joint space narrowing and subchondral sclerosis, but these patients are usually treated conservatively. Where conservative treatment fails in patients at stage 1 and 2 in Kravitz et al.'s classification, cheilectomy may be appropriate. It must be borne in mind, however, that the increased range of movement following this procedure can exacerbate symptoms, and patients should be counselled accordingly. Other surgical techniques include decompression and dorsiflexory osteotomies. Stage 3 is divided into A and B. Stage 3A symptoms include pain on movement with radiographic findings as above but include dorsal osteophytes and metatarsal head flattening. Stage 3B shows minimal joint space, subchondral cysts and clinically marked limitation of dorsiflexion, and chronic pain with all ambulation. Treatment of both stage 3 categories is by decompression osteotomies. In Stage 4 there is ankylosis, obliterated joint space, periarticular pain and often postural symptoms. Surgical treatment takes the form of joint destructive procedures such as excision arthroplasty or arthrodesis. As in hallux valgus with severe degenerative disease, in end-stage hallux rigidus, arthrodesis remains the definitive treatment with excision interposition arthroplasty in the elderly, sedentary patient.

18.3.3 Bunionette Deformity (Tailor's Bunion)

This is a deformity of the 5th ray involving the metatarsal and metatarsophalangeal joint and is essentially the mirror image of hallux valgus. It does, however, have some different aetiological factors, and unlike hallux valgus, deformity within the metatarsal shaft is often a feature.

Several aetiologies have been cited in this deformity including hypermobility of the 5th ray, in isolation or in association with excessive subtalar joint pronation, laxity of the transverse metatarsal ligament, splay foot deformity and valgus bowing of the metatarsal (Coughlin and Mann 1993). As with hallux valgus, tailor's bunions are exacerbated by inappropriate footwear.

Conservative treatment consists of local protection of the prominent joint and in-shoe orthoses to control hypermobility where indicated.

Plain radiographs are usually sufficient to facilitate the surgical planning. Charting of standard weight-bearing AP films should include the 5th metatarsophalangeal angle, the 4th–5th intermetatarsal angle and the degree of metatarsal bowing. Coughlin has described three types of bunionette deformity based on radiographic findings. Type I involves hypertrophy of the metatarsal head alone. Type II features valgus bowing of the 5th metatarsal, and in type III there is an increased 4th–5th intermetatarsal angle (7–8 deg is normal).

Although excisional arthroplasties and simple bumpectomy have been utilised for this condition, metatarsal osteotomies sometimes in conjunction with phalangeal osteotomy are usually required to adequately address the deformity. These include capital displacement, diaphyseal and proximal osteotomies. As with surgical correction of hallux valgus, the choice of procedure should take into consideration the underlying angular and rotational pathology and address this with biomechanical principles in mind to reduce postoperative complications such as recurrence and transfer metatarsalgia.

18.3.4 Other Toe Deformities

Acquired deformities of the 2nd to 5th toes have a reported incidence of up to 20%. They are typically described as fixed or flexible deformities in the sagittal plane at the metatarsophalangeal (MTP) and proximal (PIP) or distal interphalangeal (DIP) levels. Some component of the coronal and/or transverse plane may also be present and can complicate the surgical management. The most common examples of lesser toe deformities include claw toe, hammer toe, mallet toe and overlapping toe.

Plain weight-bearing anteroposterior, lateral and oblique films are usually sufficient to evaluate these deformities. Occasionally, stress views and arthrograms are helpful to demonstrate the degree of instability and distinguish between intra- and extraarticular causes.

Conservative treatment consists of local protection of the toes which may necessitate modified footwear or in-shoe orthoses if a biomechanical cause is suspected. In some cases simply compromising on the choice of footwear is all that is required.

Surgery of a lesser toe deformity will generally involve soft-tissue techniques or arthrodesis/arthroplasty depending on the age of the patient, the degree of flexibility and underlying cause. In the absence of neuromuscular causes, we tend to avoid PIP or DIP arthrodesis and perform a modification of DuVries excision arthroplasty. This interposes the extensor apparatus into the deficit caused by the excision of the head of the phalanx. In our experience this creates less shortening and more stability postoperatively. It is usually necessary to include an MTP extensor tenotomy and capsulotomy where there is dorsal contracture at this level. When interphalangeal arthrodesis is indicated, we try to avoid fixation with external K-wires by taking advantage of the recent technology in small cannulated systems to maintain fixation internally. Modifications to these procedures may of course be necessary where the deformity lies in more than one plane, e.g.adducto-varus 5th toe.

18.3.5 Sesamoid Pathology

These two ossicles are situated under the first metatarsal head and lie in the medial and lateral slips of the flexor hallucis brevis (FHB) tendon. There are also attachments of the adductor hallucis into the lateral sesamoid and abductor hallucis for the medial sesamoid. They are separated by a 'crista' on the plantar surface of the metatarsal head and articulate with it. Their function is to dissipate impact forces, increase the mechanical advantage of the FHB tendon and offer protection of the FHB.

Disorders of the sesamoids include inflammation (sesamoiditis) (Fig. 18.22), fracture (including stress fracture), osteochondrosis, avascular necrosis and arthrosis of the metatarsal-sesamoid articulation (Leventen 1991). Pain under the first metatarsal head is the presenting symptom. There may be a history of injury or an increase in activity levels or increase in shoe heel elevation. The plantar declination angle of the first metatarsal may also be increased as observed in the cavus foot.

Swelling and tenderness to palpation localised to the affected sesamoid are evident clinically. An equal incidence of involvement between the medial and lateral sesamoids is reported (Leventen 1991), although in my experience, the medial one is more commonly involved. There may be an associated hyperkeratotic skin lesion reflecting a localised increase in pressure. Pain exacerbated by dorsiflexion of the great toe is an occasional finding and is suspicious for stress fracture. Obviously, any true joint pathology should be excluded.

Sesamoiditis is an example of an overuse syndrome initially producing an inflammatory reaction in the surrounding soft tissue. The syndrome is now thought to encompass other pathologies and may represent the natural history of the condition. The initial stress reaction progresses to produce true stress fracture or avascular necrosis. MRI findings and histology following excision would seem to confirm this theory.

Fractures of the sesamoids should be differentiated from bi- or multipartite sesamoids. Multiple centres of ossification may occur with resultant multipartite bones. The medial sesamoid is more commonly affected, with one report noting an incidence of 31% (Dobas and Silvers 1997). On plain radiographs an irregular border between the fragments is suggestive of fracture. Differentiation from a stress fracture is more difficult, with pain on traction of the FHB being clinically helpful, but imaging is usually diagnostic.

Arthrosis at the sesamoid-metatarsal articulation is usually the result of deformity of the first ray, often in association with hallux valgus. The combination of primus metatarsus varus and valgus at the metatarsophalangeal joint leads to subluxation of the sesamoids. The analogy with incorrect tracking of the patella can be made with subsequent degenerative changes on the articular cartilage.

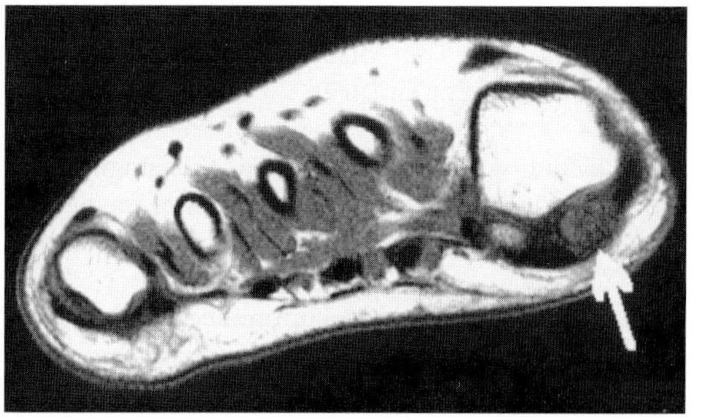

Fig. 18.22. Coronal T1-weighted image with loss of marrow signal in the medial sesamoid indicating sesamoiditis

Treatment of sesamoiditis by conservative methods includes foot orthoses to address the underlying biomechanical dysfunction and to offload the affected sesamoid. Non-steroidal anti-inflammatory drugs (NSAIDS) and other anti-inflammatory modalities may also help. In cases of stress fracture, a period of immobilisation in a walking cast may be necessary. Surgery is indicated for intractable cases, usually due to symptomatic pseudarthrosis. Excision of one or more fragments or the whole sesamoid has been described (Coughlin 1990). Complications of sesamoidectomy have also been well documented (Aper et al. 1994, 1996). The sequelae of muscle imbalance producing deformity of the first metatarsophalangeal joint are the main factors in these complications.

18.3.6 Osteochondrosis of the Metatarsal (Freiberg's Disease)

The second metatarsal is the one most frequently affected by this condition, with an increased incidence among women (Smillie 1957). The average age of presentation is 13 years. Aetiological factors include repetitive minor trauma, mechanical overload (Gauthier and Elbaz 1979) and compressive force compromising the diaphyseal arteries (Stanley et al. 1990). The onset of avascular necrosis from whatever cause is a consistent finding in the true juvenile form of the disease.

Five stages of pathology have been proposed, which can also be discerned radiographically (Gauthier and Elbaz 1979).

Stage 1. Radiographs are normal at this stage which intraoperatively demonstrates sclerosis of the opposing cancellous surfaces with an ischaemic epiphysis.

Stage 2. Revascularisation commences with consequent bone resorption. The central area of the dorsal metatarsal head starts to collapse into the metaphysis. Radiographically, this stage is seen as joint space widening and flattening of the dorsal aspect of the head and discrete sclerosis of the epiphysis.

Stage 3. Further collapse of the central portion of the metatarsal head with protrusion of the medial and lateral borders is characteristic of this stage. The plantar aspect of the metatarsal head remains intact. This represents further flattening and widening of the metatarsal head on plain radiographs together with lytic lesions and sclerosis of the epiphysis.

Stage 4. The collapse of the central area extends to the point where the remaining intact plantar fragment is also destroyed. Joint space narrowing is now visible radiographically, with increased flattening of the head and possible loose body formation.

Stage 5. Joint space narrowing, hypertrophy of the metatarsal head osteophyte formation, and irregularity of the proximal phalanx are all radiographic features of this stage. Cortical thickening of the metatarsal shaft may be noted, which probably represents a compensatory stress reaction.

The patient presents with pain localised to the affected joint. Depending on the stage of disease, there will be restricted joint dorsiflexion and activity-related pain. There may be a history of trauma or increase in activity or alteration in style of footwear. In later stages, increased joint bulk is clinically obvious, with severe joint pain on movement.

Treatment is often not instigated until radiographic changes are noted, by which time the pathology may be irreversible. Conservative management consists of off-loading pressure from the affected metatarsal head and addressing any underlying biomechanical anomaly, e.g. excessive pronation, which usually involves prescription orthoses. Surgical treatment aims to restore a functional, pain-free joint. The methods will vary according to the stage of the pathology. Where articular cartilage is still well preserved, cheilectomy and minimal metatarsal head debulking only may be sufficient. Stage 3 levels of disease may respond to dorsiflexion osteotomy as described by Gauthier and Elbaz (1979), providing sufficient plantar cartilage is available. Other joint-preserving procedures have been described, including shortening osteotomies to decompress the joint (Smith et al. 1991) and bone grafting techniques. Metatarsal head resection has a high complication rate and should not be considered. Other forms of excision arthroplasty also contravene the principle of joint preservation but may be realistically the only alternative in end-stage disease, although improvement in joint replacement technology, e.g.ceramic implants, may be a viable option in the future.

References

Aper RL, Saltzman CL, Brown TD (1994) The effect of hallux sesamoid excision on the effective movement of the flexor hallucis brevis. Foot Ankle Int 15:462–470

Aper RL, Saltzman CL, Brown TD (1996) The effect of hallucal sesamoid excision on the flexor hallucis longus moment arm. Clin Orthop 325:209–217

Bellemans J, Reynders-Frederix PA, Stoffelen D, Broos PL, Fabry G (1993) Os trigonum and soleus tertius anomaly. Acta Orthop Belg 59:412–415

Berkowitz JF, Kier R, Rudicel S (1991) Plantar fasciitis: MR imaging. Radiology 179:665–667

Bertolotto M, Perrone R, Martinoli C, Rollandi GA, Patetta R, Derchi LE (1995) High resolution ultrasound anatomy of normal Achilles tendon. Br J Radiol 68:986–991

Bottger BA, Schweitzer ME, El-Noueam KI, Desai M (1998) MR imaging of the normal and abnormal retrocalcaneal bursae. AJR Am J Roentgenol 170:1239–1241

Carl A, Ross S, Pea E (1988) Hypermobility in hallux valgus. Foot Ankle 8:264–270

Clancy W, Heiden E (1997) Achilles tendonitis treatment in the athlete. Foot Ankle Clin 2:429–438

Coughlin M (1990) Instruction course lectures.

Coughlin MJ (1995) Juvenile hallux valgus: aetiology and treatment. Foot Ankle Int 16:682–697

Coughlin MJ, Mann RA (1993) Surgery of the foot and ankle, 6th edn. Mosby, St Louis

Deutsch AL, Lund PJ, Mink JH (1997) MR imaging and diagnostic ultrasound in the evaluation of Achilles tendon disorders. Foot Ankle Clin 2:391–409

Digiovanni BE (1997) Achilles tendinitis and posterior heel disorders. Foot Ankle Clin 2:411–428

Dobas DC, Silvers MD (1997) The frequency of the bipartite sesamoids of the first metatrsophalangeal joint. J Am Podiatry Assoc 67:880–882

Ferkel RD, Fasulo GJ (1994) Arthroscopic treatment of ankle injuries. Orthop Clin North Am 25:17–32

Ferkel RD, Karzel RP, Del Pizzo W, Friedman MJ, Fischer SP (1991) Arthroscopic treatment of anterolateral impingement of the ankle. Am J Sports Med 19:440–446

Fowler A (1945) Abnormality of the calcaneus as a cause of painful heel. Br J Surg 32:494–498

Gauthier G, Elbaz R (1979) Freiberg's infraction: a subchondral bone fatigue fracture. Clin Orthop 142:93–95

Gazdag AR, Cracchiolo AR (1997) Rupture of the posterior tibial tendon. Evaluation of injury of the spring ligament and clinical assessment of tendon transfer and ligament repair. J Bone Joint Surg Am 79:675–681

Gill LH, Kiebzak GM (1996) The outcome of non surgical treatment for plantar fasciitis. Foot Ankle Int 17: 527–532

Gottschalk FA, Sallis JG, Beighton PH, Solomon L (1980) A comparison of the prevalence of hallux valgus in three South African populations. S Afr Med J 57:355–357

Gould M (1997) Direct repair of the posterior tibial tendon. Foot Ankle Clin 2:275–287

Grogan D, Walling A, Ogden J (1990) Anatomy of the os trigonum. J Paediatr Orthop 10:618–622

Haglund P (1928) Beitrag zur uliwik der Achilesse have. Z Orthop Chir 49:49

Harris O (2000) Endoscopic release of the plantar fascia. Arthroscopy 16:290–298

Hedrick MR, McBryde AM (1994) Posterior ankle impingement. Foot Ankle Int 15:2–8

Helal B (1990) Cobb repair for tibialis posterior tendon rupture. J Foot Surg 29:349–352

Jacobson JA (1999) Musculoskeletal sonography and MR imaging. A role for both imaging methods. Radiol Clin North Am 37:713–35

Johnson KA (1989) Tibialis posterior tendon dysfunction. Clin Orthop 239:196–206

Kainberger F, Fialka V, Breitenseher M, Kritz H, Baldt M, Czerny C, Imhof H (1996) Differential diagnosis of diseases of the Achilles tendon. A clinico-sonographic concept. Radiologe 36:38–46

Karasick D, Schweitzer ME (1996) The os trigonum syndrome: imaging features. AJR Am J Roentgenol 166:125–129

Kravitz M (1994) Progressive staging classification of hallux rigidus. Lower Extremity 1:55–66

Leventen EO (1991) Sesamoid disorders and treatment. Clin Orthop 269:236–240

Lipscomb P, Kelly P (1955) Injuries of the extensor tendons in the distal part of the leg & ankle. J Bone Joint Surg Am 37:1206–1213

Liu SH, Mirzayan R (1993) Posteromedial ankle impingement. Arthroscopy 9:709–711

Liu SH, Nuccion SL, Finerman G (1997) Diagnosis of anterolateral ankle impingement. Comparison between magnetic resonance imaging and clinical examination. Am J Sports Med 25:389–393

Lundberg A, Svensson OK, Bylund C, Selvik G (1989) Kinematics of the ankle foot complex. III. Influence of leg rotation. Foot Ankle 9:304–309

Mann RA (1983) Acquired flat foot in adults. Clin Orthop 181: 46–51

Myerson MS (1996) Acquired adult flatfoot deformity. J Bone Joint Surg Am 78:780–792

Nesse E, Finsen V (1994) Poor results after resection for Haglund's heel:analysis of 35 heels in 23 patients after 3 years. Acta Orthop Scand 65:107–109

Ogilvie Harris DJ, Mahomed N, Demaziere A (1993) Anterior impingement of the ankle treated by arthroscopic removal of bony spurs. J Bone Joint Surg Br 75:437–440

Parkes JC Jr, Hamilton WG, Patterson AH, Rawles JG Jr (1980) The anterior impingement syndrome of the ankle. J Trauma 20:895–898

Piggott M (1960) The natural history of hallux valgus in adolescence and early adult life. J Bone Joint Surg Br 42: 749–760

Puddu G, Ippolito E, Postacchinni F (1976) A classification of Achilles tendon disease. Am J Sports Med 4:145–150

Reynaert P, Gelen G, Geens G (1994) Arthroscopic treatment of anterior impingement of the ankle. Acta Orthop Belg 60:384–388

Riepert T, Drechsler T, Urban R, Schild H, Mattern R (1995) Frequency, age dependence and sex distribution of calcaneal spurs – analysis of x-ray morphology in 1027 Central European patients. Rofo Fortschr Geb Rontgenstr Neuen Bildgebenden Verfahren 162:502–505

Rubin G, Witton M (1963) Plantar calcaneal spurs. Am J Orthop 5:38–41

Schweitzer ME, Karasick D (1994) MRI of the ankle and hindfoot. Semin Ultrasound CT MR 15:410–422

Sim-Fook L, Hodgson AR (1958) A comparison of foot forms among the non-shoe and shoe-wearing Chinese populations. J Bone Joint Surg Am 40:1058–1062

Smillie M (1957) Freiberg's Infraction (Kohler's second disease). J Bone Joint Surg Br 39:580

Smith TWD, Stanley D, Rowley DI (1991) Treatment of Freiberg's disease. J Bone Joint Surg Br 73:129–134

Stanley D, Betts RP, Rowley DI (1990) Assessment of aetiologic factors in the development of Freiberg's disease. J Foot Surg 29:444–447

Stephens MM (1994) Haglund's deformity and retrocalcaneal bursitis. Orthop Clin North Am 25:41–46

Strehle (1997) The non operative treatment of plantar fasciitis: early results of a prospective randomised treatment study. In: European Foot and Ankle Societies Congress, Paris

Talbot M (1998) Assessing sesamoid subluxation in hallux valgus. Foot Ankle Int 19:547–554

Torg JS, Torg E (1987) Overuse injuries in sport. The foot. Clin Spoorts Med 6:291–320

Wakeley CJ, Johnson DP, Watt I (1996) The value of MR imaging in the diagnosis of the os trigonum syndrome. Skeletal Radiol 25:133–136

Zadek I (1939) An operation for the cure of Achillo bursitis. Am J Surg 43:542–547

19 Sesamoid Pathology

W. B. Morrison, H. P. Ledermann, and M. E. Schweitzer

CONTENTS

19.1 Introduction

A number of pathological entities affect the sesamoid bones of the foot (Coughlin 1990; Jahss 1981; Leventon 1991). The disease processes are modified by the chronic, repetitive stress associated with ambulation; the sesamoid bones are exposed to tremendous compression and traction forces, particularly during the push-off phase of the gait cycle. The combination of causative factors results in an overlap of clinical presentations and a spectrum of disease, the end-point of which is osteoarthritis. Since these disorders may be difficult to separate clinically, radiologic tests are often employed to distinguish between them (Karasick and Schweitzer 1998; Taylor et al. 1993). Radiologic findings may also overlap, and it may be difficult to differentiate between the primary disease and superimposed secondary pathology. This chapter will examine the major categories of disease affecting the sesamoid bones and their appearance on various imaging studies.

19.2 Anatomy

Knowledge of the anatomy of the hallux-sesamoid complex (Fig. 19.1) is essential for understanding the diseases that affect it. The medial (tibial) and lateral (fibular) sesamoid bones are positioned inferior to the first metatarsal head. Their inferior surface is rounded, and the superior surface is faceted, articulating on grooves in the metatarsal head. The sesamoid bones glide over the inferior surface of the metatarsal head during flexion and extension of the metatarsophalangeal (MTP) joint. A smooth gliding motion is facilitated by the morphology of the grooves and articular cartilage present on the metatarsal head and the sesamoids. Therefore, processes that alter the position or tracking of the sesamoids or result in cartilage loss can cause pain and secondary osteoarthritis. The sesamoid bones are incorporated into the MTP joint capsule, and any articular disease affecting the first MTP joint will also affect the MTS joint. This also makes the sesamoid bones susceptible to injury during episodes of capsular trauma, such as that caused by hyperextension injury of the MTP joint. The sesamoid bones are stabilized by their capsular location and metatarsal articulation. Additional stabilization is provided by an intersesamoid ligament that extends between them preventing excess separation (Jahss 1981), as well as the sesamoid-phalangeal ligament complex (Richardson 1987). However, this stable position under the first metatarsal head also makes

W. B. Morrison, MD; H. P. Ledermann, MD;
M. E. Schweitzer, MD
Thomas Jefferson University Hospital, Department of Radiology, 111 S. 11th St., # 3390 Gibbon, Philadelphia, PA 19107, USA

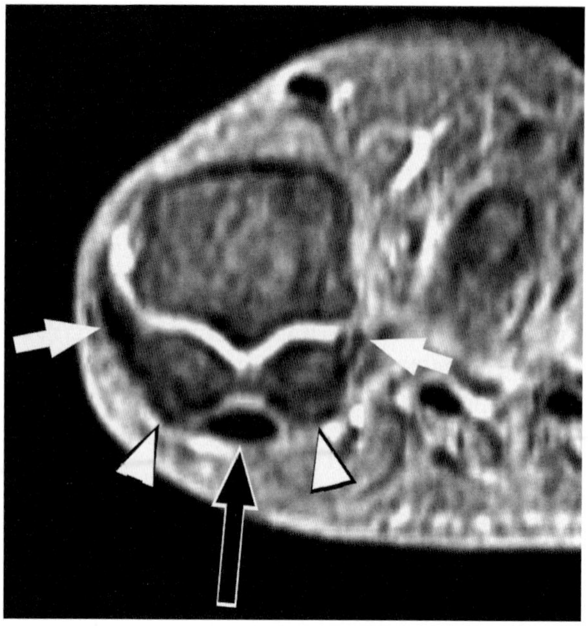

a

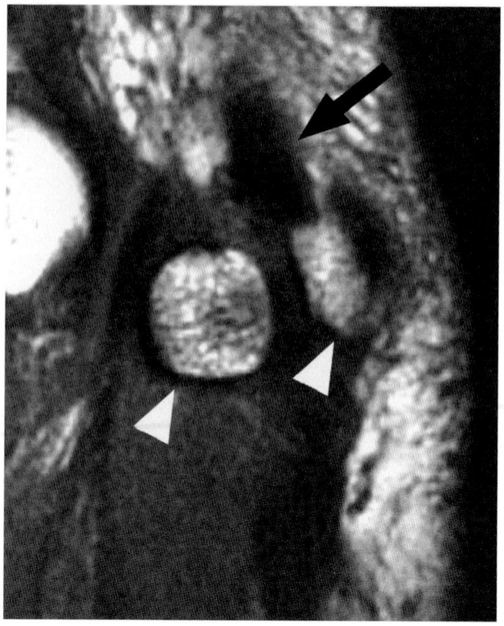

b

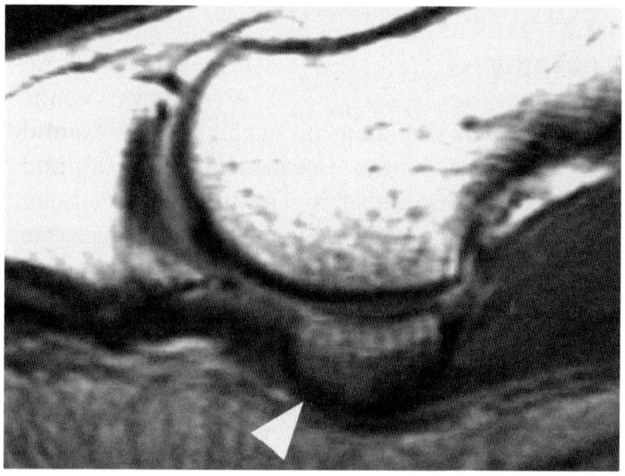

c

Fig. 19.1a–c. Normal anatomy of the hallux-sesamoid complex on MR images. **a** Coronal image shows the tibial and fibular sesamoids (*arrowheads*) articulating on the grooved surfaces of the metatarsal head; the sesamoids are connected by the intersesamoid ligament, superficial to which is the flexor hallucis longus tendon (*long arrow*). Note muscular and capsular attachments medially and laterally (*short arrows*). **b** Axial image shows the flexor hallucis longus tendon (*arrow*) passing between the sesamoid bones (*arrowheads*). **c** Sagittal image shows the normal position of the sesamoids (*arrowhead*) under the first metatarsal head

the sesamoid bones (especially the tibial sesamoid) susceptible to compressive forces during the push-off phase of the gait cycle. Forces are cushioned and dissipated somewhat by the plantar fat pad (Richardson 1987); loss of or migration of this fat pad in diseases such as rheumatoid arthritis and diabetes can leave the sesamoid bones relatively unprotected. The sesamoid bones are also part of the flexor complex of the first ray; the flexor hallucis longus tendon passes between the sesamoids, superficial to the intersesamoid ligament (David et al. 1989). The sesamoid bones are also attached to the conjoined tendons of the flexor hallucis brevis and abductor hallucis (attached to the tibial sesamoid) (Richardson 1987).

19.3 Modalities and Protocols

19.3.1 Radiography

Radiographs are very useful in the initial evaluation of the patient with sesamoid symptomatology (Karasick and Schweitzer 1998; Potter et al. 1992; Taylor et al. 1993). Sesamoid anatomy, morphology, and position are easily assessed. Several patterns of joint pathology in the foot can facilitate the formation of a differential diagnosis for sesamoid pathology. An AP view of the forefoot obtained in addition to a lateral image and oblique frontal views are often helpful to see the margins of the sesamoids which otherwise may be obscured by the metatarsal head. A 'sesamoid view' (Fig. 19.5a) is useful to evaluate the sesamoid position and articular surfaces (Taylor et al. 1993). This can be obtained by centering the X-ray beam as if to acquire an AP ankle image, but centered lower over the MTP joints. Dorsiflexion of the toes removes superimposed density.

19.3.2 Computed Tomography

CT is not often necessary for evaluation of the sesamoids but offers the ability to more precisely evaluate the articular surfaces, margins, fractures, erosions, and increased density which can indicate avascular necrosis (AVN) (Fleischli and Cheleuitte 1995). Images are obtained at 1 mm intervals through the forefoot, and sagittal and coronal reconstructions are made. Alternatively, the patient's knee can be flexed, the foot positioned flat against the CT table, and direct coronal images acquired.

19.3.3 Magnetic Resonance Imaging

MR imaging provides excellent visualization of the anatomy of the hallux/sesamoid complex and surrounding soft tissues and is the optimal modality for evaluation of the majority of pathologic conditions affecting this region (Karasick and Schweitzer 1998). The ability to differentiate different tissue types and identify areas of fluid and edema coupled with high resolution and the ability to image in any plane offer advantages over the other imaging modalities. The MR imaging protocol for dedicated evaluation of the sesamoids should be performed with a small surface coil and a field-of-view of no more than 12 cm (Karasick and Schweitzer 1998); however, sesamoid pathology is often detected incidentally on more comprehensive MR examinations of the foot. Acquiring slices in an interleaved fashion precludes the need for interslice gaps. T1-weighted and fast spin-echo T2-weighted images should be planned. Fat suppression should be used for T2 image acquisition, or if not available, STIR should be used to detect edema patterns. Use of gadolinium contrast is helpful when there is concern for infection, inflammatory arthropathy, or sesamoiditis; post-contrast T1-weighted spin-echo or turbo gradient-echo images should be acquired using fat suppression.

Images should be obtained in the coronal plane as well as the axial or sagittal plane. Coronal images provide the best evaluation of the metatarsal-sesamoid articulation, the plantar capsule, the intersesamoid ligament and plantar soft tissues. Axial and sagittal planes provide a longitudinal view of the sesamoids and are best for evaluation of a sesamoid fracture, bipartite situations, and pseudoarthrosis; these planes are also excellent for evaluation of the associated MTP joint. Imaging in at least two planes helps confirm suspected marrow signal abnormalities.

19.4 Pathology of the Sesamoids

19.4.1 Osteomyelitis/Septic Arthritis

Osteomyelitis of the sesamoids is best seen on MR images (Fig. 19.2). Inflammation replaces the fat signal on T1-weighted images, and edema results in high marrow signal on T2-weighted images and STIR images. Gadolinium-enhanced T1-weighted images will show high signal in the involved bone (Morrison et al. 1995). Fat suppression increases the detectability of infection on T2-weighted and post-contrast T1-weighted images (Morrison et al. 1993). Because of their superficial location on the plantar aspect of the foot, the sesamoid bones are particularly susceptible to infection spread transcutaneously (Potter et al. 1992), which typically occurs in diabetics. In this population, ulceration is common over bony prominences or areas of friction, and the first metatarsal head is the most common site of involvement. Cellulitis can spread directly to the sesamoids from an ulcer, or infection may initially involve the MTP joint and spread secondarily to the sesamoids. Often there is a sinus tract from the sesamoid to the ulcer; sinus tracts are seen as linear tracts of high T2-weighted signal in the soft tissues, with a 'tram track' pattern of enhancement (Morrison et al. 1998).Septic arthritis of the first MTP joint is common in the setting of medial forefoot ulceration; septic arthritis commonly presents on MR images with joint effusion that demonstrates thick marginal enhancement related to synovitis (Brower 1996; Graif et al. 1999). The adjacent subchondral bone often shows a thin rim of reactive edema; infection may spread from the joint into the underlying bone, including the sesamoids. In this

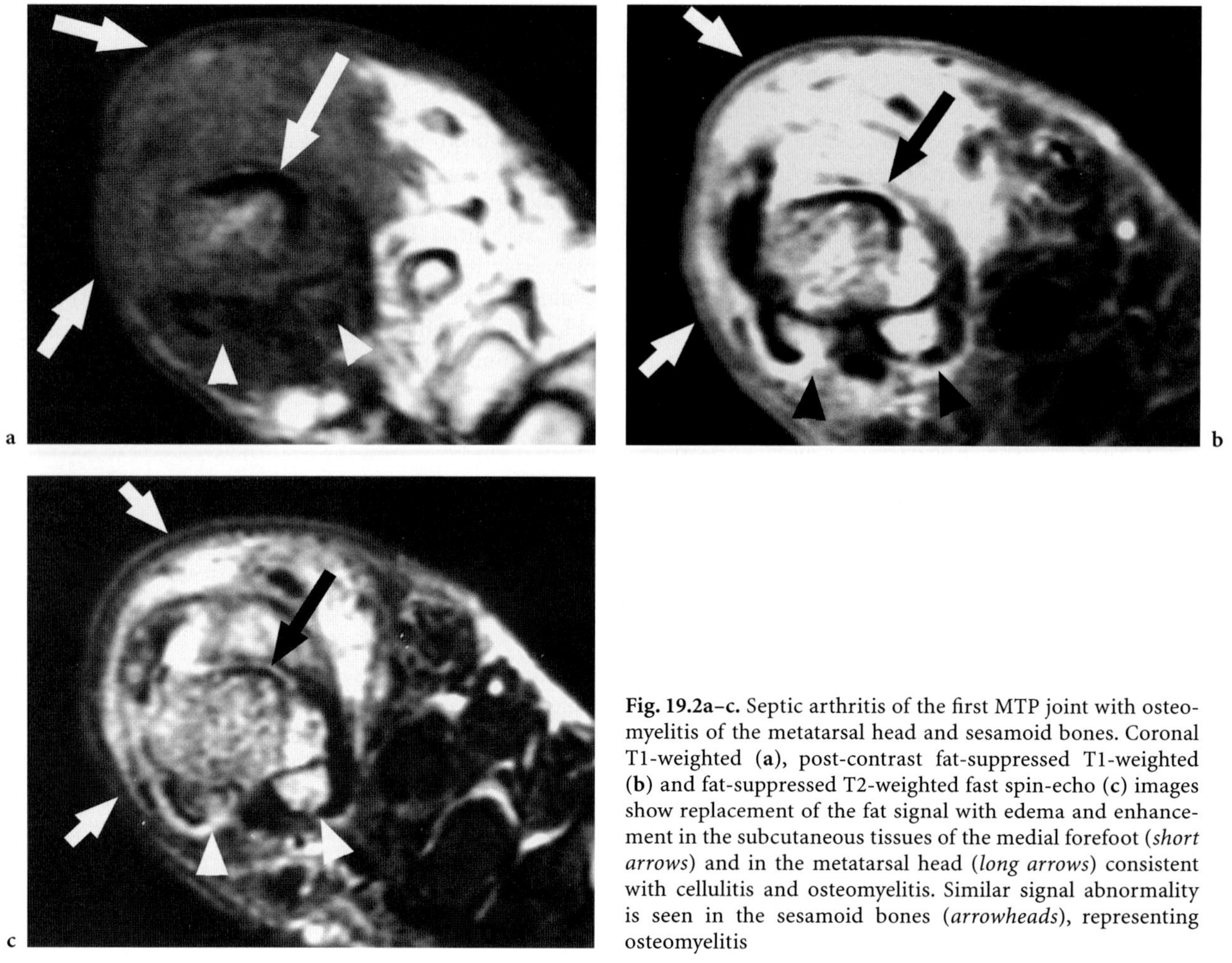

Fig. 19.2a–c. Septic arthritis of the first MTP joint with osteomyelitis of the metatarsal head and sesamoid bones. Coronal T1-weighted (**a**), post-contrast fat-suppressed T1-weighted (**b**) and fat-suppressed T2-weighted fast spin-echo (**c**) images show replacement of the fat signal with edema and enhancement in the subcutaneous tissues of the medial forefoot (*short arrows*) and in the metatarsal head (*long arrows*) consistent with cellulitis and osteomyelitis. Similar signal abnormality is seen in the sesamoid bones (*arrowheads*), representing osteomyelitis

situation, more extensive edema and enhancement will be seen in the marrow.

19.4.2 Inflammatory Arthropathies

Inflammatory arthropathies such as rheumatoid arthritis, psoriatic arthritis, and Reiter's disease may involve the sesamoid bones (Resnick et al. 1977). All can cause synovitis of the first MTP joint, the appearance of which is similar to that of septic arthritis (Fig. 19.3). A joint effusion with thick synovial enhancement is commonly seen on MR images. Synovial inflammation can cause marginal erosions and reactive edema of the sesamoids. Although the pattern of disease and differential diagnosis are facilitated by radiographic analysis, subtle erosion of the sesamoids may be more apparent on CT or MR images. Of the inflammatory arthropathies, gout can have a distinct appearance on MR images (Yu et al. 1997); intraarticular and extraarticular tophi produce masslike foci of low signal on T1-weighted and T2-weighted images (Chen et al. 1999). Extraarticular tophi are also common adjacent to the first MTP joint and can cause extrinsic erosion of the sesamoid bones. Rheumatoid arthritis in particular causes capsular and ligamentous laxity, resulting in joint deformity. The sesamoid bones may become subluxated from their sulci, especially in the setting of hallux valgus. Silastic synovitis can also cause erosion of the sesamoids (Karasick and Schweitzer 1998; Taylor et al. 1993). Silastic implants have been used to replace severely arthritic first MTP joints (DeHeer et al. 1995). Fragmentation of the implant, which is low signal on all sequences, can cause a reactive synovitis (Chan et al. 1998) and erosion of the adjacent bone, including the sesamoids. Additionally, in the postoperative setting (e.g., following hallux valgus repair), joint effusion and mild synovitis are

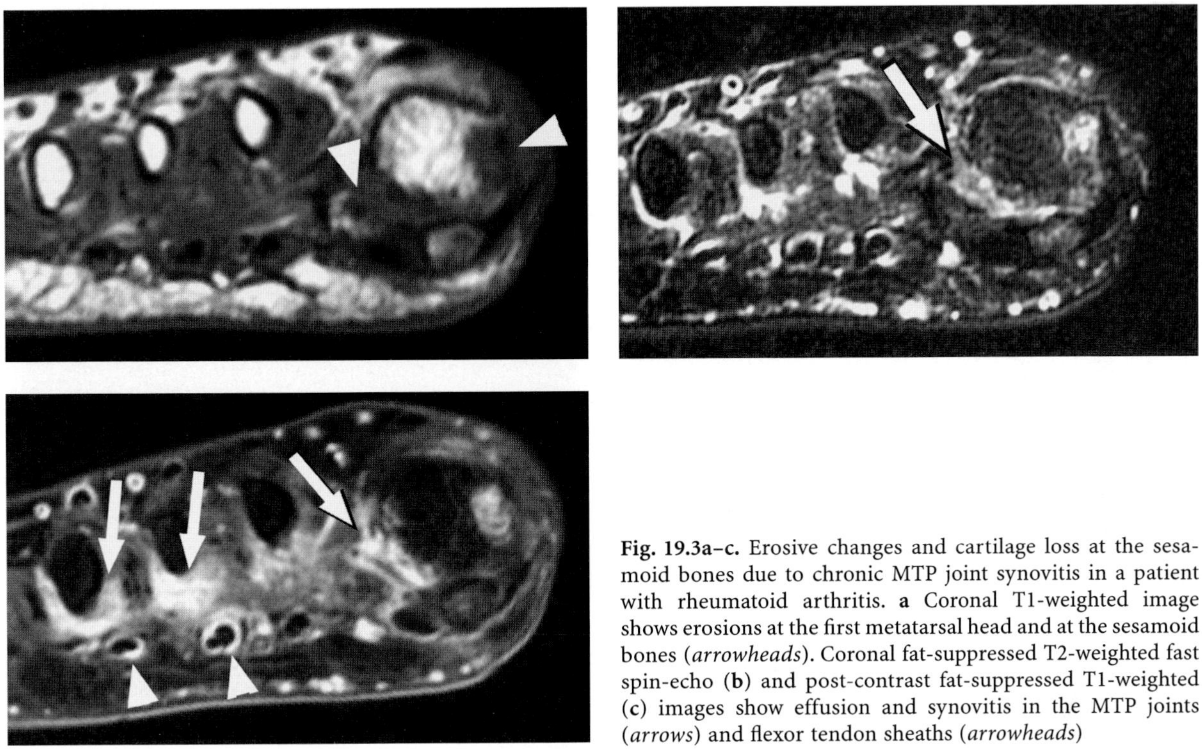

Fig. 19.3a–c. Erosive changes and cartilage loss at the sesamoid bones due to chronic MTP joint synovitis in a patient with rheumatoid arthritis. **a** Coronal T1-weighted image shows erosions at the first metatarsal head and at the sesamoid bones (*arrowheads*). Coronal fat-suppressed T2-weighted fast spin-echo (**b**) and post-contrast fat-suppressed T1-weighted (**c**) images show effusion and synovitis in the MTP joints (*arrows*) and flexor tendon sheaths (*arrowheads*)

common at the first MTP joint and may affect the associated MTS joint.

19.4.3 Osteoarthritis

Osteoarthritis is very common at the first MTP joint (Potter et al. 1992), and involvement of the MTS articulation generally mirrors the severity of the disease. At the arthritic MTS joint, initially there is loss of cartilage; associated joint narrowing may be very subtle on radiographs and CT images, but the cartilage loss is directly visualized on MR images. Subchondral cystic change is seen on both sides of the MTS joint (Fig. 19.4), and sclerosis may be present which radiographically can resemble AVN. This process can be differentiated from AVN on MR images. AVN diffusely replaces the sesamoid bone marrow on T1-weighted images (Karasick and Schweitzer 1998), whereas osteoarthritis preserves at least a portion of marrow fat signal. Osteoarthritis may also occur superimposed upon other etiologies, as an end-stage of the disease process. Processes that can accelerate the development of osteoarthritis include fracture, inflammatory arthropathy, infection, and AVN.

19.4.4 Avascular Necrosis

The sesamoid bones may be predisposed to the development of AVN because of the high loading forces they are exposed to during ambulation; the tibial sesamoid bears a disproportionate amount of force and has a reported higher incidence of AVN (Jahss 1981). Roentgenographic and CT changes with AVN (Fig. 19.5a,b) include irregularity, increased density, mottling, and fragmentation (Ogata et al. 1986; Potter et al. 1992); typically only one sesamoid bone is involved. The sclerosis is generally more extensive than would be expected from osteoarthritis and is not present on the metatarsal side of the joint. On MR images (Fig. 19.5c,d), the T2 signal can vary from low to high (Karasick and Schweitzer 1998), and the T1-weighted images help confirm the diagnosis; the T1 signal of the affected sesamoid is diffusely low in AVN with replacement of the normal marrow fat (Fleischli and Cheleuitte 1995). Unlike osteomyelitis, there is little to no surrounding soft-tissue inflammation, although often a joint effusion is present. AVN may result chronically in collapse and fragmentation of the sesamoid and secondary osteoarthritis of the MTS joint. If warranted, dynamic contrast-enhanced MR imaging can be performed to assess the viability of the bone.

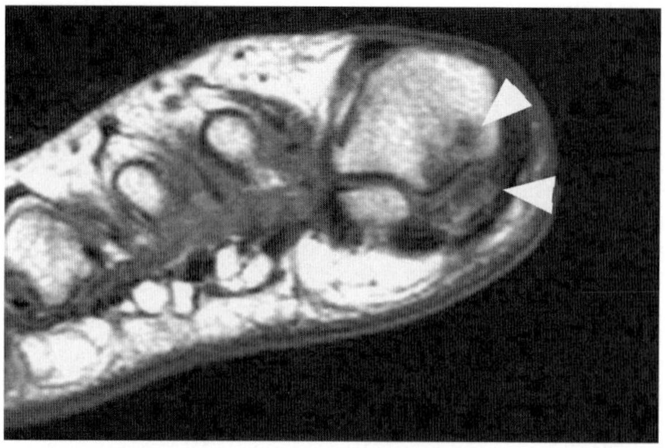
a

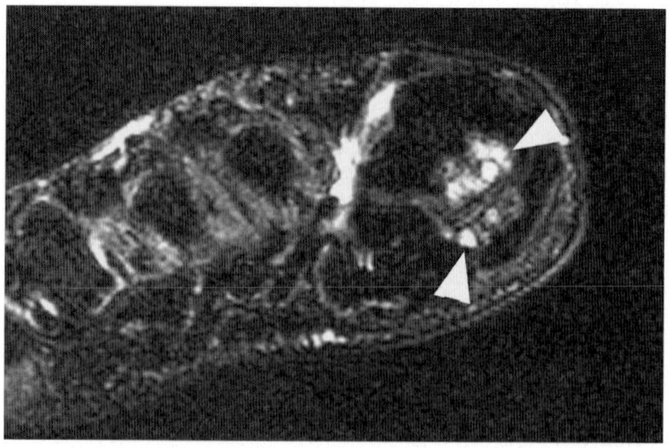
b

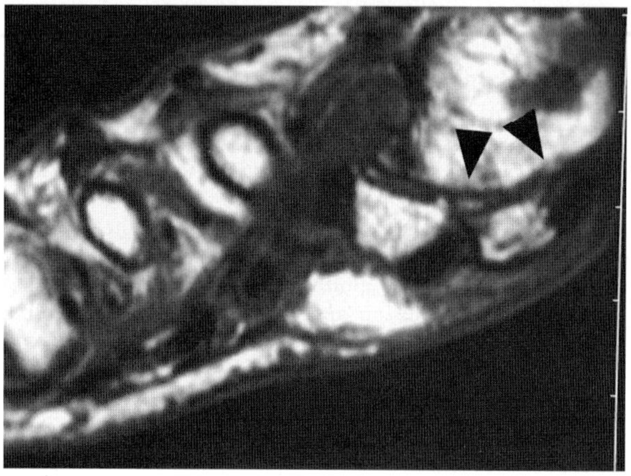
c

Fig. 19.4a–c. Osteoarthritis at the metatarsal-sesamoid joint. Coronal T1-weighted (**a**) and T2-weighted fat-suppressed (**b**) images show subchondral cysts at the tibial sesamoid which are present on both sides of the joint (*arrowheads*), consistent with osteoarthritis. **c** Coronal T1-weighted image of a different patient with hallux valgus demonstrates lateral shift of the sesamoids from their sulci (*arrowheads*) with osteophytes consistent with osteoarthritis

19.4.5 Sesamoiditis

Sesamoiditis is a painful inflammatory condition of the hallux sesamoid complex and surrounding soft tissues, thought to result from chronic repetitive stress or injury; however, the term 'sesamoiditis' has also been applied in a nonspecific fashion to describe pain associated with the sesamoids due to a variety of causes. Radiographs and CT are generally normal (Karasick and Schweitzer 1998; Taylor et al. 1993). MRI is useful to distinguish this condition (Fig. 19.6) from others such as AVN and fracture on MR images. On T1-weighted images, sesamoiditis can show a normal fat signal or low signal (Karasick and Schweitzer 1998). On T2-weighted or STIR images, sesamoiditis is seen as a diffuse high signal within the marrow of one or both sesamoids without a fracture line, whereas AVN is characterized by very low T1 and T2 signal. This pattern can, however, be difficult to differentiate from a stress response of the sesamoid; this distinction may not be important to make on MRI, since the two entities are likely to fall along the same disease spectrum caused by chronic repetitive trauma. Diffuse enhancement of the sesamoid may be seen if contrast is given; this can be useful to distinguish sesamoiditis from AVN, which would show little to no enhancement (Oloff and Schulhofer 1996).

In addition to bone marrow signal alteration, sesamoiditis may result in signal changes in the surrounding soft tissues related to inflammation (Karasick and Schweitzer 1998). Soft-tissue edema and enhancement may surround the sesamoids, and a first MTP joint effusion is commonly seen. Tenosynovitis of the flexor hallucis longus can also be seen, appearing as a fluid signal (typically a small amount) surrounding the tendon at the level of the sesamoids, and more proximally. However, it should be noted that fluid in the proximal FHL sheath is often a normal finding.

19.4.6 Stress Response/Fracture

Stress response, as noted above, is likely similar to sesamoiditis pathoetiologically (Burton and Amaker 1994). Both are caused by chronic repetitive trauma or stress and result in marrow signal altera-

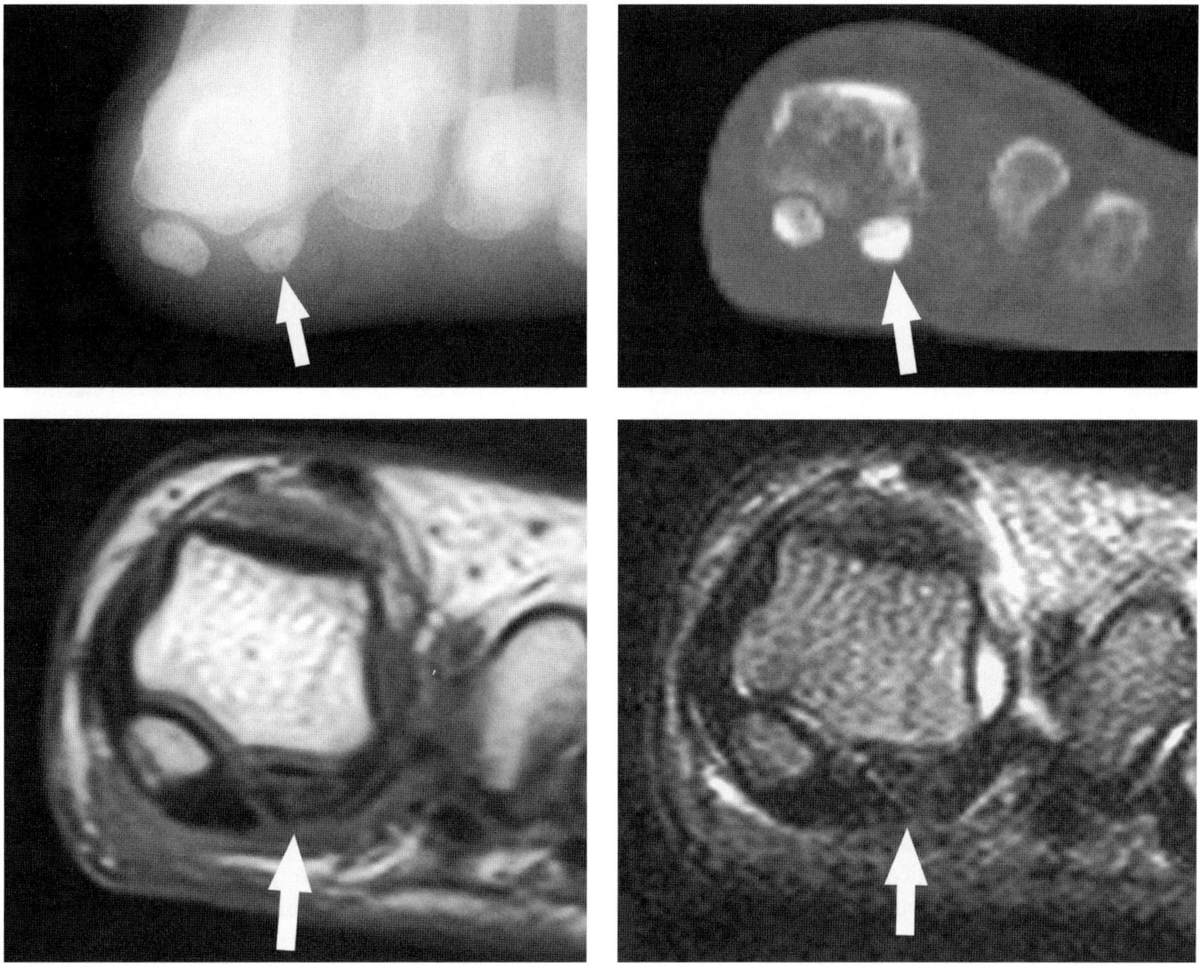

a b c d

Fig. 19.5a–d. Avascular necrosis of the fibular sesamoid. **a** Anteroposterior radiograph with the toes dorsiflexed (the 'sesamoid view') shows increased density of the fibular sesamoid (*arrow*). **b** Coronal CT image confirms the abnormal density (*arrow*). Coronal T1-weighted (**c**) and T2-weighted (**d**) images show low signal diffusely within the fibular sesamoid (*arrows*) compatible with avascular necrosis

tions within one or both sesamoids (high T2 signal, enhancement, and normal to slightly low T2 signal). When the soft-tissue inflammatory component is minimal or absent, the term 'stress response' is probably more accurate. If the stresses producing these changes are not eased, a discrete fracture line may develop, seen as a linear low signal on T1-weighted and T2-weighted images. At this point, the MR imaging appearance is identical to a subacute fracture, and only the patient's history can define the etiology. If no single traumatic event can be found, the term 'stress fracture' is applied. It is important to image the sesamoids in multiple planes so that the fracture line can be detected. This fracture line may not be visible on radiographic (Van Hal et al. 1982) or CT images, or may be perceived as a slightly increased density of one sesamoid.

19.4.7 Acute Trauma

Acute sesamoid fracture can generally be detected radiographically, like other acute fractures. However, they are often overlooked on initial inspection because of the high incidence of bipartite sesamoids, which can have a similar appearance (Potter et al. 1992). There are differentiating features that can be applied when a possible sesamoid fracture is observed on trauma radiographs. First, the bipartite sesamoid has rounded edges, whereas an acute fracture has sharp edges (Feldman et al. 1970; Taylor et al. 1993). Second, the pieces of a bipartite, when summated, are generally noticeably larger than the other sesamoid (Karasick and Schweitzer 1998). This is not the case with an acute fracture. Finally, bipartite sesamoids should not

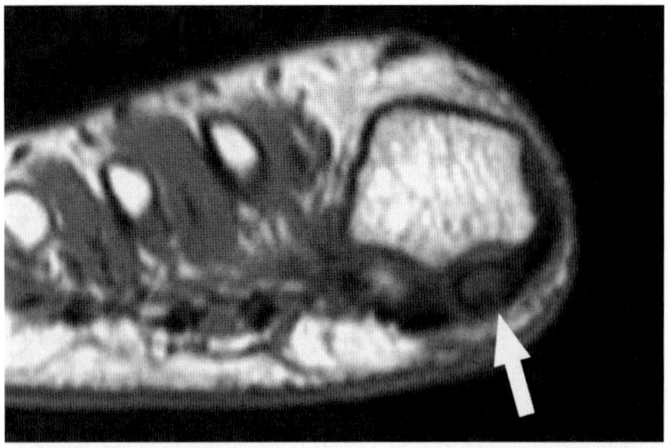
a

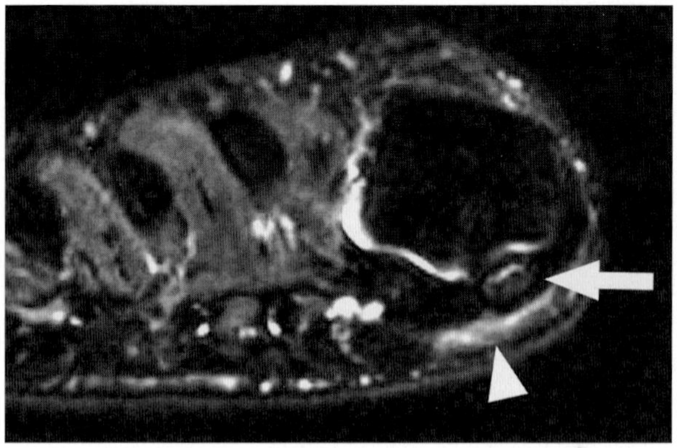
b

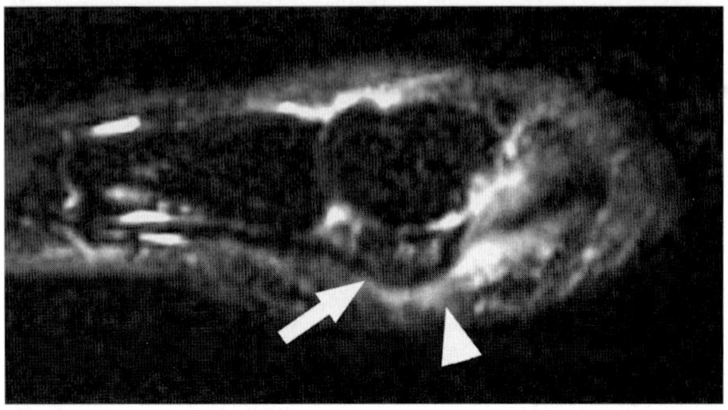
c

Fig. 19.6a–c. Sesamoiditis affecting the tibial sesamoid bone. **a** Coronal T1-weighted image shows slightly low signal in the tibial sesamoid (*arrow*). Coronal (**b**) and sagittal (**c**) T2-weighted fat-suppressed images show edema within the sesamoid (*arrows*), but there is no fracture line. There is also fluid in the MTP joint and subcutaneous edema (*arrowheads*) compatible with sesamoiditis

change over time. A short follow-up period of 5–7 days will show evolution of a fracture, initially with surrounding bone resorption and apparent widening of the fracture line, and subsequent sclerosis as the healing response progresses. Of course, if old films are available, such ambiguity is removed. Because sesamoid fractures are often overlooked on initial radiographs, patients are occasionally referred for MR imaging to explain the persistent pain (Fig. 19.7). Because of the delay in referral to MRI, the injury is nearly always subacute when imaging is performed. As noted above, the MR appearance of subacute sesamoid fracture is virtually indistinguishable from stress fracture, except for the history of a single traumatic episode. Both can show sesamoid marrow edema and normal to slightly low T1 signal, with a discrete low signal fracture line. To detect the fracture line, multiple imaging planes should be acquired, although the sagittal plane is best because most commonly the fracture line is oriented in the coronal plane. Small field-of-view images (10–12 cm) and/or thin sections facilitate detection of the fracture line.

19.4.8 Nonunion and Pseudoarthrosis

As the injury becomes chronic, undetected sesamoid fracture can lead to the development of a nonunion or pseudoarthrosis between the fragments. On radiographs, persistence of the fracture line will be seen; the edges may become rounded akin to a bipartite sesamoid, but unlike a bipartite, the size of the fragments is similar to that of the other sesamoid. Sclerosis may be seen at the margins of the fracture line (Taylor et al. 1993). On MR images, two types of nonunion can be characterized: fibrous and synovial. In a fibrous nonunion, the sesamoid fragments are connected by intermediate to low signal tissue on T1-weighted and T2-weighted images. In a synovial nonunion (or 'pseudoarthrosis'), fluid signal is seen between the sesamoid fragments. The adjacent sesamoid marrow is edematous, reflecting the chronic stress from abnormal motion between the fragments. Note that bipartite sesamoids also have intermediate to low signal tissue between the pieces, similar to a fibrous nonunion. Also, acute trauma or chronic stress can lyse this fibrous bipartite attachment, resulting in an appearance similar to that of a synovial nonunion or pseudoarthrosis.

19.4.9 Capsular/Ligamentous Injury

In acute trauma, the capsule of the first MTP joint and associated ligaments may be injured. This is

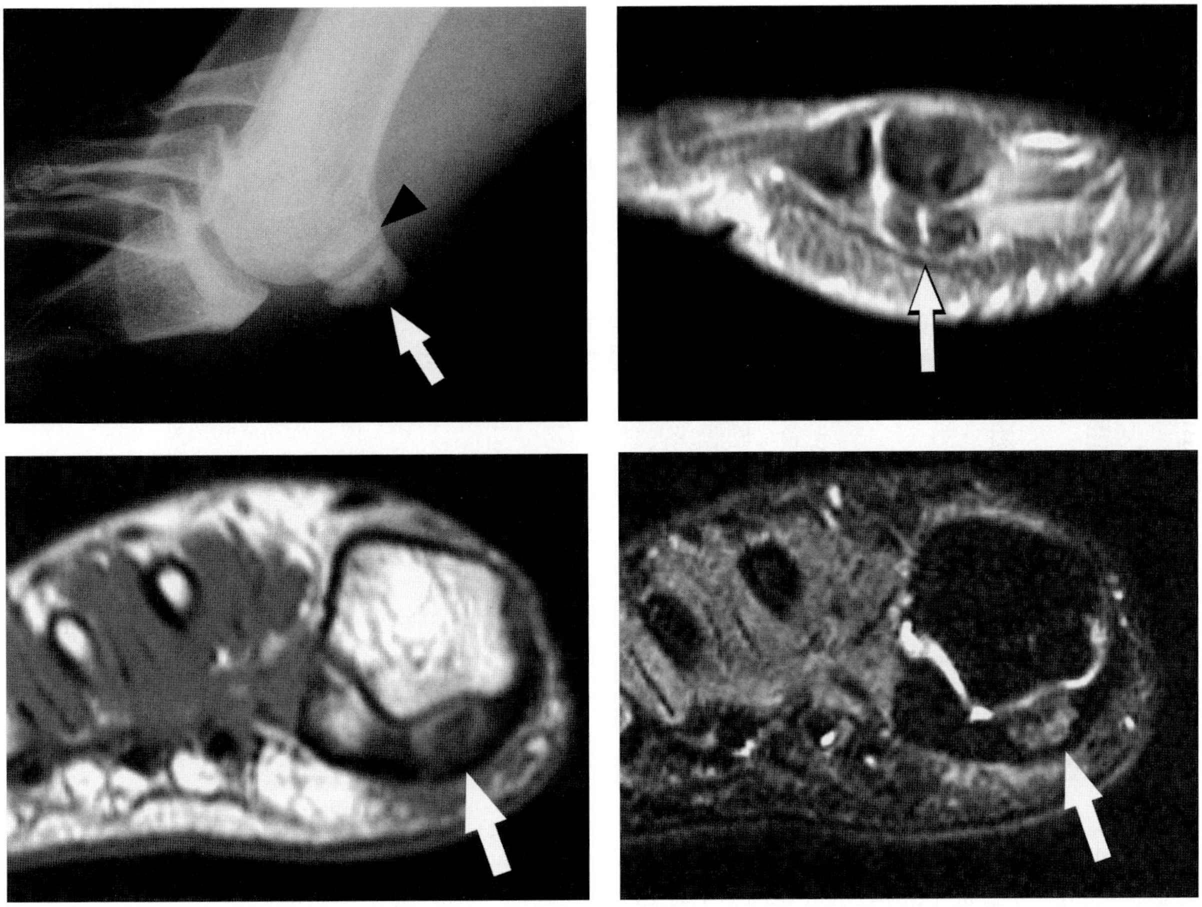

Fig. 19.7a–d. Fracture of the tibial sesamoid. **a** Lateral radiograph shows a linear lucency through the tibial sesamoid (*arrow*); note that unlike a bipartite sesamoid, the margins of the fracture are sharp, and the size of the fragments is equal to the other sesamoid (*arrowhead*). The fracture line (*arrow*) is well seen on a post-contrast sagittal T1-weighted fat-suppressed image (**b**). Coronal T1-weighted (**c**) and fat-suppressed T2-weighted (**d**) images show replacement of fat with edema in the sesamoid (*arrow*)

especially the case in hyperextension injuries to the MTP joint. The MTP joint and/or sesamoids may even transiently dislocate, resulting in a radiographic finding of soft-tissue swelling only. Slight malpositioning or separation of the sesamoids should raise the suspicion of a ligamentous injury. MR imaging (Fig. 19.8) is the optimal method for the evaluation of the capsular ligamentous complex. The intersesamoid ligament is seen on coronal images, and disruption is clearly evident, especially on T2-weighted images, with fluid penetrating through the normally low signal fibers. Disruption of this ligament results in increased separation of the sesamoids and subluxation from the sulci (Capasso et al. 1990). Similarly, disruption of the sesamoid phalangeal ligament is detectable, especially on T2-weighted images in the sagittal or axial planes. Disruption of this ligament causes the involved sesamoid to migrate proximally. Disruption of the plantar capsule, also known as 'turf toe', is a relatively common entity in high performance athletes involved in sports that require running with rapid change in speed and direction (Rodeo et al. 1990). The injury is accentuated by artificial playing surfaces (Bowers and Martin 1974). Radiographs and CT are normal. MRI shows effusion within the first MTP joint with synovitis, seen as 'dirty' fluid, or intermediate signal material within the joint. The synovium enhances brightly with gadolinium contrast. Fluid signal, edema, and enhancement extend into the plantar soft tissues adjacent to the joint, indicating capsular injury (Karasick and Schweitzer 1998). Unlike sesamoiditis, the marrow signal is normal. A similar pattern can be seen in inflammatory arthropathies such as rheumatoid arthritis, but a history of trauma and lack of erosions limit the differential diagnosis.

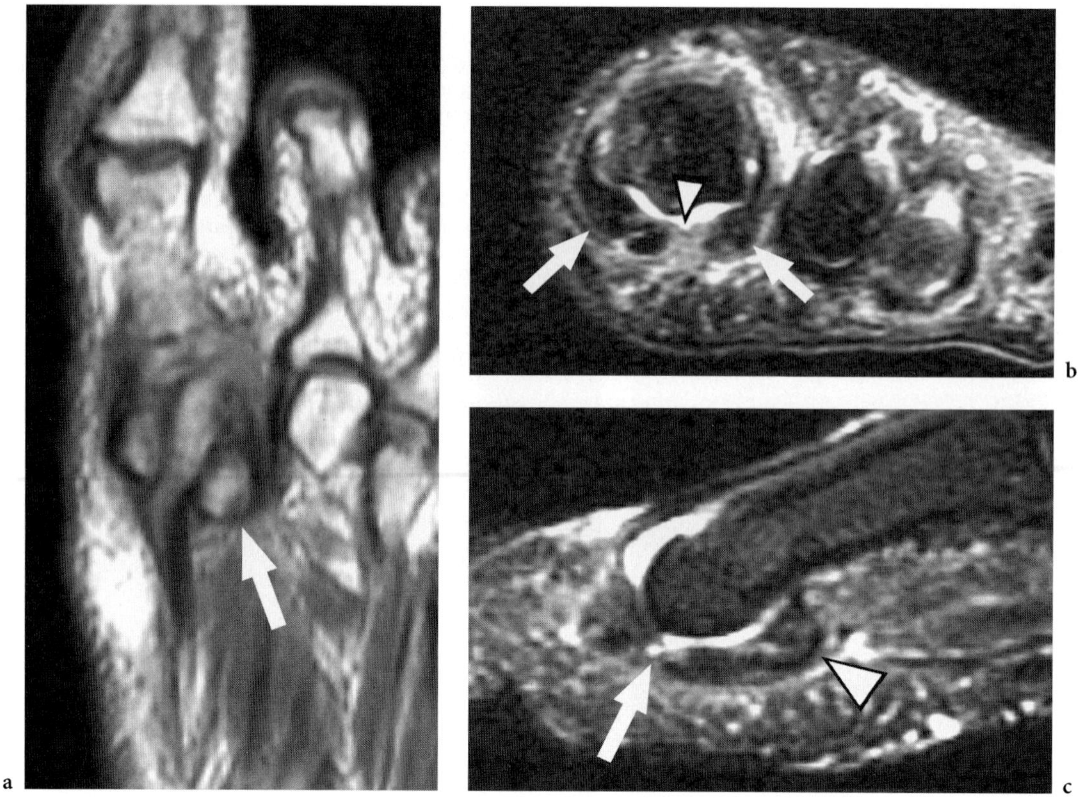

Fig. 19.8a–c. Trauma with sesamoid ligament injury. **a** After a hyperextension injury and suspected transient dislocation of the first MTP joint, an axial T1-weighted image shows abnormal separation of the sesamoids and proximal positioning of the fibular sesamoid (*arrow*). **b** Coronal fat-suppressed T2-weighted image shows tear of the intersesamoid ligament (*arrowhead*) with separation of the sesamoid bones (*arrows*) and subluxation of both from their sulci. **c** Sagittal fat-suppressed T2-weighted image shows that proximal positioning of the fibular sesamoid (*arrowhead*) is related to a tear of the sesamoid-phalangeal ligament (*arrow*)

References

Bowers KD, Martin RB (1974) Impact absorption, new and old AstroTurf at West Virginia University. Med Sci Sports 6:217–221

Brower AC (1996) Septic arthritis. Radiol Clin North Am 34: 293–309

Burton EM, Amaker BH (1994) Stress fracture of the great toe sesamoid in a ballerina: MRI appearance. Pediatr Radiol 24:37–38

Capasso G, Maffulli N, Testa V (1990) Rupture of the intersesamoid ligament of a soccer player's foot. Foot Ankle 10:337–339

Chan M, Chowchuen P, Workman T et al (1998) Silicone synovitis: MR imaging in five patients. Skeletal Radiol 27: 13–17

Chen CK, Yeh LR, Pan HB et al (1999) Intra-articular gouty tophi of the knee: CT and MR imaging in 12 patients. Skeletal Radiol 28:75–80

Coughlin MJ (1990) Sesamoid pain: causes and surgical treatment. Instr Course Lect 39:23–35

David RD, Delagoutte JP, Renard MM (1989) Anatomical study of the sesamoid bones of the first metatarsal. J Am Podiatr Med Assoc 79:536–544

DeHeer DH, Owens SR, Swanson AB (1995) The host response to silicone elastomer implants for small joint arthroplasty. J Hand Surg [Am] 20:101–109

Feldman F, Pochaczevsky R, Hecht H (1970) The case of the wandering sesamoid and other sesamoid afflictions. Radiology 96:275–283

Fleischli J, Cheleuitte E (1995) Avascular necrosis of the hallucial sesamoids. J Foot Ankle Surg 34:358–365

Graif M, Schweitzer ME, Deely D et al (1999) The septic versus nonseptic inflamed joint: MRI characteristics. Skeletal Radiol 28:616–620

Jahss MH (1981) The sesamoids of the hallux. Clin Orthop 157:88–97

Karasick D, Schweitzer ME (1998) Disorders of the hallux sesamoid complex: MR features. Skeletal Radiol 27: 411–418

Leventon EO (1991) Sesamoid disorders and treatment. Clin Orthop 269:236–240

Morrison WB, Schweitzer ME, Bock GW et al (1993) Diagnosis of osteomyelitis: utility of fat-suppressed contrast-enhanced MR imaging. Radiology 189:251–257

Morrison WB, Schweitzer ME, Wapner KL et al (1995)

Osteomyelitis in feet of diabetics: clinical accuracy, surgical utility, and cost-effectiveness of MR imaging. Radiology 196:557–564

Morrison WB, Schweitzer ME, Batte WG et al (1998) Osteomyelitis of the foot: relative importance of primary and secondary MR imaging signs. Radiology 207:625–632

Ogata K, Sugioka Y, Urano Y et al (1986) Idiopathic osteonecrosis of the first metatarsal sesamoid. Skeletal Radiol 15:141–145

Oloff LM, Schulhofer SD (1996) Sesamoid complex disorders. Clin Podiatr Med Surg 13:497–513

Potter HG, Pavlov H, Abrahams TG (1992) The hallux sesamoids revisited. Skeletal Radiol 21:437–444

Resnick D, Niwayama G, Feingold ML (1977) The sesamoid bones of the hands and feet: participators in arthritis. Radiology 123:57–62

Richardson EG (1987) Injuries to the hallucal sesamoids in the athlete. Foot Ankle 7:229–244

Rodeo SA, O'Brien S, Warren RF et al (1990) Turf-toe: an analysis of metatarsophalangeal joint sprains in professional football players. Am J Sports Med 18:280–285

Taylor JA, Sartoris DJ, Huang GS et al (1993) Painful conditions affecting the first metatarsal sesamoid bones. Radiographics 13:817–830

Van Hal ME, Keene JS, Lange TA et al (1982) Stress fractures of the great toe sesamoids. Am J Sports Med 10:122–128

Yu JS, Chung C, Recht M et al (1997) MR imaging of tophaceous gout. AJR 168:523–527

20 Tumours and Tumour-like Lesions

D. A. Ritchie, A. M. Davies, and D. Vanel

CONTENTS

D. A. Ritchie, MD
Royal Liverpool University Hospitals, Prescot Street, Liverpool, L7 8XP, UK
A. M. Davies, MD
MRI Centre, Royal Orthopaedic Hospital, Birmingham, B31 2AP, UK
D. Vanel, MD
Institut Gustave Roussy, 39 rue Camille Desmoulins, 94805 Villejuif, France

20.1 Introduction

In recent years, the management of tumours and tumour-like lesions of the foot and ankle has improved, and this is due in part to advances in imaging. The introduction of cross-sectional imaging, particularly magnetic resonance (MR) imaging, has had a major impact in tumour imaging, particularly in surgical staging. True osseous or soft-tissue neoplasms of the foot and ankle are relatively uncommon and are greatly outnumbered by tumour-like conditions. This chapter discusses the role of imaging in tumours and tumour-like conditions of the foot and ankle and is followed by an illustrated review of the various bone and soft-tissue conditions according to tissue of origin.

20.2 Imaging Tumours and Tumour-like Lesions

20.2.1 Epidemiology

Bone and soft-tissue tumours are typically classified according to the tissue of origin (Enzinger and Weiss 1995; Mirra 1989) (Tables 20.1 and 20.2). There are several series analysing tumours of the ankle and foot, but some are restricted only to the foot, and most are affected to an extent by tertiary referral patterns that skew the true incidence (Kransdorf 1995a,b; Campanacci 1990; Unni 1996; Ozdemir et al. 1997; Murari et al. 1989; Casadei et al. 1991). In a large series of 307,601 soft-tissue and bony lesions of the foot, pseudotumorous nerve lesions were by far the most common lesions, with Morton's neuromas accounting for 42.6% and traumatic neuromas accounting for 19.5% of all tumour or tumour-like conditions of the foot and ankle (Berlin 1995). Only 0.55% were due to soft-tissue malignancies, and most of these were Kaposi's sarcoma, skin tumours that do

Table 20.1. Classification of bone tumours according to tissue of origin and incidence of benign and malignant bone tumours in the foot and ankle (Unni 1996; Campanacci 1990) (in Unni's series, the classification excludes tumour-like conditions including non-ossifying fibroma, fibrous dysplasia, osteofibrous dysplasia, eosinophilic granuloma, simple bone cyst, aneurysmal bone cyst)

Tissue of origin	Benign lesion of bone (n=175, Unni; n=234, Campanacci)	Percentage of benign tumours	Primary malignant tumour of bone (n=185, Unni; n=102, Campanacci)	Percentage of malignant tumours
Bone-forming	Osteoid osteoma	29.6	Osteosarcoma (and variants)	33.4
	Osteoblastoma	5.1		
Cartilage-forming	Enchondroma	12.7	Chondrosarcoma (and variants)	18.5
	Osteochondroma	22.7		
	Chondroblastoma	4.9		
	Chondromyxoid fibroma	4.4		
Fibrous and fibrohistiocytic	Desmoplastic fibroma	<1.0	Fibrosarcoma and malignant fibrous histiocytoma	10.8
	Benign fibrous histiocytoma	<1.0		
Vascular	Haemangioma	<1.0	Angiosarcoma, haemangioendothelioma and haemangiopericytoma	4.8
	Glomus tumour	0		
	Cystic angiomatosis	0		
Haematopoietic, reticuloendothelial and lymphatic	Giant-cell tumour	16.9	Lymphoma	4.5
	Lymphangioma	0	Leukaemia	0
			Myeloma	0
			Ewing's sarcoma	28.2
Neural	Neurofibroma	0	Malignant nerve sheath tumour	0
	Neurolemmoma	0	Primitive neuroectodermal tumour	0
Fat	Lipoma	0	Liposarcoma	0
Unknown			Adamantinoma	2.8

not usually require imaging. The true incidences of benign and malignant bone tumours were 0.16% and 0.01%, respectively.

In Kransdorf's (1995b) analysis of 12,370 cases of soft-tissue sarcoma, 5.21% were located in the foot and ankle (Table 20.2). Synovial sarcoma accounted for 18.7% of cases and was the most common soft-tissue sarcoma among patients aged 5–45 years. Clear-cell sarcoma also affects young adults and was the second most common sarcoma among the 16–35 year age group. Malignant fibrous histiocytoma (16.4%) was the most common among the 45–65 year age group and Kaposi's sarcoma (11.3%) in patients over 65 years old. In Kransdorf's (1995a) series of 18,677 benign soft-tissue tumours (including some tumour-like lesions), 7.25% were located in the foot and ankle. Fibromatosis accounted for 22% of all lesions and was the most common tumour in patients aged between 5 and 75 years.

Bone tumours of the foot and ankle are uncommon, accounting for 3.25%–3.35% of all primary bone tumours (Unni 1996; Campanacci 1990). Overall, osteosarcoma and Ewing's sarcoma are the most common malignant bone tumours, with the majority found in the distal tibia and fibula (Table 20.1). In the forefoot, chondrosarcoma and Ewing's sarcoma are more common than osteosarcoma. In the foot, Ewing's sarcoma most commonly presents in the second/third decades, osteosarcoma in the fourth decade and chondrosarcoma in the fifth and sixth decades. Osteochondromas and giant-cell tumours are the most common benign bone tumours of the foot and ankle, but over 70% of these occur in the distal tibia and fibula. In the foot, osteoid osteomas are the most common tumour in

Table 20.2. Classification of soft-tissue tumours and tumour-like lesions according to tissue of origin and incidence of benign and malignant soft-tissue tumours in the foot and ankle (Kransdorf and Murphey 1997)

Tissue of origin	Benign soft-tissue tumour of foot and ankle (n=1355)	Percentage of benign tumours	Malignant soft-tissue tumours of foot and ankle (n=645)	Percentage of malignant tumours
Fibrohistiocytic	Benign fibrous histiocytoma	13.1	Malignant fibrous histiocytoma	16.4
	Juvenile xanthogranuloma	0.1	Dermatofibrosarcoma protuberans	6.0
			Atypical fibroblastoma	0.5
Fibrous	Fibroma	1.6	Fibrosarcoma	6.7
	Nodular/proliferative fasciitis	1.4		
	Fibroma of tendon sheath	1.6		
	Infantile fibromatosis	1.6		
	Calcifying aponeurotic fibroma	0.9		
	Plantar fibromatosis	16.0		
	Deep fibromatosis	6.0		
Fat	Lipoma (+ variants)	6.3	Liposarcoma	4.8
	Lipoblastoma	0.7		
Vascular and lymphatic	Haemangioma	7.3	Angiosarcoma	2.0
	Glomus tumour	0.9	Haemangioendothelioma	4.2
	Haemangiopericytoma (benign)	0.7	Haemangiopericytoma (malignant)	0.0
	Papillary endothelial hyperplasia	0.9	Kaposi's sarcoma	11.3
	Lymphangioma/ lymphangiomatosis	0.5		
Synovial	Synovial chondromatosis	0.5	Synovial sarcoma[b]	18.6
	Pigmented villonodular synovitis	3.8	Malignant GCTTS	0.15
	Giant-cell tumour of tendon sheath (GCTTS)	8.3		
Neural	Neuroma[a]	2.3	Malignant nerve sheath tumour	4.5
	Neurofibroma	4.3	Primitive neuroectodermal tumour	0.15
	Neurolemmoma	6.0	Extraskeletal Ewing's sarcoma	0.6
	Neurothekoma	0.4	Clear-cell sarcoma	7.6
	Granular-cell tumour	0.9		
Cartilage/bone-forming	Panniculitis ossificans	0.1	Extraskeletal osteosarcoma	0.6
	Extraskeletal chondroma	5.6	Extraskeletal chondrosarcoma	3.6
Muscle	Leiomyoma (including angiomyoma)	5.7	Leiomyosarcoma	7.1
	Rhabdomyoma	0.0	Rhabdomyosarcoma	1.9
Unknown	Tumoral calcinosis	0.2	Epithelioid sarcoma	2.3
	Myxoma	1.8		
Tumour-like lesions	Ganglion cyst	1.3		
	Granuloma annulare	8.1		
	Synovial cyst	0.4		

[a] The low incidence reflects the referral pattern

[b] Synovial sarcoma is a mesenchymal tumour and does not derive from synovium; however, it resembles synovial tissue on light microscopy, and therefore the name has remained

the hindfoot and enchondroma in the forefoot. Osteochondromas and osteoid osteomas tend to present in the second decade, whereas giant-cell tumours and enchondromas are more common in the third decade.

20.2.2 Imaging Techniques and Lesion Detection

Musculoskeletal tumours and tumour-like lesions usually present with swelling and/or pain. The compact structure and paucity of soft tissues around the foot and ankle often result in early presentation and easily palpable lesions.

Radiography should be the initial imaging investigation. For bone tumours, the radiograph remains the most reliable predictor of the histological nature of a tumour among all the imaging techniques, although detection depends to a degree on the radiographic technique and the size, location and aggressiveness of the lesion. Soft-tissue lesions will only be seen if they display mass effect, bone or joint involvement, or mineralisation.

Bone scintigraphy, usually with ^{99m}Tc-methylene diphosphonate, is highly sensitive but relatively nonspecific and with limited anatomical resolution. In malignant bone tumours, the main role of scintigraphy lies in the detection of metastatic disease. Scintigraphy is of limited value in the assessment of benign bone tumours but may play a significant role in the detection of osteoid osteomas.

Ultrasound (US) is an important imaging technique in the initial assessment of soft-tissue masses in the foot and ankle and is the imaging method of choice for small superficial lesions. The limited depth of the soft tissues allows the use of high-frequency probes providing high-resolution imaging. US is readily available, differentiates cystic from solid lesions and assists biopsy, while colour flow Doppler techniques allow the assessment of vascular lesions.

Computed tomography (CT) with fast high-resolution thin-slice techniques and multiplanar image reformatting is sensitive in detecting matrix mineralisation and demonstrating fine cortical detail. However, with the advent of MR imaging, CT is now of limited importance.

MR imaging now has an established role in imaging tumours and tumour-like conditions, particularly in staging. MR imaging is also the most sensitive imaging technique for lesion detection. Care should be taken in the interpretation as the sensitivity of MR imaging is such that many incidental findings are discovered which have no clinical relevance (Fig. 20.1). Appropriate coil selection and slice thickness are required for lesion coverage and high-quality images. As many structures in the foot do not lie in orthogonal planes, oblique planes may be required for optimal evaluation. Protocols vary with anatomical site and lesion extent (see Section 20.2.4, Staging).

20.2.3 Characterisation

Before assessing any imaging studies it is important to have relevant clinical information. The age of the patient is important, but it is worth noting that the age range for some foot tumours may differ from the same tumour at more proximal sites. It is also important to be aware of any pre-existing lesion or hereditary condition such as multiple enchondromatosis (Ollier's disease).

20.2.3.1 Location

Some bone tumours have a predilection for a particular bone. Osteoid osteoma and osteoblastoma commonly arise at the talar neck, and simple bone

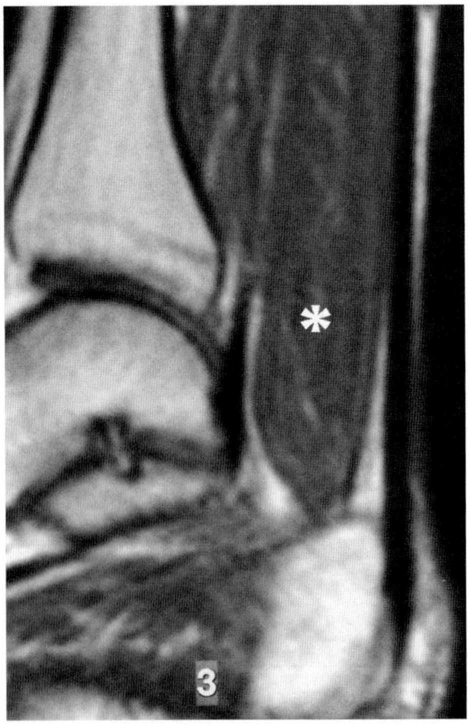

Fig. 20.1. Sagittal T1-weighted MR image showing an accessory soleus muscle – normal variant (*asterisk*) that may present as a soft-tissue mass

cysts and intraosseous lipomas in the calcaneus. The location of a tumour within a bone can also be described in transverse or longitudinal planes, but the differentiation of eccentric and central lesions in the foot in the transverse plane may be difficult due to the small cross-section of the bones. Similarly, in the longitudinal plane, since the physis of small foot bones is relatively small, differentiation of lesions into the various zones may not be possible.

However, the calcaneus has identifiable sites that correspond to the physeal zones. The calcaneal apophysis and the subarticular portions of the upper and anterior calcaneus correspond to the epiphysis equivalent zone, the bone adjacent to the metaphyseal zone, and the central calcaneus to the diaphyseal zone. Chondroblastoma frequently occurs in the apophysis posteriorly and adjacent to the posterior calcaneal facet, both epiphyseal equivalent sites. Giant-cell tumours are also found at the sites of old apophyses and occur most commonly in the anterior and posterior margins of the calcaneus. Osteoid osteoma appears most often in the subtalar region, and simple bone cysts and lipomas usually in the anterior third of the calcaneus. Of the malignant bony lesions, metastases and Ewing's sarcoma tend to occur centrally in the body and at the tuberosity of the calcaneus, but osteosarcoma has no predilection for site.

Of the soft-tissue masses, Morton's neuroma is by far the most common mass in the forefoot and typically arises in the 3rd and to a lesser extent the 2nd intermetatarsal spaces. Plantar fibromatosis is the most common lesion in the plantar region and, by definition, arises in the plantar fascia. Ganglion cysts and lipomas are the most common lesions in the midfoot and hindfoot. Soft-tissue sarcomas are less common in the forefoot.

20.2.3.2 *Radiographic Features*

It is usually possible to characterise the aggressiveness of the tumour from the radiograph, but when analysing the radiographic features in the foot, some modifications have to be borne in mind. Lesions in the foot do not have to achieve a large size to become symptomatic. The small size of many bones means that involvement of an entire bone is not uncommon. Early bone destruction and periosteal reaction are more easily detected in the small, thin tubular bones of the forefoot than in the larger bones of the midfoot and hindfoot. Intralesional mineralisation is readily detected and should suggest a lesion of osseous or cartilaginous origin. However, in the soft tissues, mineralisation may also be present in other tumour types including haemangiomas (phleboliths) and in up to one-third of synovial sarcomas.

20.2.3.3 *Cross-sectional Imaging*

Ultrasound readily distinguishes cystic from solid lesions and thus may obviate the need for further imaging. Ganglion cysts are typically homogeneous and transonic and usually have a rounded or lobulated outline. In Morton's neuroma, ultrasound typically shows an ovoid, hypoechoic mass between the metatarsal heads, but lesions smaller than 5 mm may be missed (Kaminsky et al. 1997). CT is accurate in defining the attenuation of lesions and is therefore helpful in detecting lesion mineralisation or fat. On MR imaging, as most lesions display non-specific intermediate signal intensity (similar to muscle) on T1-weighting and high signal intensity on T2-weighting, tissue characterisation based on signal intensities alone is not usually possible. In addition, the signal intensity and homogeneity will also vary with the type of tumour matrix as well as with the presence of haemorrhage and necrosis. However, some lesions may have characteristic findings. Cystic lesions such as ganglia and simple bone cysts display homogeneous low signal intensity on T1-weighting, very high signal intensity on T2-weighting, and show either no or rim enhancement. Lipomas usually have a characteristic homogeneous pattern with a signal intensity equal to that of fat on all pulse sequences. Haemangiomas also contain fatty tissue but typically also have serpentine vascular structures. Some lesions produce a low/intermediate signal intensity on both T1-weighting and T2-weighting, including pigmented villonodular synovitis (Fig. 20.2) due to haemosiderin (Bravo et al. 1996) and fibromatosis (Fig. 20.3) due to high collagen content (Morrison et al. 1994). The detection of fluid-fluid levels (sedimentation effect) in an expansile bone lesion in an adolescent is highly suggestive of an aneurysmal bone cyst (Fig. 20.4), although fluid-fluid levels may also be seen in other lesions including giant-cell tumour and chondroblastoma.

20.2.4 Staging

Further management will depend on an analysis of the imaging features in conjunction with the patient's age and clinical presentation. Some benign lesions such as

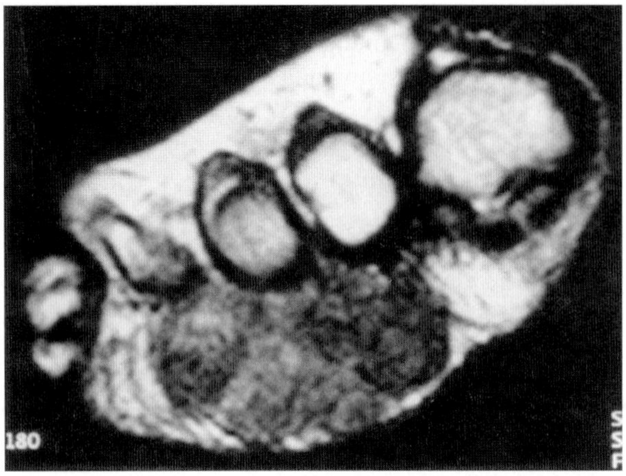

Fig. 20.2. Giant-cell tumour of the tendon sheath of flexor digitorum longus on the plantar aspect of the 3rd metatarsal bone in a 19-year-old woman. Coronal T2-weighted MR image. On T2-weighting, the lesion is moderately inhomogeneous and mainly of low/intermediate signal intensity (SI) due to the haemosiderin effect

a 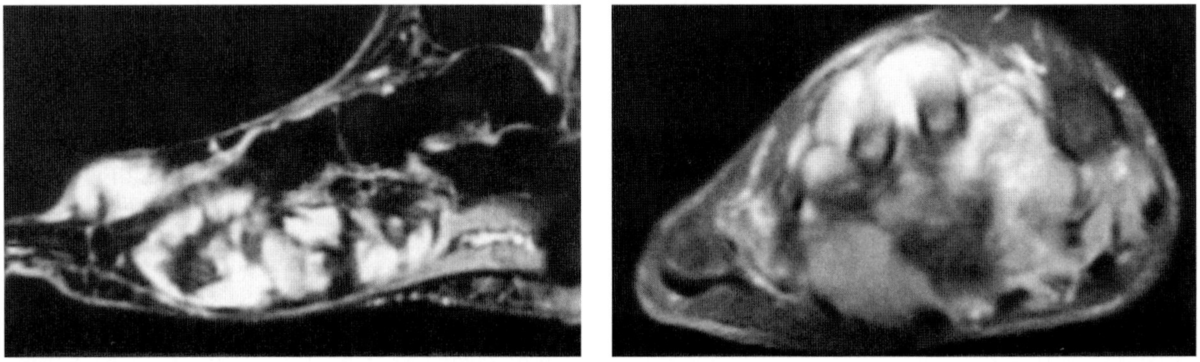 b

Fig. 20.3a, b. Aggressive fibromatosis. Sagittal STIR (**a**) and coronal postintravenous Gd-DTPA T1-weighted (**b**) MR images showing a large, ill-defined, inhomogeneous mass extending from the deep plantar soft tissues onto the dorsal aspect of the foot distally. Most of the mass displays high SI on STIR and enhances, but centrally there are several foci of non-enhancing low-SI tissue due to dense collagen

a 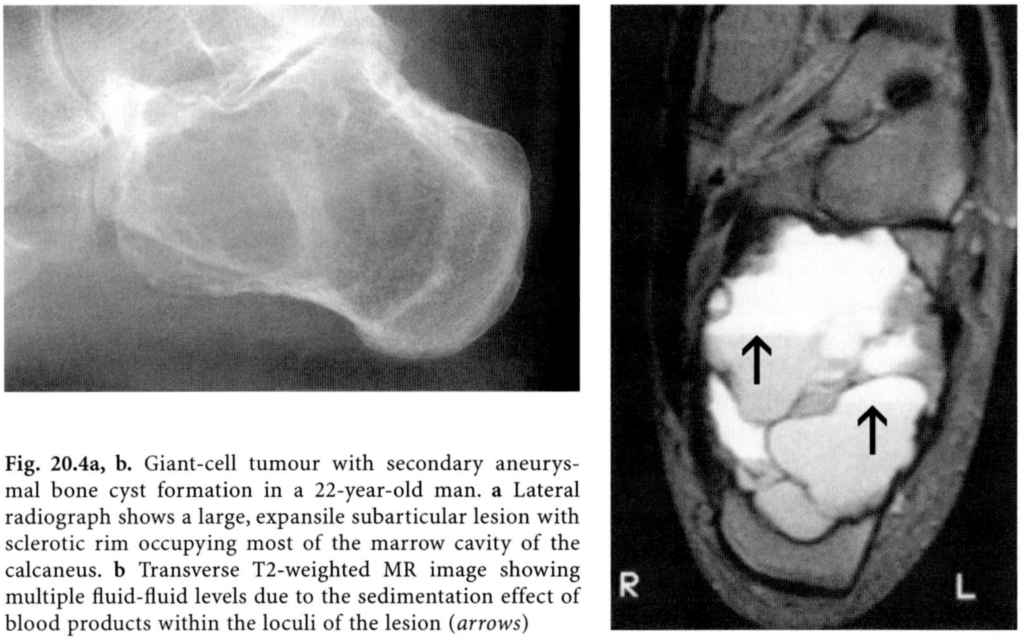 b

Fig. 20.4a, b. Giant-cell tumour with secondary aneurysmal bone cyst formation in a 22-year-old man. **a** Lateral radiograph shows a large, expansile subarticular lesion with sclerotic rim occupying most of the marrow cavity of the calcaneus. **b** Transverse T2-weighted MR image showing multiple fluid-fluid levels due to the sedimentation effect of blood products within the loculi of the lesion (*arrows*) a bone island are discovered incidentally and can be regarded as 'leave me alone' lesions that do not require further imaging, biopsy or follow-up. Other lesions such as intra-osseous lipoma might be followed up by periodic radiographic examination, whereas a simple bone cyst may require treatment. When a malignant or indeterminate lesion is suspected, local staging will be required to assess the tumour extent prior to biopsy.

The objective of surgical staging is to define the tumour in terms of histological grade and anatomical extent. Of the staging systems, the Enneking et al. (1980) system (Musculoskeletal Tumour Society) is probably the most popular one and can be applied to soft-tissue and bone sarcomas. Stage 1 lesions are classified as histologically low-grade lesions, whereas stage 2 lesions are high grade. The stages are subdivided into A and B depending on whether the lesion is intracompartmental (A) or extracompartmental (B) and is based on imaging findings. Patients with metastases at presentation are classified as stage 3, irrespective of the histological grade.

In the foot and ankle, although lesions confined to a single ray or one of the three compartments of the plantar side of the midfoot are intracompartmental, many lesions of the hindfoot and midfoot are extracompartmental due to the lack of anatomical boundaries (Anderson et al. 1999). Imaging is therefore crucial in detecting extracompartmental spread and deciding surgical management. A malignancy distal to the metatarsophalangeal joint requires ray resection, whereas lesions of the hindfoot usually require below knee amputation.

Although CT is more accurate at detecting matrix mineralisation, MRI is undoubtedly superior to CT at defining the intraosseous, soft-tissue and extracompartmental spread of tumours as well as their relationship to important neurovascular and articular structures (Bloem et al. 1988). Where an aggressive bone sarcoma of the distal tibia or fibula is suspected, a large field-of-view T1-weighted sequence of the whole bone in the longitudinal plane is required to exclude skip metastases. Compartmental anatomy is often best defined in the transverse plane. T1-weighted, fat-suppressed T2-weighted or STIR sequences all demonstrate contrast between an osseous tumour and normal marrow, although peri-tumoral oedema may obscure the tumour margin. Fat-suppressed T2-weighted or STIR sequences are required to demonstrate the soft-tissue extent. For indeterminate and aggressive lesions requiring biopsy, gadopentetate dimeglumine (Gd-DTPA)-enhanced, fat-suppressed, T1-weighted images are helpful in increasing lesion conspicuity and differentiating viable from necrotic tumour. A dynamic Gd-DTPA sequence may be useful as a baseline study in assessing the tumour response to chemotherapy.

Regarding the detection of distant metastases, CT is the best technique at present for detecting early pulmonary metastases and should be performed routinely in the initial staging of bone and soft-tissue sarcomas. Bone scintigraphy is of little value in the primary lesion but is essential in the exclusion of bony metastases.

20.2.5 Biopsy

Biopsy should not be performed until local staging has been completed. Discussion between the radiologist and orthopaedic surgeon is important in choosing the appropriate biopsy site. The biopsy should be made within a single compartment, avoiding neurovascular structures through an approach that can be resected at the definitive surgical procedure. Many authorities now accept percutaneous biopsy as the technique of choice. The technique is quick, safe and has a low risk of complications and tumour seeding. Percutaneous biopsy has an accuracy rate of over 90% in most series (Stoker et al. 1991). For soft-tissue lesions, biopsy is usually performed with a Tru-Cut needle under ultrasound guidance, whereas a trephine bone-cutting needle under fluoroscopic or CT control is usually required for bony lesions.

20.2.6 Follow-up

Neoadjuvant chemotherapy is now routinely used in almost all bone sarcomas with the exception of chondrosarcoma. Routine chemotherapy is not usually given for soft-tissue sarcomas but is used in some centres. Presurgical imaging is of value in assessing the tumour response and the timing of surgery. Radiographs are of little value in differentiating good and poor responders, and a decrease in size on cross-sectional imaging does not always allow a distinction between good and poor responders. However, on dynamic MR imaging, alterations in time-intensity curves before and after chemotherapy have been shown to correlate with the tumour response.

Following the treatment of bone tumours, lysis of the surrounding bone or bone graft should suggest local recurrence, although cystic changes may occur during healing. Where there is no mass, the

MR imaging appearances may also be confusing due to the inhomogeneity of the healing components. Both granulation tissue and recurrent tumour may enhance on static contrast MR imaging, but on dynamic MR imaging, recurrent tumour will usually give a steeper time-intensity slope than scar tissue. In the soft tissues, post-treatment changes tend to give a diffuse high signal intensity on T2-weighting without a focal mass. Seromas present high signal intensity masses on T2-weighting, but the mass itself either shows no or mild rim enhancement. Where there is diffuse or inhomogeneous enhancement within a mass, then recurrence is likely, and a biopsy should be performed. A mass that displays low signal intensity on T2-weighting may be due to scarring, but knowledge of preoperative MR characteristics is important as some lesions may display low signal intensity on T2-weighting, e.g. fibromatosis. Where there is doubt, static contrast-enhanced MR imaging will differentiate enhancing recurrent tumour from non-enhancing scar, but a dynamic sequence may be required to distinguish tumour from granulation tissue.

As most musculoskeletal sarcomas metastasise to the lung, follow-up chest radiographs are performed every 3 months for 2 years, every 6 months for a further 2 years, and then annually. CT chest and bone scintigraphy are indicated for suspected lung and bone metastases.

20.3 Bone Tumours and Tumour-like Lesions

20.3.1 Bone-Forming Bone Tumours

Osteoid osteoma is one of the most common benign tumours of the foot and ankle, with the majority found in the talus. Foot and ankle lesions account for 9%–21% of all osteoid osteomas and 18.8%–37.6% of benign bone tumours of the foot and ankle (Unni 1996; Huvos 1991; Campanacci 1990; Mirra 1989). There is a 3:1 male predominance, with the majority of patients being in the 2nd decade. Patients usually complain of a dull constant bone pain that is worse at night and relieved by salicylates, but some have presented with impingement, chronic sprains or arthropathy (Monroe and Manioli 1999). Lesions of the phalanges tend to present with swelling rather than pain (Barca et al. 1998). Most talar lesions are subperiosteal and located at the superior aspect of the talar neck (Fig. 20.5). Lesions in the calcaneus tend to be close to the subtalar joints, whereas lesions in the tubular bones occur along the shafts. In cortical lesions, radiography usually reveals a lucent or mineralised nidus with surrounding sclerosis. However, in intramedullary and subperiosteal lesions, surrounding sclerosis may be absent and the nidus occult. Bone scintigraphy may reveal the 'double density sign' where the central nidus shows greater uptake than the inflammatory response in the surrounding bone. Cross-sectional imaging is usually required for precise localisation, and at present CT is probably preferable to MR imaging. CT is more cost-effective, readily detects nidus mineralisation, and helps plan arthroscopic or percutaneous resection or CT-guided thermal ablation. On contrast-enhanced, fat-suppressed, T1-weighted MR images, the non-calcified nidi show homogeneous enhancement, whereas the calcified lesions show a ring enhancement sign (Youssef et al. 1996).

Osteoblastoma is an uncommon bone tumour but has a predilection for the foot and ankle. Foot and ankle osteoblastomas account for 8%–15.3% of all osteoblastomas and 4.0%–6.0% of benign bone tumours of the foot and ankle (Temple et al. 1998; Unni 1996; Campanacci 1990). Patient's mean age is around 24 years, with a 2:1 male predominance. Some 40% affect the talus, and half of these are in a subperiosteal location on the dorsal aspect of the talar neck. A similar preference is found with osteoid osteoma, and indeed they may be indistinguishable histologically. Although osteoid osteomas tend to be less than 1 cm in size and osteoblastomas tend to be larger than 2 cm, an arbitrary value of 1.5 cm can be used as a dividing line for lesions that are indistinguishable by all other criteria (McLeod et al. 1976). Radiologically, subperiosteal lesions are often associated with a soft-tissue mass and matrix mineralisation. Intramedullary lesions tend to have a geographic pattern of bone destruction, with variable margins and little if any mineralisation. Perilesional sclerosis is uncommon. Occasionally, lesions can be locally aggressive with infiltration of adjacent structures. The term 'aggressive osteoblastoma' is controversial; most show a tendency to recur but not to metastasise (Miyayama et al. 1993). Rarely, true osteosarcomatous transformation with metastases has been recorded (Temple et al. 1998).

Osteosarcoma of the foot and ankle only accounts for 2.3%–4.5% of all osteosarcomas, but it is one of the most common bony malignancies of the foot and ankle, accounting for 33.5% of 187 malignant bone tumours in one series (Unni 1996). Most lesions in the foot and ankle are intraosseous, osteoblastic and high

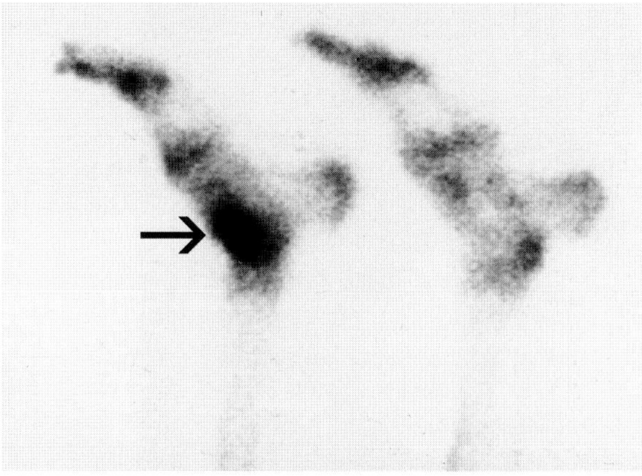

a

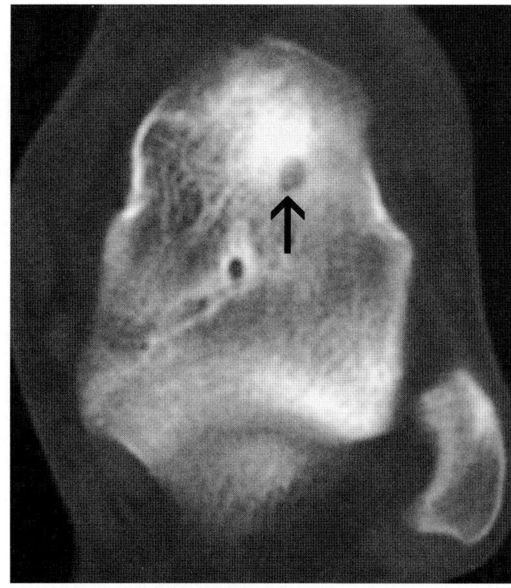

b

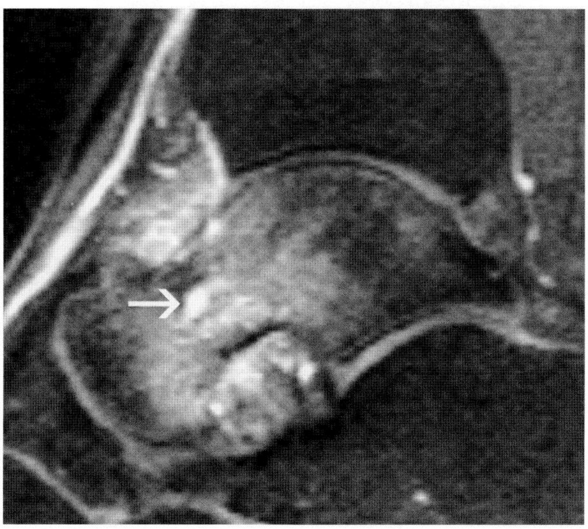

c

Fig. 20.5a–c. Recurrent osteoid osteoma of the talar neck in a 19-year-old man. Radiographs showed postsurgical changes only. **a** Bone scintigraphy shows increased uptake in the region of the right talar neck (*arrow*). **b** Transverse CT image shows a small 5-mm hypodense lesion within the medullary cavity of the talar neck (*arrow*). **c** Sagittal postintravenous Gd-DTPA T1-weighted MR images showing a small enhancing lesion (*arrow*) in the talar neck with surrounding oedema

grade. Metastatic disease is common and results in a poor prognosis of 65% mortality at 2.5 years (Choong et al. 1999). Approximately 66% are located in the distal tibia, and of the remainder, 75% are located in the tarsus and 75% of those in the calcaneus. Patients present with pain and often swelling, but the diagnosis is often delayed. In the foot, it tends to present later than osteosarcoma at other sites, with a mean age of 35 years. Radiographically, there is an aggressive moth-eaten or permeative pattern of bone destruction and usually soft-tissue extension (Fig. 20.6). Occasionally, slow-growing lesions may be expansile with well-defined margins (Lee et al. 2000). Amorphous or cloud-like mineralisation is common, and a lamellated or spiculated periosteal reaction is often present. On MR imaging, lesions typically display low to intermediate signal intensity on T1-weighting and inhomogeneous high signal intensity on T2-weighting. Mineralised foci often display low signal on all sequences. Parosteal osteosarcoma of the foot and ankle is very rare (Johnson et al. 1999).

20.3.2 Cartilage-Forming Bone Tumours

Chondroblastoma is an uncommon bone tumour that accounts for 3.8%–6.3% of benign bone tumours of the foot and ankle (Campanacci 1990; Unni 1996). In the foot, there is a male predominance of over 80%, and presentation tends to be later (mean 25.5 years) than in other parts of the skeleton (mean 17.3 years). The lesion favours an epiphyseal or subarticular location, which accounts for the high incidence in the posterior subchondral regions of the talus and calcaneus (64%) and calcaneal apophysis (36%) (Fink et al. 1997). Radiographically, lesions are typically translucent, with well-defined, often-sclerotic margins. Mineralisation is uncommon, but septation is common. Endosteal scalloping or expansion is present in almost 70% and cystic features in 50%. Subchondral fractures are frequent but often radiographically occult. On T2-weighted MR images, variable amounts of intermediate/low signal intensity tissue are commonly found and attributed

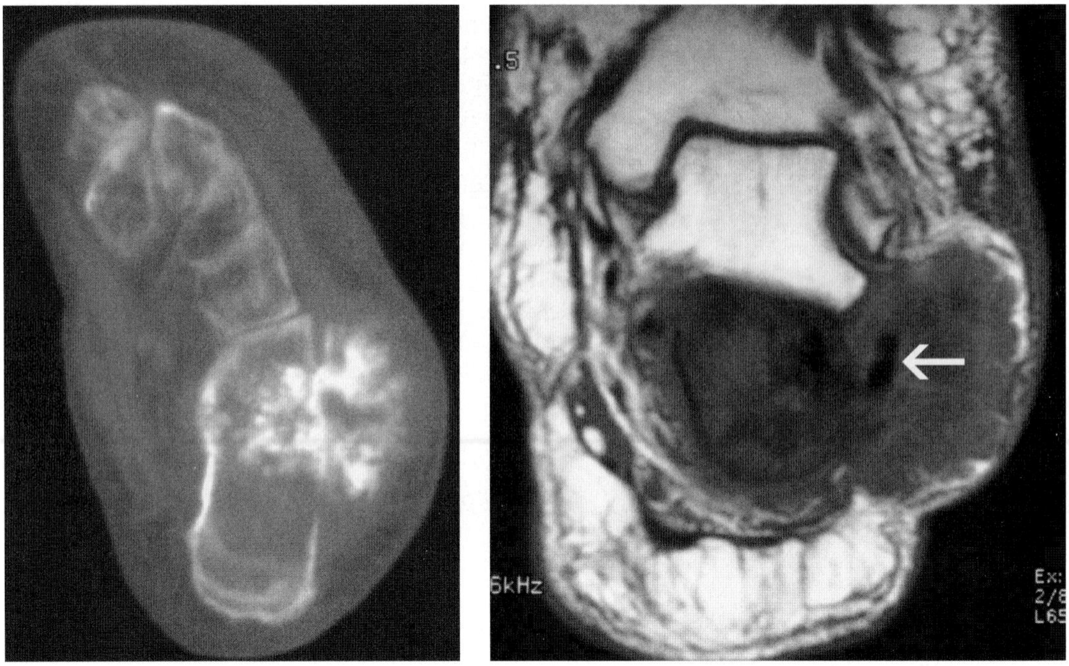

a b

Fig. 20.6a, b. Osteosarcoma of the calcaneus in a 59-year-old woman. **a** Transverse CT scan at bone settings showing an aggressive bone-forming tumour involving most of the calcaneus and infiltrating the lateral soft tissues. **b** Coronal T1-weighted MR image displaying intermediate SI from most of the mass. The rounded hypointense structures within the soft-tissue component are due to encasement of the peroneal tendons (*arrow*)

to haemosiderin, calcifications and hypercellularity of the chondroblasts. T2-weighted MR images may also reveal fluid-fluid levels due to the sedimentation effect of intralesional haemorrhage (JEE et al. 1999). Occasionally, a more aggressive appearance may be seen, which has been termed 'aggressive' or 'malignant' chondroblastoma (KYRIAKOS et al. 1985).

Enchondroma (chondroma) is a benign bony neoplasm that is much less common in the foot and ankle than the digits of the hand. However, it accounts for 9%–17.7% of benign bone tumours of the foot and ankle and is one of the most common benign bone tumours of the forefoot (UNNI 1996; CAMPANACCI 1990). Lesions usually present with a painless swelling or pathological fracture in the 3rd and 4th decades. Both sexes are affected equally. Involvement of the phalanges is more common than of the metatarsals or distal tibia and fibula, and rare in the hindfoot. Radiographs typically display a well-defined, expansile, lytic lesion that may contain punctate or stippled calcifications. Periosteal chondroma is uncommon and usually displays a rim of reactive bone (RICCA et al. 2000). Cartilage tumours often have characteristic MR appearances. On T1-weighting, unmineralised components display homogeneous low to intermediate signal intensity, but on T2-weighting, thin low signal intensity septa are noted between the lobules of high signal intensity cartilage. Following intravenous contrast, there is typically septal and peripheral enhancement. Mineralised components show low signal intensity on all sequences. The risk of sarcomatous transformation in a solitary foot lesion is very rare but may be as high as 5% for large lesions in a long bone such as the distal tibia. The risk of malignant transformation in multiple enchondromatosis is 25%, whereas in Maffucci's syndrome (enchondromatosis and soft-tissue haemangiomas), malignant transformation approaches 100%.

Osteochondroma (exostosis) is probably a developmental growth plate aberration rather than a true bone tumour but is classified with the benign chondrogenic tumours. It is one of the most common benign bone tumours of the foot and ankle, accounting for 25.7% of all benign foot and ankle tumours (UNNI 1996). However, the majority of osteochondromas of the ankle and foot are located in the distal tibia and fibula, and excluding subungual lesions, the metatarsals are most commonly involved in the foot. It is generally accepted that subungual lesions lack marrow continuity and cartilage cap and are not true osteochondromas. Most true osteochondromas present with a slow-growing, hard lump or symptoms from pressure effects on adjacent structures. Radiographically, the lesions may be sessile or pedunculated, and the cartilage cap may show variable stippled or ring-shaped calcifications.

Continued growth after maturity or pain should raise the possibility of sarcomatous degeneration, although this is very rare in solitary lesions. MR imaging is useful in excluding bursitis and allows accurate assessment of the cartilage cap. A cap thickness of less than 1 cm is likely to be benign, whereas a value greater than 2 cm is suggestive of malignant transformation. Lesions with a cap thickness of 1–2 cm are indeterminate and require biopsy. In hereditary multiple exostoses (diaphyseal aclasis), 7% of the lesions occur in the foot. Sarcomatous degeneration has a reported incidence of between 1.5% and 10%, but the true incidence is probably at the lower end of this range.

Chondromyxoid fibroma is a rare benign cartilage tumour but has a predisposition for the foot and ankle, accounting for 3.0%–6.3% of benign bone tumours at this site (Unni 1996; Campanacci 1990). There is a male predominance (1.5:1), and patients usually present in the second or third decades with discomfort and local swelling. Although the tibia is the most commonly involved bone, only 4% occur in the distal tibia and fibula (Mirra 1989). In the foot, the lesion most commonly occurs in the metatarsals, calcaneus and phalanges. Radiographs typically show a slow-growing, well-defined, expansile, osteolytic lesion often with sclerotic margins (O'Connor et al. 1996). Matrix calcification is uncommon. In the small tubular bones of the foot, lesions often extend from the metaphysis into the diaphysis or epiphysis. Occasionally, chondromyxoid fibroma can appear aggressive, mimicking a sarcoma. On MR imaging, lesions display low signal intensity on T1-weighting and hyperintense signal intensity on T2-weighting. The margin of the lesion usually displays a low signal intensity on all sequences, reflecting new periosteal bone.

Chondrosarcoma of the foot and ankle accounts for only 2.5%–4.4% of all chondrosarcomas but is the third most common bony malignancy of the foot and ankle, accounting for 17.3%–19.6% of lesions (Unni 1996; Campanacci 1990). The majority involve the distal tibia and fibula, and in the foot, lesions are most commonly found in the calcaneus, talus and metatarsals. Chondrosarcoma of the ankle and hindfoot are more likely to metastasise than phalangeal chondrosarcoma, which only rarely metastasises and behaves as a locally aggressive lesion (Bovee et al. 1999). The majority of lesions are centrally located with a geographic pattern of bone destruction, although a more aggressive permeative pattern may also be found. In a large study of 75 lesions of the foot, endosteal erosion, cortical destruction and expansion were present in over 90%, ill-defined margins and a soft-tissue mass in 80%, and mineralisation in 74% (Ogose et al. 1997). In the feet and hands, lesions are smaller than elsewhere in the skeleton, ranging between 2 and 5 cm (maximal size). On MR imaging, the signal characteristics are similar to enchondroma, although chondrosarcoma should be suspected where there is cortical destruction, periosteal reaction and soft-tissue infiltration (Hottya et al. 1999). Peripheral lesions are much less common than central lesions and usually arise from pre-existing osteochondroma rather than the periosteum (Fig. 20.7). The variants periosteal and clear-cell chondrosarcoma of the foot and ankle have been reported but are extremely rare.

20.3.3 Vascular Bone Tumours

Haemangiomas of the bones of the foot and ankle are rare, accounting for <1% of benign bone tumours of the foot and ankle (Unni 1996; Campanacci 1990). There is a wide age range and a slight female predominance. Most are asymptomatic, but some may present with pain and swelling. Radiographs usually show a well-defined, often expansile, osteolytic lesion with a coarse lattice-like trabecular pattern. They may contain detectable fat on CT and MR imaging.

Intermediate and malignant vasoformative tumours including haemangioendothelioma, haemangiopericytoma and angiosarcoma are more common in the soft tissues than bone, accounting for 2.8%–7% of malignant bone tumours and 6.2% of malignant soft-tissue tumours of the foot and ankle (Unni 1996; Campanacci 1990; Kransdorf 1995b). Haemangioendothelioma and haemangiopericytoma are usually of intermediate aggressiveness and may be benign, whereas angiosarcoma is an aggressive malignant tumour with a poor prognosis (Bakotic et al. 1999). These lesions have a wide age range and a slight male predominance in bone haemangioendotheliomas but female predominance in soft-tissue haemangioendotheliomas and haemangiopericytomas. In bony lesions, intermediate or low-grade lesions may present with lytic areas and a honeycombing appearance, whereas aggressive lesions demonstrate a permeative pattern of bone destruction and soft-tissue infiltration. In haemangioendothelioma, multicentricity is common, and the small bones of the foot may be extensively involved (Fig. 20.8) (Boutin et al. 1996). For soft-tissue lesions, imaging is usually required for lesions that may involve the deeper tissues. Radiography is usually non-specific, but the detection of prominent serpentine structures on cross-sectional imaging

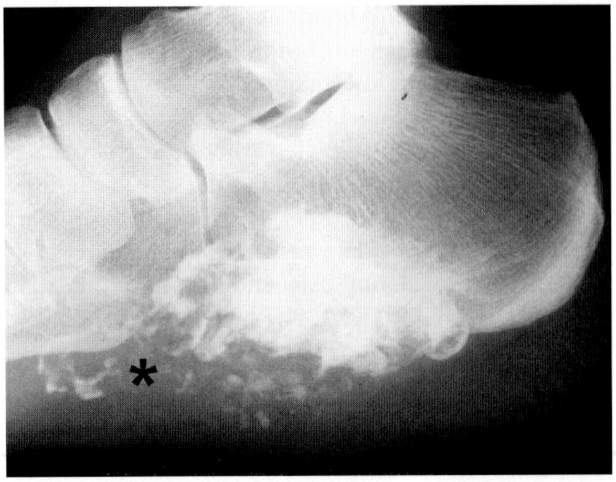

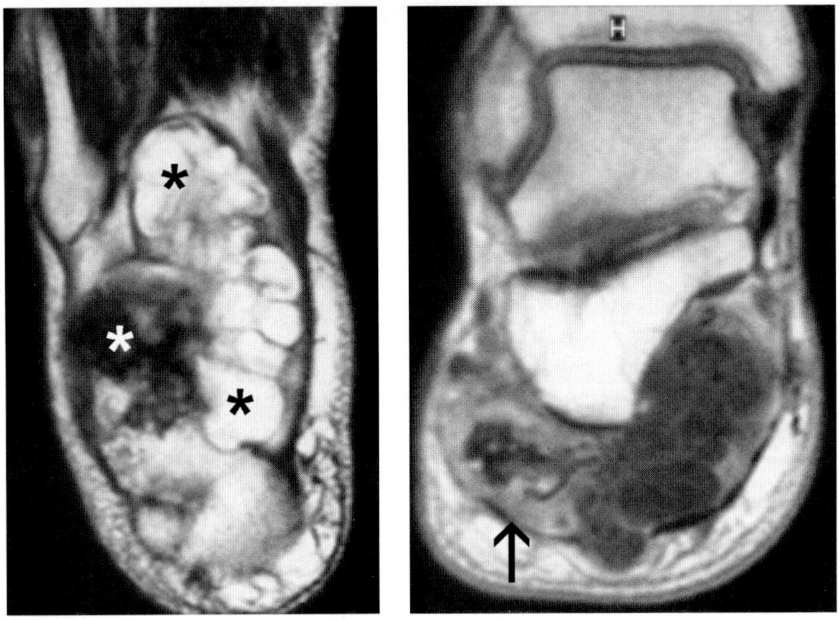

Fig. 20.7a–c. Peripheral chondrosarcoma of the calcaneus in a 43-year-old man. **a** Radiograph displays dense mineralisation over the anterior aspect of the calcaneus with punctate or stippled calcifications anteroinferiorly in keeping with a cartilage-forming tumour (*asterisk*). **b** Transverse T2-weighted MR image showing foci of low-SI mineralisation laterally (*white asterisks*) and lobules of high-SI cartilage medially (*black asterisk*). **c** Coronal postintravenous Gd-DTPA T1-weighted MR image. There is mild septal and peripheral enhancement around the lobules of low-SI cartilage (*arrow*)

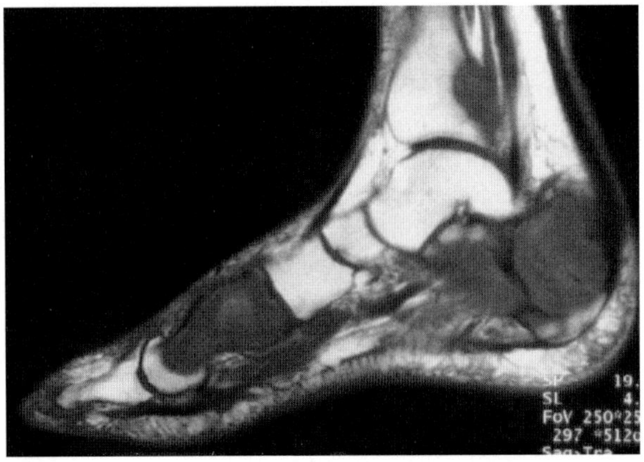

Fig. 20.8. Multifocal haemangioendothelioma in a 71-year-old woman. Sagittal T1-weighted MR image showing several nonspecific expansile lesions arising from the 1st metatarsal, calcaneus and distal tibia

should suggest the possibility of a vasoformative tumour. Ultrasound may reveal an inhomogeneous lesion containing cystic foci, and Doppler studies may reveal arteriovenous shunting. MR imaging may show prominent vessels of variable signal intensity (depending on the blood flow) and fluid-fluid levels, but unlike haemangiomas there is no fatty overgrowth. Angiography may show arteriovenous shunting, and doughnut-like lesions have been reported on bone scintigraphy (McNamara et al. 1993).

20.3.4 Fibrous and Fibrohistiocytic Bone Tumours

Non-ossifying fibroma (NOF) and *benign fibrous cortical defect* (BFCD) are histologically identical developmental anomalies that are common in the distal tibia and fibula (UNNI 1996). Although BFCDs and smaller NOFs are often incidental findings, larger NOFs may present with a pathological fracture. Radiography typically reveals an eccentric, ovoid, lytic lesion with a well-defined, sclerotic margin. Larger lesions may have a multiloculated appearance.

Cross-sectional imaging is not usually required, but MR imaging may display low signal intensity on T2-weighting due to an abundance of collagen or haemosiderin. Lesions often enhance with intravenous contrast.

Fibrous dysplasia is a relatively common developmental anomaly, but in its monostotic form, only 3.2% of lesions occur in the foot and ankle (SCHAJOWICZ 1981). In the less common polyostotic form, 73% of patients show involvement of the foot. Polyostotic disease tends to present in the first decade with pain or pathological fracture or with endocrine problems (Albright's syndrome). Monostotic disease more commonly presents in the second decade as an incidental finding or after innocuous trauma. Both forms of the disease have an equal sex distribution, although there is a predilection for girls in Albright's syndrome. Radiographs show a well-defined, expansile lesion usually with a sclerotic margin. The matrix is variable, ranging from lucent to sclerotic. MR imaging shows a hypointense or isointense signal intensity compared with muscle on T1-weighting and a variable signal intensity on T2-weighting depending on the cellularity and fibrous and mineralised components (ISEFUKU et al. 1999).

Desmoplastic fibroma is a very rare, locally aggressive, primary bone tumour that can be considered the intraosseous counterpart of fibromatosis. BOHM et al. (1996) reviewed 184 cases and found only 7.6% in the ankle and foot. Most cases present in the second and third decades, with an equal sex incidence. Lesions usually present with pain or swelling or occasionally with pathological fracture. Radiographically, a geographic pattern of bone destruction, narrow zone of transition and internal pseudotrabeculation are the most consistent features (TACONIS et al. 1994). Cortical breakthrough and soft-tissue infiltration are present in up to 48% of lesions, but periosteal reaction is uncommon. The MR features are mainly non-specific, but foci of low to intermediate signal intensity on T2-weighting are often present and reflect the fibrous, relatively acellular components of the tumour (VANHOENACKER et al. 2000).

Malignant fibrous histiocytoma and fibrosarcoma are histologically different but are discussed together as they have similar imaging appearances. Fibrosarcoma is more common than malignant fibrous histiocytoma, but together they account for 6.0%–18.9% of malignant bone tumours of the foot and ankle, and most present in the fourth and fifth decades (UNNI 1996; CAMPANACCI 1990). They most commonly occur in the ankle and hindfoot, and involvement of the forefoot is very rare. Radiographically, both lesions have a variable growth rate ranging from a geographic pattern of bone destruction to a more aggressive moth-eaten or permeative pattern with extensive bone destruction and soft-tissue infiltration (LINK et al. 1998). The lack of mineralisation helps distinguish them from osteochondroma or chondrosarcoma, although occasionally some mineralisation may be present. Lesions usually display non-specific intermediate signal intensity on T1-weighting and inhomogeneous high signal intensity on T2-weighting, although if the collagen content is high, then a predominantly lower signal intensity on T2-weighting may be noted. Foci of haemorrhage and necrosis may be present.

20.3.5 Marrow and Lymphatic Tumours of Bone

Langerhans cell histiocytosis is very rare in the foot and ankle (MIRRA 1989; CAMPANACCI 1990). Its localised form, eosinophilic granuloma, accounts for 70% of cases and heals spontaneously. Patients present between the ages of 5 and 15 years with a slight male predominance. In the early phase, lesions often have an aggressive pattern of bone destruction, with ill-defined margins and lamellated periosteal reaction simulating Ewing's sarcoma, whereas in the later healing phase they have well-defined sclerotic margins simulating a benign bone tumour. The MR imaging appearances are non-specific.

Giant-cell tumour of the foot and ankle is a locally aggressive tumour that accounts for 4.9%–6.3% of all giant-cell tumours and 14.5%–20% of benign bone tumours of the foot and ankle (UNNI 1996; CAMPANACCI 1990; MIRRA 1989). Lesions usually present with pain and swelling and often a pathological fracture. Some 80% occur in the distal tibia, with the remainder mainly in the tarsus. Calcaneal lesions are often found posteriorly at the site of the apophysis, although they may also occur in the subarticular portion of the anterior calcaneus. Lesions of the small bones of the foot tend to occur in younger patients and show a more aggressive behaviour than giant-cell tumours of large bones (BISCAGLIA et al. 2000). The majority of lesions have an ill-defined geographic pattern of bone destruction, although up to a third have a more aggressive moth-eaten pattern with cortical destruction and soft-tissue infiltration. As cystic components and haemorrhage are common, MR images typically show an inhomogeneous appearance, with foci of variable signal intensity and often fluid-fluid levels. Lesions have the potential to undergo malignant transformation, especially in recurrent disease. The very rare multicentric giant-cell tumour has a tendency to involve the feet but does not seem to carry an increased risk of pulmonary metastases (Cummins et al. 1996).

Ewing's sarcoma is a highly aggressive round-cell tumour that accounts for 23.2%–37.2% of malignant bone tumours of the foot and ankle (Unni 1996; Campanacci 1990). Lesions are most commonly found in the distal tibia and fibula and to a lesser extent the calcaneus and metatarsals. Lesions usually present with a painful swelling in the second decade. There is a slight male predominance (1.7: 1) and a shorter duration of symptoms for forefoot lesions than hindfoot lesions. Survival is much better in patients who present with localised disease and forefoot lesions. For the 50% who have metastases at presentation, the prognosis is very poor (Adkins et al. 1997). Radiographically, lesions typically show an aggressive moth-eaten or permeative pattern of bone destruction, usually with a soft-tissue mass (Fig. 20.9), although atypical features are more commonly found in the tarsal bones (Baraga et al. 2001). In particular, tarsal lesions less commonly demonstrate permeative bone destruction, periosteal reaction or soft-tissue mass. Purely osteosclerotic lesions are more common in the calcaneus. On MR imaging, lesions are usually hypointense or isointense with muscle on T1-weighting and hyperintense and inhomogeneous on T2-weighting. The lack of mineralised matrix helps differentiate it from osteosarcoma..

Primary lymphoma of the foot and ankle is rare, accounting for 0.6%–1.9% of all lymphomas and 0.4%–6.5% of all bony malignancies of the foot and ankle (Unni 1996; Campanacci 1990; Mirra 1989). Secondary involvement to the foot is also rare and usually indicates widespread disease due to red marrow reconversion. Primary lymphoma has a wide age range but usually peaks in the fifth decade and is more common in males (2:1). Lesions are more common in the distal tibia than the foot. Of the foot bones, the calcaneus is most commonly involved (Skorman and Martin 1999). Radiographically, lesions typically show an aggressive moth-eaten or permeative pattern of destruction and are predominantly lytic, although up to a third may have a mixture of lysis and sclerosis. Periosteal reaction, cortical destruction and soft-tissue extension are common. Sequestra may also be present. On MR imaging, most lesions are isointense or hypointense to skeletal muscle on T1-weighting and inhomogeneous and predominantly hyperintense on T2-weighting (White et al. 1998).

Multiple myeloma in the foot and ankle is rare, accounting for 0.13%–2.0% of all myelomas and 0.13% of all malignant bone tumours of the foot and ankle (Mirra 1989; Campanacci 1990; Unni 1996). Myeloma of the foot and ankle usually indicates widespread involvement with marrow reconversion. Solitary plasmacytoma is extremely rare in the foot, with only eight reported cases, five of which occurred in the calcaneus and talus. Radiographically, lesions

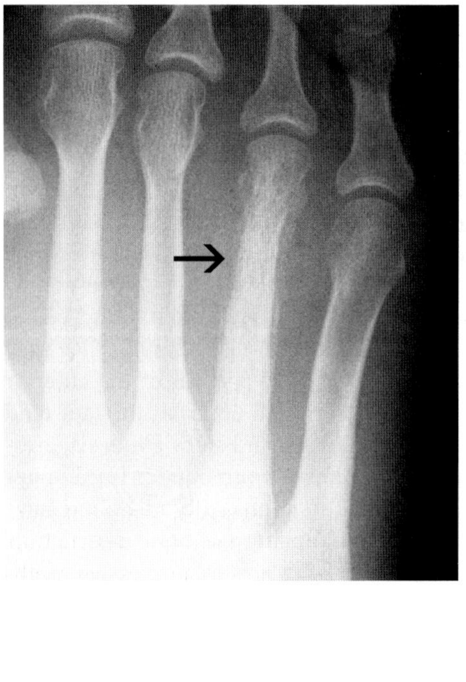

a

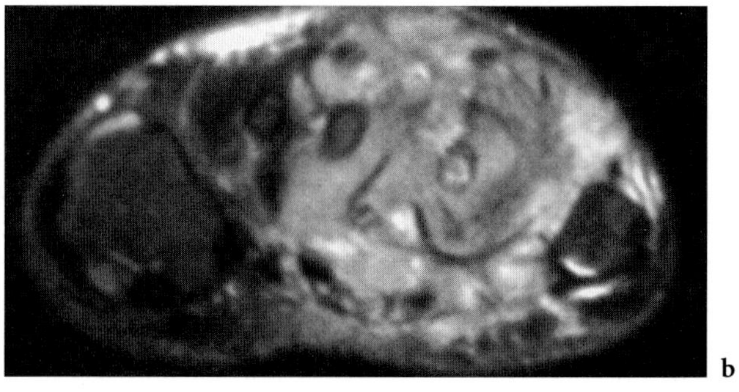

b

Fig. 20.9a, b. Ewing's sarcoma in a 23-year-old man. **a** Radiograph displaying a permeative pattern of bone destruction along the shaft of the 4th metatarsal with associated faint periosteal reaction (*arrow*). **b** Coronal T2-weighted MR image showing extensive soft-tissue involvement typical of a Ewing's sarcoma are osteolytic with a geographic pattern of bone destruction and variable margins.

Metastases to the foot and ankle are rare, with a reported incidence of <0.3% (LIBSON et al. 1987). However, it is likely that the true incidence is higher as many probably go unrecognised in disseminated disease. Primary tumours are mostly due to adenocarcinoma from the colon (17%), kidneys (17%), lung (15%), bladder (10%), and breast (10%). Occasionally, a foot or ankle metastasis may present without a known primary. In the foot, the tarsal bones are more commonly involved than the forefoot, and the majority of these occur in the calcaneus. Involvement of several foot bones is common and may result in massive bone loss (Fig. 20.10). Radiographically, 80% of metastases are purely osteolytic, but prostatic metastases are usually sclerotic, and breast, bladder and gastrointestinal primaries may be lytic, sclerotic or mixed. Although the lesions may be expansile, cortical destruction is invariably present. The MR imaging features are non-specific.

20.3.6 Bone Tumours of Lipomatous, Neural or Unknown Origin

Intraosseous lipoma is a rare benign tumour composed of mature adipose cells. However, 13%–24% of intraosseous lipomas occur in the foot and ankle, with a predisposition for the calcaneus (MILGRAM 1988; MIRRA 1989). Lesions appear most frequently in the fourth decade, show no sexual predilection and are often incidental findings. In the calcaneus, the lesion usually occurs anteriorly and is characterised by a well-defined, radiolucent lesion with a thin sclerotic rim. There may be a central calcific density representing dystrophic calcification. On MRI, the signal intensity is similar to subcutaneous fat on all sequences, although calcific foci will give a low signal on all sequences, and areas of necrosis and cyst formation will give a low signal intensity on T1-weighting and high signal intensity on T2-weighting (RICHARDSON et al. 1995).

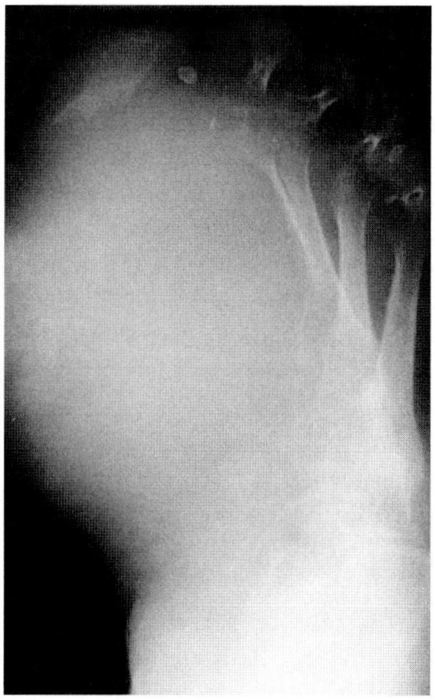

Fig. 20.10. Metastasis from colonic carcinoma. Destruction of the bones of the medial forefoot including the 1st and 2nd rays and cuneiforms with a large soft-tissue mass

Primary liposarcoma of bone is very rare and controversial but has been recorded in the calcaneus (MURARI et al. 1989).

Intraosseous neurofibroma or neurolemmoma of the foot is very rare, but cases have been reported in the phalanx and calcaneus (PYATI and SANZONE 1996; SCHAJOWICZ 1981). Radiographically, lesions are well defined and osteolytic, with multiple septations giving a multiloculated appearance.

Adamantinoma is a rare, low-grade, malignant tumour of unknown origin that has a preference for the tibia. In a large review of 200 patients, there was involvement of the distal tibia in 58 cases and the distal fibula in 9 cases (MOON and MORI 1986). Only 2 cases were recorded in the foot, one in a metatarsal and the other in a cuneiform.

20.3.7 Tumour-like Lesions of Bone

There are several lesions that may mimic bone tumours. Gout, infection, Paget's disease and stress fractures are discussed in other chapters.

Unicameral bone cyst is uncommon in the foot and ankle but does have a predilection for the calcaneus in adults. Some 2%–6.7% of simple cysts occur in the foot and ankle (MIRRA 1989; CAMPANACCI 1990). Some lesions present incidentally following minor trauma, whereas others present with chronic pain probably due to microfractures. Radiographs reveal a well-defined lytic lesion often with a sclerotic rim in the anterior third of the calcaneus. Pseudocysts can appear similar but are less well-defined, and internal trabeculations are often present (STUKENBORG-COLSMAN et al. 1999). On CT and MR imaging, lesions often display fluid characteristics, although the density and signal intensity may be greater than water due to their high protein content.

Aneurysmal bone cyst can be defined as a benign reactive lesion characterised by cyst-like walls of predominantly fibrous tissue filled with free flowing blood (Mirra 1989). Some 12.4%–16% occur in the foot and ankle (Huvos 1991; Campanacci 1990; Unni 1996). The majority of lesions are primary and occur in the 1st and 2nd decades. Later presentation should suggest an underlying lesion, most commonly a giant-cell tumour. Lesions are more commonly found in the distal tibia and fibula than in the foot. In the foot, aneurysmal bone cyst is more common in the tarsus than the metatarsals. In the initial phase, radiography shows a markedly expansile metaphyseal lytic lesion contained by a thin layer of periosteal new bone. The periosteal reaction may be occult, and the lesion may mimic an aggressive sarcoma. In the healing phase, there is maturation of the periosteal bone and consolidation of the lesion. MR imaging shows a lobulated, expansile, inhomogeneous and multiseptate lesion containing foci of variable signal depending on the age of the blood products. In the active phase, the thin rim of intact periosteal tissue gives a low signal on all sequences. MR imaging is more sensitive than CT at detecting intralesional fluid-fluid levels. In primary lesions, intravenous contrast confirms rim and septal enhancement, whereas in secondary lesions the enhancement pattern depends on the extent and nature of the underlying lesion.

Mature bone infarcts have a typical appearance, with densely mineralised foci within the medullary cavity. However, in the early stages, radiographs may show non-specific mottled bone rarefaction, sometimes with mild reactive sclerosis mimicking infection or malignancy. MR imaging is helpful as it demonstrates a central focus of high or intermediate signal surrounded by a thin, serpentine, low-signal border (Abrahim-Zadeh et al. 1998).

Giant-cell reparative granuloma is a rare, benign, reactive, intraosseous lesion with a predilection for the hands and feet. In the foot, most lesions occur in the metatarsals, and the majority present in the third decade (Ratner and Dorfman 1990). Radiographically, the lesion is typically a solitary, lytic, expanded metaphyseal lesion occasionally extending into subarticular bone and more frequently extending into the diaphysis. Extension into soft tissues is unusual unless it is located in a distal phalanx or when a pathological fracture occurs. In the differential diagnosis, giant-cell tumour tends to occur in older patients, and soft-tissue infiltration is more common.

Intraosseous ganglia are juxta-articular cystic lesions that are much less common than their soft-tissue counterparts. In a large study reviewing 213 cases in the literature, 18% were found in the medial malleolus, 3% in the lateral malleolus and 8% in the foot (Murff and Ashry 1994). Most patients present in mid-adult life with intermittent pain. Radiographs show a well-defined, non-expansile, radiolucent, juxta-articular lesion with a well-defined sclerotic margin .

Bizarre parosteal osteochondromatous proliferation (BPOP) is an uncommon tumour-like lesion that is typically found on the surfaces of the proximal phalanges and metatarsal and metacarpal bones. It is most common in the 3rd and 4th decades, has an equal sex incidence, and usually presents with a painless swelling (Harty et al. 2000). Initially, the lesion is an immature mass of mineralisation within the soft tissues with no clear osseous attachment, but as it matures, radiographs show attachment to bone with a pedunculated or sessile base (Fig. 20.11). In the differential diagnosis, there are radiological and histological similarities with parosteal osteosarcoma and florid reactive periostitis.

20.4 Soft-Tissue Tumours and Tumour-like Lesions

20.4.1 Fibrohistiocytic Soft-Tissue Tumours

Benign fibrous histiocytoma is a common benign tumour accounting for 13.1% of benign foot and ankle soft-tissue tumours (Kransdorf 1995a). It usually presents in young to middle-aged adults as a protuberant nodular mass in the skin and is multiple in up to one-third. Imaging will usually be performed in the uncommon deep variety as they may mimic a more aggressive process. On MR imaging, lesions display intermediate signal intensity on T1-weighting and an inhomogeneous variable signal intensity on T2-weighting.

Dermatofibrosarcoma protuberans is an uncommon, slow-growing, intermediate-grade malignancy that originates in the dermal layer of the skin and accounts for 6.0% of foot and ankle soft-tissue sarcomas (Kransdorf 1995b). Clinically, they are most common in the 3rd–5th decades (Cione et al. 1999). Large lesions may infiltrate deeper structures and will usually undergo imaging. Although the density and signal characteristics are non-specific on CT and MR imaging, the cutaneous components and lobular architecture of most lesions should suggest the diagnosis.

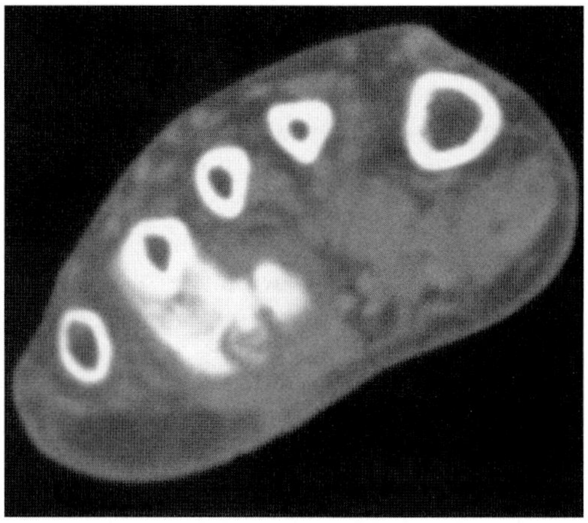

Fig. 20.11. Bizarre parosteal osteochondromatous proliferation (BPOP) in a 20-year-old woman. Coronal CT image on bone settings shows a mineralised lesion attached to the plantar surface of the 4th metatarsal. Note there is no destruction of the underlying cortex

Malignant fibrous histiocytoma is the second most common soft-tissue sarcoma in the foot and ankle, accounting for 17.3% of lesions (Kransdorf 1995b). Lesions are more common in men in the 5th–7th decades, although the rare angiomatoid type is more common in young adults (Chow et al. 1998). Clinically, the lesion presents as a non-specific, enlarging, painless mass. Radiography may reveal a soft-tissue mass and may detect mineralisations in up to 20% of cases. On MR imaging, lesions are typically inhomogeneous, with poorly defined margins and variable signal intensity depending on the different components. Myxoid change and necrosis give low signal intensity on T1-weighting and high signal intensity on T2-weighting. Fibrous tissue and mineralisation tend to give low or intermediate signal intensity on all sequences. Recent haemorrhage may give high signal intensity on all sequences, whereas fluid-fluid levels are often found with older haemorrhage. Inhomogeneous enhancement is typical.

20.4.2 Fibrous Soft-Tissue Tumours

Calcifying aponeurotic fibroma (juvenile aponeurotic fibroma) is a rare, locally aggressive but self-limiting fibroblastic lesion that is found in the palms and soles of children and adolescents (Yee et al. 1991). The majority of cases involve the deep spaces of the sole. The cellular histology, aggressive growth pattern and tendency to recur may lead to a misdiagnosis of fibrosarcoma. The imaging appearances are similar to fibromatosis.

Nodular fasciitis (pseudosarcomatous fibromatosis/fasciitis) is a benign soft-tissue lesion that is rare in the foot and ankle, accounting for only 1% of benign soft-tissue lesions of the foot and ankle (Kransdorf 1995a). On MR imaging, lesions are usually well-defined but can be irregular. Myxoid and cellular lesions display high signal intensity on T2-weighting, whereas lesions with a predominantly fibrous histology display low to intermediate signal intensity on all sequences. Lesions typically enhance.

Fibroma of the tendon sheath is an uncommon, benign, fibroblastic proliferation of the tendon sheaths that accounts for 1.6% of benign soft-tissue tumours around the ankle and foot (Kransdorf 1995a). It usually presents as a slow-growing mass and is more common in men in the 3rd–5th decades. Radiographs may demonstrate a soft-tissue mass and occasionally bony involvement. On MR imaging, lesions tend to display mainly intermediate signal intensity on both T1-weighting and T2-weighting.

Plantar fibromatosis is the most common benign soft-tissue tumour of the foot and ankle, accounting for 22.9% of lesions in Kransdorf's (1995a) series. There is a wide age range, with a mean in the fourth decade and no predilection for sex. Lesions can be multiple in up to 30% and bilateral in 20%–50%. Patients usually present with one or more firm, fixed, subcutaneous nodules measuring around 2 cm in size on the plantar side of the foot. Small lesions may remain asymptomatic, but larger, deeper, infiltrating lesions often require wide resection. Ultrasound shows a well-defined, inhomogeneous, hypoechoic mass superficial to the medial slip of the plantar aponeurosis. On MR imaging, lesions are well-defined superficially against the subcutaneous fat, but the infiltrative deep margin often blends imperceptibly with the deep aponeurosis (Morrison et al. 1994). However, the tissues deep to the aponeurosis are invaded in only 15% of patients. The signal characteristics vary with the phase of the disease. On T2-weighting, most lesions in the involutional or residual phase display only a slightly hyperintense signal intensity compared with skeletal muscle due to the high collagen content, whereas in the cellular proliferative phase, a higher signal intensity on T2-weighting is typical. Enhancement is variable and more marked in the proliferative phase (Fig. 20.3).

Fibrosarcoma is a malignant fibroblastic tumour that most commonly presents in the 5th and 6th decades. Some 6.6% of soft-tissue fibrosarcomas occur in the foot and ankle, and fibrosarcoma accounts for 6.7% of soft-tissue sarcomas of the foot and ankle (Kransdorf 1995b). The long-term prognosis is guarded, with a 5-year survival rate of less than 40%. The less common infantile fibrosarcoma usually occurs in the first 2 years of life and carries a better prognosis. Radiography may show a soft-tissue mass and occasionally bony involvement. On MR imaging, the signal characteristics are non-specific, with intermediate signal intensity on T1-weighting and inhomogeneous, intermediate signal intensity on T2-weighting.

20.4.3 Lipomatous Soft-Tissue Tumours

Lipomas are common benign lesions that only accounted for 6.3% of benign tumours of the foot and ankle in Kransdorf's series (1995a), but this is likely to be an underestimate as the lesions are often detected incidentally. The majority present in middle-aged patients as a superficial soft-tissue mass around the ankle or heel (Kirby et al. 1989). Lipomatous variants, heterogeneous lipomas and lipoblastoma are much less common but have been recorded in the foot and ankle (Fig. 20.12). Radiographically, lipomas may appear as a soft-tissue mass of low (fatty) density and rarely bone erosion (Braunschweig et al. 1992). Simple lipomas are easily diagnosed on CT and MR imaging as they are homogeneous, do not enhance, and have similar density and signal characteristics to subcutaneous fat. Simple lipomas containing various connective tissue elements; spindle-cell and pleomorphic variants of lipoma may contain foci of enhancing and non-enhancing non-lipomatous tissue that may be indistinguishable from atypical lipoma (well-differentiated liposarcoma). Angiolipoma is indistinguishable from intramuscular angioma, and both may contain serpentine structures, heterotopic bone and phleboliths. Perineural fibrolipoma rarely occurs in the foot and may be associated with macrodactylia fibrolipomatosis (Donley et al. 1996).

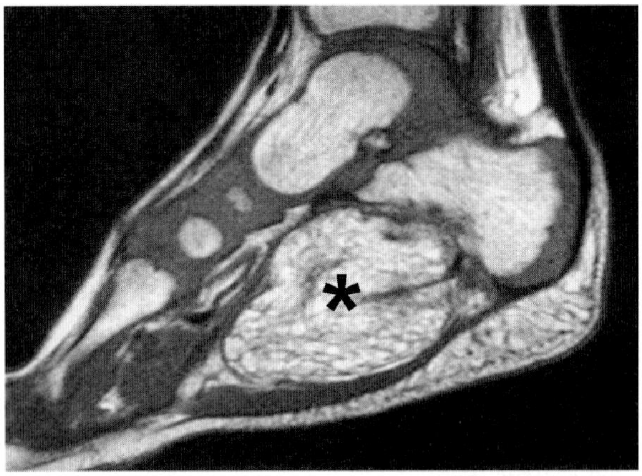

Fig. 20.12. Lipoblastoma in a 5-year-old boy. Sagittal T1-weighted MR image showing a well-defined soft-tissue mass on the plantar aspect of the hindfoot. The predominantly high SI on T1-weighting is compatible with a lipomatous lesion (confirmed on fat-suppressed images), and the reticular pattern of low SI reflects the dense collagenous septa between the fatty lobules (*asterisk*)

Liposarcoma is the second most common soft-tissue sarcoma but only accounts for 4.8% of soft-tissue sarcomas of the foot and ankle (Kransdorf 1995b). It usually presents as a painless mass in the 5th and 6th decades and is rare in children. Myxoid and well-differentiated liposarcomas are the most common subtypes and carry a better prognosis than the more aggressive round-cell, pleomorphic and dedifferentiated subtypes (Werd et al. 1995). Plain radiography may detect mineralisations in up to 10%. On MR imaging, well-differentiated lesions always contain demonstrable fat, whereas only 50% of the remainder (mainly myxoid liposarcoma) contain demonstrable fat. Well-differentiated liposarcomas tend to have thick enhancing septa or nodules, whereas lipomas have thin septa that display only slight if any enhancement.

20.4.4 Vascular Soft-Tissue Tumours

Haemangioma is a relatively common soft-tissue lesion accounting for 7.2% of benign soft-tissue tumours of the foot and ankle (Kransdorf 1995a). Symptomatic lesions tend to present in the first four decades with a swelling that may vary in size. Imaging is not usually required for superficial lesions but may be required for deep lesions. Most deep haemangiomas are of the cavernous type. Radiographs may show a soft-tissue mass that occasionally involves bone. Phleboliths are seen in nearly 50% of cavernous haemangiomas. Angiography is helpful in confirming the type and extent of the lesion and the suitability for embolotherapy (Mitty 1993). On ultrasound, appearances are variable, but lesions are usually inhomogeneous with a mixed echo pattern due to vascular and non-vascular elements (Derchi et al. 1989). Arteriovenous malformations typically demonstrate high flow on Doppler, whereas slow-flowing venous lesions may give little or no Doppler signal. On T1-weighted MR images, lesions are usually ill defined, with predominantly low/intermediate signal intensity as well as variable amounts of high signal intensity fat (Fig. 20.13). Enhancement of the non-lipomatous components is variable. On T2-weighting, lesions display very high signal intensity from the vascular components separated by low signal intensity fibrous elements and fat if fat-suppression techniques are used. The vessels have a characteristic serpentine or circular appearance depending on the imaging plane and path of the vessel. The fast-flowing blood of an arteriovenous malformation results in flow voids on all sequences. A cavernous haemangioma often contains slow-flowing blood or pooling within dilated venous channels that give high signal intensity foci on T1-weighting and phleboliths that give low signal intensity on all sequences.

Glomus tumours are uncommon benign tumours of the foot that arise from neuromyoarterial glomus bodies and are usually located in the deepest layer of the dermis of the nail bed. Patients are usually women between the ages of 20 and 40 years and present with pain and cold sensitivity. Examination may reveal a characteristic small, red-blue, superficial nodule. US may show a small hypoechoic mass, but subungual lesions may be overlooked (Fornage 1998). On MR imaging, lesions are usually around 4 mm in size, encapsulated, homogeneous and display high signal intensity on T2-weighting and marked enhancement (Drape et al. 1996). The signal intensity on T1-weighting is variable depending on the histological variations of the lesion. High-resolution MR imaging is more sensitive at detecting bone erosions than plain radiography.

Intermediate and malignant vasoformative soft-tissue tumours are discussed in the section on vascular bone tumours.

Kaposi's sarcoma has a strong predilection for the foot and is by far the most common soft-tissue malignancy of the foot (Berlin 1995). Although classified as a vascular sarcoma, it is almost always located within the cutaneous tissues and is usually regarded as a skin tumour. AIDS-related Kaposi's sarcoma usually occurs in young adults and carries a poor prognosis, whereas the chronic form of Kaposi's sarcoma (often associated with lymphoreticular neoplasms) presents in later life and has a better prognosis. There is 2:1 male predominance. Imaging is only required for deep lesions, and the appearances are

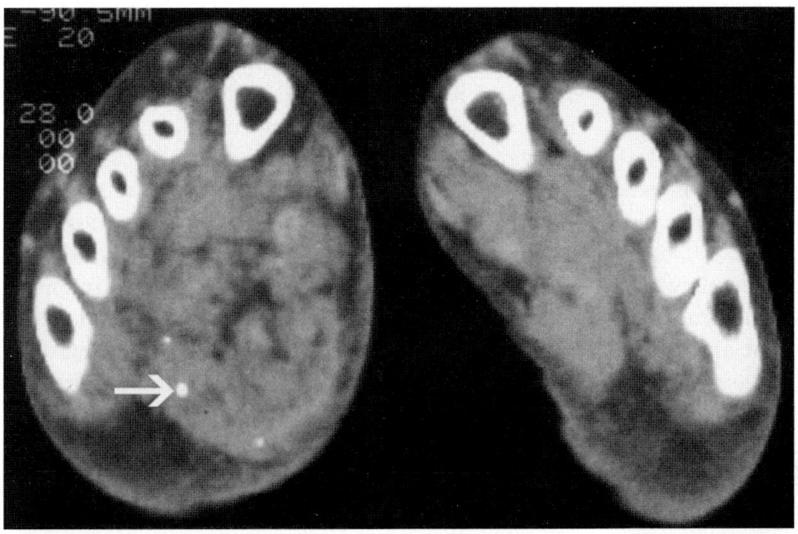
a

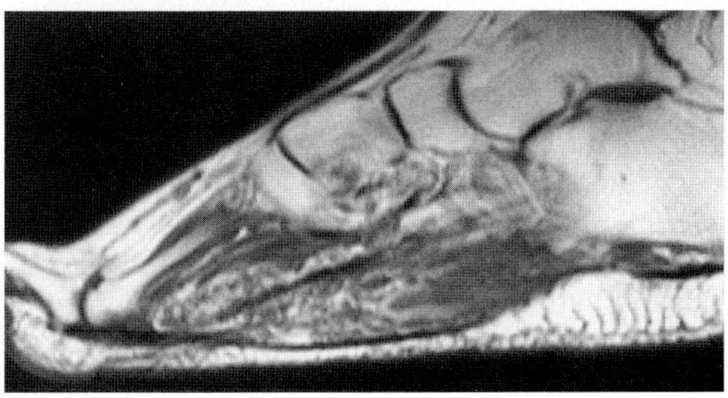
b

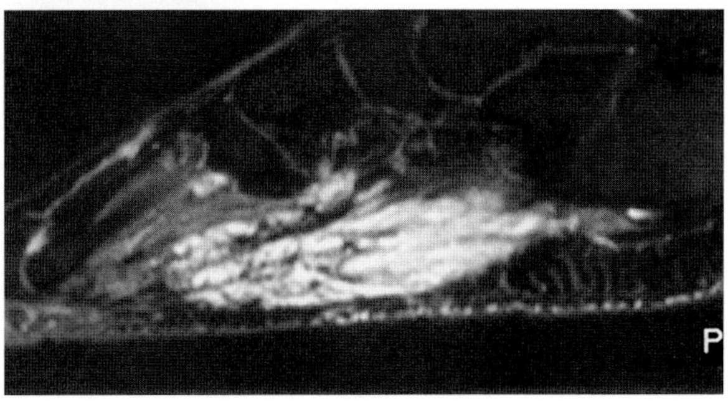
c

Fig. 20.13a–c. Soft-tissue haemangioma on the plantar aspect of the foot. **a** Transverse CT image shows a mainly soft-tissue density mass containing foci of low-density fat and three small, well-defined calcifications in keeping with phleboliths (*arrow*). Sagittal T1-weighted (**b**) and STIR (**c**) MR images showing an ill-defined inhomogeneous mass of predominantly intermediate SI on T1-weighting and high SI on the STIR image. Note multiple foci of fat (high on T1-weighting, low on STIR) and serpentine structures of low SI corresponding to prominent vessels similar to the intermediate and malignant vasoformative tumours.

20.4.5 Synovial Tumours

Synovial osteochondromatosis is rare, accounting for only 0.5% of benign soft-tissue tumours around the foot and ankle (Kransdorf 1995a). Synovial metaplasia produces multiple, round, intrasynovial, cartilaginous nodules that may ossify. It is more common in men and presents in middle age with joint swelling if intra-articular and a soft-tissue mass if extra-articular. The disease is progressive, and secondary osteoarthritis in joints is common. Radiographs may show a soft-tissue mass with variable mineralisation, and well-defined bony erosions and scalloping are occasionally seen. Loose bodies are usually smooth and round or oval shaped and are often of similar size, although a dominant nodule may be present. On MR imaging, non-mineralised lesions give an intermediate signal intensity on T1-weighting and a very high signal intensity on T2-weighting (Kramer et al. 1993). Differentiation from synovial fluid can be achieved by using intravenous Gd-DTPA as the nodules enhance if they are attached to and derive a vascular supply from the synovium. However, the majority of cases contain foci of low signal intensity on both T1-weighting and T2-weighting due to calcification of cartilaginous nodules. Ossified nodules containing fatty marrow are less common. Chondrosarcomatous degeneration is very rare but has been reported in the ankle (Ontell and Greenspan 1994).

Pigmented villonodular synovitis is a term given to a proliferative tumour-like disorder of the synovium of joints or tendon sheaths. In the foot and ankle, localised extraarticular *giant-cell tumour of the tendon sheath* (GCTTS) is the most common form of the condition, accounting for 8.3% of all benign soft-tissue tumours of the foot and ankle, whereas the localised or diffuse intraarticular form accounts for only 3.8% (Kransdorf 1995a). Patients usually present in early/middle adulthood with a slow-growing nodular soft-tissue mass related to a tendon sheath or joint capsule or mechanical joint pain. Radiographs typically show an unmineralised soft-tissue density opacity, normal bone density and often corticated erosions. On MR imaging, haemosiderin-laden synovial tissue exerts a paramagnetic effect that shortens T1 and T2 relaxation times, resulting in low/intermediate signal intensity on both T1-weighted and T2-weighted sequences (Fig. 20.2) (Bravo et al. 1996). On gradient-echo (GE) sequences, the effect is exaggerated due to increased magnetic susceptibility. This results in areas of very low signal intensity and 'blooming' artefact on T2-weighted GE sequences. Typically, lesions show marked enhancement following intravenous contrast administration. The uncommon diffuse extra-articular variant of GCTTS is a rare, locally aggressive neoplasm in the foot and ankle with significant recurrent and occasionally malignant potential (Somerhausen and Fletcher 2000).

Synovial sarcoma is the most common soft-tissue sarcoma in the foot and ankle, accounting for 18.7% of lesions (Kransdorf 1995b). It appears most usually in patients aged 6–45 years, and the sex incidence is equal. It commonly presents with a mass arising from the tendons, tendon sheaths or bursal structures. Small lesions may be homogeneous, well-defined and slow growing and mistakenly passed off as benign (Blacksin et al. 1997). Fewer than 10% are intra-articular, but articular spread from juxta-articular sites is common in the foot and ankle. Favourable factors include age <25 years, size <5 cm, prominent mineralisation and no histological evidence of poor differentiation, and the estimated 5-year survival rate is 60% (Bergh et al. 1999). Metastatic disease is mainly pulmonary (90%), and 25% have metastases at presentation. Radiographs may show a well-defined, round or lobulated, soft-tissue mass. Calcifications are found in up to 30% of cases and vary from fine stippling to dense opacities. On MR imaging, lesions are typically characterised by a fairly well-defined, lobulated, inhomogeneous, juxta-articular mass. On T1-weighting, lesions usually display low/intermediate signal intensity, although small foci of high signal intensity intratumoral haemorrhage are common. On T2-weighting, a heterogenous pattern of variable signal intensity is typically found in most lesions. Due to their periarticular position, 50% of lesions are contiguous with bone, and up to 20% cause pressure erosion or frank infiltration (Fig. 20.14). Small calcifications may be missed on MR imaging.

20.4.6 Neural Soft-Tissue Tumours

Morton neuroma is a very common non-neoplastic lesion of the forefoot due to perineural fibrosis of a plantar digital nerve. Lesions usually present with a burning sensation and most commonly involve the 3rd and to a lesser extent the 2nd intermetatarsal

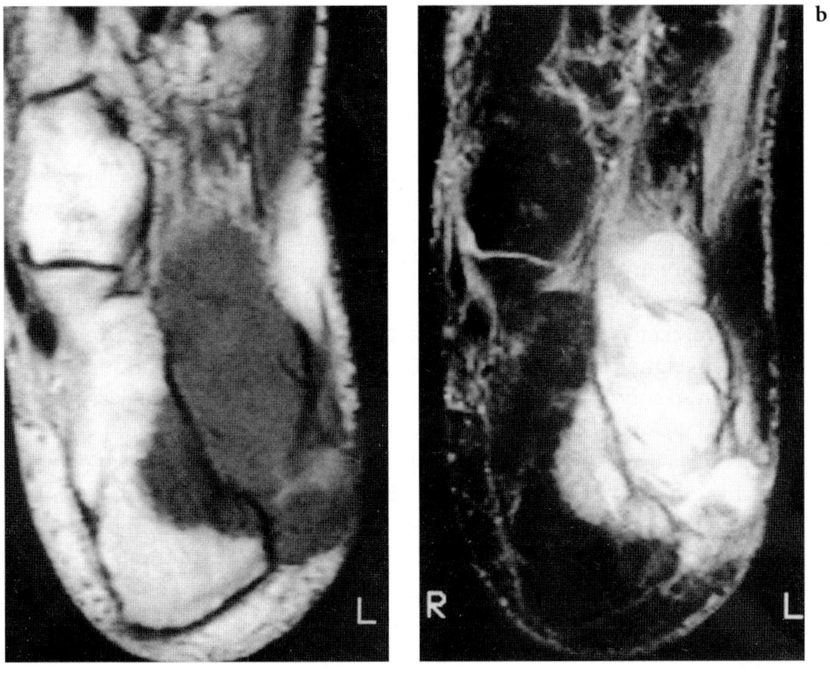

Fig. 20.14a, b. Synovial sarcoma of the hindfoot in a 70-year-old woman. Transverse T1-weighted (**a**) and STIR (**b**) MR images of an ill-defined mass on the medial aspect of the hindfoot infiltrating the calcaneus

spaces. There is a marked propensity in women, although the lesion is common in asymptomatic patients (Zanetti et al. 1997). Ultrasound typically shows an ovoid, hypoechoic mass between the metatarsal heads, but lesions smaller than 5 mm may be missed (Kaminsky et al. 1997). On MR imaging, lesions typically display low signal intensity on both T1-weighting and T2-weighting, high or intermediate signal intensity on STIR, and may enhance with intravenous gadolinium contrast administration. However, most authorities agree that lesions are best shown on T1-weighted images (Fig. 20.15). Associated fluid collections in the intermetatarsal bursae are common, but collections with a transverse diameter of 3 mm or less can be considered physiological. A more favourable clinical outcome can be expected after surgical intermetatarsal neurectomy when a Morton neuroma has a transverse measurement larger than 5 mm on MRI scans (Biasca et al. 1999).

Benign nerve sheath tumours are relatively uncommon in the foot and ankle, with neurofibroma accounting for 2.2% and schwannoma for 5.4% of benign soft-tissue tumours of the ankle and foot (Kransdorf 1995a). *Schwannomas* (neurolemmomas) are well-encapsulated tumours that arise from the Schwann cells of the nerve sheath and contain cellular and myxoid elements. As they grow, schwannomas displace the nerve fibres eccentrically and thus can be surgically removed without sacrificing the nerve. *Neurofibromas* are nonencapsulated lesions that separate the nerve fibres and cause fusiform enlargement of the nerve. Resection of the lesion requires sacrifice of the nerve. Benign nerve sheath tumours usually present with a soft-tissue mass that may cause pain or neurological symptoms (Beggs 1997). Schwannomas tend to present later (20–50 years) than neurofibromas (20–30 years). Plexiform neurofibromas are pathognomonic of neurofibromatosis type 1. Between 3% and 13% of patients with neurofibromatosis will develop a malignant peripheral nerve sheath tumour, whereas malignant transformation of a solitary neurofibroma is rare and of schwannoma is extremely rare (Michelson and Sinclair 1994). Plain radiography may show a soft-tissue mass, and mineralisation is uncommon.

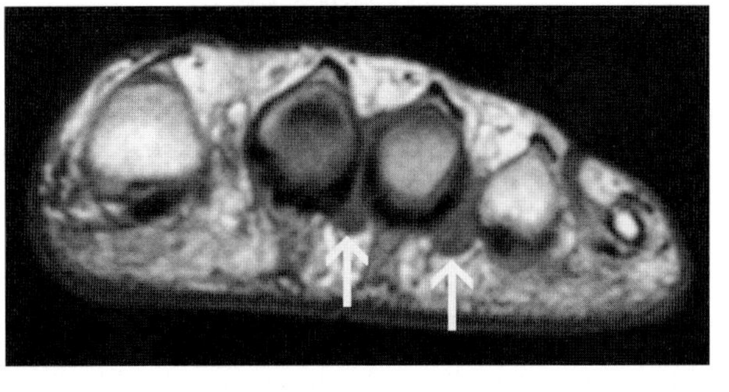

Fig. 20.15. Coronal T1-weighted MR image showing two small, well-defined, intermediate SI lesions at the 2nd/3rd and 3rd/4th interspaces due to Morton's neuromas (*arrows*)

On ultrasound, neurofibroma is fairly well defined and elongated along the nerve axis, whereas schwannoma is a sharply defined, eccentric mass often with cysts. On CT, both schwannoma and neurofibroma are usually hypodense to muscle. On MR imaging, both lesions are homogeneous and isointense or slightly hyperintense to muscle on T1-weighting and strongly enhance with intravenous Gd-DTPA. On T2-weighting, both lesions are mainly hyperintense but show inhomogeneity with foci of variable signal intensity. On T2-weighting, the target sign describes the low signal intensity fibrous central component against the high signal peripheral myxoid component and is more commonly seen in neurofibroma than schwannoma (Fig. 20.16). A fibrous pseudo-capsule, cystic change, necrosis and haemorrhage are all more common in schwannoma than neurofibroma. However, attempts to differentiate schwannoma from neurofibroma in the small nerves of the foot and ankle are usually unsuccessful.

Malignant peripheral nerve sheath tumours (MPNST) account for 4.5% of all soft-tissue sarcomas around the foot and ankle, and up to 70% are associated with neurofibromatosis type 1 (Kransdorf 1995b). It is clear that most, if not all, MPNST in NF1 patients arise from pre-existing neurofibromas. MPNST presents earlier in NF1 patients (mean 28.7 years) than in non-NF1 patients (mean 34.0 years) with a soft-tissue mass that may cause neurological symptoms in the affected nerve. Sudden enlargement of a pre-existing neurofibroma is an ominous finding suggestive of malignant transformation. Imaging features are non-specific, and differentiation from benign nerve sheath tumours may be difficult. Ultrasound and CT show irregular, inhomogeneous masses with necrotic and cystic foci and occasionally calcification. On MR imaging, lesions are often irregular and larger than 5 cm, although in the foot and ankle lesions tend to present earlier. Lesions are typically inhomogeneous, particularly on T2-weighting due in part to haemorrhage, necrosis, cystic change and mineralisation.

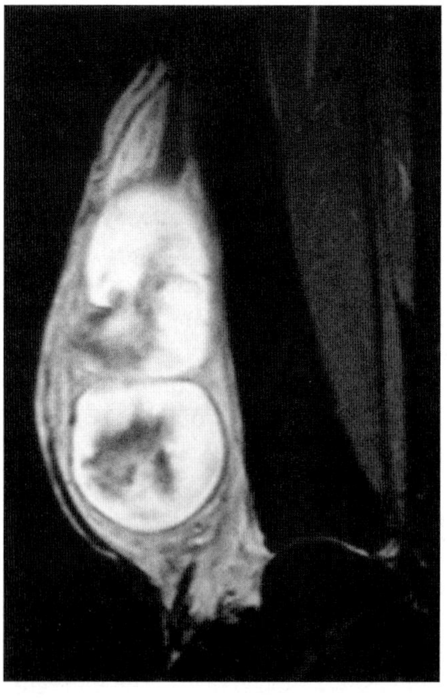

Fig. 20.16. Neurofibroma over the anterior lower leg in a 25-year-old man with neurofibromatosis. Sagittal STIR MR image showing a large inhomogeneous mass, the central component of which is divided into two loculi, both displaying low SI centrally and high SI peripherally – the 'target' sign. This reflects the predominantly fibrous component centrally and myxoid component peripherally. Note the diffuse neurofibromatous tissue around the large mass

Although *clear-cell sarcoma* (malignant melanoma of soft parts) is rare (1% of all soft-tissue sarcomas), the foot and ankle are relatively common sites of occurrence, accounting for 8% of all foot and ankle soft-tissue sarcomas (Kransdorf 1995b). It most commonly appears in the 2nd–4th decades, is more common in women, and usually presents with a mass arising from a tendon, ligament or aponeurosis. Clear-cell sarcoma usually metastasises to lungs, bone and lymph nodes and has a poor prognosis, with 56% mortality at 4 years and 80% at 10 years.

Radiographs usually show a non-specific, unmineralised soft-tissue mass. Osseous involvement is infrequent (De Beuckeleer et al. 2000). On MR imaging, the majority of lesions are well defined and homogeneous and thus may give a false impression of a benign lesion. On T1-weighting, most lesions are slightly hyperintense compared with muscle, reflecting a high melanin content in the lesion. Similarly, the low/intermediate signal intensity on T2-weighting in some cases may be due to the 'melanin' effect, but most cases display high signal intensity on T2-weighting. This probably reflects either low melanin content, high extracellular water content or other factors including the type of stromal tissue. Moderate to strong enhancement is typical.

Primitive neuroectodermal tumour (PNET)/ extraskeletal Ewing's sarcomas are very rare, accounting for only 0.75% of malignant soft-tissue masses about the ankle and foot (Kransdorf 1995b). Lesions appear hypoechoic on ultrasound and hypodense with respect to muscle on CT. On MR imaging, lesions have variable margins and non-specific features with low to intermediate signal intensity on T1-weighting and high signal intensity on T2-weighting. Lesions enhance avidly, and haemorrhage may be present.

20.4.7 Cartilage/Bone-Forming Soft-Tissue Tumours

Extraskeletal chondromas are uncommon lesions but have a propensity for the extremities and account for 5.6% of all benign soft-tissue tumours of the foot and ankle (Kransdorf 1995a). They are most commonly found in men in the 4th–6th decades, and typically present with a slow-growing soft-tissue mass usually measuring less than 3 cm. They may be attached to various structures including tendon sheaths and joint capsules. Radiographs may show a soft-tissue mass containing mineralisation in up to 70%. The uncalcified cartilaginous components of the lesions display intermediate signal intensity on T1-weighting and very high signal intensity on T2-weighting, whereas the mineralised components display low signal intensity on all sequences.

Extraskeletal chondrosarcoma is uncommon, accounting for 3.6% of malignant soft-tissue tumours of the foot and ankle (Kransdorf 1995b). The myxoid and mesenchymal subtypes show minimal cartilage formation and are much commoner than the very rare well-differentiated subtype. Patients are usually middle-aged and present with a soft-tissue mass. The low-grade myxoid type rarely shows mineralisation, whereas the more aggressive mesenchymal variant shows cartilage calcification in over 50%. On MR imaging, lesions tend to appear ill-defined and inhomogeneous. Myxoid components typically display foci of very high signal intensity on T2-weighting, whereas the mineralised components of mesenchymal lesions display signal voids on all sequences.

Extraskeletal osteosarcoma is a rare, aggressive, malignant mesenchymal osteoid-forming neoplasm accounting for only 0.6% of malignant soft-tissue tumours of the foot and ankle (Kransdorf 1995b). Plain radiographs show dense cloud-like mineralisation in 50%. MR imaging shows an ill-defined, inhomogeneous lesion with predominantly intermediate signal intensity on T1-weighting and high signal intensity on T2-weighting. Mineralised foci result in low signal intensity on all sequences.

20.4.8 Muscle Tumours

Leiomyoma is a uncommon, benign, smooth-muscle tumour that only accounts for 5.7% of benign tumours and tumour-like lesions of the foot and ankle (Kransdorf 1995b). Deep lesions are much less common than superficial lesions but may mimic a sarcoma and therefore are more likely to be imaged. Deep leiomyomas are more prone to regressive changes including fibrosis and mineralisation. The mineralisation varies from small flecks to large clumps of calcification and is readily shown on radiographs or CT. On MR imaging, lesions are typically inhomogeneous, with foci of low signal on all sequences.

Leiomyosarcoma accounts for 7.1% of foot and ankle soft-tissue sarcomas (Kransdorf 1995b). Patients most commonly present with a painless, slow-growing mass in the 5th–6th decades. Rarely, leiomyosarcoma may arise in the wall of a vessel (Begin et al. 1994). Radiography may show a soft-tissue mass and bony involvement, but calcifications are rare. CT may show foci of decreased attenuation due to necrosis and cystic change. MR imaging typically shows a non-specific, inhomogeneous, enhancing mass with necrosis, although more superficial lesions tend to be small, well-defined and homogeneous.

Rhabdomyosarcoma is the most common childhood malignancy of soft tissue but only accounts for 1.9% of foot and ankle soft-tissue sarcomas (Kransdorf 1995b). The alveolar subtype is more common than the embryonic subtype in extremity lesions and tends to occur in an older age group (10–25 years) than the embryonic subtype (0–15 years). Radiography may show a non-specific soft-tissue mass and bony involvement in up to 24% (Suzuki et al. 1997). MR imaging shows an ill-defined, inhomogeneous, non-specific mass, isointense on T1-weighting and hyperintense on T2-weighting. Prominent vascularity, intralesional haemorrhage and necrosis are typical of the alveolar subtype and explains its inhomogeneous enhancement. On the other hand, embryonic lesions are less necrotic and display a more homogeneous enhancement pattern.

20.4.9 Soft-Tissue Tumours of Unknown Origin

Idiopathic tumoral calcinosis is a tumour-like lesion that is rare in the foot and ankle. Patients usually present in the first two decades with a slow-growing, juxta-articular, soft-tissue mass that may ulcerate and drain chalky-like material (Slomovitz et al. 1990). Similar appearances may be seen in various metabolic disorders including chronic renal failure. Radiographs demonstrate well-defined, juxta-articular, lobulated, calcific masses with linear radiolucencies and fibrous septations that may occasionally erode bone. CT may show a uniformly calcified mass or cystic lesion with calcific walls and fluid-fluid levels. On MR imaging, lesions show low signal intensity on all sequences but may have diffuse or focal areas of high signal intensity on T2-weighting if the lesions are inflammatory or contain fluid.

Myxomas are small lesions typically located in the subcutaneous tissues of the dorsal aspect of the foot. Imaging is only required for the less common indeterminate deep intramuscular lesions. There is a peak presentation in the 5th–7th decades. Ultrasound typically shows a well-defined hypoechoic or transonic lesion, although occasionally some internal echoes may be present. On MR imaging, lesions are well-defined, homogeneous and hypointense on T1-weighting and markedly hyperintense on T2-weighting. Enhancement is variable.

Epithelioid sarcoma is an uncommon soft-tissue sarcoma that only accounts for 2.3% of malignant soft-tissue tumours about the foot and ankle (Kransdorf 1995b). It presents in young adults, more commonly men, with a hard, slow-growing, soft-tissue mass. Metastatic spread most commonly involves the lymphatic system and to a lesser extent the lungs. Plain radiographs may show a soft-tissue mass containing speckled calcifications or ossification. On MR imaging, the majority show non-specific intermediate signal intensity on T1-weighting and high signal intensity on T2-weighting, but some also display evidence of haemorrhage. Haemorrhagic tumours are more aggressive and appear to metastasise more commonly and earlier than non-haemorrhagic lesions.

20.4.10 Tumour-like Lesions of Soft Tissues

Ganglia are common lesions found over the dorsal aspect of the foot and around the hindfoot and ankle. They usually arise from the surface of joint capsules or tendon sheaths but rarely communicate with these structures and are not lined by synovium. Patients present with a painless mass most commonly in the 3rd or 4th decades. Ultrasound typically demonstrates a homogeneous unilocular or multilocular transonic cystic lesion, often with pseudopodia extending towards a joint. MR imaging usually demonstrates a well-defined homogeneous lesion of low signal intensity on T1-weighting and very high signal intensity on T2-weighting. However, if the protein content is high, then the signal intensity on T1-weighting may be isointense with muscle. Peripheral enhancement may occur.

Granuloma annulare is a benign, inflammatory dermatosis that is most commonly found around the foot and ankle. The subcutaneous form is usually seen in children and presents with a rapidly growing nodule. Lesions tend to regress over time but may progress to a more generalised form and may recur following excision (Davids et al. 1993). Ultrasound shows an ill-defined mass hypoechoic to subcutaneous fat. MR imaging reveals an ill-defined mass that is hypointense on T1-weighting and hypointense or isointense on T2-weighting.

Epidermal inclusion (infundibular) cysts are common superficial lesions that probably occur as a result of traumatic implantation of epidermal cells into dermal tissue (Fisher et al. 1998). They are most common in the 4th decade. In the foot, lesions often arise in the plantar or medial aspect of the head of the 1st metatarsal bone. Radiography may demonstrate a mass with bony erosion. On ultrasound, lesions are well defined and hypoechoic but may contain small echogenic foci due to keratin clusters. On MRI, lesions typically display low signal intensity on T1-weighting and high signal intensity on T2-weighting, although the hypointense keratin clusters may result in an inhomogeneous appearance.

Myositis ossificans is a benign, mineralising, intramuscular mass that is usually post-traumatic but rarely occurs in the foot (De Maeseneer et al. 1997).

Subcutaneous *rheumatoid nodules* and *mycetoma* are discussed elsewhere.

References

Abrahim-Zadeh R, Klein RM, Leslie D et al (1998) Characteristics of calcaneal bone infarction: an MR imaging investigation. Skeletal Radiol 27:321–324

Adkins CD, Kitaoka HB, Seidl RK et al (1997) Ewing's sarcoma of the foot. Clin Orthop 343:173–182

Anderson MW, ThomasTemple H, Dussault RG et al (1999) Compartment anatomy: relevance to staging and biopsy of musculoskeletal tumours. Am J Roentgenol 173: 1663–1671

Bakotic BW, Robinson M, Williams M, et al (1999) Aggressive epithelioid hemangioendothelioma of the lower extremity: a case report and review of the literature. J Foot Ankle Surg 38:352–358

Baraga JJ, Amrami KK, Swee RG et al (2001) radiographic features of Ewing's sarcoma of the bones of the hands and feet. Skeletal Radiol 30:121–126

Barca F, Acciaro AL, Recchioni MD (1998) Osteoid osteoma of the phalanx: enlargement of the toe. Two case reports. Foot Ankle Int 19:388–393

Beggs I (1997) Pictorial review: imaging of periperal nerve tumours. Clin Radiol 52:8–17

Begin LR, Guy P, Mitmaker B (1994) Intramural leiomyosarcoma of the dorsal pedal vein: a clinical mimicry of ganglion. Foot Ankle Int 15:48–51

Bergh P, Meis-Kindblom JM, Gherlinzoni F et al (1999) Synovial sarcoma: identification of low and high risk groups. Cancer 85:2596–2607

Berlin SJ (1995) Statistical analysis of 307,601 tumors and other lesions of the foot. J Am Podiatr Med Assoc 85: 699–703

Biasca N, Zanetti M, Zollinger H (1999) Outcomes after partial neurectomy of Morton's neuroma related to preoperative case histories, clinical findings and findings on magnetic resonance imaging scans. Foot Ankle Int 20:568–575

Biscaglia R, Bacchini P, Bertoni F (2000) Giant cell tumor of the bones of the hand and foot. Cancer 88:2022–2032

Blacksin MF, Siegel JR, Benevenia J et al (1997) Synovial sarcoma: frequency of nonaggressive MR characteristics. J Comput Assist Tomogr 21:785–789

Bloem JL, Taminiau AHM, Eulderink F et al (1988) Radiologic staging of primary bone sarcoma: MR imaging, scintigraphy, angiography, and CT correlated with pathologic examination. Radiology 169:805–810

Bohm P, Krober S, Greschniok A et al (1996) Desmoplastic fibroma of the bone. A report of two patients, review of the literature, and therapeutic implications. Cancer 78:1011–1023

Boutin RD, Spaeth HJ, Mangalik A et al (1996) Epithelioid haemangioendothelioma of bone. Skeletal Radiol 25:391–395

Bovee JV, Van der Heul RO, Taminiau AH, et al (1999) Chondrosarcoma of the phalanx: a locally aggressive lesion with minimal metastatic potential: a report of 35 cases and a review of the literature. Cancer 86:1724–1732

Braunschweig IJ, Stein IH, Dodwad MIM et al (1992) Case report 751: spindle cell lipoma causing marked bone erosion. Skeletal Radiol 21:414–417

Bravo SM, Winalski CS, Weissman BN (1996) Pigmented villonodular synovitis. Rad Clin North Am 34:311–326

Campanacci F (1990) Bone and soft tissue tumours. Springer, Vienna New York

Casadei R, Ferraro A, Ferruzzi A et al (1991) Bone tumors of the foot: epidemiology and diagnosis. Chir Organi Mov 76:47–62

Choong PF, Qureshi AA, Sim FH et al (1999) Osteosarcoma of the foot: a review of 52 patients at the Mayo Clinic. Acta Orthop Scand 70:361–364

Chow LT, Allen PW, Kumta SM et al (1998) Angiomatoid malignant fibrous histiocytoma: report of an unusual case with highly aggressive clinical course. J Foot Ankle Surg 37:235–238

Cione JA, Lynn B, Boylan J (1999) Dermatofibrosarcoma protuberans. A rare case involving the pediatric foot. J Am Podiatr Med Assoc 89:419–423

Cummins CA, Scarborough MT, Enneking WF (1996) Multicentric giant cell tumor of bone. Clin Orthop 322:245–252

Davids JR, Kolman BH, Billman GF et al (1993) Subcutaneous granuloma annulare: recognition and treatment. J Pediatr Orthop 13:582–586

De Beuckeleer LH, De Schepper AM, Vandevenne JE et al (2000) MR imaging of clear cell sarcoma (malignant melanoma of the soft parts): a multicenter correlative MRI-pathology study of 21 cases and literature review. Skeletal Radiol 29:187–195

De Maeseneer M, Jaovisidha S, Lenchik L et al (1997) Myositis ossificans of the foot. J Foot Ankle Surg 36:290–293

Derchi LE, Balconi G, De Flaviis L et al (1989) Sonographic appearances of hemangiomas of skeletal muscle. J Ultrasound Med 8:263–267

Donley BG, Neel M, Mitias HM (1996) Neural fibrolipoma of the foot: a case report. Foot Ankle Int 17:712–713

Drape JL, Idy-Peretti I, Goettmann S et al (1996) Standard and high resolution magnetic resonance imaging of glomus tumors of toes and fingertips. J Am Acad Dermatol 35: 550–555

Enneking WF, Spanier SS, Goodman MA (1980) A system for the surgical staging of musculoskeletal sarcoma. Clin Orthop 153:106–120

Enzinger F, Weiss S (1995) Soft tissue tumours, 3rd edn. Mosby, St Louis

Fink BR, Temple HT, Chiricosta FM et al (1997) Chondroblastoma of the foot. Foot Ankle Int 18:236–242

Fisher AR, Mason PH, Wagenhals KS, et al (1998) Ruptured plantar epidermal inclusion cyst. AJR Am J Roentgenol 171:1709–1710

Fornage BD (1998) Glomus tumors in the fingers: diagnosis with US. Radiology 167:183–185

Harty JA, Kelly P, Niall D, O'Keane JC, Stephens MM (2000) Bizarre parosteal osteochondromatous proliferation (Nora's lesion) of the sesamoid: a case report. Foot Ankle Int 21:408–412

Hottya GA, Steinbach LS, Johnston JO et al (1999) Chondrosarcoma of the foot: imaging, surgical and pathological correlation of three new cases. Skeletal Radiol 28:153–158

Huvos AG (1991) Bone tumors: diagnosis, treatment and prognosis, 2nd edn. Saunders, Philadelphia

Isefuku S, Hatori M, Ehara S et al (1999) Fibrous dysplasia arising from the calcaneus. Tohoku J Exp Med 189:227–232

Jee WH, Park YK, McCauley TR (1999) Chondroblastoma: MR characteristics with pathologic correlation. J Comput Assist Tomogr 23:721–726

Johnson K, Davies AM, Mangham DC et al (1999) Parosteal osteosarcoma of a metatarsal with intramedullary invasion. Skeletal Radiol 28:111–105

Kaminsky S, Griffin L, Milsap J et al (1997) Is ultrasonography a reliable way to confirm the diagnosis of Morton's neuroma? Orthopedics 20:37–39

Kirby E, Shereff M, Lewis M (1989) Soft tissue tumors and tumor-like lesions of the foot: an analysis of 83 cases. J Bone Joint Surg 71A:621–626

Kramer J, Recht M, Deely DM et al (1993) MRI appearance of idiopathic synovial osteochondromatosis. J Comput Assist Tomogr 17:772–776

Kransdorf MJ (1995a) Benign soft-tissue tumors in a large referral population: distribution of diagnosis by age, sex, and location. AJR Am J Roentgenol 164:395–402

Kransdorf MJ (1995b) Malignant soft-tissue tumors in a large referral population: distribution of diagnoses by age, sex, and location. AJR Am J Roentgenol 164:129–134

Kransdorf MJ, Murphey MD (1997) Imaging of soft-tissue tumors. WB Saunders Co. Philadelphia, pp 3–35

Kyriakos M, Land VJ, Penning HL et al (1985) Metastatic chondroblastoma. Report of a fatal case with a review of the literature on atypical, aggressive, and malignant chondroblastoma. Cancer 55:1770–1789

Lee EY, Seeger LL, Nelson SD et al (2000) Primary osteosarcoma of a metatarsal bone. Skeletal Radiol 29:474–476

Libson E, Bloom RA, Husband JE et al (1987) Metastatic tumours of bones of the hand and foot. A comparative

review and report of 43 additional cases. Skeletal Radiol 16:387–392
Link TM, Haeussler MD, Poppek S et al (1998) Malignant fibrous histiocytoma of bone: conventional X-ray and MR imaging features. Skeletal Radiol 27:552–558
McLeod RA, Dahlin DC Beabout JW et al (1976) The spectrum of osteoblastoma. Am J Roentgenol 126:321–335
McNamara D, Beauregard GC, Lemieux RJ (1993) Scintigraphic ‚doughnut sign' on skeletal imaging due to a hemangioendothelioma of bone. J Nucl Med 34:297–300
Michelson JD, Sinclair M (1994) Sarcomatous degeneration of neurofibromatosis presenting in the foot. Foot Ankle Int 15:400–403
Milgram JW (1988) Intraosseous lipomas: radiologic and pathologic manifestations. Radiology 167:155–160
Mirra JM (1989) Bone tumours. Clinical, radiologic and pathologic correlations. Lea and Febiger, Philadelphia
Mitty HA (1993) Musculo neoplasms: role of angiography in diagnosis and intervention. Semin Intervent Radiol 10: 317–313
Miyayama H, Sakamoto K, Ide M et al (1993) Aggressive osteoblastoma of the calcaneus. Cancer 71:346–353
Monroe MT, Manoli A Jr (1999) Osteoid osteoma of the lateral talar process presenting as a chronic sprained ankle. Foot Ankle Int 20:461–463
Moon NF, Mori H (1986) Adamantinoma of the appendicular skeleton – updated. Clin Orthop Relat Res 204:215–237
Morrison WB, Schweitzer ME, Wapner KL et al (1994) Plantar fibromatosis: a benign aggressive neoplasm with a characteristic appearance on MR images. Radiology 193: 841–845
Murari T, Callaghan J, Berry B et al (1989) Primary benign and malignant osseous neoplasms of the foot. Foot Ankle 10:68–80
Murff R, Ashry HR (1994) Intraosseous ganglia of the foot. J Foot Ankle Surg 33:396–401
O'Connor PJ, Gibbon WW, Hardy G et al (1996) Chondromyxoid fibroma of the foot. Skeletal Radiol 25:143–148
Ogose A, Unni KK, Swee RG, et al (1997) Chondrosarcoma of small bones of the hands and feet. Cancer 80:50–59
Ontell F, Greenspan A (1994) Chondrosarcoma complicating synovial chondromatosis: findings with magnetic resonance imaging. Can Assoc Radiol J 45:318–323
Ozdemir HM, Yildiz Y, Yilmaz C et al (1997) Tumors of the foot and ankle: analysis of 196 cases. J Foot Ankle Surg 36:403–408
Pyati PS, Sanzone AG (1996) Intraosseous neurilemoma of the calcaneus. Orthopedics 19:353–355
Ratner V, Dorfman HD (1990) Giant-cell reparative granuloma of the hand and foot bones. Clin Orthop 260:251–258
Ricca RL Jr, Kuklo TR, Shawen SB et al (2000) Periosteal chondroma of the cuboid presenting in a 7-year-old-boy. Foot Ankle Int 21:145–149
Richardson AA, Erdmann BB, Beier-Hanratty S et al (1995) Magnetic resonance imagery of a calcaneal lipoma. J Am Podiatric Med Assoc 85:493–496
Schajowicz F (1981) Tumors and tumor-like lesions of bones and joints. Springer, Berlin Heidelberg New York
Skorman SE, Martin R (1999) Primary lymphoma of the calcaneus with recurrence in the distal tibia: a case report. J Foot Ankle Surg 38:278–282
Slomovitz M, Nixon B, Mott RC (1990) Tumoral calcinosis of the foot: case report and literature review. J Foot Surg 29: 278–283
Somerhausen NS, Fletcher CD (2000) Diffuse-type giant cell tumor: clinicopathologic and immunohistochemical analysis of 50 cases with extraarticular disease. Am J Surg Pathol 24:479–492
Stoker DJ, Cobb JP, Pringle JS (1991) Needle biopsy of musculoskeletal lesions. A review of 208 procedures. J Bone Joint Surg [Br] 158:498–500
Stukenborg-Colsman C, Wulker N, Wirth CJ (1999) Cystic bone lesions of the calcaneus: a report of five cases. Foot Ankle Surg 5:33–38
Suzuki Y, Ehara S, Shiraishi H, et al (1997) Embryonal rhabdomyosarcoma of foot with expansive growth between metatarsals. Skeletal Radiol 26:128–130
Taconis WK, Schutte HE, van der Heul RO et al (1994) Desmoplastic fibroma of bone: a report of 18 cases. Skeletal Radiol 23:283–288
Temple HT, Mizel MS, Murphey MD et al (1998) Osteoblastoma of the foot and ankle. Foot Ankle Int 19:698–704
Unni K (1996) Dahlin's bone tumors: general aspects and data on 11,087 cases, 5th edn. Lippincott-Raven, Philadelphia
Vanhoenacker FM, Hauben E, De Beuckeleer LH et al (2000) Desmoplastic fibroma of bone: MRI features. Skeletal Radiol 29:171–175
Werd MB, DeFronzo D, Landsman AS et al (1995) Myxoid liposarcoma of the ankle. J Foot Ankle Surg 34:465–474
White LM, Schweitzer ME, Khalili K et al (1998) MR imaging of primary lymphoma of bone: variability of T2-weighted signal intensity. AJR 170:1243–1247
Yee DY, Mott RC, Nixon BP (1991) Calcifying aponeurotic fibroma. J Foot Surg 30:279–283
Youssef BA, Haddad MC, Zahrani, et al (1996) Osteoid osteoma and osteoblastoma: MRI appearances and the significance of ring enhancement. Eur Radiol 6:291–296
Zanetti M, Strehle JK, Zollinger H (1997) Morton neuroma and fluid in the intermetatarsal bursae on MR images of 70 asymptomatic volunteers. Radiology 203:516–520

21 Orthopaedic Hardware

T. H. Berquist

CONTENTS

21.1 Introduction

There are numerous surgical approaches (internal fixation using wires, pins, staples, plates and screws; external fixation; arthroplasty) for the treatment of disorders affecting the foot and ankle. Appropriate use of imaging procedures and diagnostic injections is important for the treatment planning.

T.H. Berquist, MD, FACR
Professor of Radiology, Director for Education, Mayo Foundation, Mayo Clinic, 4500 San Pablo Road, Jacksonville, FL 32224, USA

Postoperative imaging plays a significant role in evaluating the surgical results and assessing potential complications. This chapter will review preoperative and postoperative imaging of common orthopedic procedures used for fracture reduction, fusion, reconstruction, and arthroplasty.

21.2 Preoperative Imaging

The selection of appropriate imaging procedures depends upon the underlying disorder (trauma, arthrosis, joint deformity, etc.) and the surgical procedure that may be performed (Berquist 1995).

21.2.1 Routine Radiography

Routine film/screen or computed radiography (CR) remains the primary screening technique for osseous and articular disorders of the foot and ankle. Standing AP and lateral views of the foot and ankle are critical, if tolerated by the patient, to obtain appropriate preoperative measurements (Berquist 2000). The mortise view of the ankle is important to assess symmetry of the talus.

Stress views of the ankles are performed using varus and valgus stress in the coronal plane and anteroposterior stress in the sagittal plane. Normal talar tilt may approach 25° in hypermobile ankles, so both ankles must be examined for comparison. A talar tilt of >5° suggests a ligament injury. Anteroposterior talar shift >2.5 mm indicates an anterior talofibular ligament tear (Morrey et al. 1986).

There are numerous special views for the foot. However, fluoroscopic positioning allows optimal alignment for spot views of the area or areas of interest (Berquist 2000).

21.2.2
Computed Tomography

The complex anatomy of the foot and ankle may require CT for complete evaluation of complex fractures or articular anatomy when arthrodesis is a consideration. Thin section (<3 mm) studies can be reformatted in coronal and sagittal planes to optimize the anatomic information. One-millimeter sections are used when three-dimensional (3D) reconstruction is required (Berquist 2000; Morrey et al. 1986).

21.2.3
Ultrasonography

Ultrasonography is useful for evaluating soft-tissue injury (ligament, tendon) and certain vascular disorders. Ultrasonography is readily available and inexpensive compared with CT or magnetic resonance (MR) imaging (Berquist 2000).

21.2.4
Radionuclide Scans

Radionuclide bone scans are useful for the detection of subtle fractures, infection, and other complications, such as reflex sympathetic dystrophy. Specific isotopes will be noted later when the possible complications of surgical procedures are reviewed.

21.2.5
Magnetic Resonance Imaging

MR imaging is useful for the detection and staging of soft-tissue injuries, detection of subtle osseous and articular trauma or arthrosis, and for evaluating complications such as nonunion, infection, and avascular necrosis. Metal artifact is expected after surgical fixation or arthroplasty. However, local image distortion does not always obscure the area of interest. Screws cause the most significant local image distortion. The type of device used and its composition (fewer artifacts with titanium) are important when considering whether MR imaging is appropriate.

In most cases, spin-echo or fast spin-echo T1-weighted and T2-weighted sequences in two planes are adequate for lesion detection and characterization. Special sequences or contrast (gadolinium)-enhanced images are useful in selected cases (Berquist 2001; Rosenberg et al. 2000).

21.2.6
Interventional Techniques

Arthrography, tenography, and diagnostic and therapeutic injections are all useful techniques. Additional information regarding ligament and tendon disorders and pain localization are useful in treatment planning and confirming the clinical diagnosis (Berquist 1993; Jaffee et al. 2001; Khoury et al. 1995). Techniques can be performed using fluoroscopic or ultrasound guidance.

21.3
Postoperative Imaging/Complications

Postoperative evaluation is important to assess the surgical results and confirm suspected complications. Complications vary with the extent of the procedure and instrumentation used. For example, complications seen with internal fixation may be significantly different than complications associated with external fixation (Behrens 1980, 1989; Helm 1990; Moekel et al. 1991).

For purposes of discussion, we will consider trauma, arthrodesis, arthroplasty, and forefoot deformities separately.

21.3.1
Trauma

The management of fractures and dislocations is accomplished by closed reduction whenever possible. However, surgical intervention using internal or external fixation devices is common in the foot and ankle. The treatment options vary with the location, extent of injury, patient expectations, patient activity, and overall clinical status plus surgical preference.

21.3.1.1
Ankle Fractures

Most ankle fractures occur with inversion or eversion forces. Lateral rotation and axial loading may also occur (Berquist 1995; Marsh et al. 1995). Fractures that are displaced (>2 mm), high fibular fractures (>5 cm above the joint line), and pilon fractures (involve the tibial articular surface) most often require fixation (Gourineni et al. 1999; Vander Greind et al. 1996).

External fixation is not commonly employed except for complex distal tibial fractures (Wyrsch et al. 1996)

(Fig. 21.1). Medial malleolar fractures that are displaced >2 mm are often internally fixed with malleolar screws or wires. Fibular fractures may be reduced with plate and screws (Fig. 21.2) (BERQUIST 1995).

Complications following ankle fractures are common. In adults, 30%–40% develop arthritis regardless of the treatment method (Fig. 21.3). The incidence of arthrosis increases with pilon fractures and when the syndesmosis is poorly reduced, leading to chronic instability (BERQUIST 1995; MORREY et al. 1986) (Fig. 21.4).

Nonunion or malunion may occur with poor reduction of implant failure (Fig. 21.4). Medial malleolar avulsions are more prone to nonunion (GOURINENI et al. 1999). In children, growth plate deformity and leg length discrepancy may occur (BERQUIST 1995). Table 21.1 summarizes the possible complications of ankle fractures.

21.3.1.2 Hindfoot Fractures

Calcaneal fractures account for 60% of foot fractures. Talar fractures comprise only 6% of foot fractures (MORREY et al. 1986; SANDERS 2000). In adults, 75% of calcaneal fractures are intraarticular. Fragmentation and articular deformity are most effectively demonstrated with CT in the axial and coronal planes (Fig. 21.5). Treatment should reestablish articular alignment, particularly the posterior facet (Böhlers angle, normal 20°–40°), and the normal calcaneal width must be maintained. Reconstruction plates and screws (Fig. 21.5) are commonly used to achieve these goals (SANDERS 2000). More recently, cement augmentation has been advocated to increase the stability and compressive strength (THORDARSON et al. 1999).

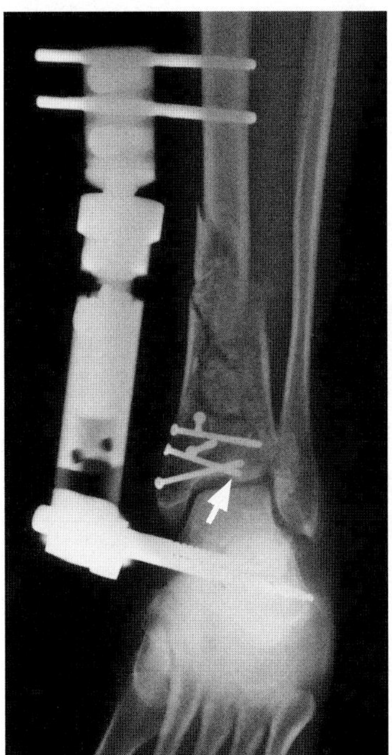

Fig. 21.1. Complex open distal tibial fracture with partially threaded screws to restore the articular surface (note persistent step-off, *arrow*) and external Orthofix fixator

Talar neck fractures that are displaced also require screw or wire fixation (MORREY et al. 1986) (Fig. 21.6). Talar fracture complications included delayed union (15%), nonunion (4%), and avascular necrosis. The last is particularly common after displaced talar neck fractures (BERQUIST 1995).

Chronic pain is common after calcaneal fractures. It may be related to arthrosis nerve entrapment or tendon impingement. CT (Fig. 21.7) is best for evaluating fracture reduction even in the presence of orthopedic implants. Diagnostic injections are useful when considering arthrodesis to relieve symptoms (BERQUIST 1993; KHOURY et al. 1995).

21.3.1.3 Midfoot and Forefoot Fractures

The midfoot consists of the lesser tarsal bones (navicular, cuboid, and three cuneiforms). Isolated tarsal fractures without joint and ligament involvement are uncommon.

Tarsometatarsal dislocations are referred to as Lisfranc injuries. Multiple patterns have been described. CT may be required to assess the extent of injury and plan the course of treatment if internal fixation is required.

Metatarsal fractures are common and usually result from direct trauma from a heavy object striking the foot. Fractures of the 5th metatarsal base may be due to avulsion from pull of peroneus brevis. Fractures of the proximal 5th metatarsal shaft are more problematic and require internal fixation using a long screw (Fig. 21.8). Other forefoot fractures are treated with closed reduction in most cases. If reduction cannot be maintained, K-wire, screw, or miniplate and screw fixation may be required.

Complications of midfoot and forefoot fractures include malunion, nonunion, or painful arthrosis. The last may require arthrodesis for treatment. Selection of fusion sites can be confirmed with preoperative diagnostic anesthetic injections (BERQUIST 1993; KHOURY et al. 1995).

Fig. 21.2a–d. Ankle fractures with internal fixation. AP (**a**) and lateral (**b**) radiographs of a healed ankle fracture with Rush rod in the fibula and single cortical screw for medial malleolar fixation. The joint space is normal. Mortise and AP views (**c**) and lateral view (**d**) of a complex tibial articular (pilon) fracture fixed with two partially threaded cancellous screws. The articular surface is restored (compare to Fig. 21.1). There is a syndesmotic screw (*arrow*) to reduce the syndesmosis. The fibular fracture is reduced with a 1/3 tubular plate and cortical screws with a lag screw across the fracture (*open arrow*)

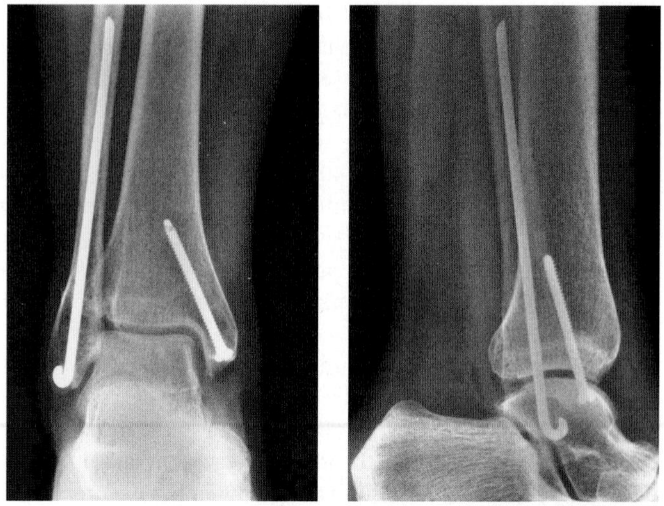

a b

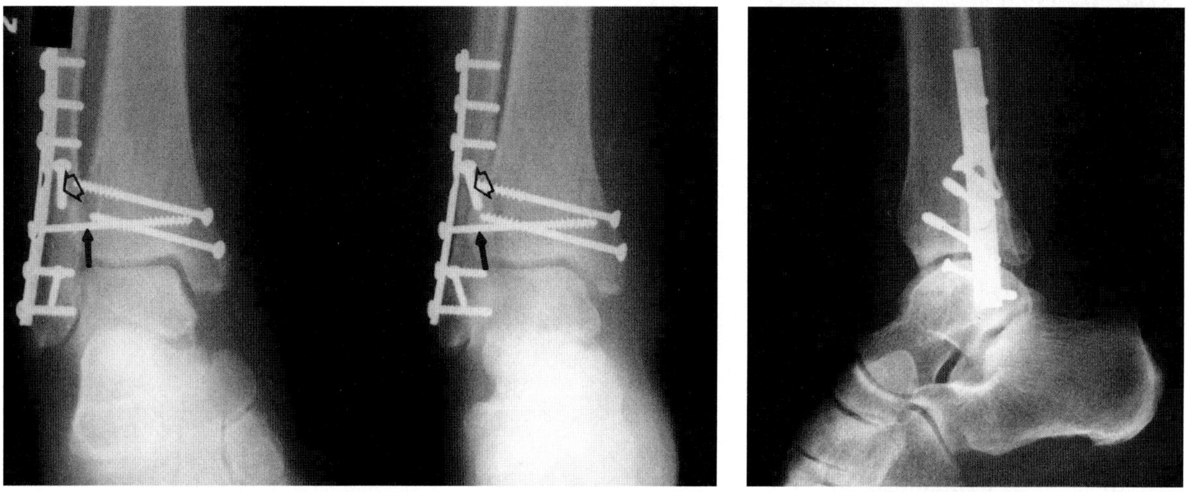

c d

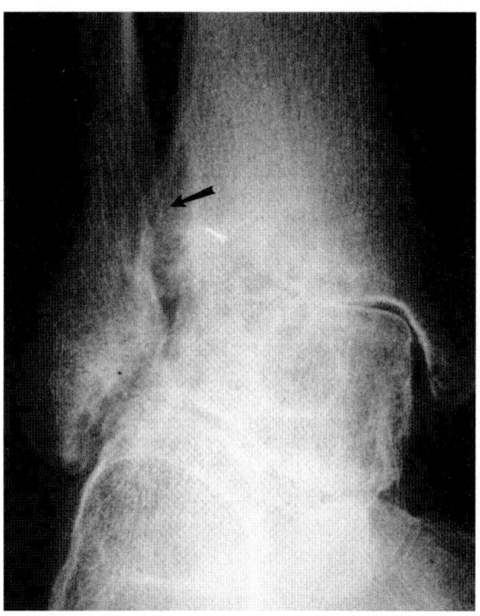

Fig. 21.3. AP radiograph after ankle fracture demonstrates marked joint space loss and talar tilt with widening of the syndesmosis (*arrow*)

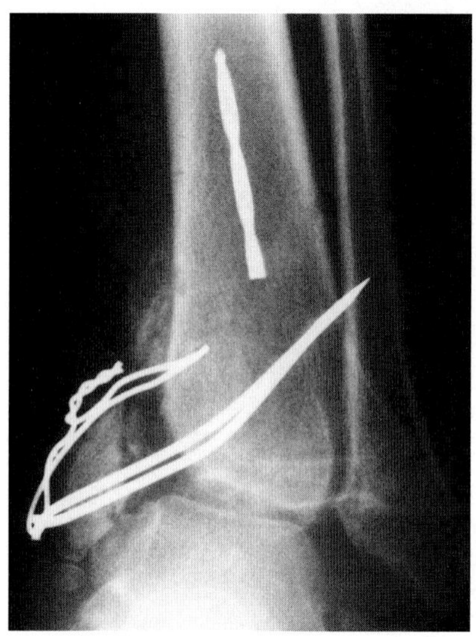

Fig. 21.4. Old nonunited medial malleolar fracture with obvious subluxation and failed K-wire and tension band fixation

Fig. 21.5a–e. Calcaneal fracture. Axial (**a**) and coronal (**b**) CT images clearly demonstrate the articular involvement with widening and shortening of the calcaneus. **c** Lateral radiograph shows loss of Böhler's angle (15°, normal 20°–40°). Reconstruction plate and cortical screws restored the calcaneal width and length, and Böhler's angle is improved on postoperative lateral (**d**) and axial (**e**) radiographs

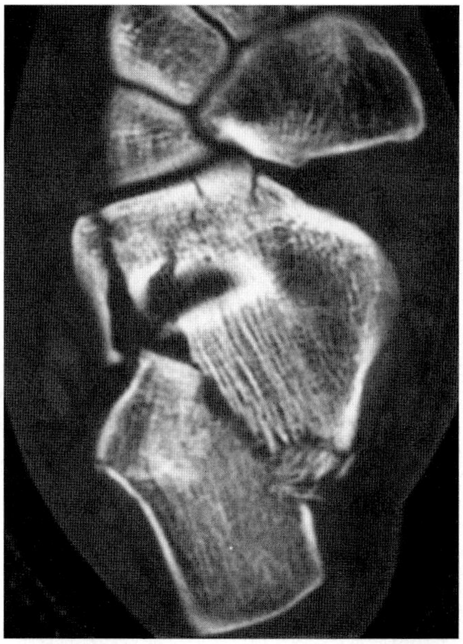

a

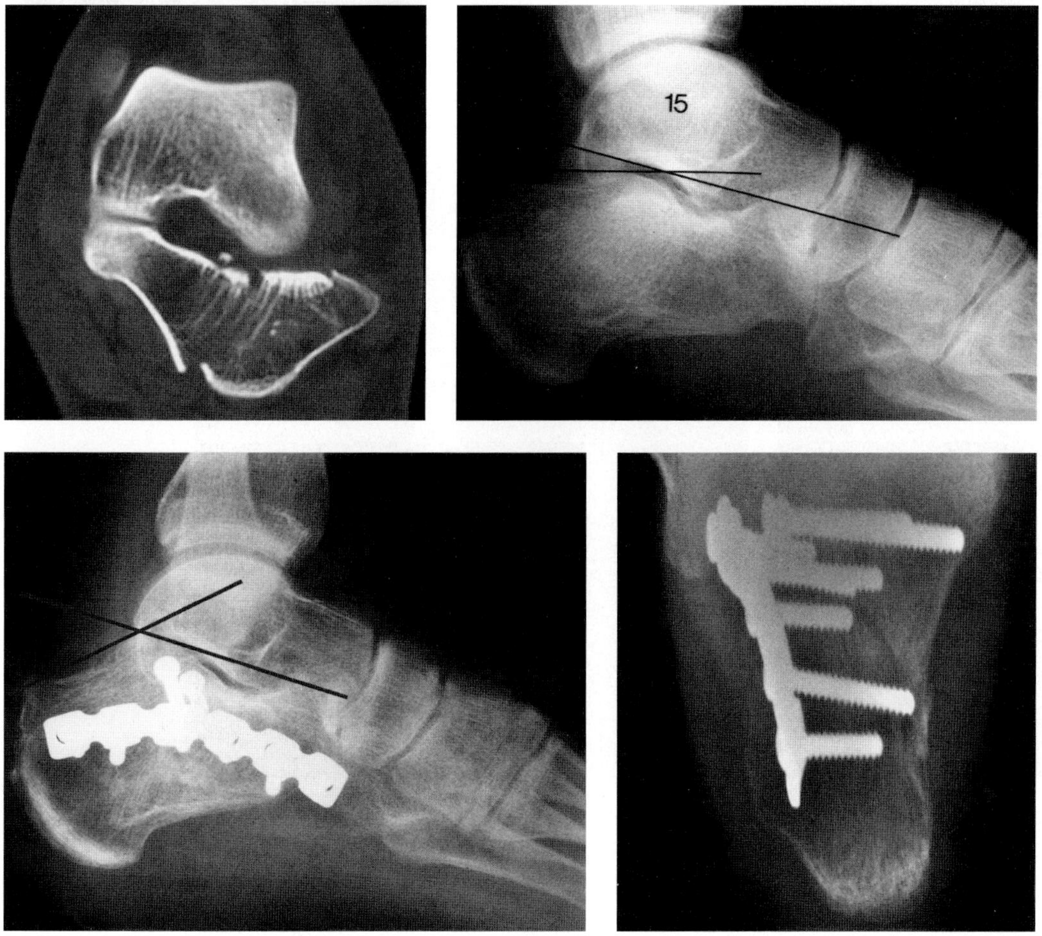

b c

d e

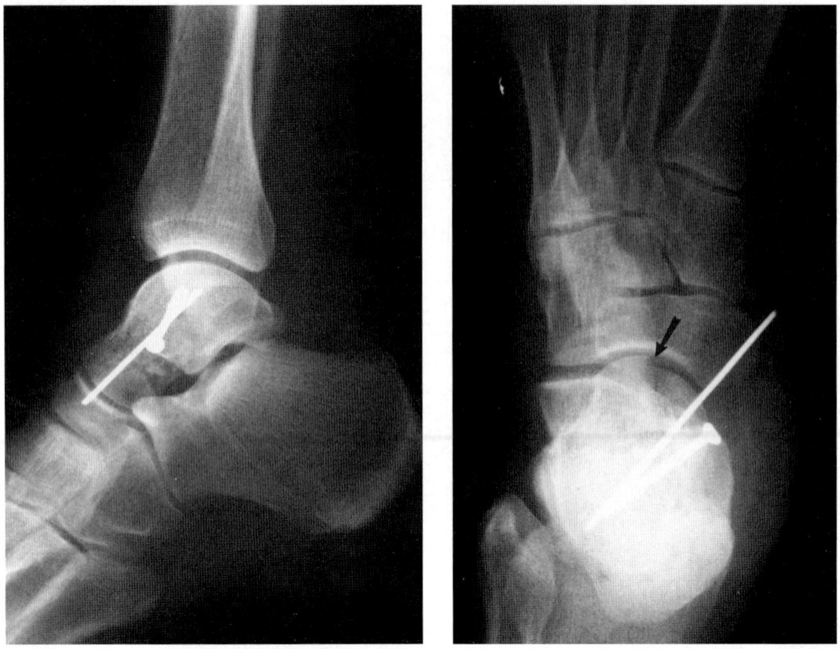

a b

Fig. 21.6a,b. Displaced talar neck fracture. Lateral (**a**) and AP (**b**) radiographs show K-wire and screw fixation. There is residual articular deformity (*arrow*) in the talar head

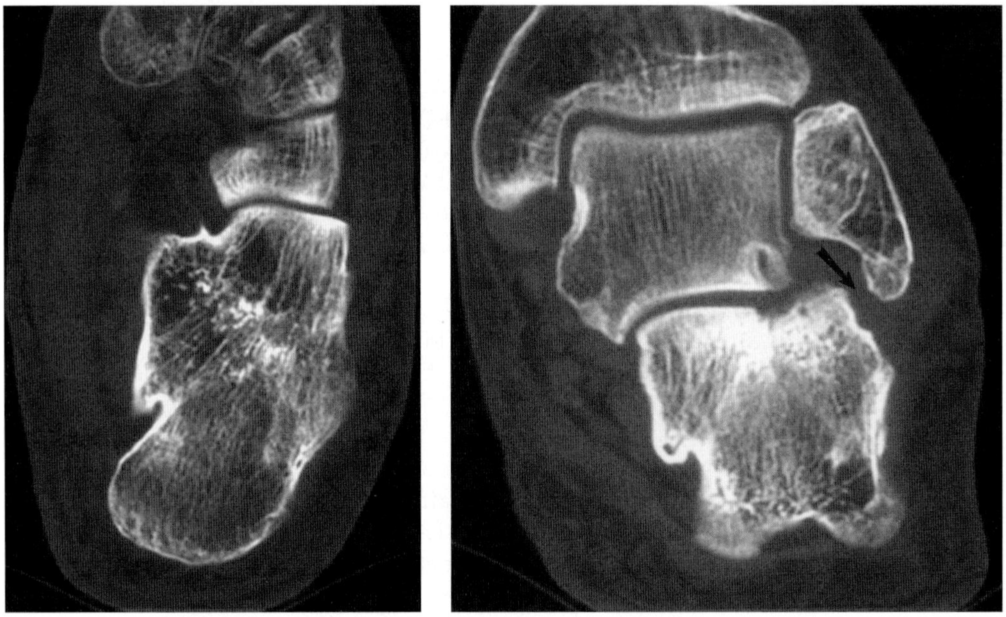

a b

Fig. 21.7a,b. Old healed calcaneal fracture. Axial (**a**) and coronal (**b**) CT images demonstrate residual shortening and calcaneal widening (**a**) and joint arthrosis and subluxation (**b**). There is also fibular abutment (*arrow*)

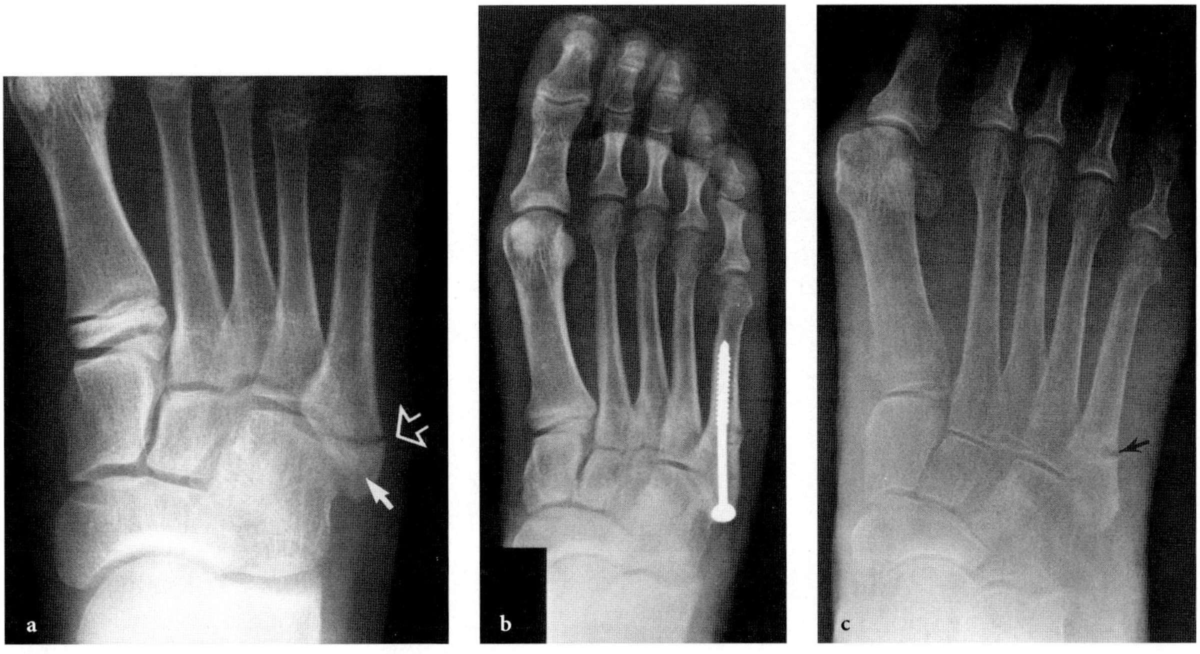

Fig. 21.8a–c. Fifth metatarsal base fractures. **a** AP view of a typical avulsion fracture (*open arrow*) and parallel epiphysis (*arrow*). **b** Jones's fracture with screw fixation. **c** Jones's fracture with sclerotic margins due to nonunion (*arrow*)

Table 21.1. Ankle fracture complications (Berquist 1995; Gourineni et al. 1999; Lindenfeld et al. 1996)

Osteoarthritis
Chronic instability
Nonunion
Malunion
Physeal deformity
Leg length discrepancy
Reflex sympathetic dystrophy
Adhesive capsulitis
Infection
Neurovascular injury

21.3.2 Arthrodesis

Arthrodesis may be used in the ankle or foot to restore activity and reduce pain (Anderson et al. 1997; Cracchiola 1990). Indications are similar for the foot and ankle. However, the surgical approaches differ based upon anatomic regions.

21.3.2.1 Ankle Arthrodesis

Ankle arthrodesis in adults is most commonly performed for osteoarthritis, post-traumatic arthritis, rheumatoid arthritis, failed arthroplasty, and neoplasms (Cracchiola 1990; Kitaoka and Romners 1992).

Preoperative imaging (see Section 21.2) is important for selecting among the numerous surgical fixation options (Fig. 21.9). Both external and internal fixation systems have been advocated.

External fixation may be preferred following failed arthrodesis or failed ankle arthroplasty (DeCoster et al. 1986; Kitaoka and Romners 1992; Smith et al. 1990). Patients with osteopenia or requiring large bone grafts may also be better served with external fixation approaches (Malarkey and Buiski 1991) (Fig. 21.10).

Internal fixation is typically accomplished using plates, screws, and bone grafts. Compression arthrodesis is performed using a lateral approach and fibular osteotomy (Fig. 21.9). The fibula is used as a bone graft with oblique screws placed across the prepared articular surfaces of the tibia and talus. The foot is maintained in a neutral to slight plantar flexed position (Berquist 1995) (Fig. 21.9).

The complications of ankle arthrodesis vary with the type of procedure and patient compliance. Healing typically occurs in 3–6 months. Higher complication rates are noted in patients with previous surgery (Fig. 21.10), rheumatoid arthritis, or diabetes mellitus. Table 21.2 summarizes the possible complications.

Nonunion occurs more commonly (21%) with external fixation than with internal fixation (5%) (Moekel et al. 1991). Serial radiographs are useful

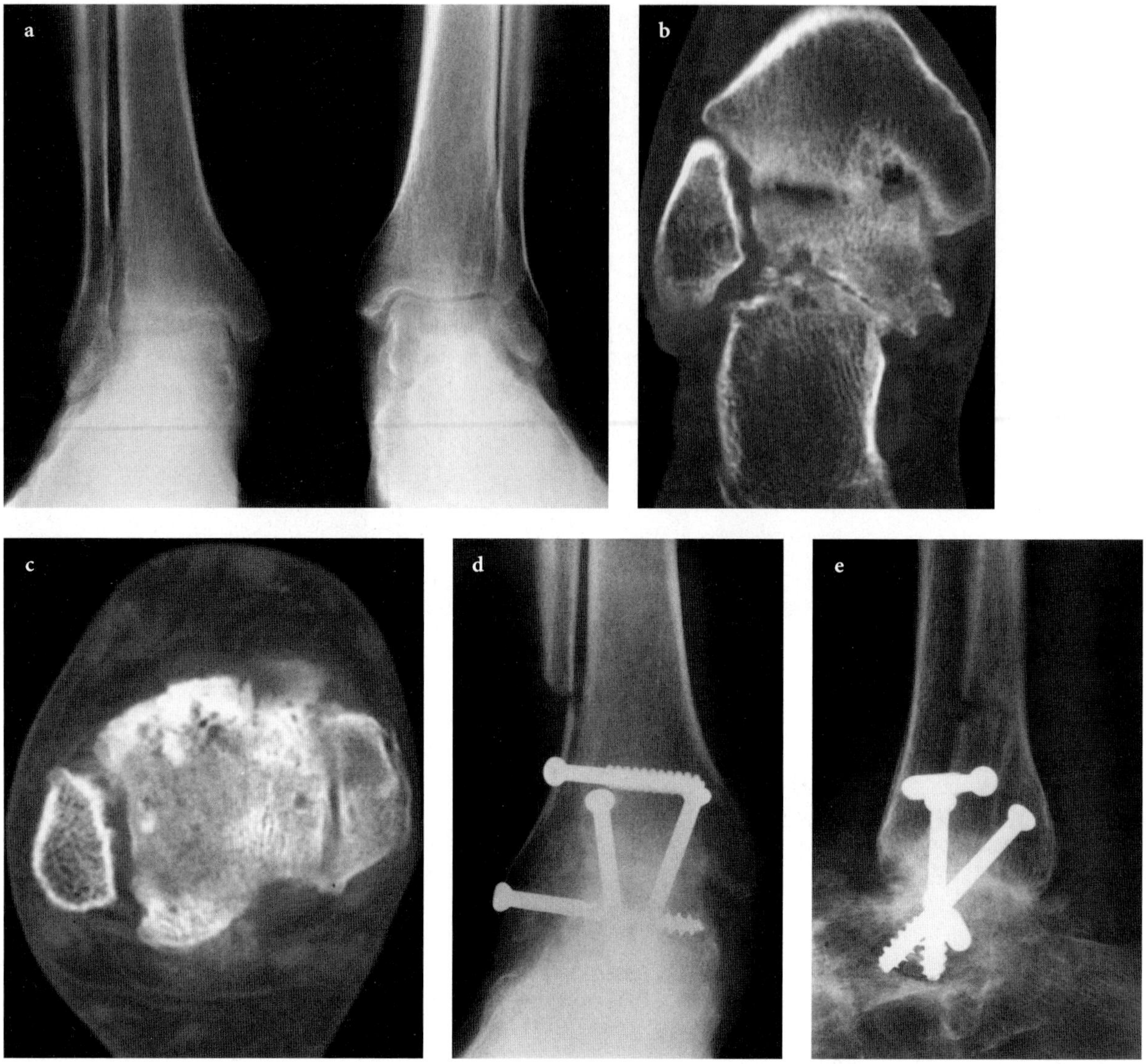

Fig. 21.9a–e. Posttraumatic arthrosis treated with ankle arthrodesis. Standing AP radiograph (**a**) and coronal (**b**) and axial (**c**) CT images demonstrate marked tibiotalar and subtalar arthrosis. Postoperative AP (**d**) and lateral (**e**) radiographs show a fibular osteotomy with screw fixation of the prepared tibiotalar joint

Table 21.2. Ankle arthrodesis complications (Berquist 2000; Frey et al. 1994; Helm 1990; Kitaoka and Patzer 1998; Moekel et al. 1991)

Nonunion
Malunion/loss of position
Infection:
Deep
Superficial
Wound sloughs
Subtalar arthrosis
Implant failure

to follow healing and detect indications of delayed or nonunion such as lucency around external fixation pins or screws (Fig. 21.11). CT or MR imaging is also useful in selected cases (Berquist 1995).

Infections may be deep or superficial. The incidence of superficial infection is 4%–18%, pin tract (external fixation) infection 9%–18%, and deep infection 5%–60%. Deep infection is most common in patients with rheumatoid arthritis, diabetes mellitus, and open wounds (Berquist 1995; Moekel et al. 1991). Radionuclide scans (combined technetium and indium or technetium-labeled white blood cells) or MR imaging may be useful when infection is suspected.

a 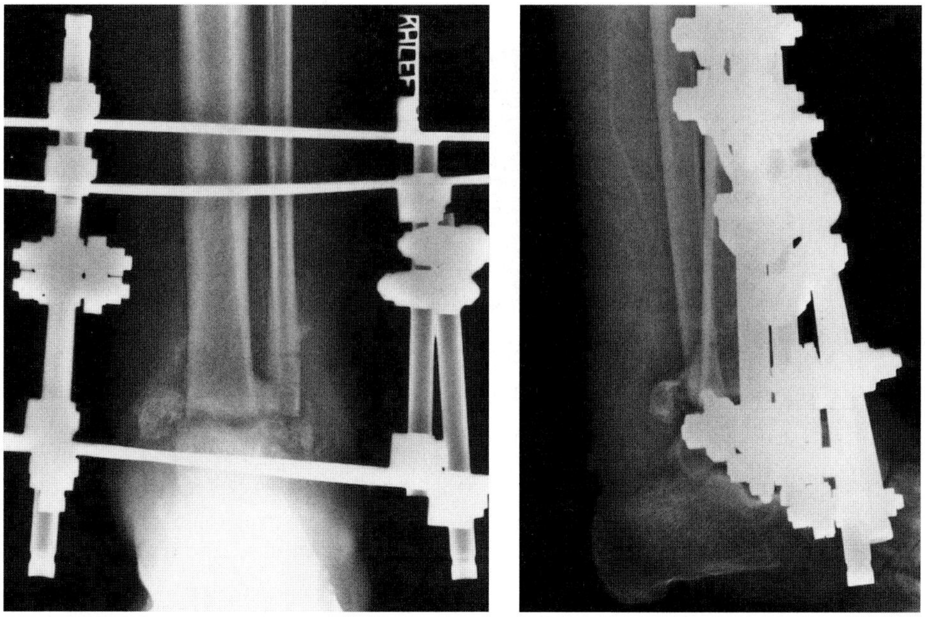 b

Fig. 21.10a,b. Failed arthrodesis with external fixation frame seen on AP (a) and lateral (b) radiographs

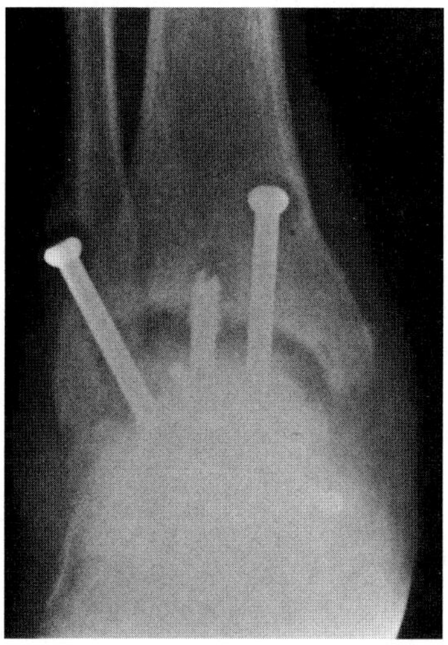

Fig. 21.11. AP radiograph on an infected nonunited ankle arthrodesis. Note the lucency around the screws and the wide irregular tibiotalar joint

Serial radiographs are usually effective for evaluating hardware failure, fractures, and other complications (Berquist 1995).

21.3.2.2
Hindfoot Arthrodesis

Triple arthrodesis (talonavicular, talocalcaneal, and calcaneocuboid) was originally performed in pediatric patients with polio and congenital foot deformities. To date, selected arthrosis of one or more joints is commonly performed in adults as well. Indications are similar to ankle arthrodesis except that posterior tibial dysfunction, congenital deformities, and neurotrophic arthritis are added to the list of indications (Grace 1996; Wertheimer 1990).

Surgical approaches vary; however, external fixations are not commonly used compared with ankle arthrodesis. Internal fixation with cancellous screws or staples and bone grafting of the prepared joint spaces are preferred (Berquist 1995). Subtalar fusion rates approach 100%, and those for triple arthrodesis 90% (Berquist 2000).

Complications are similar to ankle arthrodesis. Arthrosis of adjacent unfused joints is common. Nonunion is reported in 17%, wound infections in 11%, and tibiofibular impingement in 5% (Graves et al. 1993).

21.3.2.3
Midfoot and Forefoot Arthrodesis

Indications for midfoot and forefoot arthrodesis are similar to those described above. Surgical techniques are designed to prepare the articular surfaces and apply screws, miniplates and screws, or staples for fixation (Fig. 21.12). Complications do not differ significantly from ankle and hindfoot arthrodesis.

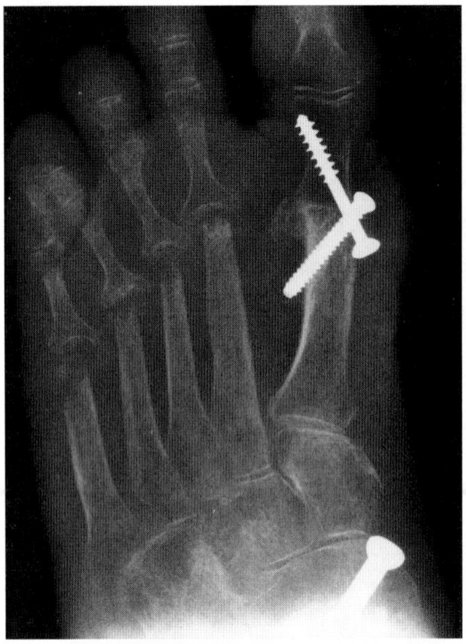

a

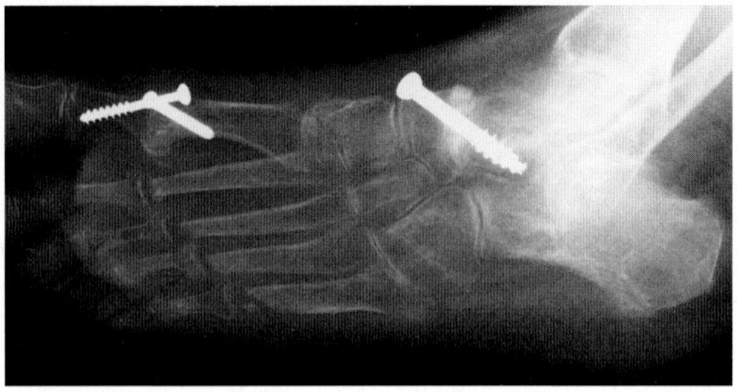

b

Fig. 21.12a,b. AP (**a**) and oblique (**b**) radiographs demonstrate osteopenia with resection arthroplasties of the 2nd–5th MTP joints and arthrodesis of the 1st MTP and talonavicular joints with screw fixation

21.3.3 Arthroplasty

Arthroplasty is performed on the ankle and metatarsophalangeal joints. The procedure is more frequently considered in the ankle.

21.3.3.1 Ankle Arthroplasty

Ankle arthroplasty was developed to provide a functional pain-free joint as an alternative to arthrodesis (Kitaoka and Patzer 1995) (Fig. 21.13). Early results were unsatisfactory, with failure rates of 38% (Johnson 1991).

Numerous improvements have been made since the 1970s. Today, components are classified by their design. Some systems allow only flexion and extension (constrained), while others permit some degree of motion in other directions (unconstrained). Most systems are configured using metal and polyethylene, but ceramic components are also available (Kitaoka and Patzer 1995; Pyevich et al. 1998). Components may be used with or without cement (Takakura et al. 1990).

At our institution, a recent report by Kitaoka and Patzer (1995) showed survival rates of 79%, 65%, and 61% for implants at 5, 10, and 15 years, respectively. Higher failure rates were noted in patients with previous surgical procedures and those who were younger than 57 years of age.

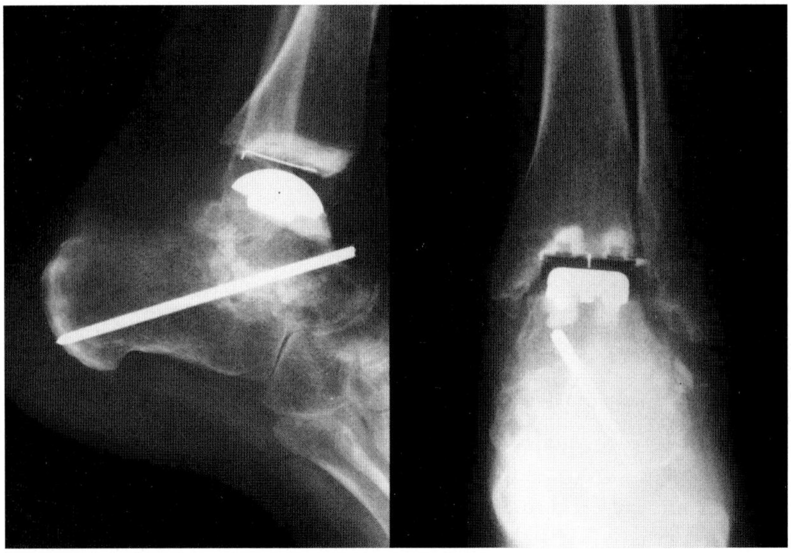

Fig. 21.13. Lateral and AP radiographs of a cemented ankle arthroplasty. There is also subtalar arthrodesis

Contraindications include previous arthrodesis, failed arthroplasty, and talar avascular necrosis (Johnson 1991).

Possible complications of ankle arthroplasty are summarized in Table 21.3. As with other arthroplasty procedures, loosening and infection are significant complications. The incidence of deep infection for ankle arthroplasty is 2.7%–3.5% (Johnson 1991). Pain may be due to loosening or impingement. The latter usually occurs over time with component subsidence (Fig. 21.14) (Berquist 1995).

Serial radiographs are most useful for the routine screening of potential complications. Stress views are useful for evaluating impingement and instability. Combined technetium-99 m and indium-111 or technetium-labeled white cell scans are useful for evaluating infection. Joint aspiration is also useful in this setting (Berquist 2000).

21.3.3.2 *Metatarsophalangeal Arthroplasty*

Metatarsophalangeal (MTP) joint arthroplasty is most commonly performed on the great toe but may also be used on the lesser toes (Coughlin and Mann 1993; Cracchiola et al. 1988; Stockley et al. 1989). Like ankle arthroplasty, MTP joint arthroplasty was developed as an alternative to cheilectomy, resection arthroplasty, and arthrodesis (Swanson et al. 1979).

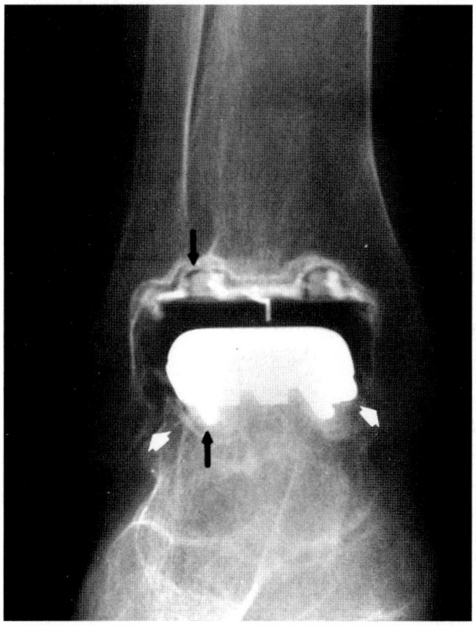

Fig. 21.14. AP radiograph of the ankle demonstrates lucency (*black arrows*) due to loosening and malleolar abutment (*white arrows*) on the talus

Table 21.3. Ankle arthroplasty complications (Johnson 1991; Kitaoka and Patzer 1995; Pyevich et al. 1998)

Delayed wound healing
Loosening
Deep infection
Tibiofibular impingement
Instability

Indications for great toe arthroplasty include hallux valgus, hallux rigidus, rheumatoid arthritis, and failed surgical procedures. Lesser toe arthroplasty may be indicated for Freiberg's disease, subluxation, and rheumatoid arthritis (Cracchiola et al. 1988; Berquist 1995).

MTP arthroplasty components may be single- or double-stemmed silicone implants or metal and polyethylene components (Cracchiola et al. 1992; Granberry et al. 1991; Swanson et al. 1979) (Fig. 21.15).

The complications of MTP joint arthroplasties are similar to ankle implant problems (Fig. 21.16). However, the correlation of radiographic features and clinical problems is less useful. Implants may appear distorted without associated clinical findings (Granberry et al. 1991). Serial radiographs are still the most useful follow-up imaging technique (Berquist 1995).

21.3.4 Digital Deformities

There are numerous approaches for the surgical correction of hallux and lesser toe deformities. The two most common hallux deformities are hallux valgus with bunion deformity and hallux rigidus. Lesser toe deformities include claw toe, hammer toe, and other digital deformities (Coughlin and Mann 1993; Eustace et al. 1993; Johnson et al. 1979).

21.3.4.1 *Hallux Valgus (Bunion)*

With hallux valgus, one sees lateral deviation of the great toe, medial deviation of the first metatarsal, and in some cases, hypermobility or instability of the cuneiform 1st metatarsal articulation (Berquist 2000). The 1st metatarsal may be rotated and the sesamoids deviated laterally (Eustace et al. 1993). The deformity is classified as mild (MTP angle = 20°, 1st–2nd intermetatarsal angle = 11°, sesamoids anatomic

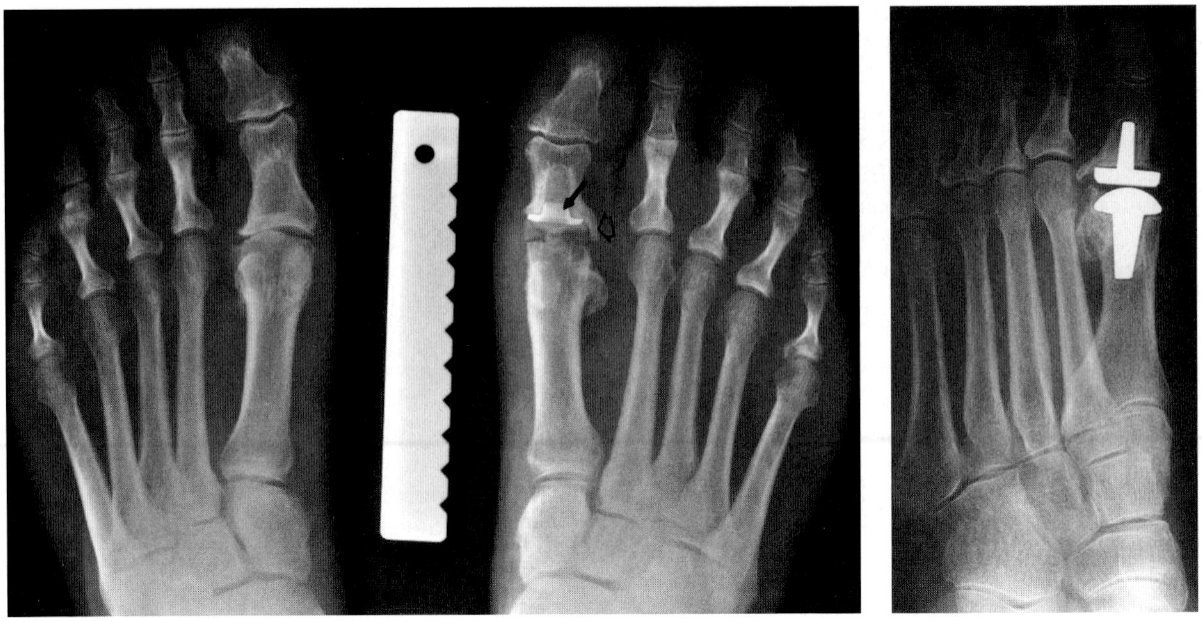

a b

Fig. 21.15a,b. Metatarsophalangeal arthroplasty. **a** Standing AP radiograph of the feet with hallux rigidus on the left and a double-stemmed silicone implant on the right with a metal grommet (*arrow*) to protect the articular surface. Note the heterotopic bone forming laterally (*open arrow*). **b** Metal implants with surrounding lucency due to loosening

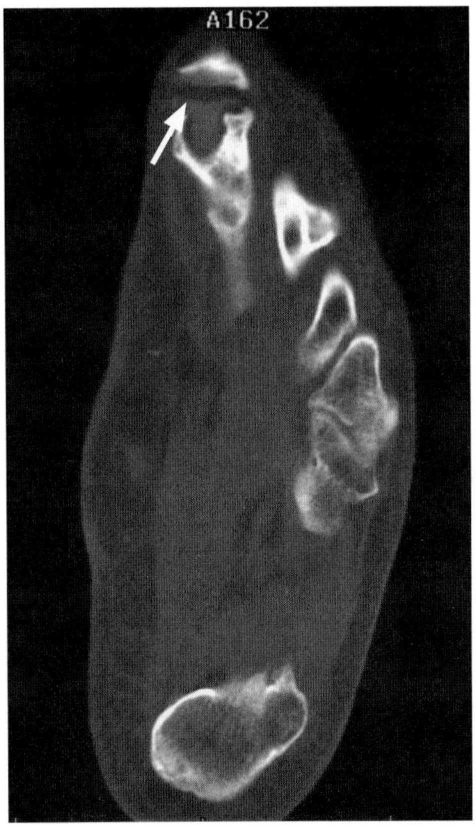

Fig. 21.16. CT image of a loose, fractured (*arrow*) silicone implant

or mildly subluxed), moderate (MTP angle 20°–40°, 1st–2nd intermetatarsal angle 11°–18°, lateral sesamoid subluxed), severe (MTP angle >40°, 1st–2nd intermetatarsal angle >40°, 1st–2nd intermetatarsal angle >18°, 1st–2nd toe overlap, large medial prominence, and lateral sesamoid dislocated) (Berquist 2000) (Fig. 21.17). Measurements are obtained on standing AP and lateral views.

Surgical correction may be accomplished with 1st metatarsal osteotomy, proximal phalangeal osteotomy, bunion resection, and soft-tissue repair. K-wire or screw fixation may be used to secure the osteotomy sites (Fig. 21.18) (Berquist 1995).

Complications vary with patient status and the type of procedure. Standing AP and lateral radiographs are essential to monitor the degree of correction and to serve as a baseline for recurrence or complications (Berquist 1995). The most common complications include loss of reduction, malunion, or nonunion of osteotomies (Fig. 21.19). Avascular necrosis of the metatarsal head and hallux varus (11%) may also occur (Berquist 2000; Johnson et al. 1979). Serial radiographs are usually adequate to evaluate complications. CT is useful to evaluate bone stock before revision surgery. MR imaging is useful for evaluating nonunion tendon shift and avascular necrosis (Berquist 1995).

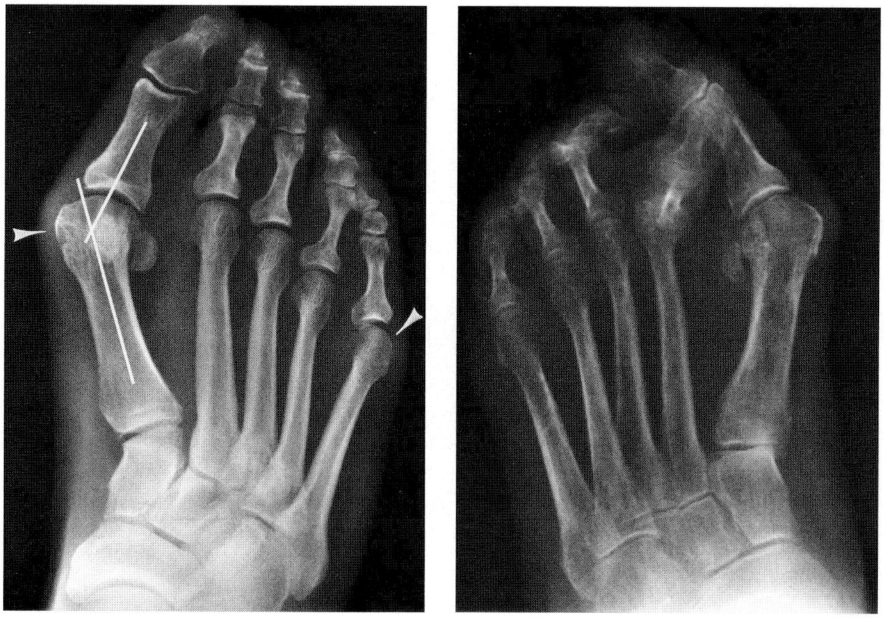

a b

Fig. 21.17a. Standing AP radiograph demonstrating moderate hallux valgus (*lines*) with medial prominence (*medial arrowhead*) and bunionette deformity (*lateral arrowhead*). **b** Standing AP radiograph shows marked hallux valgus with crossed toe deformity

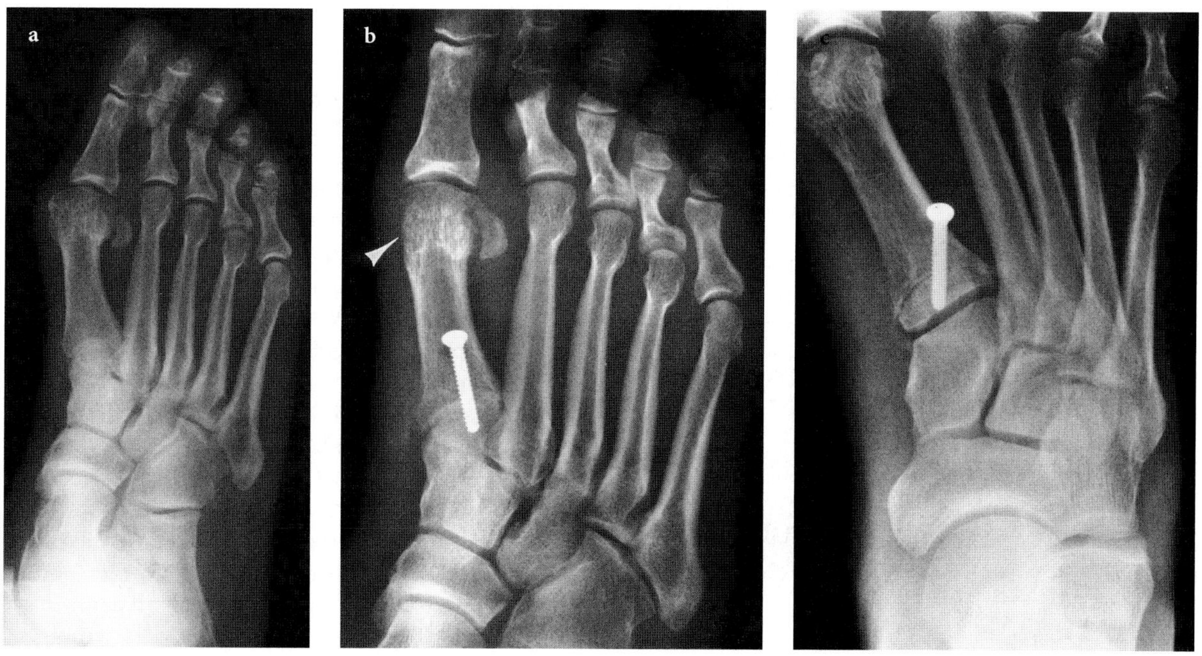

Fig. 21.18a–c. Oblique preoperative radiograph (**a**) and oblique (**b**) and PA (**c**) postoperative images show improved hallux orientation, resection of the prominence (*arrowhead*) and screw fixation of the 1st metatarsal osteotomy

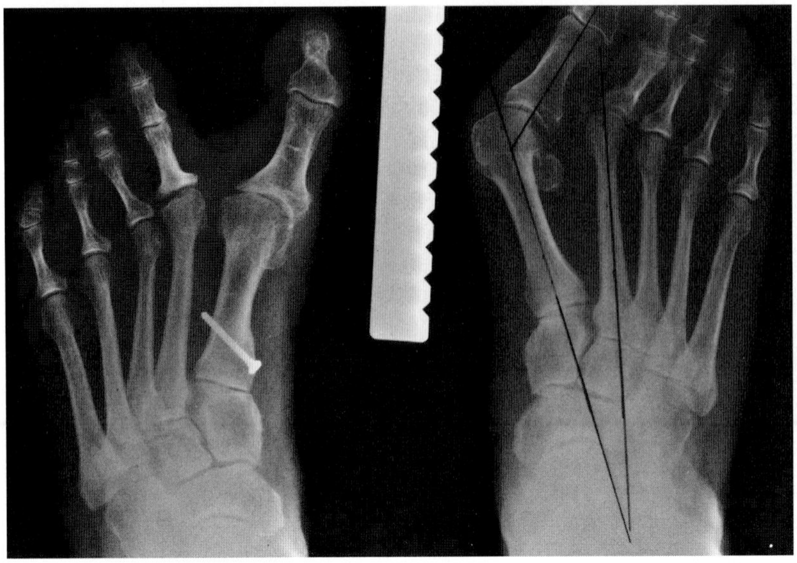

Fig. 21.19. Standing AP radiograph of the feet show hallux valgus on the right with over correction and hallux varus on the left

21.3.4.2 Hallux Rigidus

Hallux rigidus is a painful disorder of the first MTP joint with prominent osteophytes and a limited range of motion. Symptoms are usually unilateral and may be related to previous trauma (Berquist 2000) (Fig. 21.15a).

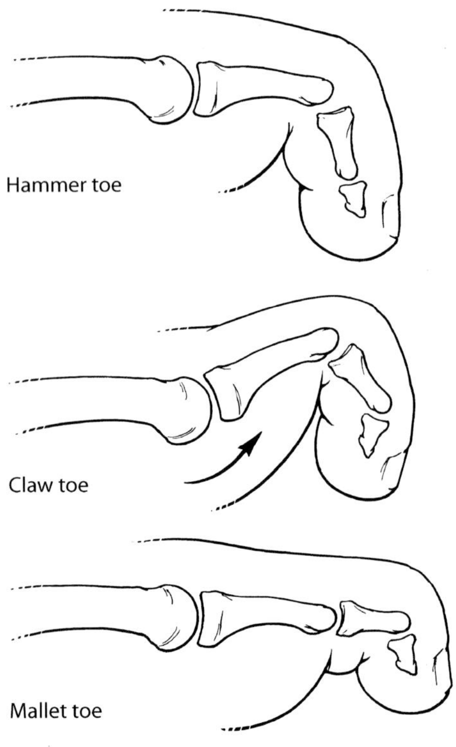

Fig. 21.20. Illustration of lesser toe deformities

The treatment may involve osteophyte resection (dorsal cheilectomy), soft-tissue interposition, or arthrodesis.

21.3.4.3 Lesser Toe Deformities

Lesser toe deformities are usually diagnosed clinically. Radiographs are used for surgical planning. Lesser toe deformities (Fig. 21.20) are summarized below (Coughlin and Mann 1993).

- Curly toe deformity (overlapping toes): Children.
  Proximal interphalangeal (PIP) joint is flexed with lateral rotation and varus deformity.
- Overlapping 5th toe: Bilateral and familial
  Fifth toe is adducted over the 4th toe.
- Hammer toe:
  Flexion of the PIP joint and hyperextension of the proximal phalanx. Typically bilateral and most often involves the 2nd toe.
- Claw toe:
  Hyperextension of the MTP joint and flexion at the PIP joint. Typically affects all four lesser toes bilaterally.
- Mallet toe:
  Flexion of the distal IP joint. Typically the 2nd toe, similar to hammer toe deformity.

Treatment may be conservative, but this is typically ineffective. Therefore, resection arthroplasty with K-wire fixation (Fig. 21.21) is often required (Coughlin and Mann 1993).

Complications include loss of reduction and subluxation. Infection is uncommon.

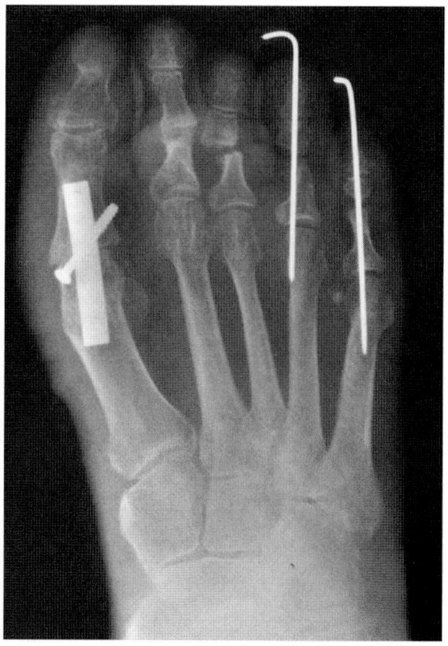

Fig. 21.21. Standing AP radiograph of the right foot shows plate and screw arthrodesis of the great toe with lesser toe resection arthroplasties to correct claw toe deformity. The 4th and 5th digits are fixed with K-wires

Bunionette deformities are similar to the great toe bunion deformity, but they involve the lateral foot (Coughlin 1991). The condition is related to footwear. Patients are more often symptomatic when the 4th–5th metatarsal angle is increased (normal 6°, range 3°–11°).

Treatment includes resection of the eminence, soft-tissue repair, and osteotomy. Complications include overcorrection, loss of reduction, and infection (Coughlin and Mann 1993).

Serial radiographs are usually adequate for the detection of complications. MR imaging may be required when infection is suspected (Berquist 2000).

References

Anderson JG, Coetzoe C, Hansen ST (1997) Revision ankle fusion using internal compression arthrodesis with screw fixation. Foot Ankle Int 18:300–309

Behrens F (1980) General theories and principles of external fixation. Clin Orthop 241:15–23

Behrens F (1989) A primer on fixation devices and configurations. Clin Orthop 251:5–14

Berquist TH (1993) Diagnostic and therapeutic injections as an aid to musculoskeletal diagnosis. Semin Intervent Radiol 10:326–343

Berquist TH (1995) Imaging atlas of orthopedic appliances and prostheses. Raven, New York

Berquist TH (2000) Radiology of the foot and ankle, 2nd edn. Lippincott / Williams and Wilkins, Philadelphia

Berquist TH (2001) MRI of the musculoskeletal system, 4th edn. Lippincott / Williams and Wilkins, Philadelphia

Coughlin MJ (1991) Treatment of bunionette deformity with longitudinal osteotomy and distal soft tissue repair. Foot Ankle 11:195–203

Coughlin MJ, Mann RA (1993) Lesser toe deformities. In: Mann RA, Coughlin MJ (eds) Surgery of the foot and ankle, 6th edn. Mosby-Year Book, St Louis, pp 341–412

Cracchiola A III (1990) Surgical arthrodesis for foot and ankle pathology. Instr Course Lect 39:49–63

Cracchiola A III, Kitaoka HB, Leventen EO (1988) Silicone implant arthroplasty for second metatarsophalangeal joint disorders with and without hallux valgus deformities. Foot Ankle 9:10–18

Cracchiola A III, Weltmer JB, Lian G et al (1992) Arthroplasty of the first metatarsophalangeal joint with a double-stemmed silicone implant. J Bone Joint Surg 74A:552–563

DeCoster T, Alvarez R, Trevino S (1986) External fixation of the foot and ankle. Foot Ankle 7:40–48

Eustace S, O'Bryne J, Stack J et al (1993) Radiographic features enable assessment of first metatarsal rotation. The role of pronation in hallux valgus. Skel Radiol 22:153–156

Frey C, Halikies NM, Vu-Rose T et al (1994) A review of ankle arthrodesis. Pre-disposing factors to non-union. Foot Ankle Int 15:581–584

Gourineni P, Knuth AE, Nuber GF (1999) Radiographic evaluation of the position of implants in the medial malleolus in relation to the ankle joint space. Anteroposterior compared with mortise radiographs. J Bone Joint Surg 81A: 364–369

Grace DL (1996) The surgical management of the rheumatoid foot. Br J Hosp Med 56:473–480

Granberry WM, Noble PC, Bishop JO et al (1991) Use of hinged silicone prostheses for replacement arthroplasty of the first metatarsophalangeal joint. J Bone Joint Surg 73A:1453–1459

Graves SC, Mann RA, Graves KV (1993) Triple arthrodesis in older adults. J Bone Joint Surg 75A:355–362

Helm R (1990) The results of ankle arthrodesis. J Bone Joint Surg 72B:141–143

Jaffee NW, Gilula LA, Wissman RD et al (2001) Diagnostic and therapeutic ankle tenography: outcomes and complications. AJR 176:365–371

Johnson KA (1991) Total ankle arthroplasty. In: Morrey BF (ed) Joint Replacement arthroplasty. Churchill Livingstone, New York, pp 1173–1182

Johnson KA, Cofield RH, Morrey BF (1979) Chevron osteotomy for hallux valgus. Clin Orthop 142:44–47

Khoury, El-Khoury GY, Saltzman CL (1995) Intra-articular foot and ankle injections to identify the source of pain before arthrodesis. AJR 167:669–673

Kitaoka HB, Romners DW (1992) Arthrodesis for failed ankle arthroplasty. Arthroplasty 7:277–289

Kitaoka HB, Patzer GL (1995) Clinical results after Mayo total ankle arthroplasty. J Bone Joint Surg 78A:1658–1664

Kitaoka HB, Patzer GL (1998) Arthrodesis for treatment of the ankle and osteonecrosis of the talus. J Bone Joint Surg 80A:370–379

Kleinberg S (1932) Operative cure of hallux valgus and bunions. Am J Surg 15:75–81

Laird L (1990) Silastic arthroplasty of the great toe. A review of 228 implants using the double-stemmed implant. Clin Orthop 255:268–272

Lindenfeld TN, Bach BR, Wojtys EM (1996) Reflex sympathetic dystrophy and pain dysfunction in the lower extremity. J Bone Joint Surg 78A:1936–1944

Malarkey RF, Buiski JC (1991) Ankle arthrodesis with calandruccio frame and bimaleollar on lay grafting. Clin Orthop 268:44–48

Marsh JL, Bunar S, Nepola JV et al (1995) Use of an articulated external fixator for fractures of the tibial plafond. J Bone Joint Surg 77A:1498–1509

Moekel BH, Patterson BM, Inglis AE et al (1991) Ankle arthrodesis: A comparison of internal and external fixation. Clin Orthop 268:78–83

Morrey BF, Caso JF, Johnson KA et al (1986) Foot and ankle. In: Berquist TH (eds) Imaging of orthopedic trauma and surgery. Saunders, Philadelphia, pp 407–498

Pyevich MT, Saltzman CL, Callaghan JJ et al (1998) Total ankle arthroplasty: a unique design. J Bone Joint Surg 80A:1410–1420

Rosenberg ZS, Beltran J, Bencardino JT (2000) MR imaging of the foot and ankle. Radiographics 20: 5153–5179

Sanders R (2000) Displaced intra-articular fractures of the calcaneus. J Bone Joint Surg 82A:225–250

Smith SR, Morgan CG, Pinder IM (1990) Results and complications of ankle arthrodesis. J Bone Joint Surg 72B:530

Stockley I, Betts RP, Getty CJ et al (1989) A prospective study of forefoot arthroplasty. Clin Orthop 248:213–218

Swanson AB, Lunsden RM, Swanson G (1979) Silicone implant arthroplasty of the great toe. A review of flexible hinge implants. Clin Orthop 142:30–43

Takakura Y, Tanaka Y, Sugimoto K et al (1990) Ankle arthroplasty: a comparative study of cemented and uncemented ceramic prosthesis. Clin Orthop 252:209–216.

Thordarson DB, Hedman TD, Yetkinler DN et al (1999) Superior compressive strength of a calcaneal fracture construct augmented with remoldable cancellous bone cement. J Bone Joint Surg 81A:239–246

Vander Greind R, Michelson JD, Bone LB (1996) Fractures of the ankle and distal part of the tibia. J Bone Joint Surg 78A: 1772–1783

Wertheimer SJ (1990) Role of epiphysodesis in the management of deformities of the foot and ankle. J Foot Surg 29: 459–462

Wyrsch B, McFerran, McAndrew M et al (1996) Operative treatment of fractures of the tibial plafond. J Bone Joint Surg 78A:1646–1657

22 Sequelae of Torture

H. Vogel

CONTENTS

22.1 Introduction

Diagnostic imaging frequently shows the extent of bony and soft-tissue trauma and helps confirm the aetiology of injuries experienced by torture victims. It can be used to plan subsequent management and has potential legal implications in that it may provide substantive proof that torture has indeed occurred (Vogel 1999). Imaging must show both bones and the soft tissues, with particular emphasis on the ligaments, tendons and fascia (aponeuroses). The principal forms of torture involving the foot and ankle which the individual may have had the misfortune to experience are as follows:

- falaca
- electric torture
- toe-screws
- palmatoria

In addition, specific entities such as the 'lotus foot' and bullet wounds, the latter a variant of 'knee-capping', will be reviewed. The findings may be classified into early and late features according to the time elapsed since the violence was applied.

H. Vogel, MD
Professor, Department of Radiology, Albers-Schönberg Institut für Strahlendiagnostik, Allgemeines Krankenhaus St. Georg, Lohmühlenstrasse 5, 20099 Hamburg, Germany

22.2 Early Findings

Imaging analysis in the acute phase is rare. Obviously, this can be explained by the circumstances. Often the victim is held in custody until the visible external traces of torture have disappeared; or even if the victim has been set free, he/she is usually frightened by their horrific experience and will hesitate to seek diagnosis or treatment, let alone documentation. This is especially true when torture is being tolerated by the state in general, or even actually performed by government agencies, and when doctors and medical institutions are considered to be an active part of the system that applies the torture, or at least that they are controlled or obliged to report when treating victims. Nevertheless, there have been isolated reports objectively documenting the findings in victims of recent torture, for example from Turkey (Lök 1994).

22.2.1 Falaca

Falaca, otherwise known as falanga, is the term applied to beating of the foot and is the most frequently observed form of torture to the foot and ankle. The beating is applied particularly, but not exclusively, to the sole of the foot and is seen all too frequently in victims from the Middle East, most notably Turkey and Iraq. Falaca produces oedema, haematoma, fractures, ruptures of ligmaments and tendons, and fascial damage (Lie and Skjeie 1996; Rasmussen and Skylv 1992). Shortly after the torture, the clinical findings alone are usually diagnostic. Radiographs can confirm or exclude fractures and enable an estimate of the time interval since the torture was applied. In my experience the fractures involve the toes, the ankle, the calcaneus and the metatarsal bones, a pattern found when the feet were fixed during the beating (Meier and Andersen 1985; Rasmussen et al. 1982). Fractures of the lateral malleolus seem to be an exception. Nevertheless, the lower leg near the ankle is also often involved.

Generalised swelling is the predominant clinical feature. CT, MR imaging and ultrasound can furnish important additional findings (Fig. 22.1). They allow evaluation of the underlying soft tissues. Bone scintigraphy can verify that beating has occurred, when clinical examination and radiographs fail to show anything (Fig. 22.2). Increased activity can be demonstrated months and even years later, long after any oedema and haematoma have resolved (Lök 1994). Initially, increased activity is due to the beating itself. In the long term the falaca alters the biomechanics of the foot, resulting in flatfoot and/or splayfoot deformity. Bone scintigraphy shows the reaction of bone due to unusual degenerative changes induced by altered weight-bearing. MR imaging demonstrates similar findings, revealing bone marrow oedema.

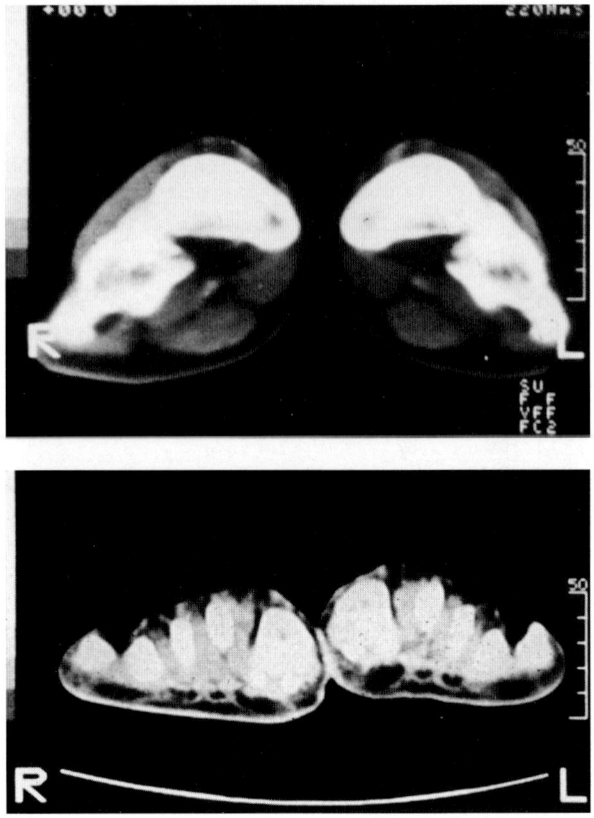

Fig. 22.1a,b. Victims of falaca. **a** Soft-tissue swelling due to oedema and haematoma shortly after the beating. **b** Flatfoot and splayfoot deformity in the chronic stage

22.2.2 Electric Torture

Electric or E-torture of the feet has rarely been documented. If E-torture is applied, the electrode is usually placed in the interdigital space in order to hide the entrance of the electric current. The point of entry of the electric current, however, can be identified by a circumscribed focus of tissue necrosis. To prove E-torture, this area can be excised locally for microscopic evaluation.

In severe cases the electric current provokes muscular contractures, sometimes causing fractures and ruptures of ligaments as well as bone necrosis. Radiographs will reveal the fractures, and ultrasound or MR imaging, the muscle contractures and soft-tissue oedema.

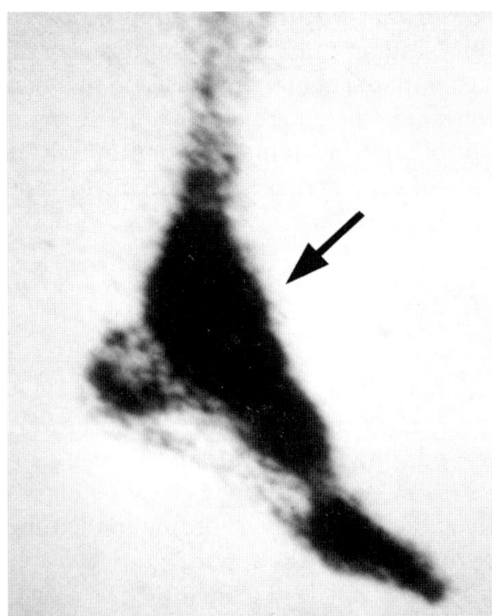

Fig. 22.2. Bone scintigraphy after falaca showing increased activity

22.2.3 Injuries Due to Bullets and Explosives

Knee-capping was a form of punishment introduced by paramilitary groups operating in the Northern Ireland province of the United Kingdom approximately 30 years ago. It implies a close range shot usually with a hand firearm across the front of the knee. However, with the improved experience of the surgeons and rehabilitation reducing the morbidity of this injury, other joints were shot in addition to the knee, such as the ankle joint (Fig. 22.3); in an extreme case, both knees, both ankles and both elbow joints were shot.

Radiographs will show the bullet and/or metallic fragments, the destruction of bone and to a limited degree of the soft tissues, and are used for the legal

a b

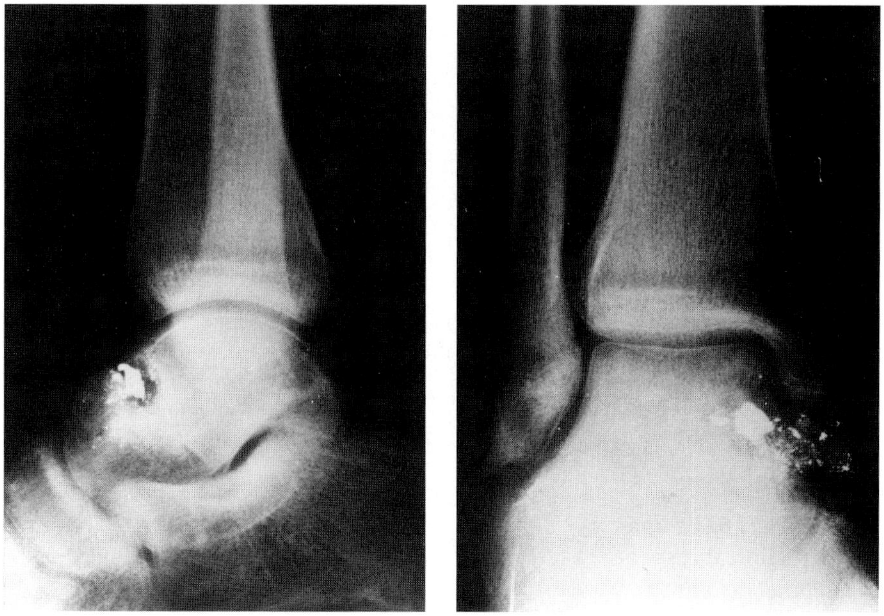

Fig. 22.3a,b. Victim of 'knee capping' from Northern Ireland showing a low-velocity bullet injury to the ankle. This individual was also shot in the other ankle and both knees

documentation of the injury (Fig. 22.3). Low-velocity bullets frequently remain in the patient, and the destruction is limited to the path of the bullet. Clinical inspection soon after injury shows smoke discoloration of the skin if the firearm was close to or even touching the skin, which is, obviously, not detectable radiographically.

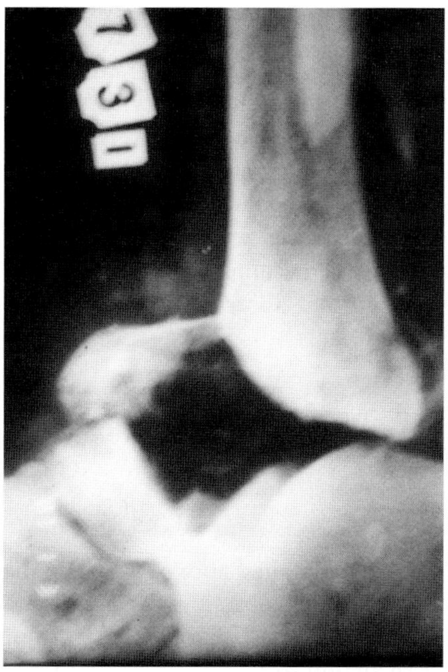

Fig. 22.4. High-velocity bullet injury to the ankle producing a large bone defect

Fragmentation of the bullet and the location of the fragments away from the path of the bullet need to be documented, including tiny pinpoint-like bullet fragments ('dots'). These indicate high-energy transfer, characteristic for high-velocity bullets with an enlarged area of destruction. High-velocity bullets move two to three times the speed of sound. Upon impact, they produce a hypersonic shockwave which propagates conically in the tissues. The tip of the cone is the point of the bullet's entry. The cone itself marks the area of destruction, which means that the destruction is far larger than the path of the bullet. The bullet's exit is recognisable by the larger-sized defect. Large parts of the bone can be ejected (Fig. 22.4), or the bone can be reduced to multiple small fragments within the cone of destruction.

In the acute assessment of vascular injuries, angiography will show the degree of the damage and possible collateral circulation. This is particularly applicable to injuries sustained from stepping on land mines. This type of injury mechanism can usually be determined by its characteristic pattern of destruction.

22.3 Late Findings

Late findings are malalignment and pseudoathrosis of bones and, after injuries to the ligaments alone, again malalignment and unusual or premature degenerative changes. Malalignment requires a precise analysis.

Flatfoot and splayfoot deformity are typical sequelae of falaca (Fig. 22.1). Soft-tissue contractures can be documented with MR imaging (HAYES 1997; SAVNIK et al. 2000). It is worth noting that a good physiotherapist, experienced in treating the victims of torture, can recognise these contractures clinically with great certainty. He/she is thus able to furnish the same information without recourse to imaging for both falaca and E-torture. A court of law, however, may find a visual record more persuasive than the verbal testimony of an expert witness.

22.3.1 Toe Screws

The degree of destruction of the toes has to be analysed and documented by combined clinical inspection and imaging (Fig. 22.5). The applied instruments are reminiscent of the medieval 'thumbscrew'. It is easy to imagine that instruments like the 'petite guillotine' can be applied to the toes. The petite guillotine is typically applied to amputate fingers or part of a finger (VOGEL 1997). It was originally developed under the regime of the Shah of Iran and is reputedly still in use, even today.

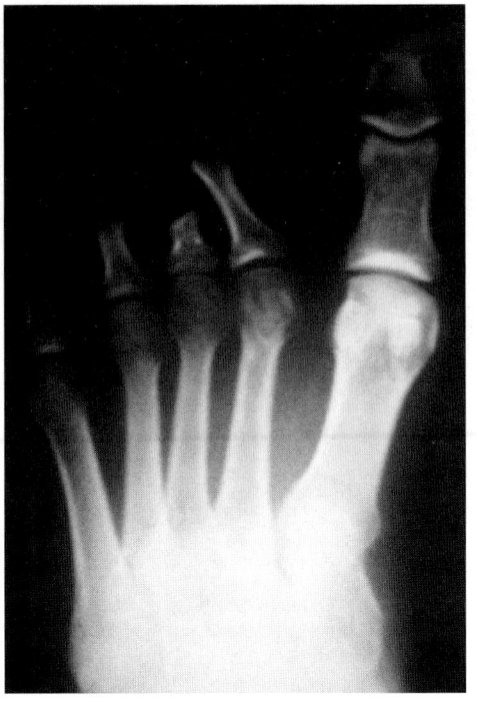

Fig. 22.5. Severe bone destruction due to the application of toe screws

22.3.2 Palmatoria

Palmatoria is the term applied to blunt trauma (beating) to the tibia. Victims of palmatoria come from Guinea Bissao. Abnormal thickening of the cortical bone resulting from subperiosteal bleeding and infractions can easily be demonstrated on radiographs. By the way, this may be an important concurrent finding on radiographic examinations of the ankle, obtained for other reasons in torture victims. If the beating has been less focussed, which happens in palmatoria as well as in falaca, and which also depends on whether the feet have been fixed or not, fractures of the ankle (more often the lateral ankle) can be observed.

22.3.3 Lotus Foot

Cultural pressures may result in individuals experiencing 'trauma' which in other countries might be considered no less than a form of torture. An example from China, no longer practised, is the so-called lotus foot. During the last decades of Imperial China, the feet of newborn female babies were made smaller by binding the forefoot under the presumption that a smaller foot was more beautiful, and that it was also a sign of wealth, indicating that this girl did not need to work to support herself or her family. The binding of the foot was probably done with the full consent of the parents or even by the parents themselves. Fatal outcomes due to inflammation induced by the toenails growing into the sole of the foot are reported. Two cases I observed revealed two different procedures: one showed the binding of the forefoot towards the heel, the other a lateral compression of the forefoot (Fig. 22.6).

22.4 Conclusions

All the imaging features detailed above and all forms of torture and maltreatment mentioned constitute a general review of the subject. The precise nature of torture varies from region to region, and regrettably new forms are being added. They all illustrate the potential extent of man's inhumanity to man.

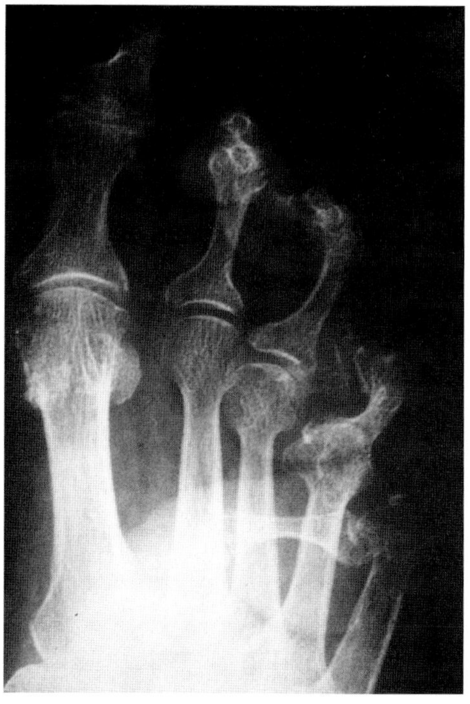

Fig. 22.6. Lotus foot. The forefoot is narrowed by lateral binding, resulting in atrophy of the little toe

Acknowledgements. The images used in this chapter were originally collected for a project on 'X-ray diagnosis of violence' (VOGEL 1997). We reviewed the archives of the rehabilitation centers for torture victims in Europe in Copenhagen (IRCT, Dr. Genefke, Dr. Rasmussen), Izmir (Dr. Veli Lök), Paris (Avre, Dr. Jaffe), Stockholm (Prof. Johannson), of medical centers in countries in which torture and maltreatment occur, in countries with war and civil war (Prof. Montani, Croatia; Dr. Laird, Northern Ireland), and personal collections (China, Dr. Bao; Hamburg, Dr. Michalik). I acknowledge my colleagues for their dedication and courage.

References

Hayes E (1997) MRI illustrates history of torture. Diagn Imaging Eur 13:17

Lie B, Skjeie H (1996) Torture-related injuries: a medical challenge. Diagnosis and treatment of Falanga victims. Tidsskr Nor Laegeforen 116:1073–1075

Lök V (1994) Communication. International Torture Meeting (organized by the national centers for rehabiltation of victims of torture), Istanbul

Meier J, Andersen JG (1985) Sclerosing of the calcaneus following phalanga torture. Ugeskr Laeger 147:4206–4207

Rasmussen F, Henriksen OB, Rasmussen OV, Sakelleriades PD (1982) Aseptic necrosis of bone following phalanga torture. Ugeskr Laeger 114:1165–1166

Rasmussen OV, Skylv G (1992) Sings of falanga torture (letter). Lancet 340:725

Savnik A, Amris K, Rogind H, Prip K, Danneskiold-Samsoe B, Bojsen-Moller F, Bartels EM, Bliddal H, Boesen J, Egund N (2000) MRI of the plantar structures of the foot after falanga torture. Eur Radiol 10:1655–1659

Skylv G (1994) Falanga: diagnosis and treatment of late sequelae. Torture [Suppl] 36–41

Vogel H (1997) Gewalt im Röntgenbild (x-ray diagnosis of violence). Ecomed, Landsberg

Vogel H (1999) Imaging helps unveil torture's dark secrets. Diagn Imaging Eur 37:22–28

Subject Index

List of Contributors

Thomas D. Berg, MD
Department of Radiology
University of Iowa Hospitals & Clinics
Iowa City, IA 52242
USA

Thomas H. Berquist, MD, FACR
Professor of Radiology,
Director of Education
Mayo Foundation
Mayo Clinic
4500 San Pablo Road
Jacksonville, FL 32224
USA

Stefano Bianchi, MD
Division of Radiodiagnosis and Interventional Radiology
Hôspital Cantonal Universitaire de Geneve
Rue Micheli-du-Crest 24
1211 Geneva 14
Switzerland

S. Leon Burrows, MD
Professor, Department of Radiology
University of Iowa Hospitals & Clinics
Iowa City, IA 52242
USA

Victor N. Cassar-Pullicino, LRCP, MRCS, MD, DMRD, FRCR
Consultant Radiologist
Department of Radiology
The Robert Jones & Agnes Hunt Orthopaedic
and District Hospital
Oswestry, Shropshire SY10 7AG
UK

Vijay P. Chandnani MD
Department of Radiology
Grant Medical Center (JWH, VPC)
111 S. Grant Avenue
Columbus, OH 43215
USA

Mark Cobby, MD
Department of Radiology
Frenchay Hospital
Frenchay Park Road
Bristol BS16 1LE
UK

A. Mark Davies, MD
Consultant Radiologist
The MRI Centre
Royal Orthopaedic Hospital
Birmingham B31 2AP
UK

Brian J. DeMichaelis, MD
Department of Radiology
University of Iowa Hospitals & Clinics
Iowa City, IA 52242
USA

George Y. El-Khoury MD
Professor, Department of Radiology
University of Iowa Hospitals & Clinics
Iowa City, IA 52242
USA

J. Mark Elliott, MRCPI, FRCR
Consultant Radiologist
Department of Radiology
Musgrave Park Hospital
Stockman's Lane
Belfast BT9 7JB
UK

Scott J. Erickson, MD
Department of Radiology
Froedtert East Clinics - 2nd Floor
9200 West Wisconsin Avenue
Milwaukee, WI 53226-3596
USA

Jean Garcia, MD
Division of Radiodiagnosis and Interventional Radiology
Hôspital Cantonal Universitaire de Geneve
Rue Micheli-du-Crest 24
1211 Geneva 14
Switzerland

Harry K. Genant MD
Professor of Radiology, Medicine, Epidemiology
and Orthopaedic Surgery
Department of Radiology
University of California San Francisco
San Francisco, CA 94143-0628
USA

Amilcare Gentili, MD
Professor of Radiology
UCSD Thornton Hospital, Department of Radiology
9300 Campus Point Drive, 7756
La Jolla, CA 92037
USA

Andrew J. Grainger, MRCP, FRCR
Consultant Musculoskeletal Radiologist
Department of Radiology
Freeman Hospital
High Heaton
Newcastle upon Tyne NE7 7DN
UK

J. Walter Helgason, MD
Department of Radiology
Grant Medical Center (JWH, VPC)
111 S. Grant Avenue
Columbus, OH 43215
USA

Siegfried Hofmann, MD
Orthopedic Hospital Stolzalpe
8852 Stolzalpe
Austria

Herwig Imhof, MD
Professor, Universitätsklinik für Radiodiagnostik
Klinische Abteilung fur Osteologie
Allgemeines Krankenhaus
Währinger Gürtel 18-20
1090 Wien
Austria

Jeremy P. R. Jenkins, MBChB, FRCP, DMRD, FRCR
Department of Clinical Radiology
Manchester Royal Infirmary
Oxford Road
Manchester, M13 9WL
UK

Franz Kainberger, MD
Professor, Universitätsklinik für Radiodiagnostik
Klinische Abteilung fur Osteologie
Allgemeines Krankenhaus
Währinger Gürtel 18-20
1090 Wien
Austria

Allen Katz, MD
Department of Radiology
Froedtert East Clinics - 2nd Floor
9200 West Wisconsin Avenue
Milwaukee, WI 53226-3596
USA

Josef Kramer, MD, PhD
Institut für CT & MR Diagnostik
Am Schillerpark
Rainerstrasse 6-8
4020 Linz
Austria

Grahame Lavis, BSc (Hons) FpodA FChS
Associate Specialist Podiatrist
Nuffield Orthopaedic Centre
Windmill Lane
Oxford OX3 7LD
UK

Hans Peter Ledermann, MD
Department of Radiology
Thomas Jefferson University Hospital
132 S. 10th Street – 1096 Main Building
Philadelphia, PA 19107
USA

Carlo Martinoli, MD
Istituto di Radiologia
Università di Genova
Largo R Benzi 1
16100 Genova
Italy

Eugene G. McNally, FRCR, FRCPI
Consultant Musculoskeletal Radiologist
Department of Radiology
Nuffield Orthopaedic Centre
Windmill Lane
Oxford OX3 7LD
UK

William B. Morrison, MD
Department of Radiology
Thomas Jefferson University Hospital
111 S. 11th St. 3390 Gibbon
Philadelphia, PA 19107
USA

Stefan Nehrer, MD
Professor, Universitätsklinik für Orthopädie
Klinische Abteilung fur Osteologie
Allgemeines Krankenhaus
Währinger Gürtel 18-20
1090 Wien
Austria

Michael Recht, MD
Cleveland Clinic Foundation
Diagnostic Radiology
Musculoskeletal Section
9500 Euclid Avenue
Cleveland, OH 44195-5145
USA

Peter Renton, FRCR
Consultant Radiologist
Royal National Orthopaedic Hospital
London W1W 5AQ, and
University College London Hospitals
London WC1E 3BG
UK

David A. Ritchie, MD
Department of Radiology
Royal Liverpool University Hospital
Prescot Street
Liverpool L7 8XP
UK

Leanne L. Seeger, MD
Professor, Department of Radiological Sciences
200 UCLA Medical Plaza
Suite 165 - 57
Los Angeles CA 90095-6952
USA

Mark E. Schweitzer, MD
Department of Radiology
Thomas Jefferson University Hospital
111 S. 11th , # 3390 Gibbon
Philadelphia, PA 19107
USA

Bernhard Tins, MD, Dipl. Phys., FRCR
Department of Radiology
The Robert Jones & Agnes Hunt Orthopaedic
& District Hospital
Oswestry
Shropshire, SY10 7AG
UK

Prudencia N.M. Tyrrell, MD
Consultant Radiologist
Department of Diagnostic Imaging
The Robert Jones & Agnes Hunt Orthopaedic
and District Hospital
Oswestry, Shropshire SY10 7AG
UK

Daniel Vanel, MD
Department of Radiology
Institut Gustave Roussy
39 rue Camille Desmoulins
94805 Villejuif
France

Hermann Vogel, MD
Professor, Department of Radiology
Albers-Schönberg Institut für Strahlendiagnostik
Allgemeines Krankenhaus St. Georg
Lohmühlenstrasse 5
20099 Hamburg
Germany

Iain Watt, MD
Department of Clinical Radiology
Bristol Royal Infirmary
Marlborough Street
Bristol BS2 8HW
UK

Richard William Whitehouse, MD
Department of Clinical Radiology
Manchester Royal Infirmary
Oxford Road
Manchester, M13 9WL
UK

Joseph S. Yu, MD
Associate Professor of Radiology
Chief, Musculoskeletal Division
Department of Radiology
The Ohio State University Medical Center
S-255 Rhodes Hall
450 W. 10th Avenue
Columbus, OH 43210
USA

MEDICAL RADIOLOGY Diagnostic Imaging and Radiation Oncology

Titles in the series already published

DIAGNOSTIC IMAGING

Innovations in Diagnostic Imaging
Edited by J. H. Anderson

Radiology of the Upper Urinary Tract
Edited by E. K. Lang

The Thymus - Diagnostic Imaging, Functions, and Pathologic Anatomy
Edited by E. Walter, E. Willich, and W. R. Webb

Interventional Neuroradiology
Edited by A. Valavanis

Radiology of the Pancreas
Edited by A. L. Baert, co-edited by G. Delorme

Radiology of the Lower Urinary Tract
Edited by E. K. Lang

Magnetic Resonance Angiography
Edited by I. P. Arlart, G. M. Bongartz, and G. Marchal

Contrast-Enhanced MRI of the Breast
S. Heywang-Köbrunner and R. Beck

Spiral CT of the Chest
Edited by M. Rémy-Jardin and J. Rémy

Radiological Diagnosis of Breast Diseases
Edited by M. Friedrich and E.A. Sickles

Radiology of the Trauma
Edited by M. Heller and A. Fink

Biliary Tract Radiology
Edited by P. Rossi

Radiological Imaging of Sports Injuries
Edited by C. Masciocchi

Modern Imaging of the Alimentary Tube
Edited by A. R. Margulis

Diagnosis and Therapy of Spinal Tumors
Edited by P. R. Algra, J. Valk, and J. J. Heimans

Interventional Magnetic Resonance Imaging
Edited by J. F. Debatin and G. Adam

Abdominal and Pelvic MRI
Edited by A. Heuck and M. Reiser

Orthopedic Imaging
Techniques and Applications
Edited by A. M. Davies and H. Pettersson

Radiology of the Female Pelvic Organs
Edited by E. K.Lang

Magnetic Resonance of the Heart and Great Vessels
Clinical Applications
Edited by J. Bogaert, A. J. Duerinckx, and F. E. Rademakers

Modern Head and Neck Imaging
Edited by S. K. Mukherji and J. A. Castelijns

Radiological Imaging of Endocrine Diseases
Edited by J. N. Bruneton in collaboration with B. Padovani and M.-Y. Mourou

Trends in Contrast Media
Edited by H. S. Thomsen, R. N. Muller, and R. F. Mattrey

Functional MRI
Edited by C. T. W. Moonen and P. A. Bandettini

Radiology of the Pancreas
2nd Revised Edition
Edited by A. L. Baert
Co-edited by G. Delorme and L. Van Hoe

Emergency Pediatric Radiology
Edited by H. Carty

Spiral CT of the Abdomen
Edited by F. Terrier, M. Grossholz, and C. D. Becker

Liver Malignancies
Diagnostic and Interventional Radiology
Edited by C. Bartolozzi and R. Lencioni

Medical Imaging of the Spleen
Edited by A. M. De Schepper and F. Vanhoenacker

Radiology of Peripheral Vascular Diseases
Edited by E. Zeitler

Diagnostic Nuclear Medicine
Edited by C. Schiepers

Radiology of Blunt Trauma of the Chest
P. Schnyder and M. Wintermark

Portal Hypertension
Diagnostic Imaging-Guided Therapy
Edited by P. Rossi
Co-edited by P. Ricci and L. Broglia

Recent Advances in Diagnostic Neuroradiology
Edited by Ph. Demaerel

Virtual Endoscopy and Related 3D Techniques
Edited by P. Rogalla, J. Terwisscha Van Scheltinga, and B. Hamm

Multislice CT
Edited by M. F. Reiser, M. Takahashi, M. Modic, and R. Bruening

Pediatric Uroradiology
Edited by R. Fotter

Transfontanellar Doppler Imaging in Neonates
A. Couture and C. Veyrac

Radiology of AIDS
A Practical Approach
Edited by J.W.A.J. Reeders and P.C. Goodman

CT of the Peritoneum
Armando Rossi and Giorgio Rossi

Magnetic Resonance Angiography
2nd Revised Edition
Edited by I. P. Arlart, G. M. Bongratz, and G. Marchal

Pediatric Chest Imaging
Edited by Javier Lucaya and Janet L. Strife

Applications of Sonography in Head and Neck Pathology
Edited by J. N. Bruneton in collaboration with C. Raffaelli and O. Dassonville

Imaging of the Larynx
Edited by R. Hermans

3D Image Processing
Techniques and Clinical Applications
Edited by D. Caramella and C. Bartolozzi

Imaging of Orbital and Visual Pathway Pathology
Edited by W. S. Müller-Forell

Pediatric ENT Radiology
Edited by S. J. King and A. E. Boothroyd

Radiological Imaging of the Small Intestine
Edited by N. C. Gourtsoyiannis

Imaging of the Knee
Techniques and Applications
Edited by A. M. Davies and V. N. Cassar-Pullicino

Perinatal Imaging
From Ultrasound to MR Imaging
Edited by Fred E. Avni

Radiological Imaging of the Neonatal Chest
Edited by V. Donoghue

Diagnostic and Interventional Radiology in Liver Transplantation
Edited by E. Bücheler, V. Nicolas, C. E. Broelsch, X. Rogiers, and G. Krupski

Radiology of Osteoporosis
Edited by S. Grampp

Imaging and Intervention in Abdominal Trauma
Edited by R. F. Dondelinger

Imaging of the Foot and Ankle
Techniques and Applications
Edited by A. M. Davies, R. W. Whitehouse, and J. P. R. Jenkins

Interventional Radiology in Cancer
Edited by A. Adam, R. F. Dondelinger, and P. R. Mueller

Imaging of the Pancreas
Cystic and Rare Tumors
Edited by C. Procacci and A. J. Megibow

Intracranial Vascular Malformations and Aneurysms
From Diagnostic Work-Up to Endovascular Therapy
Edited by M. Forsting

Imaging Pelvic Floor Disorders
Edited by C. I. Bartram and J. O. L. DeLancey
Associate Editors: S. Halligan, F. M. Kelvin, and J. Stoker

High Resolution Sonography of the Peripheral Nervous System
Edited by S. Peer and G. Bodner

Radiology Imaging of the Ureter
Edited by F. Joffre, Ph. Otal, and M. Soulie

Springer

MEDICAL RADIOLOGY Diagnostic Imaging and Radiation Oncology

Titles in the series already published

RADIATION ONCOLOGY

Lung Cancer
Edited by C.W. Scarantino

Innovations in Radiation Oncology
Edited by H. R. Withers and L. J. Peters

Radiation Therapy of Head and Neck Cancer
Edited by G. E. Laramore

Gastrointestinal Cancer – Radiation Therapy
Edited by R.R. Dobelbower, Jr.

Radiation Exposure and Occupational Risks
Edited by E. Scherer, C. Streffer, and K.-R. Trott

Radiation Therapy of Benign Diseases
A Clinical Guide
S.E. Order and S. S. Donaldson

Interventional Radiation Therapy Techniques – Brachytherapy
Edited by R. Sauer

Radiopathology of Organs and Tissues
Edited by E. Scherer, C. Streffer, and K.-R. Trott

Concomitant Continuous Infusion Chemotherapy and Radiation
Edited by M. Rotman and C. J. Rosenthal

Intraoperative Radiotherapy – Clinical Experiences and Results
Edited by F. A. Calvo, M. Santos, and L.W. Brady

Radiotherapy of Intraocular and Orbital Tumors
Edited by W. E. Alberti and R. H. Sagerman

Interstitial and Intracavitary Thermoradiotherapy
Edited by M. H. Seegenschmiedt and R. Sauer

Non-Disseminated Breast Cancer
Controversial Issues in Management
Edited by G. H. Fletcher and S.H. Levitt

Current Topics in Clinical Radiobiology of Tumors
Edited by H.-P. Beck-Bornholdt

Practical Approaches to Cancer Invasion and Metastases
A Compendium of Radiation Oncologists' Responses to 40 Histories
Edited by A. R. Kagan with the Assistance of R. J. Steckel

Radiation Therapy in Pediatric Oncology
Edited by J. R. Cassady

Radiation Therapy Physics
Edited by A. R. Smith

Late Sequelae in Oncology
Edited by J. Dunst and R. Sauer

Mediastinal Tumors. Update 1995
Edited by D. E. Wood and C. R. Thomas, Jr.

Thermoradiotherapy and Thermochemotherapy

Volume 1:
Biology, Physiology, and Physics

Volume 2:
Clinical Applications
Edited by M.H. Seegenschmiedt, P. Fessenden, and C.C. Vernon

Carcinoma of the Prostate
Innovations in Management
Edited by Z. Petrovich, L. Baert, and L.W. Brady

Radiation Oncology of Gynecological Cancers
Edited by H.W. Vahrson

Carcinoma of the Bladder
Innovations in Management
Edited by Z. Petrovich, L. Baert, and L.W. Brady

Blood Perfusion and Microenvironment of Human Tumors
Implications for Clinical Radiooncology
Edited by M. Molls and P. Vaupel

Radiation Therapy of Benign Diseases
A Clinical Guide
2nd Revised Edition
S. E. Order and S. S. Donaldson

Carcinoma of the Kidney and Testis, and Rare Urologic Malignancies
Innovations in Management
Edited by Z. Petrovich, L. Baert, and L.W. Brady

Progress and Perspectives in the Treatment of Lung Cancer
Edited by P. Van Houtte, J. Klastersky, and P. Rocmans

Combined Modality Therapy of Central Nervous System Tumors
Edited by Z. Petrovich, L. W. Brady, M. L. Apuzzo, and M. Bamberg

Age-Related Macular Degeneration Current Treatment Concepts
Edited by W. A. Alberti, G. Richard, and R. H. Sagerman

Radiotherapy of Intraocular and Orbital Tumors
2nd Revised Edition
Edited by R. H. Sagerman, and W. E. Alberti

Clinical Target Volumes in Conformal and Intensity Modulated Radiation Therapy
A Clinical Guide to Cancer Treatment
Edited by V. Grégoire, P. Scalliet, and K. K. Ang

Biological Modification of Radiation Response
Edited by C. Nieder, L. Milas, and K. K. Ang

Palliative Radiation Oncology
R. G. Parker. N. A. Janjan, and M. T. Selch

Springer

Printing and Binding: Stürtz AG, Würzburg